ECG in Emergency Medicine and Acute Care

ECG in Emergency Medicine and Acute Care

Theodore C. Chan, MD
Associate Professor of Clinical Medicine
Department of Emergency Medicine
University of California, San Diego
San Diego, California

William J. Brady, MD
Associate Professor of Emergency Medicine and Clinical Internal Medicine
Vice Chair, Department of Emergency Medicine
University of Virginia School of Medicine
Charlottesville, Virginia

Richard A. Harrigan, MD
Associate Professor of Emergency Medicine
Temple University Hospital and School of Medicine
Philadelphia, Pennsylvania

Joseph P. Ornato, MD
Professor and Chairman
Department of Emergency Medicine
Virginia Commonwealth University Medical Center
Richmond, Virginia

Peter Rosen, MD
Senior Lecturer
Department of Medicine
Harvard University
Beth Israel/Deaconess Hospital
Boston, Massachusetts

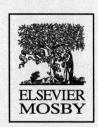

ELSEVIER
MOSBY

The Curtis Center
170 S Independence Mall W 300E
Philadelphia, Pennsylvania 19106

ECG IN EMERGENCY MEDICINE AND ACUTE CARE   ISBN 0-323-01811-4
Copyright © 2005, Elsevier Inc.

Library of Congress Cataloging-in-Publication Data

ECG in emergency medicine and acute care/[edited by] Theodore C. Chan—[et al.].—1st ed.
    p. ; cm.
    Includes bibliographical references.
    ISBN 0-323-01811-4
    1. Electrocardiography. 2. Cardiovascular emergencies. I. Chan, Theodore C.
    [DNLM: 1. Electrocardiography—methods. 2. Emergency Medicine—instrumentation.
    WG 140 E1715 2005]
    RC683.5.E5E246 2005
    616.1'207547—dc22   2003071094

Acquisitions Editor: Todd Hummel
Developmental Editor: Carla Holloway
Publishing Services Manager: Frank Polizzano
Senior Project Manager: Natalie Ware
Design Coordinator: Karen O'Keefe Owens

Printed and bound by CPI Group (UK) Ltd, Croydon, CR0 4YY

Transferred to digital print 2012

I would like to thank Peter Rosen, my friend and mentor, for his inspiration and encouragement. A lifetime of thanks is due to my parents, Eva and Lun Chan, whose guidance and example set me on my path. Finally, I would like to thank my wife, Diana, and our children, Taylor James and Lauren, for their understanding, flexibility, support, and love, which have helped me keep perspective on what is truly important in life.
TCC

I would like to thank my wife, King, for her support, guidance, love, and patience; my children, Lauren, Anne, Chip, and Katherine, for their love; my parents, Joann and Bill Brady, for all they've done and continue to do; the Emergency Medicine Residents at the University of Virginia, for their devotion to our patients and Emergency Medicine; and to my co-editors, for their support, understanding, guidance, and, most of all, their friendship.
WJB

To my parents, Tom and Ruth Harrigan, thank you for being all that you are, which is more than you know. To Noreen, thank you so much for selflessly giving the time, support, and patience necessary to complete this project. To Quinn and Kelly, thank you for being the perfect answer to what is important.
RAH

I would like to dedicate this book to the family of Emergency Medicine practitioners, residents, and students who strive to provide the highest quality care to our patients with cardiovascular disease.
JPO

I would like to add my thanks to my coeditors whose labor and erudition have helped to keep me educated, and whose efforts will translate into much improved care of patients who rely on our knowledge.
PR

Editors

Theodore C. Chan, MD, FACEP, FAAEM
Associate Professor of Clinical Medicine,
Assistant Clinical Director,
Department of Emergency Medicine,
University of California, San Diego,
San Diego, California
>*8: Tachydysrhythmias, 10: P Wave, 11: PR Interval
>and Segment, 16: U Wave, 27: Pacemakers: Normal
>Function, 28: Pacemakers: Abnormal Function,
>37: Myopericarditis, and 49: Toxicology Section:
>Introduction*

William J. Brady, Jr., MD, FACEP, FAAEM
Associate Professor and Vice Chair,
Department of Emergency Medicine,
Associate Professor,
Department of Internal Medicine,
University of Virginia School of Medicine,
Charlottesville, Virginia;
Medical Director, Life Support Learning Center
University of Virgina Health System,
Charlottesville, Virginia
>*7: Bradydysrhythmias, 13: ST Segment, 14: T Wave,
>20: Atrioventricular Block, 25: Preexcitation Syndromes,
>34: Acute Myocardial Infarction: Confounding Patterns,
>40: Benign Early Repolarization, 47: Long QT Syndromes,
>and 71: The Prehospital 12-Lead Electrocardiogram*

Richard A. Harrigan, MD, FAAEM
Associate Professor of Emergency Medicine,
Temple University Hospital and School of Medicine,
Philadelphia, Pennsylvania
>*6: Dysrhythmias at Normal Rates, 9: Abnormal Axis,
>12: QRS Complex, 15: QT Interval, 20: Atrioventricular
>Block, 30: Atrioventricular Dissociation, 55: Tricyclic
>Antidepressant Agents, and 62: Pneumothorax*

Joseph P. Ornato, MD, FACP, FACC, FACEP
Professor and Chairman,
Department of Emergency Medicine,
Virginia Commonwealth University Medical Center,
Richmond, Virginia
>*75: Body Surface Mapping*

Peter Rosen, MD, FAAEM
Senior Lecturer, Department of Medicine,
Harvard University, Beth Israel/Deaconess Hospital,
Boston, Massachusetts;
Visiting Professor,
Department of Emergency Medicine,
University of Arizona School of Medicine,
Tucson, Arizona;
Attending Emergency Physician,
Beth Israel/Deaconess Hospital,
Boston, Massachusetts;
Attending Emergency Physician,
St. John's Hospital, Jackson, Wyoming

Contributors

Douglas S. Ander, MD
Associate Professor,
Department of Emergency Medicine,
Emory University School of Medicine,
Atlanta, Georgia
38: Myocarditis

Tom P. Aufderheide, MD, FACEP
Professor of Emergency Medicine,
Department of Emergency Medicine,
Medical College of Wisconsin,
Milwaukee, Wisconsin
*71: The Prehospital 12-Lead Electrocardiogram,
73: QT Dispersion, and 74: Electrocardiographic
Predictive Instruments*

Alexander B. Baer, MD
Clinical Instructor, Department of Emergency Medicine,
University of Virginia Health System,
Charlottesville, Virginia
56: Other Sodium Channel Blocking Agents

James Dave Barry, MD
Faculty Emergency Medicine Physician,
Emergency Department, Brooke Army Medical Center,
San Antonio, Texas; Staff Emergency Medicine Physician,
San Antonio Uniformed Services Health Education
    Consortium Emergency Medicine Residency,
San Antonio, Texas
51: Beta-Adrenergic Blocking Agents

Todd J. Berger, MD
Assistant Professor, Assistant Residency Director,
Department of Emergency Medicine,
Emory University, Atlanta, Georgia;
Attending Physician,
Department of Emergency Medicine,
Grady Memorial Hospital,
Atlanta, Georgia
66: Acute Rheumatic Fever

James D. Bergin, MD
Associate Professor of Medicine,
Department of Medicine,
University of Virginia,
Charlottesville, Virginia
44: Cardiac Transplant

Steven L. Bernstein, MD
Assistant Professor, Department of Emergency Medicine,
Albert Einstein College of Medicine, Bronx, New York;
Attending Physician, Department of Emergency Medicine,
Montefiore Medical Center,
Bronx, New York
*64: Neurologic and Neuromuscular Conditions,
65: Rheumatologic/Immunologic Disorders*

Thomas P. Bleck, MD, FCCM
Louise Nerancy Eminent Scholar in Neurology and
    Professor of Neurology, Neurological Surgery, and
    Internal Medicine,
Department of Neurology,
University of Virginia, Charlottesville, Virginia;
Director, Neuroscience Intensive Care Unit,
University of Virginia,
Charlottesville, Virginia
64: Neurologic and Neuromuscular Conditions

Ioliene Boenau, MD
Assistant Director,
Emergency Medicine Residency Program,
Eastern Virginia Medical School,
Norfolk, Virginia
29: Sick Sinus Syndrome

Michael J. Bono, MD, FACEP
Associate Professor of Emergency Medicine,
Department of Emergency Medicine,
Eastern Virginia Medical School,
Norfolk, Virginia; Associate Program Director,
Emergency Medicine Residency Program,
Department of Emergency Medicine,
Eastern University Medical School,
Norfolk, Virginia
36: Cardiomyopathy

Kenneth J. Bramwell, MD
Director, Pediatric Emergency Medicine,
Emergency Medicine of Idaho,
St. Luke's Regional Medical Center,
Boise, Idaho
5: The Pediatric Electrocardiogram

Joseph S. Bushra, MD

Adjunct Assistant Professor,
Department of Emergency Medicine,
Temple University School of Medicine,
Philadelphia, Pennsylvania; Attending Physician,
Department of Emergency Medicine,
The Lankenau Hospital, Wynnewood, Pennsylvania
2: The Normal Electrocardiogram and Its Interpretation

Taylor Y. Cardall, MD

Emergency Physician, Department of Emergency Medicine,
Scottsdale Healthcare, Scottsdale, Arizona
27: Pacemakers: Normal Function, and 28: Pacemakers: Abnormal Function

Leslie S. Carroll, MD, ABMT

Assistant Professor, Department of Emergency Medicine,
Temple University, Philadelphia, Pennsylvania
54: Antipsychotic Agents and Lithium

Richard F. Clark, MD

Professor, Department of Medicine,
University of California, San Diego,
San Diego, California;
Director, Division of Medicine Toxicology,
University of California, San Diego Medical Center,
San Diego, California; Medical Director,
California Poison Control System, San Diego Division,
San Diego, California
53: Other Cardioactive Agents

M. Todd Clever, MD

Medical College of Wisconsin,
Milwaukee, Wisconsin
71: The Prehospital 12-Lead Electrocardiogram

Francis L. Counselman, MD, FACEP

EVMS Distinguished Professor of Emergency Medicine,
Department of Emergency Medicine,
Eastern Virginia Medical School, Norfolk, Virginia;
Chairman and Program Director,
Department of Emergency Medicine,
Eastern Virginia Medical School, Norfolk, Virginia
43: Pericardial Effusion

Wendy M. Curulla, MD

Instructor, Department of Emergency Medicine,
Eastern Virginia Medical School, Norfolk, Virginia
29: Sick Sinus Syndrome

Kurt R. Daniel, DO

Chief Resident, Department of Internal Medicine,
Wake Forest University, Winston-Salem, North Carolina
59: Pulmonary Embolism

Brian F. Erling, MD

Chief Resident, Department of Emergency Medicine,
University of Virginia, Charlottesville, Virginia
1: Standard 12-Lead Electrocardiogram: Principles and Techniques, 31: Waveform Genesis in Acute Coronary Syndrome, and 46: Cardiac Trauma

Timothy C. Evans, MD

Associate Professor of Emergency Medicine,
Program Director,
Department of Emergency Medicine,
Virginia Commonwealth University Medical Center,
Medical College of Virginia, Richmond, Virginia
35: Ventricular Hypertrophy

Jeffrey D. Ferguson, MD, NREMT-P

Department of Emergency Medicine,
University of Virginia Health System,
Charlottesville, Virginia;
Charlottesville-Albemarle Rescue Squad,
Charlottesville, Virginia
71: The Prehospital 12-Lead Electrocardiogram

Renee Yvette Friday, MD, MPH, FAAP, FACC

Assistant Professor of Pediatrics,
Department of Pediatric Cardiology,
University of Texas Medical Branch Galveston,
Galveston, Texas
48: Congenital Heart Disease

J. Lee Garvey, MD

Medical Director, Chest Pain Evaluation Center,
Department of Emergency Medicine,
Carolinas Medical Center,
Charlotte, North Carolina
70: Serial Electrocardiography and ST Segment Trend Monitoring

Paolo M. Gazoni, MD

Assistant Professor,
Department of Emergency Medicine, Virginia
Commonwealth University Health System,
Richmond, Virginia
35: Ventricular Hypertrophy

Christopher R. George, MD

Senior Resident, Department of Emergency Medicine,
Medical College of Wisconsin,
Milwaukee, Wisconsin
74: Electrocardiographic Predictive Instruments

Chris A. Ghaemmaghami, MD

Associate Professor of Emergency Medicine and
   Internal Medicine,
Department of Emergency Medicine,
University of Virginia, Charlottesville, Virginia
60: Chronic Obstructive Pulmonary Disease

W. Brian Gibler, MD
Professor and Chairman, Department of Emergency Medicine,
University of Cincinnati College of Medicine,
Cincinnati, Ohio;
Director, Center for Emergency Care,
University Hospital, Cincinnati, Ohio
Foreword

Melody C. Graves, DO
Senior Resident, Department of Emergency Medicine,
Medical College of Wisconsin, Milwaukee, Wisconsin
73: QT Dispersion

Glenn C. Hamilton, MD
Professor and Chair, Department of Emergency Medicine,
Wright State University School of Medicine,
Dayton, Ohio
33: Acute Coronary Syndromes: Regional Issues

Richard J. Harper, MS, MD
Assistant Professor, Department of Emergency Medicine,
Oregon Health and Sciences University, Portland, Oregon;
Chief of Emergency Medicine,
Emergency Medicine Service, Portland-VAMC,
Portland, Oregon
4: Electrode Misplacement and Artifact, 41: Ventricular Aneurysm, and 42: Valvular Disorders

Katherine L. Heilpern, MD
Associate Professor and Vice Chair for Academic Affairs,
Department of Emergency Medicine,
Emory University School of Medicine,
Atlanta, Georgia
38: Myocarditis, 39: Endocarditis, and 66: Acute Rheumatic Fever

Robert S. Hoffman, MD
Associate Professor,
Departments of Emergency Medicine and Medicine,
New York University School of Medicine,
New York, New York;
Director, New York City Poison Center,
Department of Health and Mental Hygiene,
New York, New York
57: Cocaine and Other Sympathomimetics

Christopher P. Holstege, MD
Director, Division of Medical Toxicology,
Assistant Professor, Department of Emergency Medicine,
University of Virginia, Charlottesville, Virginia
50: Digitalis, and 56: Other Sodium Channel Blocking Agents

Lawrence Isaacs, MD, FACEP, FAAEM
Assistant Professor (Adjunct) of Emergency Medicine,
Department of Emergency Medicine,
Temple University School of Medicine,
Philadelphia, Pennsylvania;

Attending Physician,
Lourdes Medical Center of Burlington County,
Willingboro, New Jersey
30: Atrioventricular Dissociation

Timothy G. Janz, MD, FACEP, FCCP
Professor, Department of Emergency Medicine,
Wright State University School of Medicine,
Dayton, Ohio
33: Acute Coronary Syndromes: Regional Issues

Sharone Jensen, MD
Attending Physician, Our Lady of Lourdes Medical Center,
Camden, New Jersey
26: Ventricular Tachycardia and Ventricular Fibrillation

David J. Karras, MD
Associate Professor of Emergency Medicine, Associate Chair for Academic Affairs and Director of Research,
Department of Emergency Medicine,
Temple University School of Medicine,
Philadelphia, Pennsylvania
67: Miscellaneous Infectious Syndromes: Lyme Carditis, Human Immunodeficiency Virus-Associated, and Chagas Disease

Varnada A. Karriem-Norwood, MD
Assistant Professor of Emergency Medicine,
Assistant Medical Director, Grady Emergency Care Center,
Department of Emergency Medicine, Emory University,
Atlanta, Georgia; Assistant Medical Director,
Emergency Care Center, Grady Memorial Hospital,
Atlanta, Georgia
39: Endocarditis

A. Antoine Kazzi, MD, FAAEM
Vice Chair and Associate Professor of Clinical Emergency Medicine,
Department of Emergency Medicine,
University of California, Irvine, Orange, California
24: Other Supraventricular Tachydysrhythmias

Mark A. Kirk, MD
Director, Medical Toxicology Fellowship,
Department of Emergency Medicine, University of Virginia,
Charlottesville, Virginia
50: Digitalis

Jeffrey A. Kline, MD
Director of Research, Department of Emergency Medicine,
Carolinas Medical Center, Charlotte, North Carolina;
Associate Professor, Department of Emergency Medicine,
University of North Carolina, Chapel Hill,
North Carolina
59: Pulmonary Embolism

Michael C. Kontos, MD
Associate Director, Acute Cardiac Care, Assistant Professor,
Departments of Internal Medicine (Division of Cardiology),
Emergency Medicine, and Radiology,
Virginia Commonwealth University, Richmond, Virginia
  72: The Electrocardiogram and Stress Testing

Brian Korotzer, MD
Assistant Chief, Department of Internal Medicine,
Kaiser Permanente, Bellflower, California;
Assistant Clinical Professor of Medicine,
David Geffen School of Medicine at UCLA,
Los Angeles, California
  61: Pulmonary Hypertension

John R. Lindbergh, MD
Assistant Professor of Emergency Medicine,
Emergency Department, University of Virginia,
Charlottesville, Virginia; Emergency Physician,
Emergency Department, Martha Jefferson Hospital,
Charlottesville, Virginia
  25: Preexcitation Syndromes

Binh T. Ly, MD
Assistant Clinical Professor,
Department of Emergency Medicine,
University of California, San Diego Medical Center,
San Diego, California
  52: Calcium Channel Antagonists

Marcus L. Martin, MD
Professor and Chair,
Department of Emergency Medicine,
University of Virginia, Charlottesville, Virginia
  40: Benign Early Repolarization

John Matjucha, MD
Department of Emergency Medicine,
Newark Beth Israel Medical Center,
Newark, New Jersey
  65: Rheumatologic/Immunologic Disorders

Amal Mattu, MD
Co-Director, Emergency Medicine/Internal Medicine
Combined Residency, Director of Academic Development,
Emergency Medicine Residency,
University of Maryland School of Medicine,
Baltimore, Maryland
  21: Intraventricular Conduction Abnormalities

Nancy L. McDaniel, MD
Associate Professor of Pediatric Cardiology,
Department of Pediatrics, University of Virginia,
Charlottesville, Virginia
  48: Congenital Heart Disease

Bryon K. McNeil, MD
Attending Physician, Emergency Department,
Christi Regional Medical Center, Wichita, Kansas
  62: Pneumothorax

Moss Mendelson, MD
Associate Professor, Department of Emergency Medicine,
Eastern Virginia Medical School, Norfolk, Virginia
  45: Dextrocardia

Steven R. Offerman, MD
Assistant Professor, Division of Emergency Medicine and
    Clinical Toxicology,
University of California Davis,
Sacramento, California
  52: Calcium Channel Antagonists

Sonal M. Patel, MD
Clinical Fellow, Department of Gastroenterology,
Beth Israel Deaconess Medical Center,
Boston, Massachusetts
  *68: Electrocardiographic Manifestations of
  Gastrointestinal Diseases*

Andrew D. Perron, MD, FACEP, FACSM
Residency Program Director,
Department of Emergency Medicine,
Maine Medical Center, Portland, Maine
  *1: Standard 12-Lead Electrocardiogram: Principles and
  Techniques, and 31: Waveform Genesis in Acute
  Coronary Syndrome*

Jesse M. Pines, MD, MBA
Lecturer, Department of Emergency Medicine,
University of Pennsylvania School of Medicine,
Philadelphia, Pennsylvania
  47: Long QT Syndromes

Sridevi R. Pitta, MBBS
Department of Emergency Medicine,
Department of Internal Medicine,
Wayne State University, Detroit, Michigan
  69: Additional Lead Electrocardiograms

Marc L. Pollack, MD, PhD
Research Director, Department of Emergency Medicine,
York Hospital, York, Pennsylvania
  34: Acute Myocardial Infarction: Confounding Patterns

Christopher F. Richards, MD
Associate Professor, Department of Emergency Medicine,
Oregon Health and Sciences University, Portland, Oregon;
Chief, Acute Clinical Care,
Department of Emergency Medicine,
Oregon Health and Sciences University,
Portland, Oregon
  *4: Electrode Misplacement and Artifact, and
  42: Valvular Disorders*

Robert L. Rogers, MD
Assistant Professor and Program Director,
Emergency Medicine/Internal Medicine Combined Residency,
University of Maryland School of Medicine,
Baltimore, Maryland
  21: Intraventricular Conduction Abnormalities

Pamela A. Ross, MD
Assistant Professor, Clinical,
Departments of Emergency Medicine and Pediatrics,
University of Virginia Health System,
Charlottesville, Virginia
48: Congenital Heart Disease

Joshua G. Schier, MD
Assistant Professor, Department of Emergency Medicine,
Emory University School of Medicine,
Atlanta, Georgia;
Medical Toxicology Attending,
Emory/CDC Medical Toxicology Fellowship,
Georgia Poison Control Center, Atlanta, Georgia
57: Cocaine and Other Sympathomimetics

Aaron B. Schneir, MD
Assistant Professor, Department of Emergency Medicine,
University of California, San Diego Medical Center,
San Diego, California
53: Other Cardioactive Agents

George M. Shumaik, MD
Clinical Professor of Medicine,
Department of Emergency Medicine,
University of California, San Diego School of Medicine,
San Diego, California;
Medical Director, Department of Emergency Medicine,
University of California, San Diego Medical Center,
San Diego, California
58: Electrolyte Abnormalities

Stephen W. Smith, MD, FACEP
Associate Professor of Emergency Medicine,
Department of Emergency Medicine,
University of Minnesota School of Medicine,
Minneapolis, Minnesota
32: Acute Coronary Syndromes: Acute Myocardial Infarction and Ischemia

Teresa L. Smith, MD
Clinical Assistant Professor,
Michigan State University College of Human Medicine,
Kalamazoo, Michigan;
Medical Director, Adult Neurology,
Bronson Methodist Hospital, Kalamazoo, Michigan
64: Neurologic and Neuromuscular Conditions

Sarah A. Stahmer, MD
Associate Professor, Department of Emergency Medicine,
Robert Wood Johnson/UMDNJ Medical School,
Camden, New Jersey;
Program Director, Department of Emergency Medicine,
Cooper Hospital/University Medical Center,
Camden, New Jersey
26: Ventricular Tachycardia and Ventricular Fibrillation

Jacob W. Ufberg, MD
Assistant Residency Program Director,
Department of Emergency Medicine,
Temple University School of Medicine,
Philadelphia, Pennsylvania
17: Bradycardia and Escape Rhythms, 18: Sinus Pause/Sinus Arrest, and 19: Sinoatrial Exit Block

Edward Ullman, MD
Attending Physician, Department of Emergency Medicine,
Beth Israel Deaconess Medical Center,
Boston, Massachusetts
68: Electrocardiographic Manifestations of Gastrointestinal Diseases

Michael J. Urban, MD
Senior Resident, Department of Emergency Medicine,
Medical College of Wisconsin, Milwaukee, Wisconsin
71: The Prehospital 12-Lead Electrocardiogram

Robert A. VerNooy, MD
Electrophysiology Fellow,
Department of Internal Medicine,
Cardiovascular Division,
University of Virginia Health System,
Charlottesville, Virginia
44: Cardiac Transplant

Gary M. Vilke, MD
Associate Professor of Clinical Medicine,
Department of Emergency Medicine,
University of California, San Diego Medical Center,
San Diego, California
3: Variants of Normal

Robert P. Wahl, MD
Assistant Professor (Clinical Educator),
Department of Emergency Medicine,
Wayne State University/Detroit Medical Center,
Detroit, Michigan;
Emergency Medicine Residency Program Director,
Department of Emergency Medicine,
Wayne State University/Detroit Medical Center,
Detroit, Michigan
69: Additional Lead Electrocardiograms

David A. Wald, DO
Director of Undergraduate Medical Education,
Assistant Professor of Emergency Medicine,
Department of Emergency Medicine,
Temple University School of Medicine,
Philadelphia, Pennsylvania; Attending Physician,
Department of Emergency Medicine,
Temple University Hospital,
Philadelphia, Pennsylvania
63: Endocrine and Metabolic Disorders

Christopher J. Ware, MD
Department of Emergency Medicine,
Temple University School of Medicine,
Philadelphia, Pennsylvania
17: Bradycardia and Escape Rhythms

Wayne Whitwam, MD
Fellow, Division of Cardiology,
Department of Emergency Medicine,
Wayne State University School of Medicine,
Detroit, Michigan;
Fellow, Division of Cardiology,
Department of Internal Medicine, Harper Hospital,
Detroit, Michigan
32: Acute Coronary Syndromes: Acute Myocardial Infarction and Ischemia

Saralyn R. Williams, MD, FACMT, FACEP
Associate Clinical Professor of Medicine,
Department of Medicine,
University of California, San Diego,
San Diego, California
51: Beta-Adrenergic Blocking Agents

Hubert Wong, MD, RDMS, FACEP
Director of Emergency Ultrasound,
Department of Emergency Medicine,
Loma Linda University Medical Center,
Loma Linda, California
24: Other Supraventricular Tachydysrhythmias

Keith Wrenn, MD
Professor and Program Director,
Department of Emergency Medicine,
Vanderbilt University School of Medicine,
Nashville, Tennessee
22: Atrial Fibrillation and Atrial Flutter, and 23: Wandering Atrial Pacemaker and Multifocal Atrial Tachycardia

Jeffrey S. Young, MD, FACS
Associate Professor of Surgery and Health
   Evaluation Sciences,
Department of Surgery,
University of Virginia Health System,
Charlottesville, Virginia;
Director, Trauma Center,
Department of Surgery,
University of Virginia Health System,
Charlottesville, Virginia
46: Cardiac Trauma

Robert J. Zalenski, MD, MA
Professor, Department of Emergency Medicine,
Wayne State University School of Medicine,
Detroit, Michigan;
Attending Physician, Department of Medicine,
John D. Dingell Veterans Hospital,
Urgent Care Center,
Detroit, Michigan
69: Additional Lead Electrocardiograms

Foreword

It is only fitting that this textbook, **ECG in Emergency Medicine and Acute Care,** edited by Drs. Chan, Brady, Harrigan, Ornato, and Rosen, essentially commemorates the 100-year anniversary of the discovery of the electrocardiogram by Willem Einthoven in 1903. A Dutch physician and scientist, Dr. Einthoven used a string galvanometer to obtain a 3-lead ECG. Within 15 years, James Bryan Herrick, M.D., of Chicago, used the electrocardiogram to support his theory for myocardial infarction. The electrocardiogram became widely used after this demonstration of its usefulness, serving as one of the support pillars for the evolving field of Cardiology. Essentially unchanged after the expansion of the original 3-lead ECG with augmented limb and precordial leads to the 12-lead tracing used routinely in care today, the electrocardiogram is arguably the most powerful diagnostic tool available to the clinician caring for patients in the emergency setting.

For emergency physicians, and any clinicians caring for patients in the emergency department or acute care setting, the 12-lead electrocardiogram provides a highly reproducible, easily archived, low-cost diagnostic test that provides diagnostic and prognostic information for a large variety of disease processes which commonly impact patients. The electrical activity of the heart is uniquely perturbed not only by diseases involving the heart, such as congenital abnormalities and acute coronary syndromes, but also by abnormalities in other organ systems, such as the brain and lungs; infectious processes, such as myocarditis and pericarditis; metabolic disorders, such as hyperkalemia and hypocalcemia; as well as toxic ingestions. Emergency physicians take care of a large population of undifferentiated patients presenting to Emergency Departments across the United States and the world each year—over 108 million in the US alone—with electrocardiograms obtained on many of these patients, particularly those who are severely ill or injured. A definitive textbook such as this one, which describes the normal electrocardiogram in detail and characterizes essentially every disease process which impacts the 12-lead electrocardiogram tracing, serves as a wonderful read and an invaluable reference for real-time care of patients.

The authors and editors have constructed an exhaustive evaluation of all aspects of the 12-lead electrocardiogram. In the first chapters, the normal ECG of the child and adult is described in detail, followed by information regarding the ECG in abnormal states with a discussion of the pathophysiology responsible for waveform disturbance. The cardiac researcher will enjoy this scholarly discussion of the chemical origins of many of the electrical derangements seen on the surface cardiac tracing. The middle portion of the text focuses on the electrocardiographic manifestations of disease, diseases of the heart and contiguous structures, and impact of toxicology and systemic diseases on the electrocardiogram. It is from here that the practicing clinician will derive the most enjoyment and benefit from this textbook. For the emergency physician attempting to gain a more thorough understanding of a pathological condition, or to use this important information to understand a patient's condition and treat the individual in real time in the Emergency Department, this book will prove extremely helpful. Finally, the last chapters in the book will provide details on state-of-the-art advances in techniques for performing the electrocardiogram, such as 15-lead electrocardiography, and technological advances such as body surface mapping which will be of interest to the clinician and cardiac researcher alike.

For an area of significant concern to emergency physicians, the electrocardiographic evaluation of acute coronary syndromes including unstable angina, non-ST-segment elevation myocardial infarction and ST-segment elevation myocardial infarction, is provided in comprehensive detail. The **ECG in Emergency Medicine and Acute Care** textbook rightly focuses on this critical area. The 12-lead electrocardiogram triggers the treatment of patients with ST-segment elevation myocardial infarction using thrombolytic therapy or literally brings a cardiologist and the entire cardiac catheterization laboratory team into the hospital at night to open an occluded coronary artery by percutaneous coronary intervention. Diagnosis and prognosis for patients with non-ST-segment elevation acute coronary syndrome are based on electrocardiographic findings. Potent anti-thrombotic therapies such as heparin and low molecular weight heparin, and anti-platelet therapies such as clopidogrel and glycoprotein IIb/IIIa receptor inhibitors, are administered to the patient with acute coronary syndrome based on electrocardiographic findings of ST-segment depression or transient ST-segment elevation. The 12-lead electrocardiogram is the first diagnostic tool used by the clinician taking care of these patients and clearly the most important early in the course of a patient's illness.

Finally, it is perhaps most indicative of the advancement of Emergency Medicine as a specialty over the last 35 years that a sub-specialty textbook such as **ECG in Emergency Medicine and Acute Care** has been written and, I anticipate, will be widely used. This book is written and edited by emergency physicians for emergency physicians, specifically to address the issues associated with emergent and urgent care of the patient presenting to the emergency setting or for clinicians caring for patients in an office or other acute care setting. Our discipline of Emergency Medicine has become inundated by an expanding scientific knowledge necessary for evidence-based practice. The diagnosis and treatment of patients in the Emergency Department has subsequently become exceedingly complex. Clinicians and researchers alike in our field need exhaustive textbooks such as this one to help provide the pathophysiological and clinical basis for our practice, to answer questions regarding a fundamental diagnostic tool, the electrocardiogram. The editors and authors are to be congratulated for their efforts. This textbook helps to set a new standard for future sub-specialty books in Emergency Medicine.

W. BRIAN GIBLER, M.D.

Preface

We have developed a textbook which offers what we think is a new approach to learning about the ECG. It is not intended to replace any of the excellent existing textbooks on the topic that have been relied upon for years for the instruction of health care providers. It is written, however, not from the cardiologists' perspective, but from that of the many practicing clinicians who provide acute care and encounter ECG findings that are challenging, perplexing, or intriguing. This book stresses the differential diagnostic approach to these ECG findings, and also gives due emphasis to not only ischemic heart disease, but also to the many everyday non-coronary disease states affecting the ECG.

The textbook is divided into four sections:

- **Section I** instructs the reader on the normal ECG in both adults and children. Variants of normal, as well as practical issues, such as electrode misplacement and artifact, are also discussed here.
- **Section II** approaches the ECG from the perspective of differential diagnosis. This method is applied to all components of the ECG: the various abnormalities in rhythm, electrical axis, and waveform morphology that are encountered every day in clinical practice. We see this as having real-time clinical utility. The reader can consult this section when faced with a variety of findings; for example, ST segment elevation, narrow complex tachycardia, QRS axis deviation, and prolongation of the QT interval.

- **Section III** provides a thorough review of the many disease states that affect the ECG. While an emphasis is placed on acute coronary syndrome and dysrhythmia, the reader can use this section to find the many disease entities that impact upon the ECG and quickly review the clinical features as well as the associated ECG findings.
- **Section IV** moves beyond the 12-lead ECG, and highlights the various electrocardiographic-based technologies and techniques applicable to emergency and acute care. Established approaches such as the additional-lead ECG and ST segment monitoring are reviewed in detail, as well as newer methods, including body surface mapping and predictive instruments.

While this textbook can be applied at the bedside to an individual patient's ECG, we hope it also will be used in self-instruction and board-preparation, or simply while trying to better the knowledge base from which we draw as we care for our patients. This book is intended to supplement clinical judgment, to remind the reader of significant changes, and to help sort out confusing clinical entities. We owe our thanks to the wide range of practicing acute care and emergency physicians who have contributed to this project.

THE EDITORS

Acknowledgments

The creation of a new textbook such as this requires the support, hard work, and guidance of many individuals. First and foremost, we thank our contributors who have given us their expertise, valuable time, and effort in producing this textbook. Each has provided his or her own perspective, insight, and focus in making this book relevant to the practice of electrocardiography in Emergency Medicine and Acute Care – without them this text would not exist.

We owe many thanks to Judith Fletcher, Todd Hummel, Natalie Ware, Joan Nikelsky, and Carla Holloway of Elsevier for their dedication, encouragement, and attention to detail. Without their support and understanding, this project would never have gotten off the ground.

Special thanks are due to Maegan Heflin Carey of the University of California, San Diego, whose editing assistance, commitment, and hard work were essential in keeping us on schedule to complete this text. She, in many ways, was another editor for this text.

THE EDITORS

Contents

Introduction

Cardiac muscle tissue is unique in its ability to generate regular electrical impulses that produce rhythmic cardiac contractions. These impulses can be measured and recorded at the body surface. Developed nearly 100 years ago, the standard electrocardiogram (ECG) utilizes measuring electrodes over the chest and limbs to record this electrical activity of the cardiac cycle.

The ECG was easily the greatest advance in clinical cardiology of the early twentieth century. As a graphic recording of the electrical activity of the heart, electrocardiography is the most commonly employed noninvasive diagnostic tool in cardiology. In fact, the ECG remains the single most important initial diagnostic tool for the assessment of myocardial disease, ischemia, and cardiac dysrhythmias.

Today, electrocardiography is performed widely throughout the health care field, particularly in acute care settings such as ambulances, ambulatory clinics, emergency departments, and hospitals. Annually, nearly 100 million ECGs are recorded in the United States alone.[1]

History

The appreciation of the significance of the ECG came long before the understanding of the physiology involved in the now familiar waveform. The pioneers of the field could not have imagined the significance of their work. Beginning with Matteucci's work in 1842 on pigeon hearts, and followed by Kolliker and Muller's study of frog heart action potentials, there was recognition of the ability of the heart to produce electrical current.[2,3,4] In 1887, this animal research was applied to human subjects by Waller, who first used a capillary electrometer to demonstrate electrical activity associated with the heartbeat.

In 1903, Dutch physiologist Willem Einthoven first published his recordings of the cardiac cycle utilizing a string galvanometer device.[5] This instrument consisted of a thin silver-coated quartz filament, stretched across a magnetic field, that would move whenever an electrical current passed through the string. With electrodes placed on the limbs of an individual, Einthoven's instrument could measure differences in potential created by the electrical activity of the heart. These measurements were enlarged and recorded photographically producing the first rudimentary ECG.[6]

Einthoven's instrument laid the basis for modern clinical electrocardiography. He described the standard limb lead ECG utilizing bipolar electrodes. He established standards for recording rate and amplitude. Einthoven was the first to describe five separate electrical deflections, termed P, Q, R, S, and T, establishing basic ECG nomenclature.[7] Einthoven won the Nobel Prize in medicine in 1924 for his invention, and according to historian John Burnett, his recording machine was "probably the most sophisticated scientific instrument in existence when it was first invented."[8]

Einthoven limited most of his work to the laboratory, not venturing into the clinical arena. After visiting with Einthoven, Thomas Lewis recognized the potential clinical utility of the ECG machine and undertook numerous clinical investigations with the device. Utilizing the ECG machine, he determined that atrial fibrillation was due to a "circus conduction" involving the auricle of the heart. Lewis published his clinical work on electrocardiography in his landmark texts, "The Mechanisms of the Heart Beat" in 1911 and "Clinical Electrocardiography" in 1913.[9,10] He became the leading authority on electrocardiography in his day and was instrumental in developing the clinical applications of this new technology.[6]

Clinical use of the ECG machine, however, was limited by its large size. After World War I, the development of smaller, portable bedside ECG recording machines led to their rapid dissemination into the clinical setting. In the early 1930s, Francis Wood and Charles Wolferth first reported the use of ECGs in patients presenting with complaints of chest pain.[6] Along with Frank Wilson, their work also led to the development of the unipolar "exploring" electrode lead, which measured electrical activity anywhere in the body with a central zero potential terminal as a reference. These leads formed the basis for the standard precordial leads.[11]

In 1938, the American Heart Association, in conjunction with the Cardiac Society of Great Britain, established the standard 6 precordial chest electrode positions (V_1-V_6).[12] These precordial leads, along with Einthoven's original bipolar limb lead system (I, II, III) and the augmented unipolar limb leads developed by Emmanual Goldberger (aVR, aVL, and aVF) in 1942, established the standard 12-lead ECG utilized today.[13]

Since the mid 1900s, low-cost electrocardiography machines have been widely available. A number of improvements and advances have been made to the technology. These include instantaneous recording that allows multiple leads to be recorded simultaneously, as well as improvements in the graphical recording systems of the machines. The advent of the computer age has led to smaller machines with memory storage, as well as computer-assisted interpretation of standard ECGs.[6,14] These developments, however, have not altered the basic design and operation of the first ECG machine developed by Einthoven a century ago.

Today, numerous situations in the Emergency Department (ED) may require an electrocardiographic evaluation. The ECG may be obtained to evaluate a specific complaint such as chest pain—a complaint-based indication; alternatively, the clinician may obtain an ECG based upon a specific presentation, such as syncope or status post cardiac arrest, or a system-based indication, as in the "rule-out myocardial infarction" protocol or operative clearance. Within a given diagnosis, the ECG may perform many functions. For instance, in the chest pain patient, the ECG is used to help establish the diagnosis of acute coronary syndrome or, alternatively, some other non-coronary ailment. Moreover, it is used to select appropriate therapy, determine the response to ED-delivered treatments, establish the correct inpatient disposition location, and help predict risk of both cardiovascular complication and death.

References

1. Greenfield Jr, JC: Electrocardiography. In Wyngaarden JB, Smith LH, Bennet JC (eds): Cecil Textbook of Medicine, 19th ed. Philadelphia: Saunders, 1991.
2. Dunn MI, Lipman BS: Lipman-Massie: Clinical Electrocardiography. Chicago: Year Book Medical Publishers, 1989.
3. Coumel P, Garfein OB: Electrocardiography: Past and Future. New York: The New York Academy of Sciences, 1990.
4. Burch GE, DePasquale NP: A History of Electrocardiography. Chicago: Year Book Medical Publishers, 1964.
5. Einthoven W: The string galvanometer and the human electrocardiogram. Proc Kon Akademie voor Wetenschappen 1903;6:107–115.
6. Fye WB: A history of the origin, evolution, and impact of electrocardiography. American Journal of Cardiology 1994;73(13):937–949.
7. Henson JR: Descartes and the ECG lettering series. J Hist Med Allied Sci 1971;26:181–186.
8. Burnett J: The origins of the electrocardiograph as a clinical instrument. Med Hist Supple 1985;5:53–76.
9. Lewis T: The Mechanisms of the Heart Beat. London: Shaw & Sons, 1911.
10. Lewis T: Clinical Electrocardiography. London: Shaw & Sons, 1913.
11. Kossmann CE: Unipolar electrocardiography of Wilson: a half century later. Am Heart J 1985;110:901–904.
12. Barnes AR, Pardee HEB, White PD, et al: Standardization of precordial leads: supplementary report. Am Heart J 1938;15:235–239.
13. Goldberger E: A simple, indifferent, electrocardiographic electrode of zero potential and a technique of obtaining augmented, unipolar, extremity leads. Am Heart J 1942;23:483–492.
14. Macfarlane PW: A brief history of computer-assisted electrocardiography. Meth Inf Med 1990;29:272–281.

Abbreviations

ACS	acute coronary syndrome		mm	millimeter
AMI	acute myocardial infarction		msec	millisecond
APB	atrial premature beat		mV	millivolts
AV	atrioventricular		MVT	monomorphic ventricular tachycardia
BBB	bundle branch block		NSIVCD	nonspecific intraventricular conduction delay
BER	benign early repolarization		NSR	normal sinus rhythm
bpm	beats per minute		PAC	premature atrial contraction
CAD	coronary artery disease		PE	pulmonary embolism
CNS	central nervous system		PJC	premature junctional contraction
COPD	chronic obstructive pulmonary disease		PSVT	paroxysmal supraventricular tachycardia
CV	cardiovascular			
CVA	cerebrovascular accident		PVC	premature ventricular contraction
dL	deciliter		PVT	polymorphic ventricular tachycardia
EAD	extreme axis deviation		QT$_C$	corrected QT interval
ECG	electrocardiogram/electrocardiographic		RA	right atrium/right atrial
ED	emergency department		RAA	right atrial abnormality
GI	gastrointestinal		RAD	right axis deviation
HIV	human immunodeficiency virus		RBBB	right bundle branch block
IVCA	intraventricular conduction abnormality		RV	right ventricle/right ventricular
LA	left atrium/left atrial		SA	sino-atrial
LAA	left atrial abnormality		STE	ST segment elevation
LAD	left axis deviation		SVT	supraventricular tachycardia
LAFB	left anterior fascicular block		TdP	torsades de pointes
LBBB	left bundle branch block		UA	unstable angina
LPFB	left posterior fascicular block		VPB	ventricular premature beat
LV	left ventricle/left ventricular		VT	ventricular tachycardia
LVH	left ventricular hypertrophy		WAP	wandering atrial pacemaker
MAT	multifocal atrial tachycardia		WCT	wide QRS complex tachycardia
mEq	milli-equivalents		WPW	Wolff-Parkinson-White syndrome
MI	myocardial infarction			

Terminology

ECG LEAD TERMINOLOGY

Precordial leads:	V_1-V_6
Right precordial leads:	V_1-V_2
Mid-precordial leads:	V_3-V_4
Left precordial leads:	V_5-V_6
Limb leads:	I, II, II, aVR, aVL, aVF
Inferior leads:	II, III, aVF
Lateral leads:	I, aVL, V_5, V_6
High lateral leads:	I, aVL
Septal leads:	V_1, V_2
Anterior leads:	V_3, V_4
Anteroseptal leads:	V_1, V_2, V_3, V_4
Posterior leads:	V_7, V_8, V_9
Right-sided leads:	V_{1R}, V_{2R}, V_{3R}, V_{4R}, V_{5R}, V_{6R}

WAVEFORM MORPHOLOGIC TERMINOLOGY

ST Segment *ELEVATION* Contour

Concave. With regard to ST segment elevation, concavity means the ST segment is elevated but also cupped or coved, with the open aspect directed upward (Fig. 1*A*).

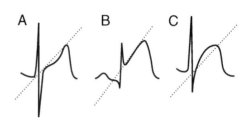

FIGURE 1 · **ST segment elevation contour.** *A,* Contour is concave. *B,* Contour is obliquely straight. *C,* Contour is convex.

Obliquely Straight. With regard to ST segment elevation, the ST segment rises without cupping or doming (i.e., without concavity or convexity), moving from QRS complex toward T wave (Fig. 1*B*).

Convex. With regard to ST segment elevation, convexity means the ST segment is elevated but also domed or humped, with the domed aspect directed upward (Fig. 1*C*).

ST Segment *DEPRESSION* Contour

Horizontal. ST segment is depressed but essentially flat.

Downsloping. ST segment is depressed and sloping in a downward direction, moving from QRS complex toward T wave.

Upsloping. ST segment is depressed and sloping in an upward direction, moving from QRS complex toward T wave.

Section I

The Normal Electrocardiogram

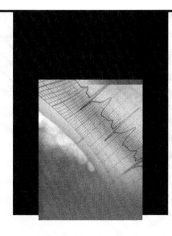

Chapter 1

Standard 12-Lead Electrocardiogram: Principles and Techniques

Brian F. Erling and Andrew D. Perron

Electrocardiographic Leads and Their Placement

Bipolar and unipolar leads are the two types of sensing electrodes used in clinical practice today. Bipolar electrodes have both a positive and a negative electrode, which are anatomically separated on the patient. These electrodes detect an electrical vector as it relates to the direction of the vector of the leads. A unipolar lead is named as such because it consists of only one reading electrode, which is positive. The utility of this type of lead was enhanced after it was discovered that removing the negative lead would augment the normal bipolar deflection. Three bipolar leads (I, II, III) and nine unipolar leads (aVR, aVL, aVF, and V_1 through V_6) make up the standard 12-lead electrocardiogram (ECG). Whereas a single-view radiograph provides some useful clinical information, more than one view is required fully to interpret the anatomy; similarly, a single-lead rhythm strip will provide some useful information, but it is useful only for reading rhythms, not the subtleties of diagnoses that require a 12-lead tracing.

The actual lead placement is a simple task, but requires precision to allow for consistency in ECG interpretation. The four limb leads are placed on their respective appendages as follows: white on the right arm (labeled RA), black on the left arm (LA), green on the right leg (RL), and red on the left leg (LL). There are many mnemonics for this; a common one is "Christmas trees below the knees. White on right and green is go." Translated, the Christmas colors (red and green) are on the lower extremities, with the green lead on the foot that pushes the gas pedal. This leaves black and white on the upper extremities with "white on right."

The precordial leads are placed in a systematic manner. The technician first locates the angle of Louis at the articulation of the manubrium with the body of the sternum, which also marks the articulation of the sternum with the second rib. Proceeding inferiorly two more ribs identifies the fourth rib. Inferior to the fourth rib is the fourth intercostal space, where leads V_1 and V_2 are placed on either side of the sternum, as shown in Figure 1-1. Proceeding inferiorly to the fifth intercostal space, lead V_4 is placed at that level along the left midclavicular line. Lead V_3 is located midway between leads V_2 and V_4. Leads V_5 and V_6 also are placed in the fifth intercostal space, lateral to lead V_4, in the anterior axillary line and the midaxillary line, respectively.

Principles of Electrophysiology

The vector concept of electrocardiography assumes that cardiac electrical activity originates in the center of the heart and is three-dimensional.[1] Each lead is a reflection of the sum of all the electrical activity as it relates to the perspective of that particular lead. The exact wave form depends on many factors, including the direction and amplitude of the electrical vector, the location and direction of the lead axis, and the distance of the electrical vector from the leads (Fig. 1-2). All vectors have magnitude, direction, and polarity. A positive vector toward a positive lead generates a positive deflection on the ECG. In cardiac electrophysiology, the vector is the mean of the sum of electrical activity at any one point in time.

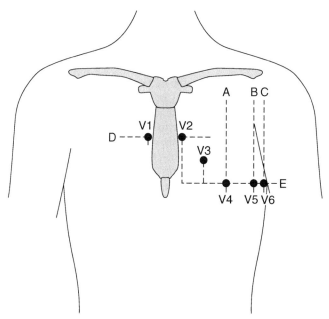

FIGURE 1-1 • Precordial lead placement. The precordial leads are placed in a systematic and precise manner. A is the midclavicular line; B is the anterior axillary line; C is the midaxillary line; D is the fourth intercostal space; and E is the fifth intercostal space.

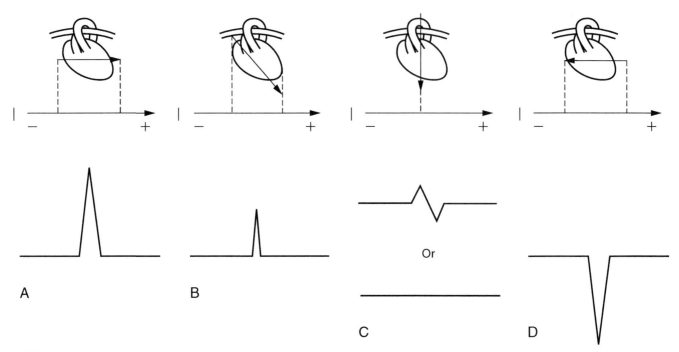

FIGURE 1-2 · Wave form generation as it relates to the depolarization vector and electrode location. The electrical wave form depends on the direction and magnitude of the depolarization vector as they relate to the vector of the electrodes. Lead I is shown by the *long arrow*. The *shorter arrow* over the heart indicates the depolarization vector. *A,* Depolarization vector occurs in same direction as lead I, producing a large-amplitude QRS complex. *B,* Depolarization vector at 45 degrees to lead I, producing a smaller QRS complex. *C,* Depolarization vector at 90 degrees to lead I, producing an isoelectric QRS complex. *D,* Depolarization vector at 180 degrees to lead I, producing a negative deflection QRS complex. (Adapted with permission from Erling B, Brady W: Basic principles and electrophysiology. In Smith SW, Zvosec D, Henry TD, Sharkey SW [eds]: The ECG in Acute MI: An Evidence-based Manual of Reperfusion Therapy. Philadelphia, Lippincott Williams & Wilkins, 2002, pp 1-5.)

The 12-lead ECG is a catalogue of tracings, each of which represents a two-dimensional view of the electrical vectors in the heart. The bipolar limb leads (I, II, III) and the unipolar augmented leads (aVL, aVR, aVF) examine the heart in the frontal plane. Einthoven's triaxial system is combined with the augmented leads to form an expanded hexaxial system, without requiring additional lead placement. The three-dimensionality of the ECG is the result of the addition of the unipolar precordial leads (V_1 through V_6), as shown in Figure 1-3.

To understand clearly the ECG and its changes, one must appreciate the cellular activity of the heart. Cardiac cells have intrinsic excitability, automaticity, conductivity, and contractility, all of which contribute to the electrical functioning of the heart. The excitability of the cells results from the familiar cellular action potential. This five-phase depolarization is shown in Figure 1-4. The resting diastolic transmembrane potential is established by the sodium–potassium adenosine triphosphatase pump during phase 4 of the action potential. This level is variable depending on the activity of this pump, and changes by anatomic location in the heart. The result is a range of resting diastolic transmembrane potentials from approximately –60 mV in the SA node to –90 mV in the contractile cells of the left ventricle. This pump establishes an electrolyte gradient, with high concentrations of potassium inside the cells opposed by high sodium concentrations outside of the cells. The cell membrane charge depends on which of the two ions can freely cross the membrane. In diastole, or phase 4, the cell membrane is more permeable to potassium,

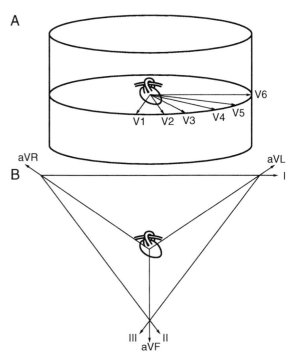

FIGURE 1-3 · The three dimensions of the 12-lead ECG. *A,* The precordial leads are shown. *B,* The hexaxial plane of the bipolar and augmented unipolar limb leads. *Arrowheads* represent positive polarity in all cases. (Adapted with permission from Erling B, Brady W: Basic principles and electrophysiology. In Smith SW, Zvosec D, Henry TD, Sharkey SW [eds]: The ECG in Acute MI: An Evidence-based Manual of Reperfusion Therapy. Philadelphia, Lippincott Williams & Wilkins, 2002, pp 1-5.)

FIGURE 1-4 · **The five phases of membrane depolarization.**
Phase 0, rapid depolarization; phase 1, overshoot; phase 2, plateau;
phase 3, repolarization; phase 4, return to resting membrane potential. Cardiac cells with automaticity are shown by the *solid line*,
whereas nonpacemaker cells are demonstrated by the *dashed line*.
(Adapted with permission from Erling B, Brady W: Basic principles
and electrophysiology. In Smith SW, Zvosec D, Henry TD, Sharkey
SW [eds]: The ECG in Acute MI: An Evidence-based Manual of
Reperfusion Therapy. Philadelphia, Lippincott Williams & Wilkins,
2002, pp 1-5.)

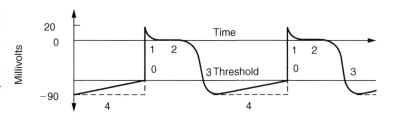

which provides for the largely negative transmembrane
potential.[2]

Automaticity is inherent in most cardiac cells because
of the slowly depolarizing sodium leak into the cell during
phase 4 (Fig. 1-4). As a result, the noncontractile pacemaker
cells are primarily responsible for the rhythmogenic nature
of the heart. The stable, or very slowly increasing,
phase 4 diastolic transmembrane potential in contractile
cells explains their relative lack of automaticity and stable
diastolic polarization. It is the polarity of the cell that results
in the electrical vectors that form the familiar QRS
complex–T wave pattern on the ECG. These vectors are also
responsible for the pathologic changes seen in the ST segment
and T waves. When the membrane potential rises enough to
cross the threshold, which can be due to phase 4 leak or
direct stimulus (either iatrogenic or from neighboring cells),
phase 0 depolarization occurs with opening of the fast sodium
channels. The transmembrane potential initially overshoots,
attaining around +20 mV in phase 1 depolarization, and then
plateaus during phase 2 at or near 0 mV. Slow calcium
channels are responsible for this plateau and serve to balance
the slow potassium efflux. It is this delay that allows for the
prolonged contraction of cardiac myocytes. The calcium
channels eventually close and potassium efflux results in
phase 3 repolarization, whereby the negative resting
membrane potential is restored.[3]

The changes in electrolyte channels and different phases
of depolarization explain why depolarization occurs, but do
not clarify exactly how this progresses on a cellular level.
After the initial stimulus, the membrane does not completely
and instantaneously depolarize the entire length of the cell;
rather, it is a three-dimensional process beginning at the point
of initial stimulus and progressing temporally toward the
opposite pole of the cell. The baseline permeability of the cell
membrane to potassium results in a continuous state of efflux,
which generates the negative electrical potential. In other
words, the outside of the cell is given a positive charge. At the
site of depolarization, the membrane becomes negative in
only that portion of the cell. As the process progresses
through the remainder of the cell, a dipole is established with
the resultant vector oriented from the depolarized (negative)
side toward the direction of the resting, and soon to be
depolarized, positive portion of the cell (Fig. 1-5). If a
positive-reading electrode were placed opposite to the origin
of depolarization, a positive electrical deflection would be
generated. This wave form would peak when the cell was

halfway depolarized, precisely when the vector would be
greatest. Under normal conditions, repolarization originates
exactly at the same point at which depolarization had begun.
It then progresses in the same direction that depolarization
occurred, from the newly repolarized (positive) side toward
the still depolarized (negative) segment. Therefore, on a
cellular level, repolarization occurs in the same direction as
depolarization, but generates a vector that is exactly
opposite.[4] This is in exact contrast to what is observed in the
clinical ECG, the reasons for which will be discussed further.
Cardiac cells depolarize adjacent cells and result in
conductivity.

On a gross level, ventricular depolarization is represented
electrocardiographically by the QRS wave. In leads oriented
with the axis of depolarization, the QRS complex has a
recognizable upright pattern. Cardiac repolarization, however,
generates a T wave vector that is normally positive, which is
distinctly opposite to the pattern observed during cellular
repolarization. The reason for this is based on a fundamental
delay in repolarization as seen in the subendocardium

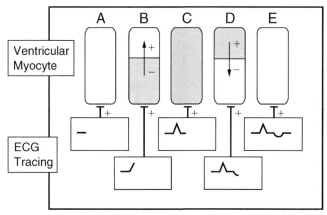

FIGURE 1-5 · **Cellular depolarization from a single reading electrode.** Progression from the resting state through cellular depolarization
and repolarization. Depolarization and repolarization progress in the
same direction, but repolarization generates a negative electrical vector.
A, Resting state, predepolarization; B, depolarizing state; C, fully depolarized; D, repolarizing state; E, resting state, postdepolarization and fully
repolarized. (Adapted with permission from Erling B, Brady W: Basic principles and electrophysiology. In Smith SW, Zvosec D, Henry TD, Sharkey SW
[eds]: The ECG in Acute MI: An Evidence-based Manual of Reperfusion
Therapy. Philadelphia, Lippincott Williams & Wilkins, 2002, pp 1-5.)

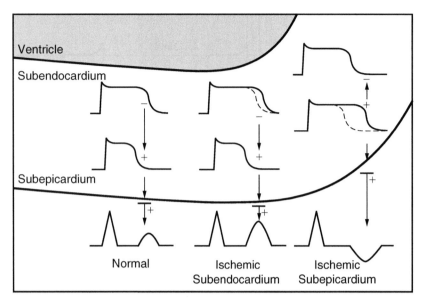

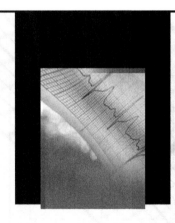

FIGURE 1-6 • **Repolarization in normal and ischemic cardiac tissue.** The intrinsic delay of the endocardium to repolarize generates a positive T wave during normal repolarization. Subendocardial ischemia augments this delay and results in hyperacute T waves. Subepicardial ischemia results in a repolarization delay in the subepicardium, which reverses the repolarization vector and inverts the T wave. (Adapted with permission from Erling B, Brady W: Basic principles and electrophysiology. In Smith SW, Zvosec D, Henry TD, Sharkey SW [eds]: The ECG in Acute MI: An Evidence-based Manual of Reperfusion Therapy. Philadelphia, Lippincott Williams & Wilkins, 2002, pp 1-5.)

compared with the subepicardium.[4] This is believed to be due to a chronic hypometabolic state in the subendocardium secondary to a chronically compromised blood supply, which results in cells behaving as if they were ischemic (Fig. 1-6). The result is a wave of repolarization that progresses from the subepicardium to the subendocardium, and moves away from the positive electrode. In other words, this wave results in a positive repolarization vector toward the positive-reading electrode, and an upright deflection on the ECG.

References

1. Chung EK: Fundamentals of Electrocardiography. Baltimore, University Park Press, 1984.
2. Dunn MI, Lipman BS, Lipman-Massie E: Clinical Electrocardiography. Chicago, Year Book, 1989.
3. Goldman MJ: Principles of Clinical Electrocardiography. Los Altos, Calif, Lange Medical, 1982.
4. Bayes de Luna A: Clinical Electrocardiography: A Textbook. New York, Futura, 1993.

Chapter 2

The Normal Electrocardiogram and Its Interpretation

Joseph S. Bushra

Interpreting the Electrocardiogram

Interpretation of the electrocardiogram (ECG) must be done systematically; all of its essential components need to be examined and synthesized into a coherent analysis. The approach presented in this chapter is not exclusive of other methods; it is a simple and tried process, however, that will accomplish the goal of rapid and accurate diagnosis.

Introduction

The heart is composed of electrical cells and mechanical cells.[1] The electrical cells are responsible for initiating and

2-1 • PACEMAKER SITES OF THE HEART

Pacemaker	Normal Rate (bpm)
Sinoatrial node	60–100
Atrioventricular node ("junctional")	40–60
Ventricle	20–40

The normal sinoatrial node has the fastest automaticity, making it the normal pacemaker of the heart. If the automaticity slows below 60 bpm, one of the other sites may assume the pacemaker role.

propagating action potentials through the heart, which, in turn, cause the mechanical cells to contract. It is essential to understand these electrical cells to determine heart rate and rhythm. The electrical cardiac cells are located in the sinoatrial (SA) node, the internodal fibers, the atrioventricular (AV) node, the bundle of His, the right and left bundle branches, and the Purkinje fibers. As with other nervous tissue in the body, these cells have both a negative resting potential and an excitation threshold. These cells are unique, however, in that their negative resting potential is not static, but slowly depolarizes to the excitation threshold at a given rate. This property gives these cells *automaticity*—the ability to initiate action potentials spontaneously.

The different parts of the conduction system of the heart have different rates of automaticity. Normally, the SA node is the fastest of these, depolarizing 60 to 100 times per minute. Thus, the SA node is the normal pacemaker in the heart, overriding the slower AV node and the ventricles (Table 2-1). The rate of SA nodal automaticity is under the influence of both the sympathetic and parasympathetic nervous systems. Sympathetic discharge can increase SA nodal automaticity far above 100/bpm in response to physiologic stress, and parasympathetic discharge can decrease SA nodal automaticity below 60/bpm in both healthy and disease states.

Rate

The heart rate is expressed in beats per minute. In the healthy heart, the atria and ventricles beat synchronously at the same rate. If dysrhythmias are present, however, these rates may not be identical and each must be calculated separately. The principles outlined in the following can be used to calculate both the atrial and ventricular rates.

To calculate the rate from the ECG, it is important to understand standard ECG paper and recording techniques. ECG paper is divided into a grid by a series of horizontal and vertical lines. Thinner lines are spaced 1 mm apart, and thicker lines mark 5-mm distances. ECG tracings are taken at a standard rate of 25 mm/sec; therefore, each thin vertical line represents 0.04 sec, and each thick vertical line represents 0.2 sec (Fig. 2-1). Knowing this, the rate can be calculated in two ways:

1. Start with a QRS complex that occurs on a thick line. Assuming that the rhythm is regular, simply count the number of thick lines to the next complex. Because each thick line represents 0.2 sec, there are 300 such lines in 1 minute. Divide 300 by the number of thick lines, and the quotient will be the rate in beats per minute. A simplification of this technique is to memorize the rates associated with

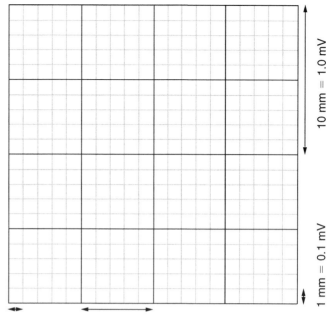

1 mm = 0.04 sec 5 mm = 0.2 sec

10 mm = 1.0 mV

1 mm = 0.1 mV

FIGURE 2-1 • **Standard ECG paper.** On the horizontal scale, thin lines are 1 mm apart, and thick lines are 5 mm apart. The standard ECG is recorded at 25 mm/sec. Vertically, 1 mm is equal to 0.1 mV; thus, 10 mm represents 1.0 mV.

corresponding numbers of thick lines. For example, as the number of thick lines from one complex to the next increases (starting at 1), the rate decreases as follows: 300, 150, 100, 75, 60, 50, 42, 38. This technique is less accurate at higher rates, and therefore one must take into account the 1-mm lines. There are 1500 thin lines in 1 minute, so dividing 1500 by the number of thin lines will give the rate in beats per minute. Plastic ECG rulers are available that greatly simplify this process.

2. The second method of calculating the rate is to count the number of complexes in 6 seconds and multiply by 10. Many brands of ECG recording paper conveniently have 3-second markings. This is the more accurate method if the rhythm is irregular.[2]

Rhythm

The SA node is the normal pacemaker of the heart. As the automaticity of the SA node causes atrial depolarization, a P wave is generated on the ECG. This impulse progresses through the AV node and conduction system to the ventricles. Ventricular depolarization generates the QRS complex on the ECG. Thus, a normal rhythm produces a P wave before every QRS complex, and a QRS complex after every P wave. If this one-to-one relationship between P waves and QRS complexes does not exist, then a dysrhythmia is present. P waves are most easily visualized in leads II and V_1.

To describe the cardiac rhythm, one must determine both the *location* of the pacemaker and its *rate*. The rhythm of the normal heart is therefore designated *normal sinus rhythm* (NSR) because it originates in the sinus node. A rapid rhythm originating in the SA node is called *sinus tachycardia*, whereas a slow rhythm originating in the SA node is called

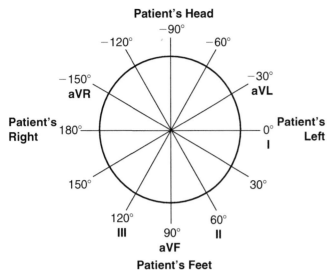

FIGURE 2-2 · **Axis.** The standard designation of axis in the coronal, or frontal plane. *Boldface type* denotes vector positivity.

sinus bradycardia. This dual designation applies to most other dysrhythmias as well.

Axis

Electrical impulses in the heart progress systematically from the SA node, through the atria, to the AV node and conduction system, then to the ventricles. The term *axis* refers to the direction of these impulses in both the coronal and the transverse planes. In general, the QRS axis is the most commonly considered, but it is useful also to inspect the axes of the P and T waves.

Understanding ECG lead placement and polarity enables the determination of axis. The limb leads enable calculation of axis in the coronal (or frontal) plane, whereas the precordial leads enable calculation of axis in the transverse (or horizontal) plane (Figs. 2-2 and 2-3). More detailed information on axis is given later in discussions of the individual waveforms of the ECG.

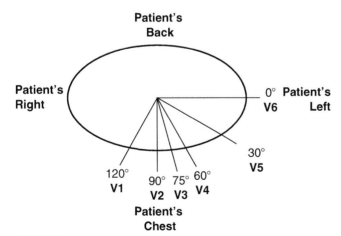

FIGURE 2-3 · **Axis.** A schematic of the designation of axis in the transverse, or horizontal, plane. These axes are much more variable than the coronal axes, and depend in large measure on the body habitus of the patient as well as precordial lead placement. *Boldface type* denotes vector positivity.

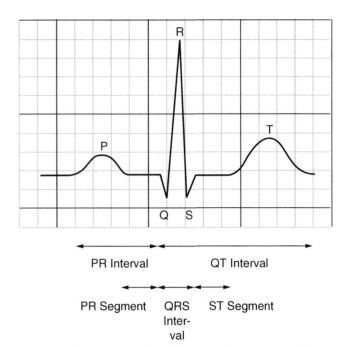

FIGURE 2-4 · **Normal ECG complex.** A normal ECG complex is shown, and waveforms, segments, and intervals are labeled.

Morphology and Intervals

A schematic of a normal ECG cycle is shown in Figure 2-4. Each of the components is explained in detail in the following sections.

P wave

Definition. The P wave corresponds to atrial depolarization. It is usually easily found just before the QRS complex; however, if the rate is rapid, the P wave may merge with the previous T wave, making it difficult to locate.

Shape. The P wave is a small, smooth, rounded wave that corresponds to the depolarization of the atria. Because of the location of the SA node in the right atrium near the superior vena cava, the right atrium depolarizes first, followed by the left atrium. Therefore, the normal direction of depolarization is leftward and inferior, yielding a positive deflection in most leads except aVR (where it is negative). Because of the right-sided placement of lead V_1, the P wave is often biphasic in this lead (and at times also in lead V_2), with the initial positive deflection reflecting right atrial depolarization, and the subsequent negative deflection reflecting left atrial depolarization[2] (Fig. 2-5).

Axis. The normal axis of the P wave is between 0 degrees and +75 degrees in the coronal plane.

Duration. The normal P wave lasts less than 0.12 sec (3 mm).

Amplitude. The P wave is normally less than 0.25 mV.

PR segment

Definition. The PR segment begins with the end of the P wave and ends with the beginning of the QRS complex.

Axis and Amplitude. The normal PR segment is isoelectric; that is, the recording returns to the baseline voltage of the

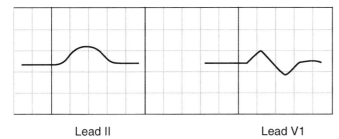

FIGURE 2-5 · P wave morphology. The normal P wave appears round and smooth in most leads, as shown in lead II here. It is often biphasic in lead V_1, with the initial positive deflection representing right atrial depolarization, and the subsequent negative deflection representing left atrial depolarization.

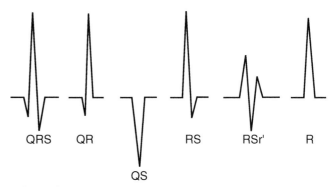

FIGURE 2-6 · QRS nomenclature. Various QRS complex morphologies and the nomenclature of the individual waves are presented. Regardless of the presence of each wave, the complex is still called a QRS complex.

preceding TP segment. Certain disease states can change the isoelectricity of this segment.

Duration. PR segment duration is discussed with the PR interval.

PR interval

Definition. The PR interval comprises the P wave and the PR segment. It represents the time required for an impulse to be conducted from the atrial fibers, through the AV node and conduction system, and to the ventricular muscle.

Duration. The normal PR interval is between 0.12 and 0.20 sec. This interval increases with age. It is also rate dependent; a faster heart rate necessitates a shorter PR interval.

QRS complex

Definition. The QRS complex represents ventricular depolarization.

Shape. The normal QRS complex is a high-amplitude, high-frequency signal on the ECG. The morphology is therefore peaked instead of rounded.

Nomenclature. Not every QRS complex has Q, R, and S waves. In fact, most do not have all three components. It is important therefore to understand the nomenclature of this complex (Fig. 2-6).

Q Wave. The designation *Q wave* refers to any initial negative deflection of the QRS complex. If the initial deflection is positive, the complex has no Q wave (it is still referred to as a QRS complex, however). If the only deflection of the complex is negative, the wave is called a QS wave.

R Wave. The first positive deflection of the QRS complex is called the **R wave**, even if it is not preceded by a Q wave.

S Wave. This designation is given to any negative deflection that is not the initial deflection (i.e., follows an R wave).

R′ Wave. Any positive deflection that follows an S wave is referred to as an *R′ wave*.

Sequence of Events. Normal ventricular depolarization begins with the activation of the interventricular septum.[3] Because this activation usually proceeds from left to right in the septum, the initial deflection of the ECG is usually rightward. This often results in a small Q wave in the leftward leads (I, II, aVL, V_4, V_5, and V_6), usually less than 0.03 sec

in duration. Q waves can also be normal in leads III and aVR, but any Q wave in leads V_1 to V_3 should be considered abnormal.[2] Depolarization then extends to the left and right ventricular myocardium. Because the left ventricular myocardium is normally larger and thicker than the right, this portion of the QRS complex is usually directed leftward and posterior, resulting in large R waves in the leftward leads. Finally, depolarization proceeds posteriorly to the left ventricular free wall, resulting in deep S waves in the anterior leads.

Axis. The different axes of the components of the QRS complex have been described previously. The summation of these vectors yields the overall QRS axis. This is determined by the relative size of both the left and right ventricles, and a change in axis from normal can be due to an increase in muscle mass in the same direction of the deviation, or a decrease in muscle mass in the opposite direction of the deviation. In the frontal plane, the normal QRS axis is between −30 degrees and +90 degrees (Fig. 2-7). QRS axis is easily determined by examining leads I, II, and aVF (Table 2-2). For the axis to be normal, the major deflection of the QRS complex must be positive in lead I and in either II or aVF (often it is positive in all three leads). Exact determination of axis in the transverse plane is more difficult, mainly because of a dependence on lead placement together with variability in body habitus between patients. In general, however, the QRS complex should be negative in lead V_1 and positive in lead V_6, with a transitional lead around V_3. The transitional lead is distinguished by having equal positive and negative deflections.

Duration. The duration, or width, of the QRS reflects the time expended during ventricular depolarization. Although there is no lower limit for the duration of the QRS, it is usually completed in less than 0.12 sec. To determine the QRS duration, measure from the onset of the first deflection to the end of the last. This may vary among leads because the onset or end of the deflection may be isoelectric in a given lead; the widest complex determines the QRS duration.

Amplitude. The amplitude of the QRS complex is variable, and may be as high as 3 mV (30 mm) in young, healthy individuals. High QRS amplitude may be an indication of a pathologic process as well. Low QRS voltage is defined as less than 0.5 mV (5 mm) in all limb leads, and less than 1.0 mV (10 mm) in all precordial leads.

R Wave Progression. As described earlier, the normal transverse axis of the QRS complex is leftward and posterior, yielding small R waves in leads V_1 and V_2, and large R waves

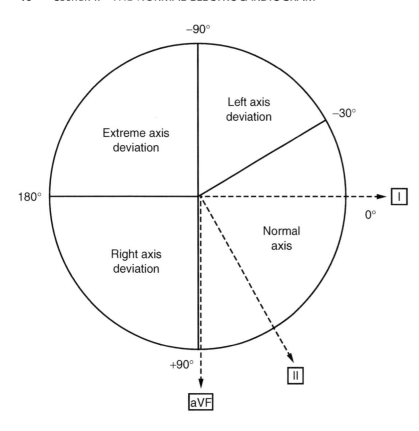

FIGURE 2-7 · **QRS axis.** Designations of frontal plane QRS axis and their relations to leads I, II, and aVF are given. (Modified from Wagner GS: Marriott's Practical Electrocardiography, 10th ed. Philadelphia, Lippincott Williams & Wilkins, 2001, p 55.)

in leads V_5 and V_6 (Fig. 2-8). Notice should be taken if the R wave progression is early or late, or does not occur at all. Progression of the R wave is associated with regression of the S wave through the precordium.

Transition Zone. As stated earlier, the precordial lead in which the QRS complex has equal positive and negative deflections is called the *transitional lead* (Fig. 2-8). As with the QRS axis in the frontal plane, the transverse axis of the QRS complex is 90 degrees, or perpendicular, to this lead; however, it is a finding that is not ordinarily expressed when reading an ECG. This lead is usually V_3 or V_4, but can vary with age and disease. Displacement of the transition zone toward the right-sided precordial leads (V_1, V_2) is termed *counterclockwise rotation,* whereas transition zone displacement toward the left-sided chest leads (V_5, V_6) is referred to

as *clockwise rotation.* This terminology can be easily remembered if the thorax is viewed in transverse section, looking up at the bottom of the heart's surface and imagining the placement of the precordial chest leads as spokes emanating out from the hub of a wheel.

Intrinsicoid Deflection. The concept of intrinsicoid deflection seeks to measure the time required from the onset of ventricular depolarization at the endocardium to the arrival of the depolarization at the epicardium. It is determined by measuring the distance from the first deflection of the initial Q or R wave

2-2 • QRS AXIS DETERMINATION USING LEADS I, II, AND aVF			
QRS Deflection			**QRS Axis**
LEAD I	**LEAD II**	**LEAD aVF**	
+	+	+	Normal
+	−	+	Normal
+	+	−	Normal
+	−	−	Left axis deviation
−	+/−	+	Right axis deviation
−	−	−	Extreme axis deviation

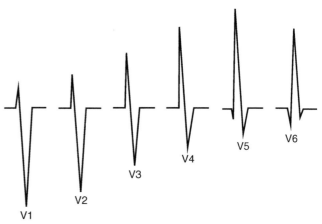

FIGURE 2-8 · **R wave progression.** The normal progression of R waves and the regression of S waves through the precordium is represented schematically. The transitional lead is V_3.

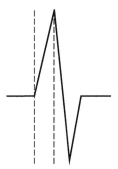

FIGURE 2-9 · Intrinsicoid deflection. The time from the onset of the QRS to the peak of the R wave in the precordium (represented by the time limited by the two *vertical broken lines*) is the intrinsicoid deflection.

to the peak of the R wave (or the nadir of the S wave in the absence of an R wave) in the precordial leads (Fig. 2-9). Normally, this occurs in less than 0.035 sec in the right precordial leads (V_1 or V_2) and less than 0.045 sec in the left precordial leads (V_5 or V_6). Thickening of the muscular wall or delay in conduction can prolong this measure.[2]

See Table 2-3 for a summary of the normal measurements of the ECG.

ST segment

Definition. The ST segment begins with the end of the QRS complex (even if there is no S wave) and ends with the beginning of the T wave.

Axis and Amplitude. Like the PR segment, the ST segment is usually isoelectric. However, many healthy people have variants in this segment of the ECG.

Duration. ST segment duration is incorporated into the discussion of the QT interval.

T wave

Definition. The T wave represents ventricular repolarization and follows the QRS complex.

Shape. Like the P wave, the T wave is usually smooth and round. The initial deflection of the T wave occurs more slowly than the return to baseline, giving the wave slight asymmetry.

Axis. T wave axis can be determined in the same way as QRS axis, as described previously. The axis of the T wave depends in large measure on the axis of the preceding QRS

complex. Repolarization is represented in the direction opposite of depolarization on the ECG. Knowing this, one would expect the T wave axis to be opposite to the QRS axis. However, depolarization occurs from endocardium to epicardium, whereas repolarization occurs from epicardium to endocardium. Thus, the QRS and T wave axes are usually similar. A precordial transitional lead may be identified for the T wave just as for the QRS complex. There may be some divergence between QRS and T axes, particularly in the precordial leads (e.g., the QRS may be negative in lead V_2 with a positive T wave), but these two axes are usually no more than 60 degrees apart.

Duration. T wave duration is discussed with the QT interval.

Amplitude. The normal amplitude of the T wave is variable. Many physiologic and pathologic factors influence its amplitude, including the amplitude of the preceding QRS complex. In general, however, T wave amplitude is less than 0.5 mV (5 mm) in the limb leads and less than 1.0 mV (10 mm) in the precordial leads.

QT interval

Definition. The QT interval is bounded by the onset of the QRS complex and the end of the T wave. It represents the time required for ventricular activation and recovery.

Duration. The duration of the QT interval varies with heart rate. Ventricular recovery must occur before the following depolarization, so as the heart rate increases, the QT interval decreases. The measurement of the QT interval must therefore be corrected for the heart rate, yielding the corrected QT interval (QT_C). The QT_C is calculated as follows (the Bazett formula):

$$QT_C = \frac{QT\ interval}{\sqrt{R\text{-}R\ interval}}$$

where the intervals are expressed in seconds. Thus, the QT interval equals the QT_C only at a heart rate of 60 bpm (where the R-R interval is 1 sec). The normal QT_C is slightly longer in women than in men, and increases with age. Many studies have been performed to define the normal range of the QT interval, with most arriving at a QT_C less than 0.44 sec.[4] As a rough assessment of QT prolongation at heart rates between 60 and 100 bpm, the QT interval should be no more

2-3 • COMPONENTS OF THE ELECTROCARDIOGRAM AND THEIR NORMAL RANGES			
ECG Component	**Axis**	**Duration (sec)**	**Amplitude (mV)**
P wave	0 to +75 degrees	≤0.12	≤0.25
PR interval	—	0.12–0.2	—
QRS complex	−30 to +90 degrees	≤0.12	>0.5 in limb leads; >1.0 in precordial leads
T wave	Within 60 degrees of QRS axis	—	—
Corrected QT interval (QT_C)	—	<0.44	—

—, not applicable.

than half the preceding R-R interval.[2] There are a few pitfalls to be avoided in measuring the QT interval. First, several leads must be examined to determine the exact end of the T wave. Second, if the rate is high, the T wave may overlap the following P wave, making determination of the end of the interval difficult. Third, if a U wave is present, it may also complicate the determination of the end of the T wave.

U wave

Definition. The U wave is a positive deflection that occasionally appears after the T wave. It is more commonly seen at slower heart rates in leads V_2 and V_4. Although its presence or absence does not signify a pathologic process, certain disease states make the U wave more prominent.

Shape. The U wave is usually smooth and round.

Axis. Normally, the U wave axis is leftward, anterior, and inferior, making it upright in all leads except aVR, and occasionally leads III and aVF.

Amplitude. The amplitude of the U wave is small, usually 5% to 25% of that of the preceding T wave.[4]

References

1. Huff J, Doernbach DP, White RD: ECG Workout, 2nd ed. Philadelphia, JB Lippincott, 1993.
2. Wagner GS: Marriott's Practical Electrocardiography, 10th ed. Philadelphia, Lippincott Williams & Wilkins, 2001.
3. Miles WM, Zipes DP: Special tests and procedures in the patient with cardiovascular disease. In Andreoli TE, Bennett JC, Carpenter CCJ, et al (eds): Cecil Essentials of Medicine, 3rd ed. Philadelphia, WB Saunders, 1993.
4. Surawicz B, Knilans TK: Chou's Electrocardiography in Clinical Practice, 5th ed. Philadelphia, WB Saunders, 2001.

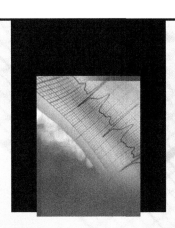

Chapter 3

Variants of Normal

Gary M. Vilke

Many electrocardiographic (ECG) findings may appear to be pathologic, but in actuality are variants of normal and do not represent a disease state. Often, these findings are noted on ECGs performed on patients with historical or clinical findings worrisome for acute disease, potentially misleading the clinician to believe that pathologic process is present when, in fact, it is not.

BENIGN EARLY REPOLARIZATION

Clinical Features

Benign early repolarization (BER), also known as early repolarization, or J point elevation, has been found in approximately 1% to 2% of the general population and 13% of emergency department (ED) patients presenting with chest pain.[1] In adult patients who use cocaine and present with chest pain, BER is found in 23% to 48%.[2]

Electrocardiographic Manifestations

ST Segment Elevation. The ST segment is minimally elevated beginning at the J point (i.e., junction of the QRS complex and the ST segment), with an upwardly concave morphology, particularly at the initial portion of the ST segment. These ST segment elevations are diffuse in distribution. Most frequently, ST segment elevation is seen in the precordial leads, ranging from V_2 to V_6, and often is greatest in V_4. The ST segment elevations range from 0.5 to 5 mm, but are usually less than 2 mm in the precordial leads and less than 0.5 mm in the limb leads.

T Waves. The T waves are usually concordant with the QRS complex and have a relatively tall amplitude and very pointed or "peaked" symmetry. The height of the T waves ranges from 5 mm in the limb leads to 6.5 mm in the precordial leads.

Tall R Waves. The R waves are tall in the left precordial leads, and there may be a rightward shift in the precordial transition zone.

ELECTROCARDIOGRAPHIC HIGHLIGHTS

Benign early repolarization

- ST segment elevation, usually from leads V_2 to V_6, ranging from 0.5 to 5 mm
- Tall T waves usually concordant with the QRS complex, ranging from 5 to 6.5 mm
- Tall R waves in the left precordial leads
- Prominent J point best seen in leads V_4 and V_5, and occasionally prominent in leads II, III, and aVF

Athlete's heart

- Sinus bradycardia (as low as 40 bpm)
- First degree atrioventricular (AV) block and second degree AV block, Mobitz type 1
- Increased R or S wave voltages
- ST segment elevation at the J point with an upwardly concave morphology
- T waves concordant with QRS complex and relatively tall
- Deep Q waves occur in up to 10% of athletes

Persistent juvenile pattern

- Inverted T waves in the right precordial leads up to a depth of 5 mm

Nonspecific T wave patterns

- T wave inversions or flattening
- QRS-T angle may be widened

ELECTROCARDIOGRAPHIC PEARLS

- In patients with cardiac risk factors or histories with concerning features, true ischemic disease often needs to be ruled out before a "normal variant" ECG diagnosis is given.
- Changes in the athletic heart's ECG are benign, but often mimic hypertrophic cardiomyopathy. A small subset has true structural cardiac disease.
- J point elevation that is concave is often a benign finding, but its presence does not rule out ischemic cardiac disease; assume the worst, especially without the help of an old ECG for comparison.

clinical presentation; in the absence of a prior ECG for comparison, it is perhaps most prudent to assume the changes are due to cardiac ischemia if the clinical scenario is suspect for that. For additional information on BER, see Chapter 40, Benign Early Repolarization.

ATHLETE'S HEART

Clinical Features

Highly trained athletes can show morphologic and functional cardiac changes, often called *athlete's heart syndrome*, that are physiologic adaptations to chronic and intensive exercise conditioning. Many of these athletes have ECGs that demonstrate a variety of changes suggesting the presence of structural cardiovascular disease, such as hypertrophic cardiomyopathy or dysrhythmogenic right ventricular cardiomyopathy. After additional evaluation, including echocardiography, these patients lack any identifiable cardiac pathologic process.[3]

Electrocardiographic Manifestations

Sinus Bradycardia. Sinus bradycardia is the most common finding in athletes, with resting heart rates that can be as low as 40 bpm. Sinus arrhythmia with or without sinus pauses of

Prominent J Point. The J point, the junction of the QRS complex and ST segment, is frequently notched or irregular; although not diagnostic of BER, this finding is highly suggestive of early repolarization. These notched J points are best seen in leads V_4 and V_5, and occasionally are prominent in the inferior leads.

Figure 3-1 is an example of BER. The ECG differential diagnosis for early repolarization includes the following: acute pericarditis, acute coronary syndrome, left bundle branch block, left ventricular hypertrophy (LVH), left ventricular (LV) aneurysm, ventricular paced rhythm, and high take-off of the ST segment. Patients should be managed in the context of

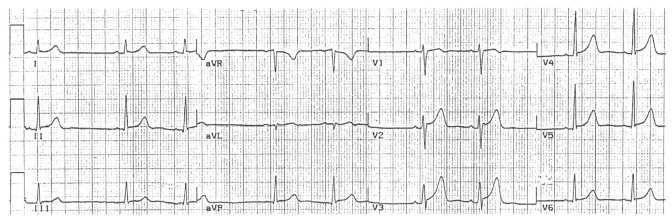

FIGURE 3-1 · **Benign early repolarization.** Note irregularity of the J point in leads II, III, aVF, and V_6 as well as the ST segment elevation with concave morphology, particularly in the precordial leads. The T waves are concordant with the QRS complex and are prominent in the precordial leads.

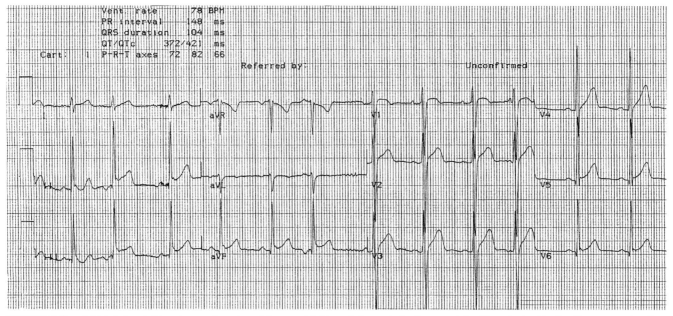

FIGURE 3-2 · Athlete's heart. Note the prominent R and S waves (similar to left ventricular hypertrophy) with upsloping J point ST segment elevations throughout the precordial leads. T waves are concordant with the QRS complex.

up to 2 seconds are also found in approximately 30% of these athletes.[4]

Heart Block. Athletes have a higher prevalence of first degree and second degree atrioventricular (AV) block compared with the general population. First degree AV block is found in up to 37% of athletes, and second-degree AV block, Mobitz type I, in 23%.[4]

Increased R or S Wave Voltages. Increases in R or S wave voltages are present in up to 80% of athletes who are engaged in endurance events. These changes may lead to the erroneous diagnosis of LVH.[4]

ST Segment Elevation. The ST segments (at the J point) may be minimally elevated with an upwardly concave morphology, particularly at the initial portion of the ST segment. These ST segment elevations are widely distributed.

Most frequently, the ST segment elevation is seen in lead V_4, but ranges from lead V_2 to V_6. Such ST segment elevation may be found in up to 30% of athletes.

T Waves. The T waves are usually concordant with the QRS complex and have a relatively tall amplitude; they are very pointed or "peaked" in shape. Numerous other altered T wave morphologies are seen, however, including flattened, biphasic, or frankly inverted T waves.[5]

Q Waves. Up to 10% of athletes may have deep Q waves, particularly in the inferior leads.[2] Figure 3-2 demonstrates some of the morphologic changes seen on the ECG of an athlete.

The ECG differential diagnosis of the morphologic changes seen with athlete's heart includes hypertrophic cardiomyopathy, LVH, acute coronary syndrome, early repolarization, LV aneurysm, and acute pericarditis.

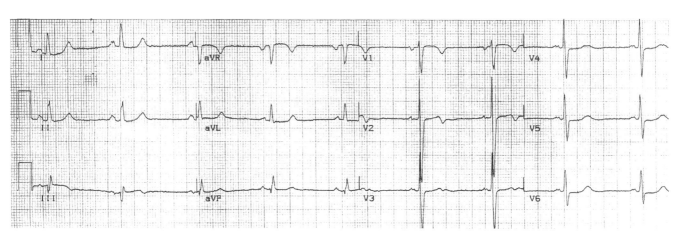

FIGURE 3-3 · Persistent juvenile pattern. Note the persistent T wave inversions in the right precordial leads, particularly V_2.

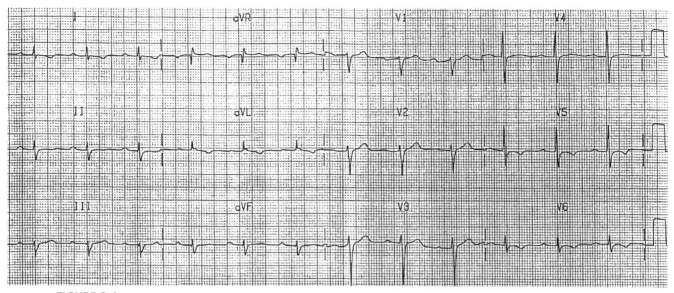

FIGURE 3-4 · **Nonspecific T wave pattern.** Note the inversions of the T waves in I, aVL, V_5, and V_6 in this otherwise healthy man.

PERSISTENT JUVENILE PATTERN

Clinical Features

Persistent juvenile pattern (PJP) is the continued presence into adulthood of T wave inversions in two or more of the right precordial leads (V_1 to V_4) that are common in infancy and childhood. PJP has been reported to be more common in blacks (11% to 12%) compared with whites (1.2%).[6]

Electrocardiographic Manifestations

The T waves of the right precordial leads (typically V_2 and V_3) are inverted in PJP, with marked inversion up to a depth of 5 mm being possible. This pattern may disappear with deep inspiration (Fig. 3-3). (For additional information, see Chapter 5, The Pediatric Electrocardiogram.)

NONSPECIFIC T WAVE PATTERNS

Clinical Features

The T wave is the one component of the ECG that can indicate underlying pathologic conditions or just be a reflection of physiologic changes in the patient. Nonspecific T wave changes that are normal variants can occur in patients at baseline, as a reaction to fear or anxiety, as a result of postprandial or postural changes, or because of hyperventilation.

Nonspecific changes have been attributed to eating a meal, and usually occur within 30 minutes of a large meal. The changes return to "normal" after a period of fasting.[7] There is a reported change in T waves in up to 11% of normal subjects with hyperventilation.[8]

Unfortunately, nonspecific changes do not always mean benign changes. In a clinical presentation that might be cardiac ischemia, and if there is no prior tracing for comparison, the nonspecific changes must be considered serious, and the patient managed as with ischemic heart disease.

Electrocardiographic Manifestations

T Wave Changes. Body position can affect T wave polarity and amplitude. For example, a semierect body position can cause diminished-amplitude or inverted T waves, particularly in the inferior leads. Postprandial changes after a large meal may include T wave flattening or inversions, particularly in leads I and II as well as V_2 to V_4. Similar changes can occur with hyperventilation (Fig. 3-4)

QRS-T Angle. The QRS-T angle (i.e., difference in number of degrees between QRS axis and T wave axis) may widen if the patient is in a more upright position.

References

1. Brady WJ, Chan TC: Electrocardiographic manifestations: Benign early repolarization. J Emerg Med 1998;17:473.
2. Hollander JE, Lozano M, Fairweather P, et al: "Abnormal" electrocardiograms in patients with cocaine-associated chest pain are due to "normal" variants. J Emerg Med 1994;12:199.
3. Pelliccia A, Maron BJ: Athlete's heart electrocardiogram mimicking hypertrophic cardiomyopathy. Curr Cardiol Rep 2001;3:147.
4. Huston P, Puffer JC, MacMillan RW: The athletic heart syndrome. N Engl J Med 1985;315:24.
5. Maron BJ, Wolfson JK, Ciro E, et al: Relation of electrocardiographic abnormalities and patterns of left ventricular hypertrophy identified by 2-dimensional echocardiography in patients with hypertrophic cardiomyopathy. Am J Cardiol 1983;51:189.
6. Gottschalk CW, Craige E: A comparison of the precordial S-T and T wave in the electrocardiograms of 600 healthy young Negro and white adults. South Med J 1956;49:453.
7. Widerlov E, Jostell KG, Claesson L, et al: Influence of food intake on electrocardiograms of healthy male volunteers. Eur J Clin Pharmacol 1999;55:619.
8. Wasserburger RH, Seibecker KL, Lewis W: The effect of hyperventilation on the normal adult electrocardiogram. Circulation 1956;13:850.

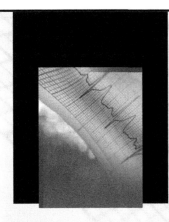

Chapter 4

Electrode Misplacement and Artifact

Richard J. Harper and Christopher F. Richards

Clinical Features

Careful use of terminology is important to the understanding of errors in technique in electrocardiographic recording. The most important of these is the confusion engendered by the use of the term *lead* for both the wires that connect to specific locations on the body and the recorded tracings on the electrocardiogram (ECG). In that context, 10 "leads" produce a 12-"lead" ECG. In this chapter we use the term *electrode* to refer to the wire that attaches the ECG machine to a specific body location and *lead* for the recording obtained by combining the data obtained from the wires.

A brief discussion of the use of electrodes to obtain the ECG is also necessary to discuss errors of ECG technique. Unlike the right arm (R arm), left arm (L arm), or left leg (L leg) electrodes, the right leg (R leg) electrode does not contribute directly to any single lead. The electrode serves as a ground but is best understood as a "drain" to eliminate voltage differences between the ECG machine and the patient. It allows the ECG machine's amplifier to eliminate the background and focus only on the voltage difference between other electrodes. In that sense, the purpose of the R leg electrode is to eliminate artifact (Personal communication, D. Brodnick, GE Marquette Inc., 2002).

Leads I, II, and III are each obtained directly by combining the output of only two limb electrodes. The unipolar augmented leads aVL, aVR, and aVF compare a single limb electrode with a "common" electrode created by combining the output of the remaining two limb electrodes. As a result, if the limb electrodes are reversed, the effect is clear and predictable in these leads. The unipolar chest electrodes use a "common" electrode obtained by the combined output of the three limb electrodes (Wilson terminal) as a basis of comparison against the single chest electrode. Reversal of limb electrodes therefore does not affect the precordial chest leads.

Electrocardiographic Manifestations

Most ECG machines in current use incorporate an algorithm for detection of common limb electrode reversals; newer technology using techniques such as neural networks promises to make detection even more sophisticated.[1] Multiple simultaneous electrode reversals are also possible but are uncommon, and the number of potential permutations exceeds the scope of this chapter. The ECG manifestations of common limb electrode reversals are reviewed in the following.

ELECTROCARDIOGRAPHIC HIGHLIGHTS

Reversed electrodes: clues to detection

L arm–R arm

- Inverted P wave and QRS complex in lead I
- Unexpected right or extreme QRS axis deviation
- Inverted P wave in lead I, together with normal precordial R wave progression (i.e., not dextrocardia)

L arm–L leg

- Lead III is upside down (may not appear abnormal)
- Leads I and II switched; aVL and aVF switched; aVR no change
- P wave is unexpectedly larger in lead I than in lead II

R arm–L leg

- P-QRS-T upside down in all leads except lead aVL
- Upright P-QRS-T in lead aVR

R leg–L leg

- Looks like normal electrode placement
- Immaterial because of similarity of potentials in lower extremities

R leg–L arm

- Lead III is practically a flat line

R leg–R arm

- Lead II is practically a flat line

L arm–L leg and R arm–R leg

- Lead I is practically a flat line
- Leads aVL and aVR are same polarity and amplitude
- Lead II is upside-down image of lead III

<table>
<tr><td>

ELECTROCARDIOGRAPHIC PEARLS

When limb electrode reversal is suspected:

- Always attempt to obtain a prior ECG for comparison.
- Repeat the ECG, checking the leads for proper placement.
- Reversal of limb electrodes produces P, QRS, and T axis shifts.

You should suspect limb electrode reversal:

- When the QRS axis is unexpectedly abnormal.
- When P waves are inverted in the limb leads—particularly lead II and lead I.
- When aVR is upright and another lead looks like aVR.
- When leads I, II, or III are a virtual flat line.

You should suspect precordial electrode reversal:

- When normal P, QRS, and T progression across the precordium is interrupted.

</td></tr>
</table>

Limb Electrode Misplacement

Although algorithms have been developed for identifying all non–R leg electrode reversals, they are often too complicated for daily use.[2] They do, however, offer two useful points to consider when there is concern about possible limb electrode reversal. The normal P wave axis in the frontal plane should lie between 0 and 75 degrees. Deviation suggests ectopic atrial rhythm, dextrocardia, or electrode reversal. Lead aVR should normally consist of inverted P, QRS, and T waves. If this is not the case, particularly if that pattern exists in another lead, electrode reversal should be suspected.

R Arm–L Arm Reversal. Arm electrode reversal is the most common error of electrode reversal and is perhaps the easiest to detect (Fig. 4-1).[3] It causes an absolute inversion of lead I wave forms; most noticeably, the P wave and QRS complex will be inverted, resulting in a right or extreme QRS axis deviation. Lead II inscribes the wave form of lead III and lead III that of lead II. Because the partial common lead is also changed, lead aVR becomes lead aVL, and vice versa. The common lead for aVF remains the combined arm electrodes

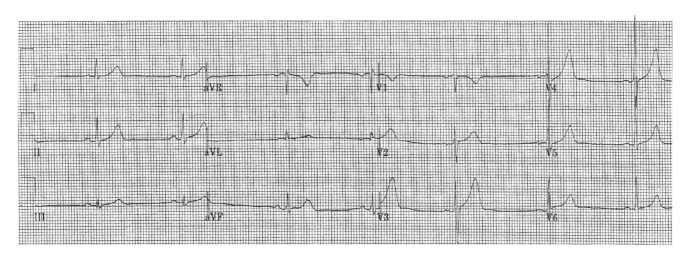

A

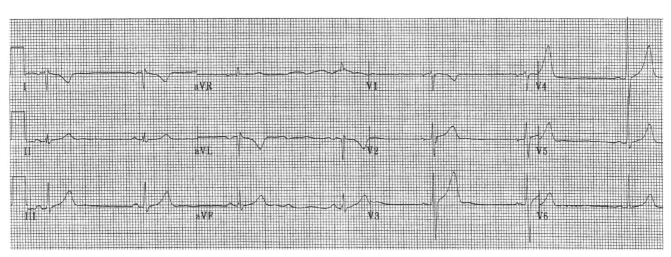

B

FIGURE 4-1 · **A, ECG obtained from a normal volunteer.** This ECG will serve as a comparison for all those in subsequent figures, except those in Figures 4-3A, 4-3B, and 4-8. **B, Arm electrode reversal.** ECG from same individual as in **A**, with left and right arm electrodes reversed. In lead I, note the P, QRS, and T wave changes, which are unexpected in a patient without dextrocardia. Note also the unusually "normal" appearance of aVR.

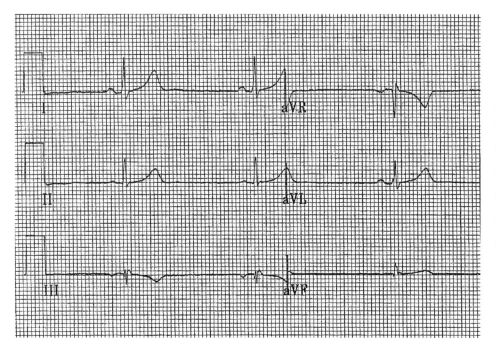

FIGURE 4-2 · L arm–L leg reversal. ECG from same individual as in Figure 4-1A, with the left arm and left leg electrodes reversed. Note that leads I and II are reversed, as are aVL and aVF. Lead aVR is unchanged, and lead III is inverted. At first glance, this tracing does not appear abnormal—without an old tracing for comparison. Note, however, that the P wave is larger in lead I than in lead II, a tip-off that L arm–L leg reversal has occurred.

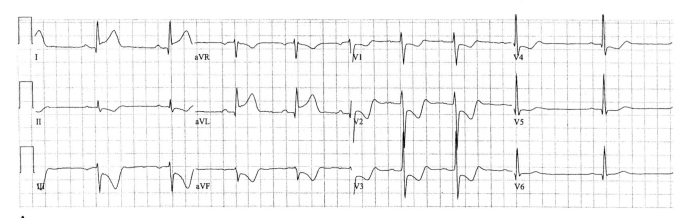

A

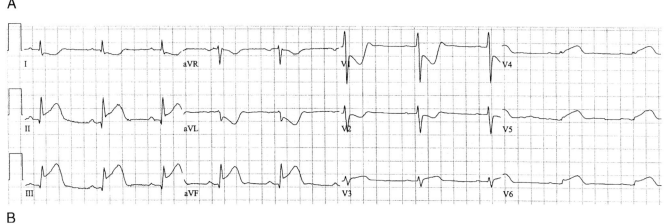

B

FIGURE 4-3 · A, L arm–L leg reversal in the setting of acute myocardial infarction. ECG showing ST elevation in leads I and aVL. This would suggest a high lateral acute myocardial infarction, with ischemic changes inferiorly (i.e., ST depression and T wave inversion)—although there is no ST elevation in V_5 or V_6. Note, however, that the P wave is larger in lead I than in lead II, a clue that on this tracing, there is L arm–L leg electrode reversal. **B, ECG from same patient with corrected limb electrode placement.** This is from the same individual as in **A**, approximately 30 minutes later. The L arm and L leg electrodes are now properly placed. As a result, ST elevation is seen in leads II, III, and aVF, and reciprocal ST depression is seen in leads I and aVL. Note also that the precordial electrodes have been repositioned across the right chest, and show evidence of concomitant right ventricular infarction (i.e., ST segment elevation in V_{3R} to V_{6R}) with posterior involvement (i.e., ST segment-T wave changes in leads V_1 to V_2).

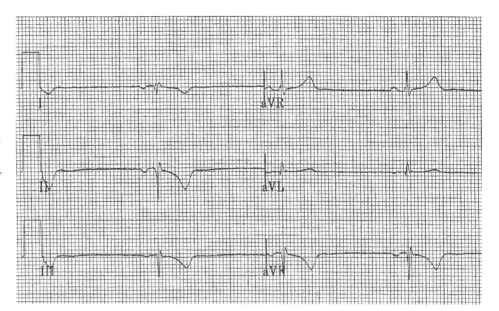

FIGURE 4-4 · R arm–L leg reversal. On this ECG, note that only lead aVL is unchanged from that in Figure 4-1A. All other nonprecordial leads appear bizarre, including the "normal" appearance of aVR.

and therefore is unchanged. The common lead for the unipolar chest leads is the combined input of the three limb electrodes, and as a result the precordial chest leads are unaffected by limb electrode reversal (see Fig. 4-1).

L Arm–L Leg Reversal.   Reversal of the L arm and L leg electrodes is more difficult to detect owing to the lack of reliable P wave inversion. Lead III is inverted by this connection. Lead I becomes lead II and lead II is lead I. Lead aVR is unchanged, whereas leads aVF and aVL are exchanged. In short, the lateral limb leads (I and aVL) are now inferior, and two of the three inferior limb leads (II and aVF) are now lateral—while the third (III) is upside down (Fig. 4-2). A helpful marker for detection is the P wave—a taller P wave in lead I compared with lead II, or a biphasic P wave in lead III with positive terminal component, suggests L arm–L leg reversal[4] (Fig. 4-3).

R Arm–L Leg Reversal.   Switching the R arm and L leg electrode inverts lead II. Lead I and III are exchanged and inverted. Although leads aVF and aVR are reversed, lead aVL is unchanged. This electrode reversal is fairly easy to detect by the upright P, QRS, and T waves in lead aVR, as well as the very abnormal QRS axis (and inverted P wave) in lead I caused by the electrode reversals (Fig. 4-4).

R Leg Reversals.   Electrode reversals involving the R leg create different patterns. Reversal of the R leg and L leg electrodes will likely go undetected, and is unimportant because there is almost no difference between the electrical potential of the legs. Reversal of the R leg electrode with either of the arm electrodes produces a characteristic and easily detectable change in the ECG. The lack of potential difference between the legs produces an asystolic, "flat line" appearance in the one limb lead that uses the L leg electrode and the

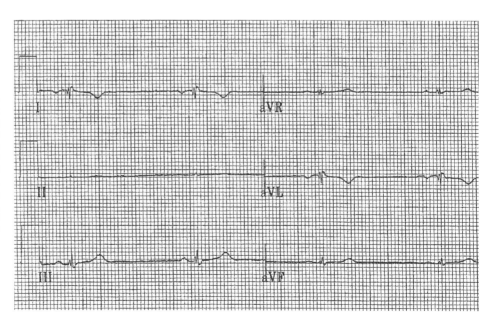

FIGURE 4-5 · R leg–R arm reversal. The characteristic "flat line" appearance in lead II signals misconnection of the R leg electrode. The point of misconnection can be deduced by remembering that the R leg electrode serves as a ground. Lead II wave forms are the result of electrical forces from the R arm position toward the L leg. Because the R arm electrode has been mistakenly replaced by the R leg electrode, there is essentially no potential difference between those two points—thus a flat line appears in lead II.

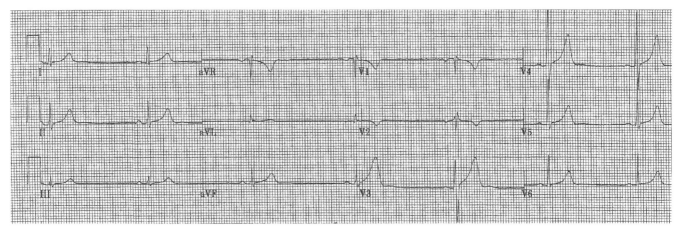

FIGURE 4-6 · **Misplacement of leads V$_1$ and V$_2$.** The appearance of a new incomplete right bundle branch block in this tracing is actually due to the fact that V$_1$ and V$_2$ were placed an interspace too high. Compare this tracing with the normal one featured in Figure 4-1A.

misconnected R leg electrode. Misconnection of the R leg electrode to the L arm makes lead III a flat line. Likewise, misconnection of the R leg electrode to the R arm causes lead II to have a flat line appearance (Fig. 4-5). Finally, placing both leg electrodes on the arms and the arm electrodes on the legs (but preserving sidedness) results in a flat line in lead I.[3]

Precordial Electrode Misplacement

Misconnection of two of the precordial electrodes interrupts the smooth transition of the R waves across the precordium and is easily detected by the careful observer. Incorrect placement of the first two precordial electrodes an interspace too high or too low may also lead to spurious recordings on the ECG. Low placement may mask incomplete right bundle branch block or right ventricular hypertrophy, and high placement may falsely suggest them (Fig. 4-6).

Artifact

ECG artifact is attributed to external (environmental) causes versus internal (patient) etiologies. Most external artifact is due to 60-Hz electrical interference; this comes from other alternating current–requiring devices in the vicinity of the patient while the tracing is recorded. Artifact can also result from a technical problem anywhere between the ECG and the patient, including the cables and their connections. Patient movement, whether involuntary (e.g., cough, hiccups, tremor, breathing) or voluntary (e.g., limb movement) is responsible for many of the internal sources of artifact.[5,6]

Electrode contact to the patient's skin can be considered an internal source of artifact. Skin impedance is minimized if the electrode is placed over an area that is not a bony prominence or pulsating artery; if hairy, the area should be clipped rather than shaven. Furthermore, drying the skin is as important as cleaning is to minimize associated artifact.[6,7] Lead artifacts may be isolated to an offending electrode by considering the leads involved (Fig. 4-7).

When movement artifact is substantial or physical considerations prevent conventional limb lead placement, the limb leads may be moved to a more proximal location. This does cause predictable changes in the ECG. Limb lead voltages may increase to a minor extent and the axis is often shifted to the right, inferiorly and posteriorly. Changes associated with acute

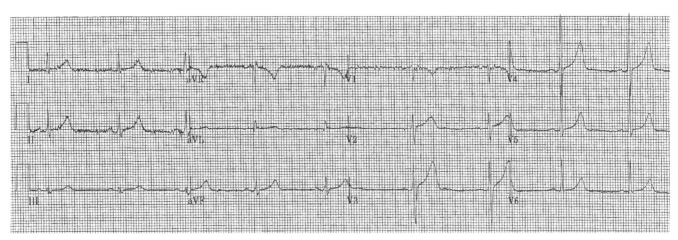

FIGURE 4-7 · **Artifact due to patient movement.** Here, the individual featured in Figure 4-1A is moving his R arm while the tracing is being recorded. The leads principally affected are, logically, I, II, and aVR because all involve the R arm electrode directly. V$_1$, as the most rightward precordial lead, is also displaying significant artifact.

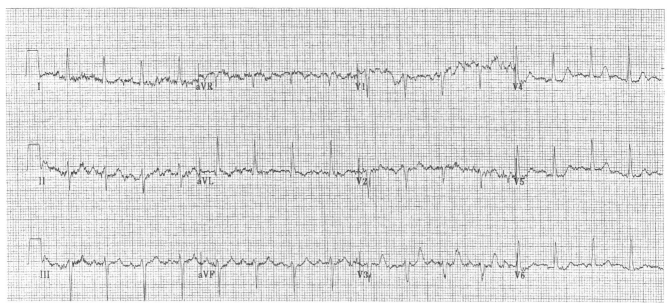

FIGURE 4-8 · **Artifact due to patient shivering.** The shivering in this mildly hypothermic patient makes P wave differentiation difficult.

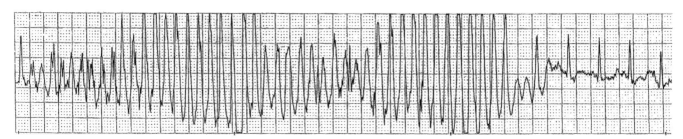

FIGURE 4-9 · **Artifact due to drug use.** This ECG rhythm strip is from a 47-year-old man with agitation from methamphetamine use. The patient's movement creates artifact mimicking the polymorphic ventricular tachycardia rhythm, torsades de pointes.

myocardial infarction (MI), particularly posterior MI, may be lost or falsely suggested. Torso positioning produces the greatest impact in the left arm because of its proximity to the myocardium.[8]

Differentiation of artifact from real abnormality is obviously important, but not always easy. The following characteristics are suggestive of artifact-induced pseudodysrhythmia as opposed to true dysrhythmia: (1) lack of symptoms or hemodynamic changes during the event; (2) appearance of "normal" ventricular complexes among dysrhythmic beats; (3) association with body movement (Figs. 4-8 and 4-9); (4) tracing baseline instability during and immediately after the apparent dysrhythmia; and (5) visible "notching" in the complexes of the pseudodysrhythmia that are synchronous with the ventricular complexes that precede and follow the apparent rhythm disturbance.[9,10]

References

1. Kors J, van Herpen G: Accurate automatic detection of electrode interchange in the electrocardiogram. Am J Cardiol 2001;88:396.

2. Ho KK, Ho SK: Use of the sinus P wave in diagnosing electrocardiographic limb lead misplacement not involving the right leg (ground) lead. J Electrocardiol 2001;34:161.

3. Surawicz B, Knilans TK: Chou's Electrocardiography, 5th ed. Philadelphia, WB Saunders, 2001.

4. Abdollah H, Milliken JA: Recognition of electrocardiographic left arm/left leg reversal. Am J Cardiol 1997;80:1247.

5. Chase C, Brady WJ: Artifactual electrocardiographic change mimicking clinical abnormality on the ECG. Am J Emerg Med 2000;18:312.

6. Surawicz B: Assessing abnormal ECG patterns in the absence of heart disease. Cardiovasc Med 1977;2:629.

7. Oster CD: Improving ECG trace quality. Biomed Instrum Technol 2000;34:219.

8. Pahlm O, Haisty WKJ, et al: Evaluation of changes in standard electrocardiographic QRS waveforms recorded from activity-compatible proximal limb lead positions. Am J Cardiol 1992;68:253.

9. Lin SL, Wang SP, Kong CW, et al: Artifact simulating ventricular and atrial arrhythmia. Jpn Heart J 1991;32:847.

10. Littman L, Monroe MH: Electrocardiographic artifact [letter]. N Engl J Med 2000;342:590.

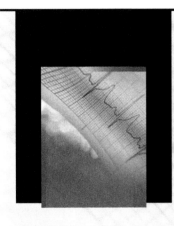

Chapter 5

The Pediatric Electrocardiogram

Kenneth J. Bramwell

Clinical Features

The electrocardiographic (ECG) changes during the first year of life reflect the switch from fetal to infant circulation, the maturation of the autonomic nervous system, and the increasing muscle mass of the left ventricle. The size of the right and left ventricles changes predictably as the neonate becomes an infant, then a child, then an adolescent. Because of the physiologic stresses on the right ventricle during fetal development, the right ventricle is larger and thicker at birth than the left ventricle. Normally, by approximately 1 month of age, the left ventricle is slightly larger. By 6 months of age, the left ventricle is twice the thickness of the right. By adolescence, the left ventricle is at least 2.5 times as thick as the right.[1]

Frequently, additional precordial leads are included on a pediatric ECG (V_{3R}, V_{4R}, and V_7). These give additional insight into the activity of the right ventricle and posterior left ventricle, which are immediately beneath these leads. This information is particularly useful for ongoing evaluation of cardiac physiology in patients with complex congenital abnormalities. In most pediatric patients, however, these leads can be ignored or covered without affecting the remainder of the ECG interpretation.

ELECTROCARDIOGRAPHIC HIGHLIGHTS

- Because of right ventricular dominance in infants, the QRS axis demonstrates a marked rightward shift with a high R/S ratio in leads V_1 and V_2, and low ratio in V_5 and V_6.
- Normal PR segment and QRS complex intervals are shorter early in infancy because of lesser cardiac muscle mass.
- With the exception of the first week of life, T wave inversion is common in children, particularly in V_1 to V_3, and is known as a *juvenile* pattern.
- Heart rates are generally higher in infants and young children, and decrease with age to adulthood.
- A QT_C interval as long as 0.49 sec is considered normal in the first 6 months of life.

Table 5-1 summarizes the significant yet normal changes that occur in cardiac physiology during the transitions from fetus to newborn, infant, child, and adolescent. The table includes age-based normal ranges for heart rate, QRS axis, PR and QRS intervals, and R and S wave amplitudes. Because such vast changes occur in the first year of life, 7 of the 12 age groupings involve the newborn and infant phases. After infancy, these changes are more subtle and more gradual as the child's ECG becomes more and more like that of the adult.

Electrocardiographic Manifestations

P Wave. The most useful leads for review of P waves are leads II and V_1. P-pulmonale or right atrial abnormality can be diagnosed in the presence of a peaked, tall P wave in lead II. In the first 6 months of life, the P wave must measure at least 3 mm to be pathologic. Thereafter, an elevation of 2 mm is adequate to establish this diagnosis.[1] P-mitrale or left atrial abnormality (LAA) can be diagnosed with a biphasic P wave in V_1 that has a terminal inferior component of one box wide and one box deep. Although LAA can also be diagnosed in the presence of a notched P wave in lead II in adults, this finding is a normal variant in approximately 25% of pediatric patients.[2]

QRS Complex. QRS complex duration is somewhat shorter than in adults, presumably because of decreased muscle mass.[2] Diagnoses of conduction disturbances must take this into account. The QRS complex is pathologically prolonged when it is longer than 0.08 sec in a patient 8 years of age or younger. In an older child or adolescent, a QRS duration of greater than 0.09 sec is also pathologic[1] (Table 5-1 and Fig. 5-1).

T Wave. The T waves in the pediatric ECG are quite variable. The change from right to left ventricular dominance in the first few days of life is reflected in the T waves.[1] The T wave is frequently upright in the first week of life throughout the precordium[2] (Fig. 5-1). Thereafter, almost all of the T waves are upright except for aVR and V_1 to V_3, where the T waves remain inverted (Figs. 5-2 and 5-3). The T waves in leads V_1 to V_3 are usually inverted from the newborn period

5-1 • AGE-RELATED NORMAL FINDINGS ON THE PEDIATRIC ECG

Age	Heart Rate, bpm (mean)	QRS Axis, degrees	PR Interval msec (mean)	QRS Duration, V₅ msec (mean)	R Wave, V₁ mm (mean)	S Wave, V₁ mm (mean)	R Wave, V₆ mm (mean)	S Wave, V₆ mm (mean)
DAYS								
<1	93–154 (123)	+59 to +193	80–160 (110)	30–70 (50)	5–26 (14)	0–23 (8)	0–11 (4)	0–9.5 (3)
1–2	91–159 (123)	+64 to +196	80–140 (110)	30–70 (50)	5–27 (14)	0–21 (9)	0–12 (4.5)	0–9.5 (3)
3–6	91–166 (129)	+77 to +193	70–140 (100)	30–70 (50)	3–24 (13)	0–17 (7)	0.5–12 (5)	0–10 (3.5)
WEEKS								
1–3	107–182 (148)	+65 to +161	70–140 (100)	30–80 (50)	3–21 (11)	0–11 (4)	2.5–16.5 (7.5)	0–10 (3.5)
MONTHS								
1–2	121–179 (149)	+31 to +113	70–130 (100)	30–80 (50)	3–18 (10)	0–12 (5)	5–21.5 (11.5)	0–6.5 (3)
3–5	106–186 (141)	+7 to +104	70–150 (110)	30–80 (50)	3–20 (10)	0–17 (6)	6.5–22.5 (13)	0–10 (3)
6–11	109–169 (134)	+6 to +99	70–160 (110)	30–80 (50)	1.5–20 (9.5)	0.5–18 (4)	6–22.5 (13)	0–7 (2)
YEARS								
1–2	89–151 (119)	+7 to +101	80–150 (110)	40–80 (60)	2.5–17 (9)	0.5–21 (8)	6–22.5 (12.5)	0–6.5 (2)
3–4	73–137 (108)	+6 to +104	90–160 (120)	40–80 (60)	1–18 (8)	0.2–21 (10)	8–24.5 (15)	0–5 (1.5)
5–7	65–133 (100)	+11 to +143	90–160 (120)	40–80 (60)	0.5–14 (7)	0.3–24 (12)	8.5–26.5 (16)	0–4 (1)
8–11	62–130 (91)	+9 to +114	90–170 (130)	40–90 (60)	0–12 (5.5)	0.3–25 (12)	9–25.5 (16)	0–4 (1)
12–15	60–119 (85)	+11 to +130	90–180 (140)	40–90 (60)	0–10 (4)	0.3–21 (11)	6.5–23 (14)	0–4 (1)

until 8 years of age. This juvenile T wave pattern, however, may persist into adolescence[1] (Fig. 5-2). T waves may remain inverted in the precordial leads up to the early teenage years (Figs. 5-2 through 5-4).

Ventricular Dominance and QRS Axis. Changes in ventricular dominance during the first year of life result in changes in the QRS axis complex, particularly across the precordium. At birth, the QRS axis is markedly rightward, the R/S ratio is high in V₁ and V₂, and the R/S ratio is low in V₅ and V₆. Over the next few months, each of these markers slowly changes to reflect the increasing muscle mass and dominance of the left ventricle. The QRS axis slowly shifts from rightward to normal. The R wave amplitude decreases in V₁ and V₂, whereas it increases in V₅ and V₆.

Heart Rate. In addition to axis changes, the heart rate decreases as these ventricles mature. The average heart rate peaks at approximately the second month of life and then gradually decreases to the adolescent and adult averages (Table 5-1).

Intervals. The PR interval and the QRS duration are relatively short in the newborn and infant phases. These intervals gradually lengthen as the cardiac muscle mass increases. During childhood, these intervals slowly approach those of

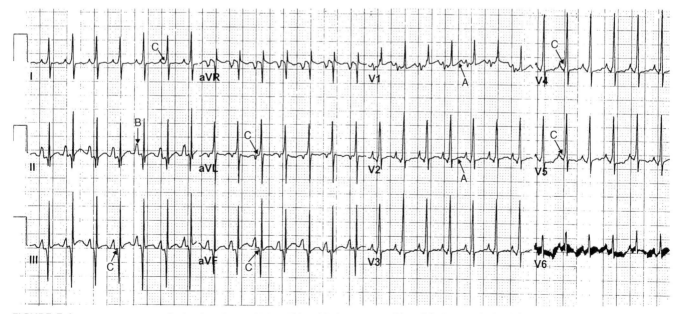

FIGURE 5-1 · **Ventricular preexcitation in a 5-day-old boy.** This ECG demonstrates (A) upright T waves in the right precordial leads (normal for age), (B) right atrial enlargement (as seen in lead II), (C) delta waves in multiple leads (indicative of ventricular preexcitation syndrome [Wolff-Parkinson-White syndrome]), and normal PR interval and QRS complex durations.

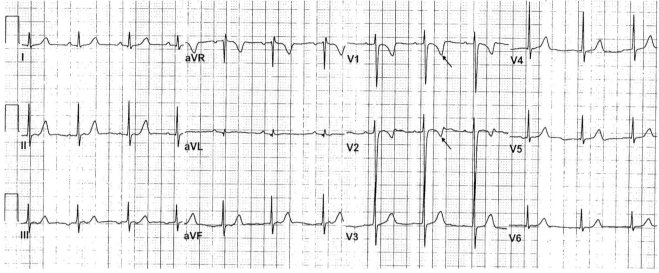

FIGURE 5-2 · **Normal ECG from a 10-year-old girl.** Note inverted T waves in leads V_1 and V_2 (*arrows*), consistent with a juvenile pattern.

the adult ECG (Table 5-1). These shorter intervals should be kept in mind when evaluating a pediatric ECG for atrioventricular (AV) blocks and bundle branch abnormalities. The corrected QT interval (QT_C) should be determined on all pediatric ECG interpretations. During the first 6 months of life, the QT_C is slightly longer and is considered normal below 0.49 sec. Thereafter, any QT_C longer than 0.44 sec is abnormal.[3]

Pathologic Conditions

Ventricular Hypertrophy. The diagnosis of right ventricular hypertrophy can be supported by various ECG findings that reflect increased mass or pressure in the right precordium. These include an R wave that is larger than the 98th percentile for age in lead V_1, an S wave that is larger than the 98th

percentile in lead V_6, an upright T wave in leads V_1 to V_3 after the first week of life, and a persistent newborn pattern of right ventricular dominance.[1] The diagnosis of left ventricular hypertrophy is, in similar fashion, supported by ECG abnormalities that suggest enlarged left ventricular muscle mass. These include an R wave that is larger than the 98th percentile in lead V_6, an S wave that is larger than the 98th percentile in lead V_1, left ventricular "strain" pattern in V_5 and V_6, and "adult" precordial R wave progression during the newborn period.[1,2]

Bundle Branch Blocks. Right bundle branch block (RBBB) can be diagnosed in the presence of pathologic QRS complex prolongation for age with normal initial forces and abnormal rightward and anterior terminal forces. Frequently, this manifests as a wide QRS complex with an rSR' pattern in leads V_1 and V_2. RBBB occurs most commonly after surgical repair of

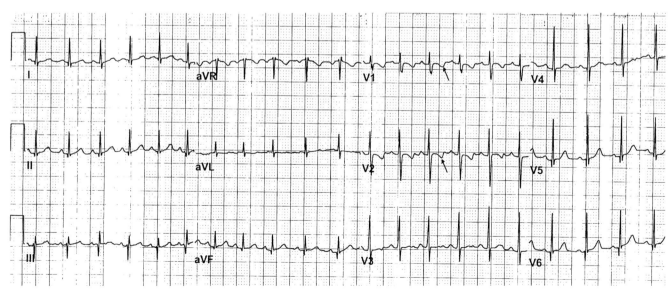

FIGURE 5-3 · **Normal ECG from a 19-month-old girl.** Note the juvenile T wave inversion (*arrows*), which is normal for age.

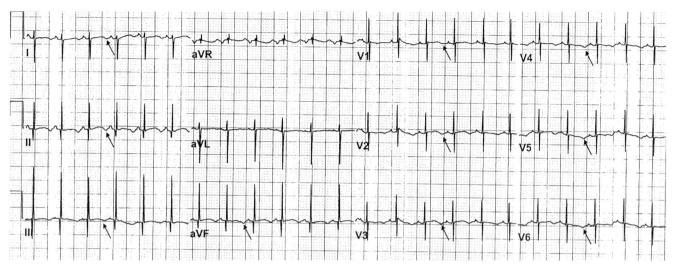

FIGURE 5-4 · ECG from a 2-day-old girl. The ECG reveals diffuse T wave flattening and slight inversion (*arrows*), which is a nonspecific finding.

congenital heart defects, especially ventricular septal defects.[1] Similarly, left bundle branch block (LBBB) can be diagnosed in the presence of a pathologically wide QRS complex with abnormal (absent) initial forces and abnormal leftward and posterior forces. This is usually best appreciated in leads V_5 and V_6. LBBB is quite rare in children. When these criteria for LBBB are met, the ECG should be carefully reviewed for Wolff-Parkinson-White syndrome because this is a more common explanation for this pattern. In both types of bundle branch block, the T waves are usually discordant from the main axis of the QRS complex. A "strain" pattern is sometimes noted wherein the ST segments are also discordant from the main QRS complex and are either elevated or depressed.

Atrioventricular Blocks.   First degree AV block can be confirmed by an ECG with a PR interval that is prolonged for age. As noted in Table 5-1, the normal PR interval duration varies with age. Second degree and third degree AV blocks are also seen on pediatric ECGs and are considered abnormal (Fig. 5-5).

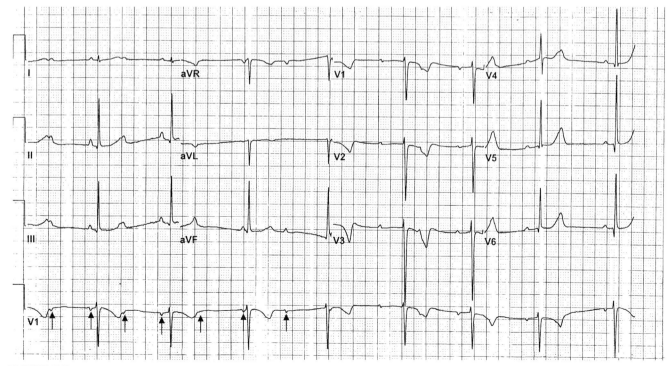

FIGURE 5-5 · Third degree AV block in a 5-year-old boy. The patient has complete heart block and a junctional escape rhythm with a rate of 49 bpm. Note the regular P waves in the rhythm strip at the bottom that are not conducted (*arrows*).

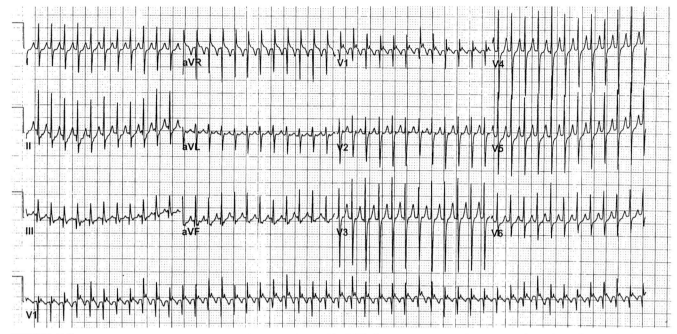

FIGURE 5-6 · **Narrow complex tachycardia in a 13-month-old boy.** The ECG shows a narrow-complex, very regular tachycardia (ventricular rate of 283 bpm), consistent with supraventricular tachycardia.

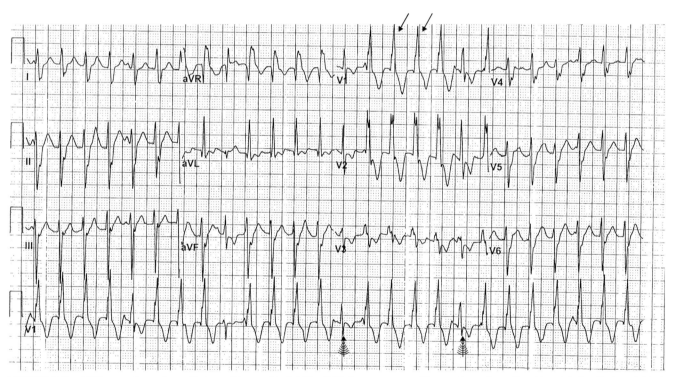

FIGURE 5-7 · **Wide complex tachycardia in an 11-year-old girl.** The ECG demonstrates a wide-complex tachycardia with a right bundle branch block morphology in lead V_1 (*plain arrows*) and occasional fusion beats (lead V_1 rhythm strip, *arrow with notches*), consistent with ventricular tachycardia.

ELECTROCARDIOGRAPHIC PEARLS

- The interpretation of the pediatric ECG is highly dependent on age.
- Because of the narrow width of the QRS complex in the pediatric ECG, ventricular tachycardia may be mistaken for supraventricular tachycardia.
- The juvenile T wave pattern can persist into early adulthood.

Supraventricular Tachycardia.   Supraventricular tachycardia (SVT; Fig. 5-6) is the most common dysrhythmia in infants and children.[1,2,4] In otherwise healthy children, SVT occurs with a frequency of between 1 in 250 and 1 in 1000 patients.[4] The ECG appearance is that of a narrow-complex, regular tachycardia with a rate between 150 and 300 bpm. P waves may not be evident because of the rapid rate. The peak age for SVT is the first 2 months of life, when approximately 40% of patients with SVT have a first episode. Most of these episodes are due to an AV reentrant mechanism.[4]

Ventricular Tachycardia.   Ventricular tachycardia (VT) is quite rare in children. The ECG in VT shows a tracing with a QRS complex that is both too fast and too wide for age. Such a tracing may also occur in cases of SVT with aberrant conduction. Similar to adult patients, it is not always clear from the ECG whether VT or SVT with aberrant conduction is present. The presence of fusion beats, capture beats, or AV dissociation favors VT (Fig. 5-7).

References

1. Allen HD, Gutgesell HP, Clark EB, Driscoll DJ (eds): Moss and Adams' Heart Disease in Infants, Children, and Adolescents, 6th ed. Philadelphia, Lippincott Williams & Wilkins, 2001.
2. Garson A Jr, Becker JT, Fisher DJ, Neish SR (eds): The Science and Practice of Pediatric Cardiology, 2nd ed. Baltimore, Williams & Wilkins, 1998.
3. Deal BJ, Wolff GS, Gelband H (eds): Current Concepts in Diagnosis and Management of Arrhythmias in Infants and Children. Armonk, NY, Futura, 1998.
4. Ziegler VL, Gillette PC (eds): Practical Management of Pediatric Cardiac Arrhythmias. Armonk, NY, Futura, 2001.

Section II
The Abnormal Electrocardiogram

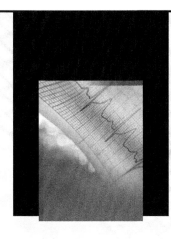

Chapter 6

Dysrhythmias at Normal Rates

Richard A. Harrigan

A normal heart rate is defined as ranging from 60 to 100 bpm in the adult, although the upper and lower limits of normal vary with conditions such as age, autonomic nervous system tone, and physical conditioning. Rhythm abnormalities may stem from the sinus node, the atrioventricular (AV) node, or virtually any other locus in the atria or ventricles.

Dysrhythmias occurring at normal rates can be deciphered by examining the *regularity* of the rhythm as well as

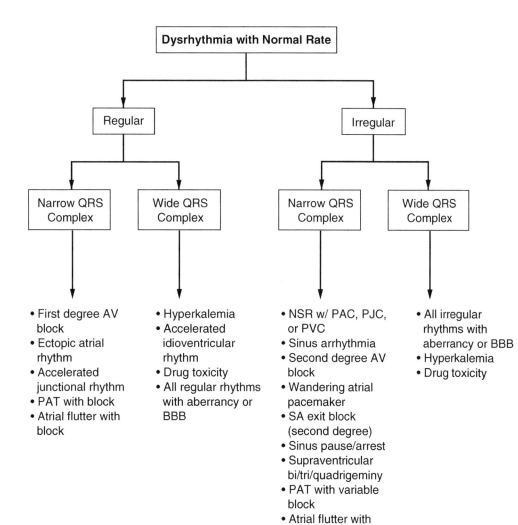

the *width of the QRS complex*. Regular rhythms imply a solitary locus of impulse activity, at the sinus node or elsewhere. Irregularity suggests that impulses are originating from a site other than the sinus node, either in competition with the sinus node (e.g., normal sinus rhythm with premature ventricular contractions), or from multiple other sites in the absence of sinus nodal impulses (e.g., atrial fibrillation). Irregularity also may arise from variable sinoatrial (SA) or AV conduction, as is the case with various "blocks" (e.g., sinus exit or SA block, AV block).

Normal ventricular depolarization is reflected by a QRS width that is less than 0.12 sec. Depolarization of the ventricle that is prolonged in duration, resulting from a number of etiologies (e.g., bundle branch block, ventricular origin of the impulse, AV conduction through an accessory pathway), manifests with QRS prolongation.

Differential Diagnosis of Dysrhythmias at Normal Rates

Regular rhythm, narrow QRS complex

Several rhythms aside from normal sinus rhythm (NSR) may occur at normal rates (60 to 100 bpm) with regular spacing of the QRS complexes. Those with narrow QRS complexes implying normal ventricular depolarization are listed in this section.

Normal Sinus Rhythm with First Degree Atrioventricular Block.   Each P wave occurs at a regular interval, and is followed by a QRS complex. The PR interval, however, is longer than 0.2 sec (Fig. 6-1).

Ectopic Atrial Rhythm.   Again, each P wave is followed by a QRS complex, and the PR interval should be normal (0.12 to 0.2 sec). Ectopic atrial rhythm differs from NSR in that the P wave morphology is different from that of the sinus P wave because of an alternative site of origin in the atrium. If the impulses originate in the lower atrium, the P waves may be inverted in the inferior leads (II, III, and aVF; Fig. 6-2), making this difficult to distinguish from an AV junctional rhythm (see next subsection).

Accelerated Junctional Rhythm.   The AV junction is a secondary pacemaker site, with an intrinsic rate of roughly 40 to 60 bpm. Accelerated junctional rhythms occur when the AV junctional rate is faster than the sinus nodal rate, are usually 70 to 130 bpm, and are seen in diseased hearts owing to such conditions as ischemia or digoxin toxicity. If these impulses capture the atria through retrograde conduction, the P wave may appear before, during, or after the QRS complex

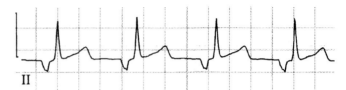

FIGURE 6-2 • **Ectopic atrial rhythm.** These atrial impulses probably originate in the low atrium because the P waves are inverted in the inferior leads (lead II shown here). This resembles a junctional rhythm, but the PR interval exceeds 0.12 sec, and thus appears to be from an ectopic atrial focus.

because the impulse originating at the AV junction may capture the ventricle before, during, or after it captures the atria (Fig. 6-3). These retrograde P waves are the clue to the source of the rhythm because they are often inverted in the inferior leads II, III, and aVF. If the P wave precedes the QRS complex, the interval should be short—less than 0.11 sec. If the AV junctional pacemaker fails to capture the atria, then the two will coexist and AV dissociation will result. The clue here is that the ventricular rate (at 70 to 130 bpm) is usually faster than the atrial rate.

Paroxysmal Atrial Tachycardia with Block.   Best known as "PAT with block," this is the classic digitoxic rhythm. The atrial rate is tachycardic, characteristically between 150 and 250 bpm. The P wave morphology differs from the sinus P waves, and is often best seen in lead V_1. With high-grade and consistent AV block (e.g., 2:1, 3:1), the QRS complexes appear at a normal rate and regular interval (Fig. 6-4).

Atrial Flutter with Block.   Atrial flutter usually features a regular atrial rate that is faster than that of atrial tachycardia (200 to 400 bpm). High-grade block, as might appear with disease or drug-modulated AV nodal conduction (e.g., 4:1), may yield a regular ventricular response in the normal range. The "sawtooth" shape of the flutter wave, best seen in lead V_1 or the inferior leads, is the key to distinguishing this rhythm (Fig. 6-5).

Regular rhythm, wide QRS complex

All of the rhythms mentioned in the preceding section may exhibit wide QRS complex morphology if there is *coexistent bundle branch block, preexcitation,* or *aberrant conduction.* The following should also be considered in the differential diagnosis of regular rhythms at normal rates with wide ventricular complexes.

Accelerated Idioventricular Rhythm.   Accelerated idioventricular rhythms are regular wide complex rhythms with

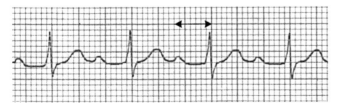

FIGURE 6-1 • **First degree atrioventricular block.** The PR interval here exceeds 0.24 sec.

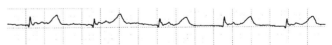

FIGURE 6-3 • **Accelerated junctional rhythm.** No P waves precede these junctional complexes, which occur at a rate higher than expected from a junctional pacemaker. The small positive deflections between the QRS complexes and their associated T waves may be retrograde P waves, seen here in lead II.

Lead VI

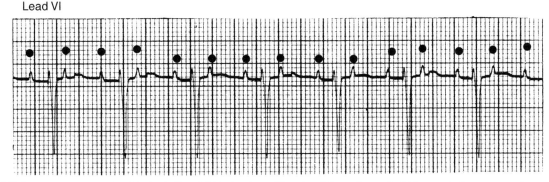

FIGURE 6-4 · **Atrial tachycardia with block.** Here 2:1 block exists, with each atrial complex marked. The ventricular rate approximates 100 bpm.

FIGURE 6-5 · **Atrial flutter with 4:1 block.** Lead II highlights the flutter waves in this tracing.

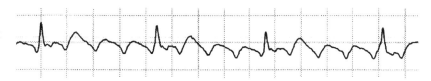

FIGURE 6-6 · **Accelerated idioventricular rhythm.** This is a regular wide-complex rhythm, with a normal rate, and without P waves. There was no evidence of bundle branch block.

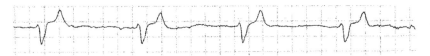

rates usually from 40 to roughly 120 bpm (Fig. 6-6). This rhythm may emerge after reperfusion following myocardial infarction, but can be associated with other types of heart disease as well as rarely with normal hearts. Clues are the regular wide QRS complexes; AV dissociation, capture beats, or fusion beats are sometimes seen, as with ventricular tachycardia.

Hyperkalemia. This electrolyte abnormality may cause widening of the QRS complex, as well as the classic peaking of the T waves that is usually evident first. Lengthening of the PR interval, and indeed in the duration of the P wave itself, may also be seen (Fig. 6-7).

Drug Toxicity. Pharmacologic agents (e.g., tricyclic antidepressants) that cause prolongation of the QRS complex at toxic levels often present with wide-complex tachycardic rhythms (see chapters in Toxicology section). However, these agents may present with wide-complex rhythms at normal rates, especially if there is a coingestion that slows the heart rate, or there is underlying heart disease.

Irregular rhythm, narrow QRS complex

Several rhythms may occur at normal rates (60 to 100 bpm) with irregular spacing of the QRS complexes. Those with narrow QRS complexes implying normal ventricular depolarization are listed in this section.

Normal Sinus Rhythm with Premature Atrial, Junctional, or Ventricular Contractions. One or more premature beats may occur on the tracing or rhythm strip; they all may be from the same focus or from a variety of foci. *Premature atrial contractions* (PACs) are characterized by P waves of a different

morphology that occur earlier than expected given the cycle length of the NSR (Fig. 6-8). The P wave morphology may be similar to the sinus P wave, or quite different, depending on the site of impulse origin in the atrium. PACs "reset" the sinus node, leading to a longer R-R interval immediately after the PAC (unless another PAC occurs). They are of little clinical significance; the patient may or may not be aware of them.

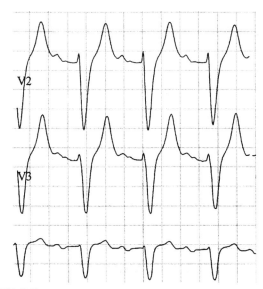

V2

V3

FIGURE 6-7 · **Hyperkalemia.** Hints to the cause of this wide-complex rhythm at a normal rate are the PR interval and QRS complex prolongation, plus the tall T waves seen in the precordial leads.

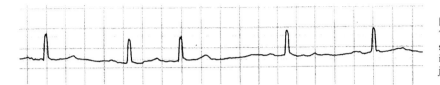

FIGURE 6-8 • **Premature supraventricular complex.** This rhythm was read as normal sinus rate with premature supraventricular beats because it is difficult to determine if the third complex is of a premature atrial or premature junctional origin.

Premature junctional contractions (PJCs) are less common than PACs, and are also of little clinical significance. They may or may not reset the sinus node. PJCs are characterized by earlier than expected QRS complexes that either are not preceded by any atrial activity, or, if the junctional impulse captures the atria, the P wave may occur before, during, or after the QRS complex. Inverted P waves in the inferior leads with a normal PR interval may be due to ectopic atrial impulses or junctional impulses. *Premature ventricular contractions* (PVCs), like PACs, are quite common, and again usually of little clinical significance, although the patient may be aware of them. PVCs are early beats emanating from the ventricle, and as such are wide-complex beats with discordant ST segment and T wave changes. Similar to PACs, they may be unifocal or multifocal. Unlike PACs, there is a "compensatory pause" after a PVC; this can be detected with calipers by "marching out" the normal QRS complexes through the PVC (the sinus node is not reset) and noting that the regular R-R interval is maintained after a pause of one beat due to the PVC (Fig. 6-9).

PACs, PJCs, and PVCs may occur in couplets (two consecutive beats), or in a "regularly irregular" pattern, such as bigeminy, trigeminy, or quadrigeminy (Fig. 6-10). Premature beats may be "blocked" (e.g., blocked PAC), wherein the atrial impulse occurs early, but the ventricle does not depolarize (i.e., there is no accompanying QRS complex) because of the ventricle's refractory period. This leads to a pause in the rhythm, and may be difficult to detect if the blocked PAC is nested in the preceding T wave.

Sinus Dysrhythmia. Here the P wave morphology does not vary, but the P-P interval does, leading to phasic variation in the cardiac cycle. Sinus dysrhythmia may be due to respiratory variation (inspiration leads to longer intervals; expiration

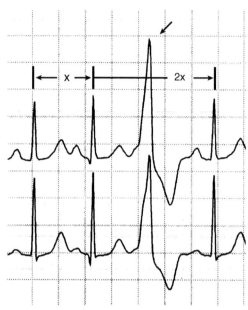

FIGURE 6-9 • **Premature ventricular contraction.** Note that the sinus rate can be "marched through" the third beat (the premature ventricular complex, marked with an *arrow*), so that the basic sinus interval ("x") is maintained.

to shorter intervals) or may be independent of respiration (Fig. 6-11). The latter is more commonly pathologic (but may be inconsequential) and is more frequently seen in the elderly.

Sinus Pause. Temporary failure of impulse generation from the SA node results in a break in the normal sinus rhythm, termed *sinus pause* (or *sinus arrest* if prolonged) (see Chapter 18, Sinus Pause/Sinus Arrest). Sinus pause results in

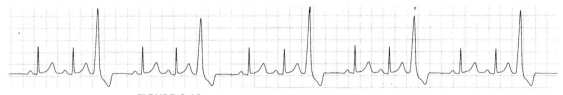

FIGURE 6-10 • **Premature ventricular contractions in trigeminy.**

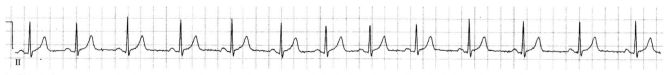

FIGURE 6-11 • **Sinus dysrhythmia.** Note the gradual lengthening and shortening of the R-R cycle; in this 19-year-old woman, it was attributable to her respiratory cycle.

FIGURE 6-12 • **Second degree atrioventricular block, Mobitz type I.** The PR interval lengthens over two beats, and then a QRS complex is "dropped" after the third P wave.

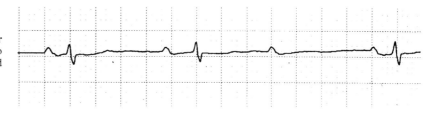

FIGURE 6-13 • **Atrial flutter with variable block.** Four flutter waves precede the second and third ventricular complexes, whereas only three precede the last complex in this lead II tracing.

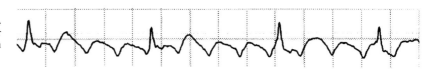

a break in the normal P-P interval that is not cyclic, as opposed to SA block (or sinus exit block; see next subsection).

Sinoatrial Block. Also termed *sinus exit block*, only second degree SA block can be detected on the surface 12-lead electrocardiogram. The key to detecting SA block is a pause in the regular rhythm due to a dropped P-QRS-T. Unlike a sinus pause, which also features a dropped P-QRS-T, type II second degree SA block characteristically has a P-P interval during the pause that is a multiple (if not perfect, nearly perfect) of the underlying sinus P-P interval. Type I second degree SA block features progressive shortening of the P-P interval until the dropped P-QRS-T. SA block may or may not be pathologic (see Chapter 19, Sinoatrial Exit Block).

Wandering Atrial Pacemaker. This term refers to three or more atrial morphologies, with each P wave still followed by a QRS complex. Physiologically, this may be due to a shift in site of origin of the atrial impulse, or to variation in impulse conduction. This finding is rarely of clinical significance.

Second Degree Atrioventricular Block. First and third degree AV blocks are usually regular rhythms, but, by definition, second degree AV block must display some irregularity because at least one QRS-T sequence is dropped with this form of conduction block (Fig. 6-12).

Paroxysmal Atrial Tachycardia with Variable Block. If PAT with block (see earlier discussion) features a block in AV conduction that is variable (i.e., not uniformly two atrial beats per one QRS, or 3:1 or the like), the rhythm will be irregular.

Atrial Fibrillation with Normal Ventricular Response. If AV nodal conduction is slowed by age, disease, or pharmacologic agents, the fibrillating atria may be associated with a ventricular response at normal rates yet at irregular intervals.

Atrial Flutter with Variable Block. Similar to PAT with block, if the ratio of atrial flutter waves to QRS complexes is variable (e.g., 4:1, then 3:1, and so forth), atrial flutter may manifest as an irregular ventricular rhythm (Fig. 6-13).

Irregular rhythm, wide QRS complex

All of the rhythms mentioned in the previous section may exhibit wide QRS complex morphology if there is *coexistent bundle branch block, preexcitation,* or *aberrant conduction.*

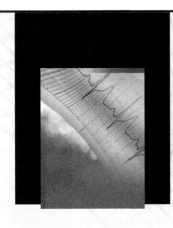

Chapter 7

Bradydysrhythmias

William J. Brady

Bradydysrhythmia occurs with a ventricular rate less than 60 beats per minute. It may result from a broad range of clinical syndromes with extremely varied pathophysiologic processes. These rhythm disturbances may result from acute coronary syndromes, chronic ischemia, pharmacologic effects, toxic issues, metabolic effects, and chronic conduction system disease. Specific mechanisms include reversible ischemia, irreversible infarction, altered autonomic influence, poisoning of the pacemaker/conduction system, metabolic effect, and chronic degeneration of the system.

Features to consider in the electrocardiographic differential diagnosis include the rate, the presence or absence of a P wave, regularity of association between the P wave and QRS complex, and width of the QRS complex. In particular, both the regularity and the width of the QRS complex are very important diagnostic considerations.

Differential Diagnosis of Bradydysrhythmia

Regular rhythm, narrow QRS complex

Sinus Bradycardia. Sinus bradycardia (Fig. 7-1) is present when the pacemaker focus is in the sinoatrial (SA) node and is diagnosed with the following criteria: (1) ventricular rate less than 60 bpm; (2) regular rhythm; (3) narrow QRS complex (note that the QRS complex may be wide if a preexisting bundle branch block is present); (4) direct P wave association with QRS complex; (5) normal P wave morphology with upright P waves in leads I and II; and (6) normal PR interval that is consistent from beat to beat.

Junctional Rhythm. If bradycardic, a junctional rhythm is considered an "escape rhythm" with a focus in the atrioventricular (AV) node (Fig. 7-2). It is diagnosed with the following criteria: (1) ventricular rate of 45 to 60 bpm; (2) regular rhythm; and (3) narrow QRS complex (note that the QRS complex may be wide if a preexisting bundle branch block is present); retrograde P waves may be seen in certain leads.

Third Degree (Complete) Atrioventricular Block. This rhythm occurs with dysfunction below the AV node in the ventricular conduction system; rarely, it is within the AV node. This rhythm occurs when the atria and ventricles are controlled by different pacemakers and are functioning independently with no atrial impulses reaching the ventricles. The atrial rhythm results from either a sinus or an ectopic pacemaker focus. The sinus rhythm is characterized by a variable rate (slow, normal, or rapid); other atrial rhythms include atrial flutter or fibrillation. The ventricular "escape" rhythms result from a focus immediately below the level of block. Rarely, no ventricular escape rhythm is seen, resulting in an asystolic arrest. Third degree AV block is diagnosed with the following criteria: (1) atrial rate greater than ventricular rate; (2) no relationship between P wave and QRS complex; (3) P waves occur in regular rhythm; and (4) QRS complexes occur in regular rhythm. The QRS complex duration and ventricular rate depend on the site of block; that is, near the His bundle the rate is greater than 40 bpm with a narrow QRS complex, and distal to His bundle, the rate is less than 40 bpm with a wide QRS complex.

Regular rhythm, wide QRS complex

Sinus bradycardia, junctional rhythm, and *third degree AV block* (Fig. 7-3) may also present with a widened QRS complex. Regarding sinus bradycardia and junctional rhythms, this widened QRS complex presentation occurs with simultaneous bundle branch block. Concerning third degree AV block, the QRS complex of the escape rhythm is frequently wide based on the location of the escape focus.

Idioventricular Escape Rhythm. An idioventricular rhythm is noted if the focus of the escape rhythm is found in the His–bundle branch system; the QRS complex is wide with a rate of 30 to 45 bpm (Fig. 7-4). Rarely, if no pacemaker site is able to assume control, complete ventricular asystole results.

Sinoventricular Rhythm. This rhythm occurs in the setting of advanced hyperkalemia with significant dysfunction of cardiac conduction (Fig. 7-5). The focus remains in the SA node, yet conduction in the atria, between the atria and ventricles, and between the ventricles is significantly disrupted, resulting in a significantly slower rate, no evidence of P waves, and a widened QRS complex.

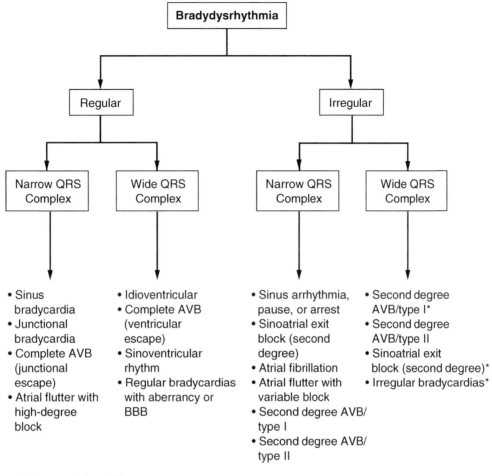

* Sinus
  bradycardia
* Junctional
  bradycardia
* Complete AVB
  (junctional
  escape)
* Atrial flutter with
  high-degree
  block

* Idioventricular
* Complete AVB
  (ventricular
  escape)
* Sinoventricular
  rhythm
* Regular bradycardias
  with aberrancy or
  BBB

* Sinus arrhythmia,
  pause, or arrest
* Sinoatrial exit
  block (second
  degree)
* Atrial fibrillation
* Atrial flutter with
  variable block
* Second degree AVB/
  type I
* Second degree AVB/
  type II

* Second degree
  AVB/type I*
* Second degree
  AVB/type II
* Sinoatrial exit
  block (second degree)*
* Irregular bradycardias*

* With co-existing BBB

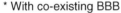

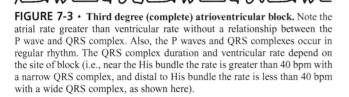

FIGURE 7-1 · Sinus bradycardia. The rate is less than 60 bpm with a normal PR interval and QRS complex duration.

FIGURE 7-2 · Junctional rhythm. Note the ventricular rate of 45 to 60 bpm with a regular rhythm and narrow QRS complex.

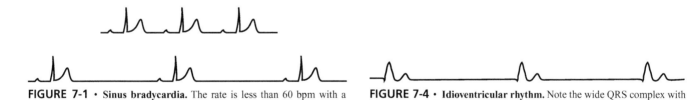

FIGURE 7-3 · Third degree (complete) atrioventricular block. Note the atrial rate greater than ventricular rate without a relationship between the P wave and QRS complex. Also, the P waves and QRS complexes occur in regular rhythm. The QRS complex duration and ventricular rate depend on the site of block (i.e., near the His bundle the rate is greater than 40 bpm with a narrow QRS complex, and distal to His bundle the rate is less than 40 bpm with a wide QRS complex, as shown here).

FIGURE 7-4 · Idioventricular rhythm. Note the wide QRS complex with a rate of 30 to 45 bpm.

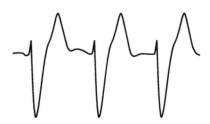

FIGURE 7-5 · Sinoventricular rhythm. Note the widened QRS complex without evidence of P wave activity.

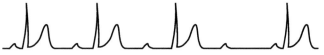

FIGURE 7-6 · **Second degree, Mobitz type I atrioventricular block.** Note the narrow QRS complex with an initially normal or prolonged "baseline" PR interval, then a progressive PR interval lengthening until an impulse is unable to reach the ventricles, resulting in a nonconducted P wave.

Irregular rhythm, narrow QRS complex

Second Degree/Mobitz Type I Atrioventricular Block. This rhythm, also known as Wenckebach AV block, occurs with dysfunction in or above the AV node (Fig. 7-6). In most instances, the rate is adequate and a progressively lengthening PR interval is noted. It is diagnosed with the following criteria: (1) a narrow QRS complex; (2) an initially normal or prolonged "baseline" PR interval; (3) progressive PR interval lengthening until an impulse is unable to reach the ventricles, resulting in a nonconducted P wave; and (4) an R-R interval pattern with grouped beating (R-R interval shortens as PR interval lengthens until a lone, nonconducted P wave appears without its associated QRS complex), producing the characteristic "grouped beating" of Wenckebach.

Second Degree/Mobitz Type II Atrioventricular Block. This rhythm, also known as non-Wenckebach AV block, occurs with dysfunction in or below the AV node (Fig. 7-7A). The "baseline" PR interval is either normal or prolonged (i.e., occurs in association with first degree AV block); the PR interval is always constant without progressive change. It is diagnosed with the following criteria: (1) a fixed PR interval; (2) a QRS complex that is usually widened (Fig. 7-7B), although it may be narrow (Fig. 7-7A); and (3) a constant PR interval until the impulse is unable to reach ventricles, resulting in a nonconducted P wave.

The magnitude of block is expressed as a ratio of P waves to QRS complexes (e.g., three P waves for two QRS complexes is a 3:2 block).

Distinguishing type I AV block from type II block is usually straightforward unless a 2:1 conduction pattern is present. The QRS complex width in Mobitz block may provide information regarding level of block, with a type II AV block usually associated with widened QRS complex escape rhythm (Fig. 7-7B).

Atrial Fibrillation/Flutter with Slow Ventricular Response. This form of bradydysrhythmia occurs with ventricular rates less than 60 bpm; criteria are otherwise unchanged for the ECG diagnoses of atrial fibrillation or flutter (see Chapter 22, Atrial Fibrillation and Atrial Flutter) (Fig. 7-8).

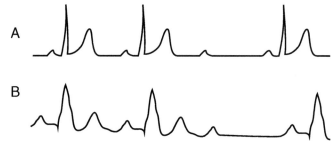

FIGURE 7-7 · **Second degree, Mobitz type II atrioventricular block with 3:2 conduction.** Note the fixed PR interval with a QRS complex that is usually widened, although it may be narrow, until the impulse is unable to reach the ventricles, resulting in a nonconducted P wave. The magnitude of block is expressed as a ratio of P waves to QRS complexes (e.g., three P waves for two QRS complexes is a 3:2 block). *A,* Narrow QRS complex. *B,* Wide QRS complex.

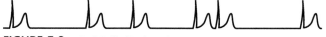

FIGURE 7-8 · **Atrial fibrillation with slow ventricular response.** Note the irregularly irregular rhythm without obvious P waves.

Sinoatrial Exit Block. SA exit block occurs when the sinus impulse does not exit the sinus nodal region and does not depolarize the atria; therefore, P waves are not seen. SA block is classified as first, second, or third degree block (similar to and not to be confused with AV nodal block). Only the second degree blocks (type I [Wenckebach] and type II) can be diagnosed by the 12-lead electrocardiogram. A second degree, type I SA block occurs with appearance of sinus pauses (i.e., no sinus node activity) of at least 3 sec associated with progressive shortening of the P-P interval until a P wave is not seen. Second degree, type II SA block is noted with the appearance of a sinus pause that is an exact multiple of the baseline P-P interval.

Irregular rhythm, wide QRS complex

Second-degree/Mobitz type I AV block, second degree/Mobitz type II AV block (Fig. 7-7B), *atrial fibrillation/flutter with slow ventricular response,* and *SA exit block* may present with a wide QRS complex owing to coexistent bundle branch block; alternatively, the site of the escape focus may also be associated with a widened QRS complex.

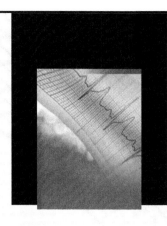

Chapter 8

Tachydysrhythmias

Theodore C. Chan

Tachycardia is defined as an increase in heart rate above the normal impulse rate based on age. An abnormally fast heart rate can result from either a primary cardiac abnormality or as a cardiac response to a primarily noncardiac abnormality or physiologic stress.

Tachycardia can originate from virtually any locus of the myocardium. There are three primary mechanisms: reentry, enhanced automaticity, and triggered activity. Reentry occurs when two functionally distinct pathways exist, allowing anterograde and retrograde conduction. Such a situation creates a circuit loop resulting in recurrent reactivation. Macroreentry circuits involve large areas of myocardium; microreentry circuits involve smaller areas, such as nodes.

Enhanced automaticity occurs when spontaneous depolarization of certain myocytes is increased. Enhanced automaticity causes tachycardia when cardiac cells at sites such as the atria, atrioventricular (AV) node, and His-Purkinje fibers depolarize at a faster rate, overcoming the normal overdrive suppression of the sinus node. Triggered activity occurs when depolarization takes place during repolarization of the myocyte (early or delayed afterdepolarization).

The keys to differentiating tachycardia are the regularity of the rhythm and width of QRS complex:

1. *Regularity*: A regular rhythm suggests a single impulse focus generating the tachycardia. An irregular tachycardia can result from premature beats, variable blocks, multiple impulse foci, or disorganized electrical activity. If the premature beats occur regularly, or the block has a consistent ratio, there may be a regular pattern to the irregularity, or a "regularly irregular" rhythm. Irregularities resulting from multiple impulse foci or disorganized electrical activity are more commonly "irregularly irregular."
2. *QRS complex width*: When ventricular depolarization occurs along the normal conduction system, ventricular activation produces a narrow QRS complex width (<0.12 sec). Activation in part or entirely outside the normal pathway usually prolongs ventricular depolarization, resulting in an abnormal, wide QRS complex (>0.12 sec). Wide complexes occur with bundle branch block (BBB), ventricular pacing, ectopic ventricular impulses, and premature ventricular activation by an accessory or aberrant pathway.

Differential Diagnosis of Tachydysrhythmias

Regular rate, narrow QRS complex

Regular narrow-complex tachycardia is defined as an abnormally fast heart rate with a normal QRS complex duration. These tachycardias are often classified as (1) AV node independent—the tachycardia is not dependent on the AV node and usually is due to automaticity or triggered activity (i.e., sinus tachycardia, atrial tachycardia); or (2) AV node dependent—the tachycardia is dependent on the AV node and usually is due to a reentry circuit involving the AV node (AV nodal reentry tachycardia [AVNRT], AV reentry tachycardia [AVRT], junctional tachycardia).

Sinus Tachycardia. Sinus tachycardia is an increased heart rate as part of a normal response to a physiologic stress. The increase is usually gradual in acceleration and deceleration, rather than sudden or "paroxysmal." Enhanced sinus node automaticity produces P waves identical to those in normal sinus rhythm (NSR) (Fig. 8-1).

Inappropriate Sinus Tachycardia. Inappropriate sinus tachycardia is a sinus tachycardia that does not occur as a response to a physiologic stress. This syndrome occurs more frequently in young women and is due to either enhanced automaticity or autonomic imbalance.

Sinus Node Reentry Tachycardia. The rare sinus node reentry tachycardia results from a microreentry circuit localized to the sinus node. The P wave is identical or similar to that of NSR and the rate is usually less than 150 bpm with a sudden onset and termination.

Atrial Tachycardias. Atrial tachycardias can occur from microreentry, macroreentry, enhanced automaticity, or triggered activity localized to atrial tissue. Although less common than other supraventricular tachycardias (SVTs), atrial tachycardias are more often associated with underlying heart disease. The heart rate varies from 120 to 250 bpm, terminating only after a QRS complex. The P wave morphology is often consistent with an ectopic focus. Because the AV node is not involved, blockade does not affect the tachycardia (although it may slow ventricular response). In fact, the presence of AV blockade during the tachycardia strongly suggests atrial tachycardia.

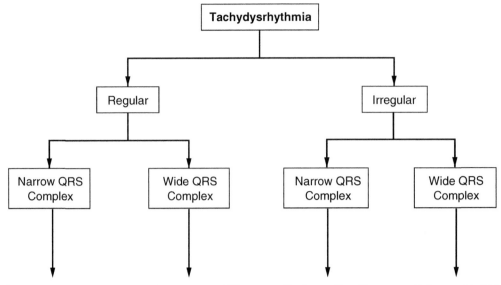

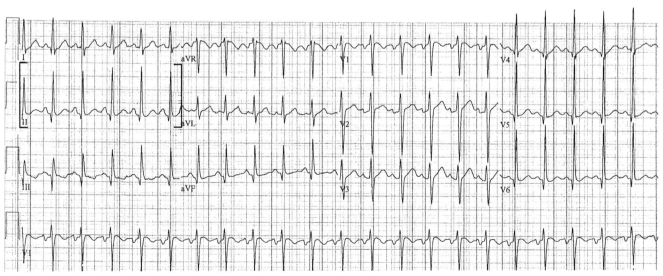

FIGURE 8-1 • **Sinus tachycardia.** Note P wave precedes every narrow QRS complex.

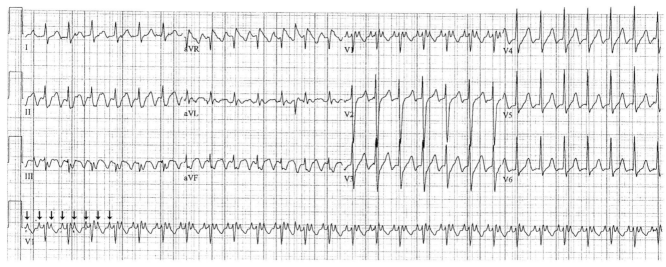

FIGURE 8-2 · Atrial flutter with 2:1 block. P waves are denoted by *arrows* and approach rates consistent with atrial flutter. The presence of the atrioventricular block slows the ventricular response, but does not affect the atrial tachycardia.

Atrial Flutter. Atrial flutter is a specific macroreentry atrial tachycardia involving a significant portion of atrial tissue, producing large, inverted flutter waves most prominent in the inferior leads (the so-called sawtooth pattern; Fig. 8-2).

Junctional Tachycardia. Junctional tachycardia results from enhanced automaticity or triggered activity localized to the AV node. In general, this activation results in a regular, narrow QRS complex tachycardia without any P waves. However, retrograde atrial activation can produce inverted P waves just before, during, or after the QRS complex.

Atrioventricular Nodal Reentry Tachycardia. AVNRT is a common cause of narrow-complex tachycardias at rates of 150 to 250 bpm, and is usually not associated with any significant structural heart disease. Resulting from microreentry localized to the AV or perinodal tissue, AVNRT is often precipitated by a premature atrial beat that is blocked down one pathway, but conducted anterograde through the other and then retrograde through the initially blocked pathway. Because the circuit involves the AV node, persistence of the tachycardia with block usually excludes AVNRT. AVNRT is difficult to distinguish from orthodromic AVRT (Fig. 8-3).

Atrioventricular Reentry (Reciprocating) Tachycardia—Orthodromic. AVRT is less common than AVNRT and occurs through macroreentry involving the normal conducting system and an accessory AV pathway. Orthodromic AVRT (most common) occurs with anterograde conduction down the normal, and retrograde conduction through the accessory pathway, producing a narrow-complex tachycardia that is very difficult to distinguish from AVNRT on the electrocardiogram (ECG). Because the AV conduction system is a component of the reentry, tachycardia in the presence of block or dissociation excludes the diagnosis. Conversely, QRS complex alternans in the setting of a regular, narrow-complex tachycardia strongly suggests AVRT.

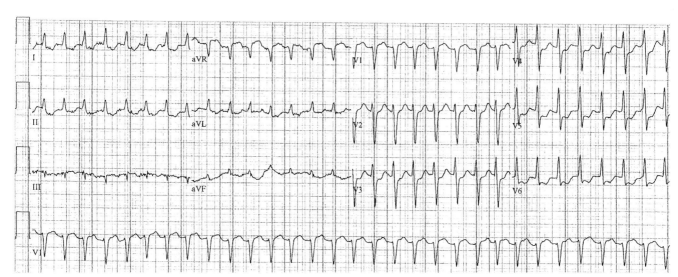

FIGURE 8-3 · Supraventricular tachycardia from atrioventricular nodal reentry tachycardia. Note the regular tachycardia with narrow QRS complexes and no preceding atrial activity.

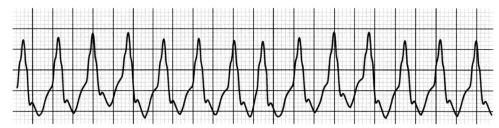

FIGURE 8-4 · **Monomorphic ventricular tachycardia (VT).** Monomorphic VT is characterized by a regular, wide QRS complex tachycardia.

Paroxysmal AVRT is associated with preexcitation syndromes, such as Wolff-Parkinson-White syndrome and Lown-Ganong-Levine syndrome. AVRT also occurs with "concealed" accessory pathways that allow only retrograde conduction (thus the potential for orthodromic AVRT), but no evidence of preexcitation (delta wave).

Fascicular Tachycardias. Fascicular tachycardia is a rare form of ventricular tachycardia (VT) associated with digoxin toxicity that produces a narrow QRS complex tachycardia because of its origin near the AV node along the fascicles.

Regular rate, wide QRS complex

Regular, wide-complex tachycardia is defined as an abnormally fast heart rate with a prolonged QRS duration. The abnormal ventricular depolarization resulting in the wide QRS complex occurs from three chief mechanisms: ectopic ventricular foci, aberrant conduction and depolarization of ventricular tissue, and preexcitation.

Although often difficult, differentiating VTs from SVTs with aberrancy or preexcitation is often critical. VT can be life-threatening and misdiagnosis can lead to inappropriate therapy with lethal consequences. A number of ECG criteria have been developed to differentiate wide-complex tachycardias of ventricular origin (VT) from those of supraventricular origin (SVT with aberrancy).

Ventricular Tachycardia—Monomorphic. VT is the most common cause of wide QRS complex tachycardias. Depolarization occurs at a focus in the ventricular tissue outside the normal conduction system, resulting in abnormal and prolonged ventricular activation. VT is defined as three or more consecutive ventricular beats at an abnormally fast rate. Nonsustained VT is defined as VT of less than 30 sec duration. Monomorphic VT results in stable wide QRS complexes that are uniform in appearance on each ECG lead. Polymorphic VT occurs when the QRS complex morphology changes with beat-to-beat variation. The most common etiology of VT is ischemic heart disease (Fig. 8-4).

Ventricular Flutter. Ventricular flutter appears as a continuous sine wave pattern with no distinction between the QRS complex, ST segment, and T waves. Ventricular flutter usually occurs at a rate in excess of 200 bpm and may be fatal if not terminated abruptly (Fig. 8-5).

Supraventricular Tachycardia with Aberrancy or Bundle Branch Block. All SVTs can result in a wide-complex tachycardia if ventricular depolarization is delayed or occurs in an abnormal fashion. The wide QRS complex occurs as a result of a delay or block in the His-Purkinje system, resulting

in abnormal ventricular activation. Aberrant conduction can be fixed and permanent, or can be functional and occur under certain circumstances, such as at higher heart rates. BBB is the most common form of aberrancy that can result in a wide-complex tachycardia (Fig. 8-6).

Tachycardia with Preexcitation. Any tachycardia in which the ventricles are fully or partially activated by an accessory pathway can produce a wide QRS complex tachycardia. A preexcited ventricle produces a short PR interval and a delta wave at the onset of the QRS complex. The degree of preexcitation depends on the relative contribution of the faster accessory pathway and the normal conduction system to ventricular activation. These pathways may not always be involved in impulse conduction (i.e., rate-related pathways). Pathway-to-pathway tachycardia occurs when two or more accessory pathways result in abnormal ventricular activation and a wide QRS complex tachycardia.

Atrioventricular Reentry (Reciprocating) Tachycardia— Antidromic. Antidromic AVRT (or preexcited tachycardia) occurs when a reentry loop is formed with the normal conducting system and the accessory AV pathway. With antidromic AVRT, impulses are conducted in an anterograde fashion down the accessory pathway and retrograde up through the AV node, producing a wide QRS complex tachycardia.

Pacemaker Tachycardia. Pacemaker tachycardia (PMT) is a reentry dysrhythmia involving a dual-chamber pacemaker with atrial sensing in which a retrograde conducted P′ wave is interpreted as a native atrial stimulus, triggering ventricular pacing, which itself generates another retrograde P′ wave, completing the circuit loop. PMT appears as a regular, ventricular-paced, wide-complex tachycardia at a rate not exceeding the maximum upper rate of the pacemaker (Fig. 8-7).

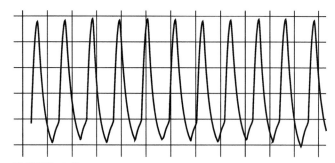

FIGURE 8-5 · **Ventricular flutter demonstrating continuous-wave patterns of ventricular activity.**

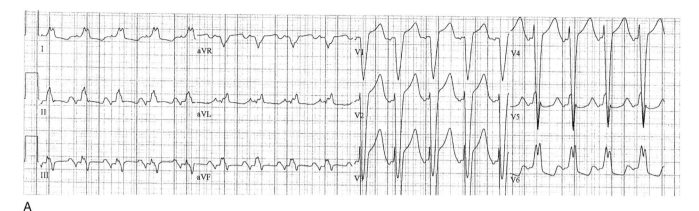

A

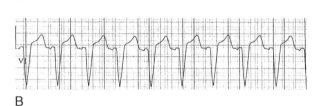

B

FIGURE 8-6 • **Supraventricular tachycardia (SVT) with bundle branch block.** Any SVT, including sinus tachycardia, will produce a wide-complex tachycardia in the presence of bundle branch block (BBB) or aberrancy. *A,* Sinus tachycardia with left BBB pattern on 12-lead ECG. *B,* Rhythm strip of the resulting wide-complex tachycardia.

Accelerated Idioventricular Rhythm. An accelerated idioventricular rhythm (AIVR) is an accelerated rhythm with a focus in the His-bundle branch system or ventricular myocardium producing a regular, wide QRS complex tachycardia at a rate faster than slow idioventricular rhythms.

Other Causes of Wide-Complex Tachycardia. There are a number of other causes of wide QRS complex tachycardias. A number of toxidromes, including cocaine intoxication, tricyclic antidepressant overdose, and procainamide overdose can result in both a tachycardia and abnormal and delayed ventricular activation, resulting in a wide-complex, regular tachycardia. Electrolyte disturbances such as hyperkalemia can result in a wide-complex tachycardia. In addition, ischemic morphologic changes associated with tachycardia and recent electrical cardioversion all can cause a wide-complex tachycardia.

Irregular rate, narrow QRS complex

Irregular, narrow-complex tachycardia is defined as an abnormally fast heart rate that is irregular with a normal

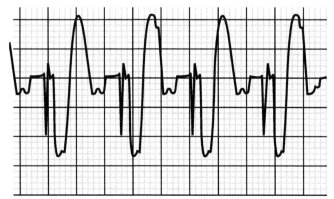

FIGURE 8-7 • **Pacemaker-mediated tachycardia.** The rhythm strip demonstrates a regular, wide-complex tachycardia from pacemaker-mediated tachycardia.

QRS duration. An irregular, narrow QRS complex rhythm can be produced by abnormal supraventricular automaticity (as with abnormal loci for impulse generation), occasional premature supraventricular impulses, and variable block of impulse conduction, usually at the AV node.

Tachycardias with Premature Beats. Narrow-complex regular tachycardias can appear irregular with any premature beat. The irregular premature beat can occur regularly (regularly irregular beat) or irregularly (irregularly irregular beat). Supraventricular premature impulses, such as premature atrial contractions (PACs) and premature junctional contractions (PJCs), result in a narrow QRS complex beat provided there is no associated aberrancy. Because they arise in ventricular tissue, premature ventricular contractions (PVCs) produce a wide QRS complex irregular beat.

Atrial Fibrillation. Atrial fibrillation (AF) is the most common cause of an irregularly irregular heart rate. AF occurs when there is no organized activation of the atrial tissue, resulting in chaotic depolarizations of atrial myocytes. On the ECG, there are no P waves present and the baseline may appear irregular as a result of this chaotic atrial electrical activity. In most cases, intermittent impulses are transmitted through the AV node, resulting in ventricular depolarization and an irregularly irregular narrow QRS complex tachycardia (provided there is no aberrancy; Fig. 8-8).

Atrial Flutter with Variable Block. With atrial flutter, atrial rates can be as high as 300 bpm. As a result, not all atrial depolarizations are transmitted through the AV node to the ventricle, resulting in block. An irregular narrow QRS complex rhythm can occur when the AV block ratio varies (most commonly between 2:1 and 3:1 AV block).

Atrial Tachycardias with Variable Block. As with atrial flutter, any atrial tachycardia or suprajunctional tachycardia can result in an irregular rhythm in the presence of variable block. In such cases, the atrial impulses may overwhelm the AV node, resulting in a variable block and an irregular, but slower rate of ventricular activation. Atrial tachycardia with variable block is associated with digitalis toxicity.

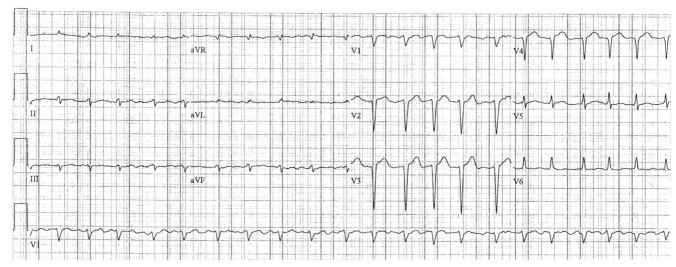

FIGURE 8-8 · **Narrow-complex tachycardia from atrial fibrillation.** Note the lack of P waves, chaotic baseline, and irregular rate.

Multifocal Atrial Tachycardia. Multifocal atrial tachycardia (MAT) occurs when there is more than one atrial focus firing independently, resulting in an irregular tachycardia. On ECG, at least three distinct P wave morphologies appear, resulting from the abnormal atrial foci. MAT can be differentiated from AF in that the baseline between abnormal P waves is isoelectric. MAT is rare, but associated with hypoxia and severe pulmonary disease (Fig. 8-9).

Irregular rate, wide QRS complex

Irregular, wide-complex tachycardia is defined as an abnormally fast heart rate that is irregular with a prolonged QRS duration. Similar to regular, wide-complex tachycardias, differentiating whether the etiology is from a ventricular dysrhythmia or of supraventricular origin is of critical importance.

Polymorphic Ventricular Tachycardia. Polymorphic VT is defined as VT in which QRS complexes vary in terms of morphology, width, and rate. On ECG, the QRS complexes appear wide with bizarre morphologies that often vary from beat to beat, and occur with an irregular fast rate.

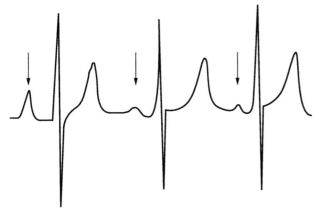

FIGURE 8-9 · **Multifocal atrial tachycardia rhythm strip showing three different P wave morphologies** (*arrows*).

Polymorphic VT can be associated with both a normal or prolonged QT interval at baseline.

Torsades de Pointes. Torsades de pointes (TdP) is a specific type of polymorphic VT in which the dysrhythmia has a cyclical pattern of alternating electrical polarity and amplitude. As a result, the QRS peaks appear to be twisting around the isoelectric baseline (Fig. 8-10). TdP occurs in the setting of abnormal repolarization manifested by a prolonged QT interval.

Ventricular Fibrillation. Ventricular fibrillation appears as chaotic, irregular, and disorganized ventricular complexes without discrete QRS complexes. With this rhythm, the myocardium is unable to generate synchronous ventricular contractions, and the rhythm can be fatal unless terminated abruptly.

Irregular Atrial or Supraventricular Tachycardias with Aberrancy or Bundle Branch Block. As noted previously, any type of dysrhythmia producing an irregular narrow-complex tachycardia can produce a wide QRS complex when there is a delay in conduction and depolarization of the ventricle, such as with BBB. The aberrancy can be permanent and present on baseline ECGs during the tachycardia, or it can be functional and present only during the tachycardia (i.e., rate related; Fig. 8-11).

Tachycardia with Preexcitation. As noted earlier, a tachycardia with preexcitation is a tachycardia in which the ventricles are fully or partially activated by an accessory pathway such that the QRS complex appears widened. With irregular tachycardias, these tachycardias appear as wide QRS complex, irregular tachycardias.

Preexcited Atrial Fibrillation and Flutter with an Accessory Pathway. Rapid atrial rhythms such as AF and atrial flutter may occur in the setting of an accessory bypass pathway. The accessory pathway provides a faster pathway for ventricular activation with less conduction delay than the normal AV conduction system. In such cases, rapid, irregular atrial impulses can cause rapid, irregular ventricular activation, resulting in a very rapid, irregular wide QRS complex tachycardia (Fig. 8-12).

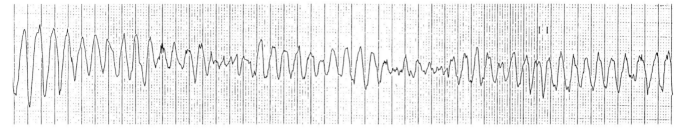

FIGURE 8-10 · Torsades de pointes. Rhythm strip of torsades de pointes demonstrates irregular, wide-complex rhythm with oscillating QRS complex amplitude and polarity.

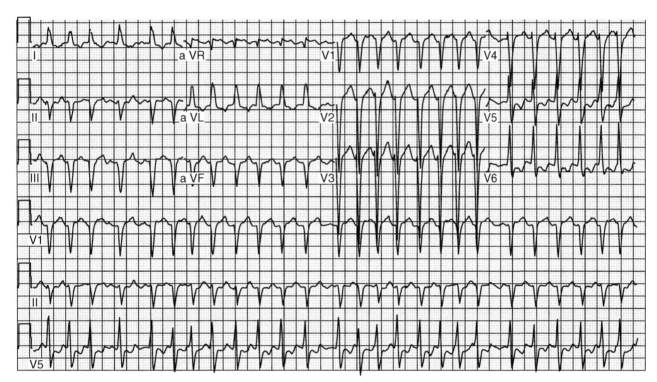

FIGURE 8-11 · Irregular tachydysrhythmias with aberrancy. Atrial fibrillation with left bundle branch block demonstrating an irregular, wide-complex tachycardia.

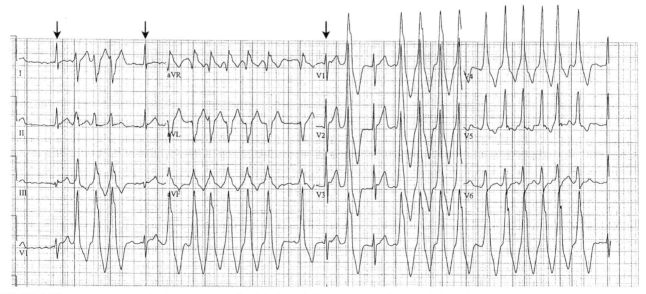

FIGURE 8-12 · Preexcited atrial fibrillation (AF). ECG and rhythm strip demonstrate AF with preexcitation and conduction down the accessory pathway, producing runs of rapid, irregular, wide-complex tachycardia. Note the intermittent narrow QRS complexes resulting from occasional normal AV conduction (*arrows*).

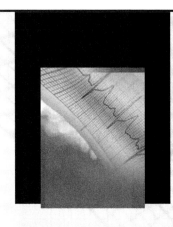

Chapter 9

Abnormal Axis

Richard A. Harrigan

Consideration of axis abnormality is usually restricted to the frontal plane QRS axis, but in fact, each waveform has a derivable axis—both in the frontal and coronal planes. The term *QRS axis* usually refers to a numeric expression of the mean QRS vector force in the frontal plane. It is formed by conjoining a reformatted version of Einthoven's triangle formed by the bipolar limb leads (I, II, and III) with the augmented unipolar limb leads (aVL, aVR, and aVF; Fig. 9-1). The result is a spoked-wheel figure with 12 points (or 6 axes, thus a hexaxial system), with 30 degrees separating each "spoke" of the figure. This figure is divided into four roughly equal quadrants (Fig. 9-2), with the following designations: (1) *normal axis*, (2) *left axis deviation*, (3) *right axis deviation*, and (4) *extreme axis deviation*. By examining the magnitude and direction of the individual QRS wave forms in the six frontal plane leads, the major vector of cardiac electrical activity can be estimated and given a numeric value expressed in degrees. This number falls within one of the four quadrants, and thus the QRS axis can be determined.

Electrocardiographic Diagnosis

QRS axis

Normal QRS axis is generally accepted to be from −30 degrees to +90 degrees, although most people are between +30 degrees and +75 degrees. Younger people have a tendency toward a more rightward axis (up to +105 degrees), whereas older individuals tend to be more leftward (−30 degrees to +90 degrees).

Left axis deviation (LAD) is defined as an axis between −30 degrees to −90 degrees; it may be seen as an isolated feature, or along with the following electrocardiographic (ECG) findings:

- *Left ventricular hypertrophy* (LVH): The presence of a leftward QRS axis may be suggestive of LVH when considered along with other findings. By itself, LAD is an insensitive indicator of LVH (see Chapter 35, Ventricular Hypertrophy).
- *Left bundle branch block* (LBBB): The finding of LAD with LBBB suggests more severe conduction system disease that involves both the fascicles and the main bundle branch.

- *Left anterior fascicular block* (LAFB): By definition, there must be LAD of −45 degrees to −90 degrees for LAFB to exist.
- *Inferior wall myocardial infarction* (MI): A dominant Q wave in the inferior leads can lead to LAD.
- *Mechanical shifts* of the heart may result in LAD, such as may occur with pneumothorax.
- *Ectopic ventricular rhythms* sometimes feature LAD. New LAD is one criterion that is suggestive of ventricular tachycardia when considering a wide-complex tachycardia of uncertain etiology.

Right axis deviation (RAD) is defined as an axis of +90 degrees to +180 degrees; it may be seen as an isolated feature, or along with the following ECG findings:

- *Right ventricular hypertrophy* (RVH): Increased right ventricular forces suggestive of RVH may be reflected in the limb leads, causing RAD. The axis is usually at least +110 degrees. RVH may exist without RAD, however, and the coexistence of LVH may confound the diagnosis of RVH and affect the final mean QRS axis (see Chapter 35, Ventricular Hypertrophy).
- *Infants and children*: RAD occurs normally in infants and children. Persistence of this into later childhood or early adulthood is more likely in tall, slender subjects.
- *Lateral wall MI*: Loss of leftward forces due to infarction may result in a rightward shift in the QRS axis, owing to the dominant Q or QS pattern seen in lead I. Confirmatory evidence would be the existence of Q waves in the lateral precordial leads (V_5 and V_6).
- *Left posterior fascicular block* (LPFB): Delayed activation of the posteroinferior part of the left ventricle causes displacement of the late QRS vectors to the right. Frontal plane QRS axis is usually greater than +120 degrees. This may be difficult to discern from RVH, however; the presence of right atrial enlargement favors the latter diagnosis. LPFB is more likely if signs of inferior or posterior wall infarction are evident.
- *Chronic obstructive pulmonary disease* (COPD): The frontal plane axis may be displaced to between +90 degrees and +110 degrees even in the absence of pulmonary hypertension.
- *Mechanical shifts*, such as may occur with pneumothorax, may result in RAD.

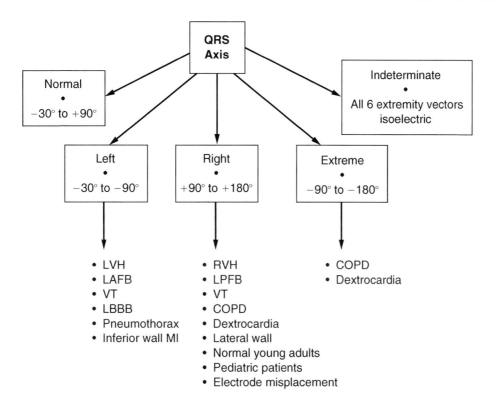

• LVH
• LAFB
• VT
• LBBB
• Pneumothorax
• Inferior wall MI

• RVH
• LPFB
• VT
• COPD
• Dextrocardia
• Lateral wall
• Normal young adults
• Pediatric patients
• Electrode misplacement

• COPD
• Dextrocardia

• *Ectopic ventricular rhythms* sometimes feature RAD. For example, healthy young individuals with ventricular tachycardia originating in the right ventricle have a morphologic pattern of LBBB in the precordial leads, yet the initial R wave in lead V_1 is broad, and the frontal plane QRS shows RAD, which would otherwise be distinctly unusual with LBBB.

• *Dextrocardia*: Mirror-image dextrocardia results in an inversion of the QRS complex in lead I; thus, this condition may result in RAD or extreme axis deviation (depending on lead aVF, which is by itself unchanged by dextrocardia). Dextrocardia also features a negative P wave in lead I, but can be differentiated from lead misplacement (see next entry) by analyzing the precordial leads. In dextrocardia, the QRS complexes diminish in size from leads V_1 to V_6 (as the leads move further away from the right-sided heart); with limb electrode misplacement, the precordial leads exhibit normal R wave progression.

• *Limb electrode misplacement*: Reversal of certain limb electrodes (e.g., the left and right arm electrodes) creates the illusion of RAD. With arm electrode reversal, as in dextrocardia (see previous entry), the P and T waves also are inverted in lead I. A "normal" appearance of the precordial leads indicates that the limb electrodes have been misplaced. Dextrocardia features smaller QRS complexes as the electrodes are placed further away from the right-sided heart (i.e., across the left side of the chest).

Extreme axis deviation is defined as an axis of −90 degrees to ±180 degrees, and is a rare finding. It can be seen with dextrocardia and other pathologic states.

Indeterminate axis exists when all six frontal plane leads feature isoelectric QRS vectors; that is, equivalent biphasic

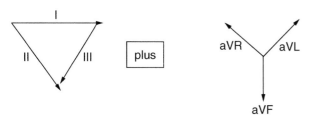

FIGURE 9-1 · **QRS axis.** Superimposing the bipolar limb leads (I, II, and III) on the augmented unipolar limb leads (aVL, aVR, and aVF) yields a hexaxial spoked-wheel figure from which frontal plane axis can be derived. Positive direction noted by *arrows*.

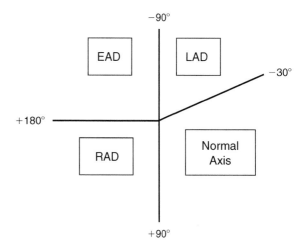

FIGURE 9-2 · **QRS axis deviation.** Frontal plane zones depicting normal QRS axis versus the various types of axis deviation. EAD, extreme axis deviation; LAD, left axis deviation; RAD, right axis deviation.

(QR or RS) complexes are found in the bipolar limb leads and the unipolar augmented leads. This can be seen as a normal variant, or may reflect an underlying pathologic process.

P wave axis

The P wave represents atrial depolarization—right atrium first, followed by the left. The two components are best demonstrated in the right precordial leads. However, as with the QRS axis, the P wave axis is determined by analyzing the P wave vectors in the limb leads. It normally lies between 0 degrees and 75 degrees, although in most cases it is between 45 degrees and 60 degrees. Thus, most ECGs feature upright P waves in leads I, II, and aVF, assuming the rhythm is normal sinus. In lead aVF, the P wave may be flattened or inverted, however. Lead III may feature a biphasic P wave; when it is biphasic, the initial deflection should be upward, whereas the terminal phase is downward. Lead aVL may display a positive or negative P wave; when it is biphasic, negative initial and positive terminal phases are expected. The P wave in lead aVR is normally inverted, conforming to the characteristic negativity of all vectors in that lead. Limb electrode misplacement may be detected by analysis of the P wave axis and detection of atypical P wave vectors (see Chapter 4, Electrode Misplacement and Artifact).

Right axis deviation (P wave), defined as a P axis greater than 75 degrees, may be seen in a number of pathologic states, including right atrial enlargement, COPD, pulmonary fibrosis, pulmonary hypertension, pulmonary embolism, left atrial ischemia, and congenital heart disease, as well as in tall, slender body habitus.

Left axis deviation (P wave), defined as a P axis less than 15 degrees, is relatively nonspecific.

T wave axis

The T wave represents repolarization of the ventricle. Normally, the principal T wave vector is directed leftward, downward, and anteriorly; the latter direction is more posterior in younger individuals. The polarity of the T wave is usually the same as the polarity of the preceding QRS complex. Thus, T waves are usually upright in leads I, II, and aVF; it may be flattened or mildly inverted in the latter, however. Like the P wave and QRS complex, it is normally negative in lead aVR. T wave vector polarity is variable in leads aVL and III. T wave axis abnormalities, both in the frontal and coronal planes, have been linked to ischemic heart disease.

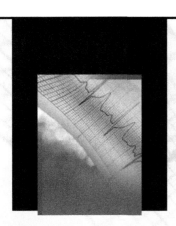

Chapter 10

P Wave

Theodore C. Chan

The P wave is the first depolarization wave encountered in the normal cardiac cycle and constitutes depolarization of both the right and left atria. Abnormalities of the P wave usually relate to changes in the atrial depolarization vector, enlargement of the atria, and changes in atrial rhythm conduction.

Because the sinoatrial (SA) node is located in the right atrium, the right atrium undergoes depolarization first, followed by the left atrium. The initial portion or ascending limb of the P wave is due to right atrial depolarization. Left atrial depolarization normally occurs 0.03 sec after the right atrium and forms the distal portion or descending limb of the P wave. The P wave is a composite of right and left atrial depolarization waves (Fig. 10-1).

ELECTROCARDIOGRAPHIC DIAGNOSIS

Normal P Wave

The maximum normal duration of the P wave is less than 0.12 sec. The P wave interval is usually shorter in duration at birth (0.05 sec) but gradually increases to normal duration by adolescence.

Morphology. The P wave is inscribed at a constant speed such that its morphology is usually smooth with little irregularity despite its composite nature. The overall morphology varies with electrocardiogram (ECG) lead depending on the axis and vectors of depolarization and repolarization.

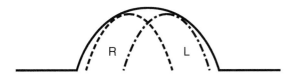

FIGURE 10-1 · **Schematic of P wave.** R represents right atrial activation and L left atrial activation. The combination of both produces the P wave.

Axis. The normal atrial activation vector is directed inferiorly and to the left, resulting in a normal P wave axis of +45 degrees to +60 degrees in the frontal plane, but it can range from 0 degrees to +75 degrees. The P wave is thus most prominent with greatest amplitude (up to 2.5 mm) in a positive deflection in lead II, and in a negative deflection in lead aVR. In the precordial plane, the initial right atrial activation is directed anteriorly to the left, followed by the later left atrial activation directed slightly posteriorly. As a result, the P wave in lead V_1 is biphasic with a prominent initial positive deflection (up to 1.5 mm), followed by a smaller terminal negative deflection (up to 1 mm). At birth and during childhood, the P wave is directed anteriorly and may be initially upright in all precordial leads, changing to the biphasic wave in lead V_1 gradually with age.

Rhythm. The P wave appearance also depends on the specific cardiac rhythm. Atrial activation originating from an ectopic focus away from the SA node, or abnormal conduction through the atria, produces an abnormal P wave morphology and axis.

Abnormal P Wave

Abnormal P waves can result from changes in P wave morphology, related axis changes, or changes in rhythm. Rhythm changes themselves may result in multiple, variable changes in P wave morphology and axis. Thus, many disease entities can result in P wave changes in morphology, axis, and rhythm combined.

Abnormal morphology

Exercise-Induced Sinus Tachycardia. Sinus tachycardias, particularly those resulting from exercise, can produce increased amplitude, resulting in taller, peaked P waves. In addition, exercise can cause a vertical axis rightward shift in P wave axis of 10 degrees to 15 degrees, such that more prominent P waves appear in leads aVF and III.

Right Atrial Abnormality. Because of the increase in the size of the right atrium in right atrial abnormality (RAA), right atrial activation increases in amplitude and duration. In lead II, the P wave increases in amplitude by greater than 2.5 mm and appears symmetrically peaked. In lead V_1, the initial positive deflection increases in amplitude by greater than 1.5 mm and can obscure the terminal negative deflection of the left atrium such that the P wave is a large positive deflection only. The overall duration of the P wave usually does not increase because the prolonged right atrial component simply encroaches temporally on left atrial activation (Fig. 10-2).

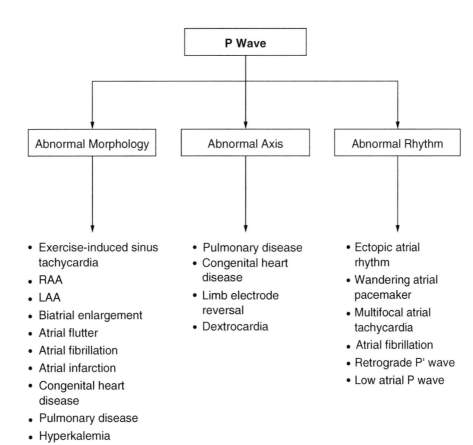

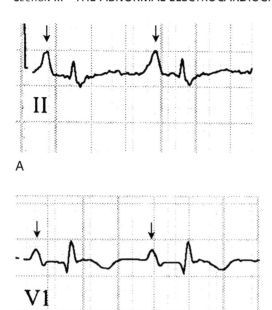

A

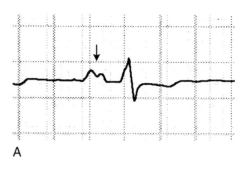

A

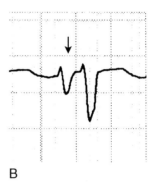

B

B

FIGURE 10-2 · Right atrial abnormality. *A*, This rhythm strip shows the increase in amplitude and "peaked" shape of the P wave in lead II (*arrows*). *B*, Note the increase in amplitude of the positive deflection (diminishing the terminal negative deflection) of the P wave in lead V₁ (*arrows*).

FIGURE 10-3 · Left atrial abnormality (LAA). *A*, The widened, notched P wave in lead I indicates that the activation of the left atrium is delayed and increased in amplitude in LAA (*arrow*). *B*, Note the increased negative terminal deflection of the P wave in lead V₁ (*arrow*).

P Pulmonale. P pulmonale refers to the tall, peaked P wave from RAA associated with acquired heart disease, usually from chronic obstructive pulmonary disease (COPD) and pulmonary disease. When associated with COPD, there is an axis shift in the P wave inferiorly because of the more vertical position of the heart, resulting in P pulmonale most commonly in leads aVF, II, and III.

P Congenitale. P congenitale refers to the tall, peaked P wave from RAA with an associated left axis deviation due to congenital heart disease (pulmonary stenosis, tetralogy of Fallot, Ebstein's anomaly).

Left Atrial Abnormality. Because of the increase in the size of the left atrium in left atrial abnormality (LAA), left atrial activation increases in amplitude and is delayed and prolonged. In the frontal leads (primarily II and I), the P wave

morphology changes to a double-peaked or notched apex. The overall duration of the P wave is greater than 0.11 sec and the distance between the two peaks is greater than 0.04 sec. In lead V₁, the negative terminal deflection becomes deeper and prolonged, occasionally resulting in a large inverted P wave. LAA is associated with a shift in the P wave axis leftward, such that the most prominent terminal P wave deflections (second peak) occur in leads I, aVL, V₅, and V₆. This notched P wave is also known as P mitrale, reflecting its left atrial etiology (Fig. 10-3).

Biatrial Abnormality. The combination of RAA and LAA result in a prolonged, wide P wave with increased amplitude. In the frontal leads, particularly the left lateral leads, the P wave appears wide and notched with markedly increased amplitude. In the precordial leads, particularly lead V₁, the initial positive deflection is taller and peaked and associated with a deep, wide, terminal negative deflection (Fig. 10-4).

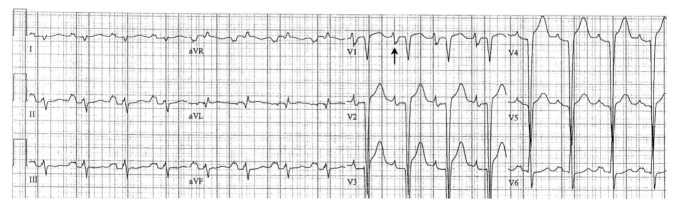

FIGURE 10-4 · Biatrial abnormality (BAA). This 12-lead ECG demonstrates P wave findings consistent with BAA: large, notched P waves in frontal, inferior, and left lateral leads. Lead V₁ shows a peaked initial positive deflection followed by a deep, wide, delayed terminal deflection (*arrow*).

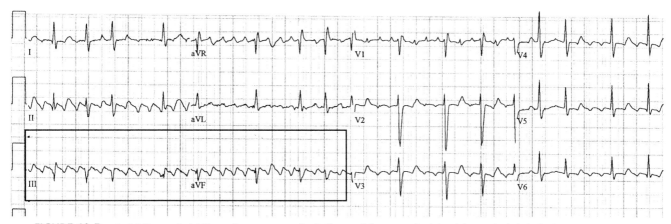

FIGURE 10-5 · **Atrial flutter.** Atrial flutter demonstrates a classic "sawtooth" pattern of atrial activity, particularly in leads III and aVF (*box*).

P Tricuspidale. P tricuspidale refers to a wide frontal plane P wave associated with biatrial abnormality (BAA) with an initial component taller than the terminal component. This finding is associated with tricuspid valve disease, as well as mitral valve disease when associated with pulmonary hypertension.

Atrial Infarction. Atrial infarction can produce marked changes in the P wave morphology from flattening to increased amplitude, as well as widening with an irregular notched or slurred appearance.

Hyperkalemia. With progressive elevation of serum potassium levels, P wave amplitude diminishes and completely disappears with levels higher than 7.5 mEq/dL.

Atrial Flutter. Atrial flutter is a specific reentry circuit loop involving a significant portion of atrial tissue, producing large, inverted flutter waves most prominent in the inferior leads (the so-called sawtooth pattern; Fig. 10-5).

Atrial Fibrillation. Atrial fibrillation occurs when there is no organized electrical depolarization of the atria, but rather a chaotic, disorganized depolarization of atrial myocytes.

There are no clear P waves on the ECG. Instead, the isoelectric baseline appears irregular because of the continuous chaotic atrial depolarizations (Fig. 10-6).

Abnormal axis

A number of the entities noted previously result in axis changes in the P wave as a result of changes in the atrial activation vector direction. These changes result in morphologic abnormalities as well as changes in specific lead prominence.

Pulmonary Disease. Lung disease can result in RAA as well as a more inferior vertical cardiac position, resulting in a rightward axis of the P wave. Prominent P waves may appear in leads aVF and III as well as II (P pulmonale).

Congenital Heart Disease. Certain congenital heart diseases can result in RAA, LAA, and leftward axis change in the P wave. P wave prominence may increase in leads I, aVL, V_5, and V_6, as occurs with P congenitale.

Limb Electrode Reversal. Errors in electrode placement can result in the appearance of P wave axis change or inversion of

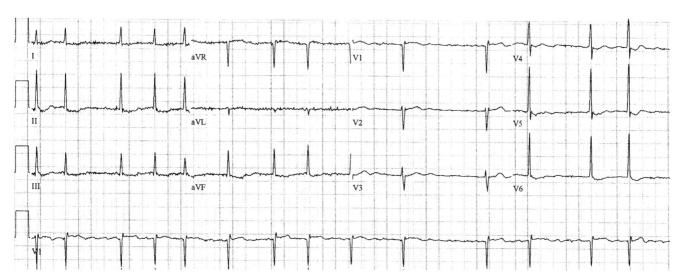

FIGURE 10-6 · **Atrial fibrillation.** Note the lack of P wave activity, chaotic baseline, and irregular rate.

normal P waves. For example, limb electrode reversal can cause a significant right axis deviation to the point that the P wave may invert in leads I and II.

Dextrocardia. Malposition of the heart can lead to axis change in the P wave. With dextrocardia, the P wave axis is shifted rightward, which may cause prominent deflections in leads III and aVR.

Other Axis Changes. As noted previously, axis changes are also associated with right QRS complex axis deviation, LAA, BAA, and exercise-induced tachycardia.

Abnormalities related to rhythm disturbances

Ectopic Atrial Rhythm. Impulses that originate in the atria at foci other than the SA node can produce abnormal P waves owing to the change in atrial conduction and activation pathway. These changes can result in morphologic, duration, and axis changes in the P wave.

Wandering Atrial Pacemaker. Wandering atrial pacemaker refers to multiple ectopic atrial foci that produce varying abnormal P wave morphologies.

Multifocal Atrial Tachycardia. Multifocal atrial tachycardia (MAT) is a specific type of wandering atrial pacemaker in which tachycardia is produced by more than one atrial focus

firing independently. The tachycardia is irregular, and at least three distinct P wave morphologies appear in any single lead. MAT is rare, but associated with hypoxia and severe pulmonary disease.

Atrial Fibrillation. Atrial fibrillation occurs when there is no organized activation of the atrial tissue, resulting in chaotic depolarizations of atrial myocytes. On the ECG, there are no P waves present and the baseline may appear irregular as a result of this chaotic atrial electrical activity.

Retrograde P Wave. Retrograde P wave (P′) activation occurs when impulses from or near the atrioventricular (AV) node activate the atria, such as occurs with junctional rhythms. The frontal plane axis is often directed toward −90 degrees and results in inverted P′ waves in leads II, III, and aVF. The P′ wave may appear as a tall, peaked positive deflection in lead V_1. For impulses arising from the AV node, the P′ wave may be buried in the QRS complex. As a result, the P′ wave may cause a small deflection of the larger ventricular activation complex or be undetectable on ECG (Fig. 10-7).

Low Atrial P Wave. On occasion, atrial impulses arising from the low atria near the AV node (such as an atrial premature beat), produce a specific morphology known as a "dome and dart" P′ wave in which there is an initial rounded, domelike deflection, followed by a sharp terminal return to baseline.

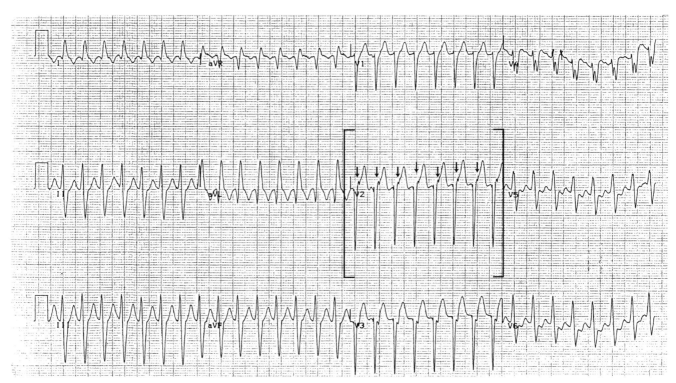

FIGURE 10-7 · Retrograde P′ wave seen in patient with supraventricular tachycardia. Note the negative deflection near the terminal portion of the QRS complex (*arrows in bracket section*).

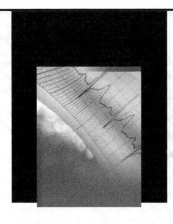

Chapter 11

PR Interval and Segment

Theodore C. Chan

The PR interval includes the atrial depolarization wave (P wave) and the initial atrial repolarization wave (Ta wave) to the start of ventricular depolarization (QRS complex). The PR interval is measured from the start of the P wave to the start of the QRS complex. In contrast, the PR segment is the portion of the PR interval from the end of the P wave to the start of the QRS complex. This segment includes the initial atrial repolarization until the Ta wave is masked by the QRS complex (Fig. 11-1).

In general, abnormalities of the PR interval relate to abnormal shortening or lengthening. Abnormalities of the PR segment relate to changes in morphologic appearance, often associated with alterations in the atrial repolarization Ta wave.

ELECTROCARDIOGRAPHIC DIAGNOSIS

Normal PR Interval and Segment

The PR interval, from the start of the P wave to the start of the QRS complex, has a normal duration of 0.12 to 0.2 sec. The duration varies with age such that the normal PR length at

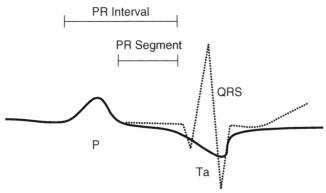

FIGURE 11-1 · PR interval. The atrial depolarization P wave (P) and repolarization Ta wave (Ta) that make up the PR interval are depicted schematically. The Ta wave is not seen because it is buried in the QRS and T complex of ventricular activation (*dotted line*). However, changes in atrial repolarization affect the morphology of the PR segment.

birth is 0.1 sec and gradually lengthens to adult duration by adolescence. In the PR segment, the Ta wave vector is usually in the opposite direction to the P wave vector (i.e., inverted in lead II, where the P wave is most prominently upright). Most of the Ta wave, however, is obscured by the QRS complex, and only the proximal portion of the Ta wave is visible (Fig. 11-1). The normal P wave downslope transitions gently into the initial Ta wave, producing a near-isoelectric terminal PR segment. This portion has been termed the *pause* between atrial activation and ventricular activation.

Abnormal PR Interval and Segment

Abnormalities in the PR interval result from abnormalities in the duration (abnormally short or long). Abnormalities in the PR segment result from alterations in morphology between the P wave and QRS complex.

Short PR interval

Exercise-Induced Sinus Tachycardia. Exercise-induced tachycardia can shorten the PR interval. This shortening is associated with a slight downsloping of the terminal segment, producing a minimal PR segment depression in leads with upright P waves.

Preexcitation. Accessory pathways, such as occur with Wolff-Parkinson-White syndrome, result in an abnormally short PR interval because of the early activation of the ventricle. On the electrocardiogram (ECG), the PR interval appears shorter owing to the delta wave of preexcitation (Fig. 11-2).

Low Ectopic Atrial Rhythms. Ectopic atrial rhythms in which the atrial impulse focus is located near the atrioventricular (AV) junction shorten the PR interval by decreasing the length of time or pause between atrial and ventricular depolarization. Because of its ectopic origin, the P wave often appears abnormal in morphology.

Atrioventricular Junctional Rhythms and Supraventricular Tachycardias. With these rhythm disturbances, atrial activation occurs in close proximity to ventricular depolarization, such that if P waves are present or visible, the PR interval appears very short.

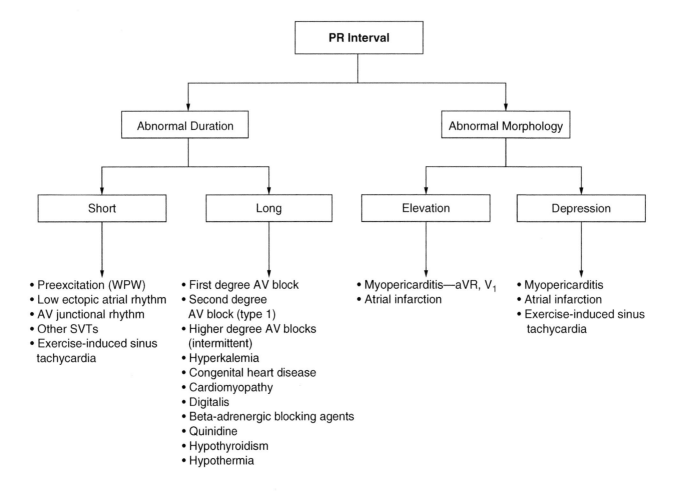

Abnormal Duration   Abnormal Morphology

Short   Long   Elevation   Depression

- Preexcitation (WPW)
- Low ectopic atrial rhythm
- AV junctional rhythm
- Other SVTs
- Exercise-induced sinus tachycardia

- First degree AV block
- Second degree AV block (type 1)
- Higher degree AV blocks (intermittent)
- Hyperkalemia
- Congenital heart disease
- Cardiomyopathy
- Digitalis
- Beta-adrenergic blocking agents
- Quinidine
- Hypothyroidism
- Hypothermia

- Myopericarditis—aVR, V_1
- Atrial infarction

- Myopericarditis
- Atrial infarction
- Exercise-induced sinus tachycardia

Other Rare Causes. Other rare causes of a short PR interval include various congenital heart conditions, certain hypertrophic cardiomyopathies, and cardiac abnormalities associated with the neurologic disorder, Friedreich's disease.

Prolonged PR interval

Aging. A slight prolongation of the PR interval has been associated with aging in adults.

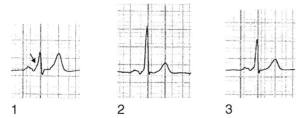

1   2   3

FIGURE 11-2 · Shortened PR interval. These three single-beat figures demonstrate a shortened PR interval from preexcitation. Note the delta wave (*arrow*) created by preexcitation of the ventricle at the start of the QRS complex.

Atrioventricular Block—First Degree. AV block and delay in atrial–ventricular impulse conduction results in prolongation of the PR interval. With first degree block, the PR interval length is greater than 0.2 sec, but each P wave is associated with a QRS complex (Fig. 11-3).

Atrioventricular Block—Second Degree. Second degree AV block results in either a progressive lengthening of the PR interval with a subsequent dropped QRS complex (type I or Wenckebach) or a constant PR interval length with an intermittent dropped QRS complex due to nonconduction of the impulse (type II) (Fig. 11-4).

Atrioventricular Block—Third Degree. With third degree AV block, the PR interval appears variable in length because of the independent nature of atrial and ventricular activity. No regular association and thus consistent PR interval pattern is seen on the ECG.

Hyperkalemia. With progressive elevation in serum potassium levels, prolongation of the PR interval may precede loss of P wave amplitude.

Congenital Heart Diseases. A number of congenital heart diseases are associated with prolongation of the PR interval.

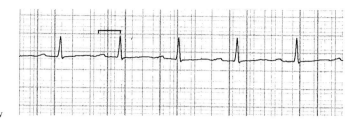

FIGURE 11-3 · PR interval prolongation. These two rhythm strips show PR interval prolongation in the setting of first degree atrioventricular block. The brackets denote the prolonged PR interval duration, which is constant.

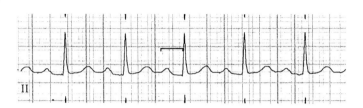

This prolongation may be related to atrial abnormalities such as left atrial enlargement, which can produce P wave prolongation and other abnormalities as well. Entities include Ebstein's anomaly, patent ductus arteriosus, ventricular septal defect, and pulmonary stenosis.

Cardiomyopathy.   Similar to congenital heart disease, certain congestive cardiomyopathies are associated with PR interval prolongation.

Medications.   Certain AV blockade medications, such as digitalis compounds and beta-adrenergic blocking agents, are associated with varying degrees of AV block. Quinidine has been associated with prolongation of the PR interval.

Other Causes.   Other causes of PR interval prolongation include hypothyroidism and hypothermia.

Abnormal PR segment morphology

The PR segment can be abnormally elevated or depressed. In assessing the PR segment, it is important to use the TP segment as baseline; otherwise, the depression may be misinterpreted as ST segment elevation.

Exercise-Induced Sinus Tachycardia.   Exercise-induced tachycardia can produce a slight downsloping and depression of the PR segment, particularly in leads with upright P waves. This change in PR segment morphology can be associated with shortening of the PR interval.

Acute Myopericarditis.   Transient, diffuse PR segment depression may be one of the earliest and most specific signs of acute myopericarditis. Depression is most prominent in leads II, V_5, and V_6. Reciprocal PR segment elevation may be seen in leads aVR and V_1 (Fig. 11-5).

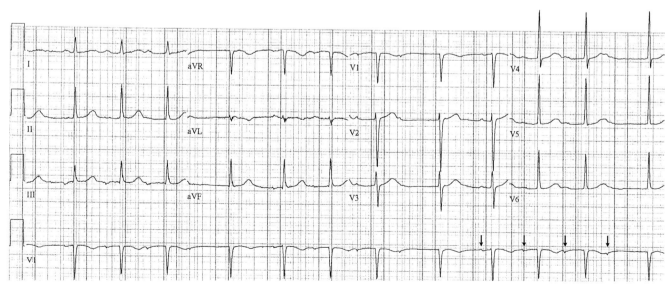

FIGURE 11-4 · PR interval prolongation. This ECG shows PR interval prolongation in the setting of a second degree atrioventricular block, type I (Wenckebach). Note the progressive lengthening of the PR interval (*arrows* denote P waves).

Atrial infarction. Atrial infarction produces abnormalities of the atrial repolarization Ta wave, which in turn produce elevation or depression of the PR segment. Elevation can be seen in leads I, V_5, and V_6, with reciprocal depression in leads V_1, V_2, II, or III. Because the normal Ta wave is directed opposite the P wave, atrial infarction should be considered when PR segment elevation is seen in leads with upright P waves. In addition, the transition from P wave to the PR segment becomes more sharply demarcated with either elevation or depression.

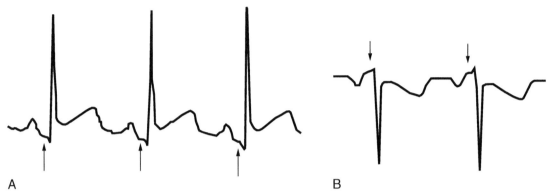

FIGURE 11-5 · **PR segment depression and elevation.** *A,* PR segment depression (*arrows*) is seen in a beat in lead II in a patient with myopericarditis. *B,* Reciprocal PR segment elevation is seen in lead aVR in a patient with myopericarditis.

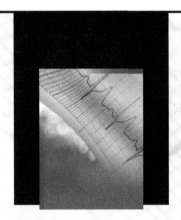

Chapter 12

QRS Complex

Richard A. Harrigan

The QRS complex is representative of ventricular depolarization. Normally, both the right and left ventricles are depolarized simultaneously. Oddly, the QRS complex may not always have a Q, an R, and an S wave, or it may have more than one R wave; this may also depend on which lead is considered.

There is some variability among the 12 standard leads with regard to QRS amplitude and duration. Absolute amplitude is important when considered in the context of the specific lead, such as with voltage criteria for ventricular hypertrophy or low voltage as may be seen with pericardial effusion. Likewise, QRS complex duration varies from lead to lead. The width of the QRS complex should be measured in the lead where it is widest; this is usually in a precordial lead, especially lead V_2 or V_3. Normally, the QRS complex varies between 0.07 and 0.11 sec in duration. There is no lower limit of normal with regard to QRS complex width.

ELECTROCARDIOGRAPHIC DIAGNOSIS

Normal Q, R, and S wave morphology

If the QRS complex begins with a negative deflection, this is called a Q wave. It is the net result of vector forces directed away from the positive electrode. If it is followed by a positive deflection (representing net forces moving toward the positive electrode), that is termed the R wave. The next negative deflection after that R wave is called the S wave. Any positive

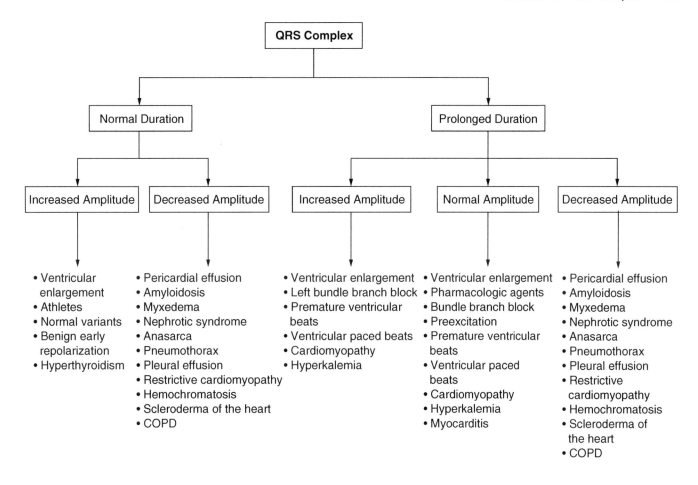

QRS Complex

Normal Duration

Prolonged Duration

Normal Duration — Increased Amplitude
- Ventricular enlargement
- Athletes
- Normal variants
- Benign early repolarization
- Hyperthyroidism

Normal Duration — Decreased Amplitude
- Pericardial effusion
- Amyloidosis
- Myxedema
- Nephrotic syndrome
- Anasarca
- Pneumothorax
- Pleural effusion
- Restrictive cardiomyopathy
- Hemochromatosis
- Scleroderma of the heart
- COPD

Prolonged Duration — Increased Amplitude
- Ventricular enlargement
- Left bundle branch block
- Premature ventricular beats
- Ventricular paced beats
- Cardiomyopathy
- Hyperkalemia

Prolonged Duration — Normal Amplitude
- Ventricular enlargement
- Pharmacologic agents
- Bundle branch block
- Preexcitation
- Premature ventricular beats
- Ventricular paced beats
- Cardiomyopathy
- Hyperkalemia
- Myocarditis

Prolonged Duration — Decreased Amplitude
- Pericardial effusion
- Amyloidosis
- Myxedema
- Nephrotic syndrome
- Anasarca
- Pneumothorax
- Pleural effusion
- Restrictive cardiomyopathy
- Hemochromatosis
- Scleroderma of the heart
- COPD

deflection that follows an S wave is referred to as an R′ wave (Fig. 12-1).

Given that each QRS complex may not have all three waves, or may even have an extra positive deflection (R′ wave), there are a number of possible combinations of these waves. If no positive deflection follows the initial negative deflection, there is only a single negative deflection, termed a QS complex (Fig. 12-2). The Q wave may be followed by an R wave without an S wave, resulting in a QR complex (Fig. 12-3). If the first deflection is positive, and is followed by a lone negative deflection, it is termed an RS complex (Fig. 12-4, Table 12-1).

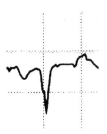

FIGURE 12-2 · QS complex. Here seen in lead V₁, a single negative deflection characterizes the QS complex.

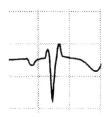

FIGURE 12-1 · rSr′ complex. This complex from lead V₁ in a patient with incomplete right bundle branch block demonstrates two positive deflections (r and r′ waves, respectively) separated by a negative deflection (S wave).

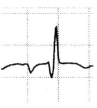

FIGURE 12-3 · QR complex. This QR complex in lead V₁ is indicative of right ventricular hypertrophy in this patient with pulmonary hypertension.

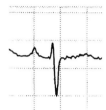

FIGURE 12-4 · RS complex. From the same patient as Figure 12-3; this rS complex in lead I contributed to this patient's rightward QRS axis deviation, giving further credence to the ECG diagnosis of right ventricular hypertrophy.

Q wave amplitude is usually less than 0.4 mV (or four small boxes on the grid), or less than 25% of the height of the R wave. In lead III, Q waves are acceptable up to 0.5 mV, and the 25% guideline does not necessarily hold. *Q wave duration* is normally less than 0.03 sec (just under one small box on the grid) in the limb leads and leads V_5 and V_6, except in leads III and aVR, where it can be wider (because of the rightward orientation of the positive aspect of these leads). Lead III may feature nonpathologic Q waves as wide as 0.04 or rarely 0.05 sec. Any Q wave appearing in leads V_1 to V_3 is considered pathologic, and lead V_4 may feature a nonpathologic Q wave up to 0.02 sec.

The absence of Q waves in the lateral leads (especially leads V_6 and I) suggests left bundle branch block. The presence of Q waves of pathologic dimensions as described previously suggests myocardial infarction, ventricular enlargement, or abnormal ventricular conduction.

R wave amplitude is maximal in the leads that parallel in direction (and polarity) the major QRS axis vector (in the frontal and coronal planes). Larger R waves are at times seen as a normal variant in younger individuals. They may also be seen in ventricular enlargement and left anterior and left posterior fascicular blocks (see Chapter 21, Intraventricular Conduction Abnormalities, and Chapter 35, Ventricular Hypertrophy). Lead V_4 usually features the largest precordial R wave in a normal heart; R waves normally get progressively larger across the precordium as the leads overlie the bigger left ventricle. *R wave duration* should be considered within the context of QRS complex width (see later).

S wave amplitude is usually largest in leads aVR and V_2; S waves normally get progressively smaller across the precordium as the leads overlie the larger left ventricle. Larger-than-expected S waves are seen with ventricular enlargement and in intraventricular conduction delays (see Chapters 21, Intraventricular Conduction Abnormalities, and 35, Ventricular Hypertrophy). *S wave duration* should be considered within the context of QRS complex width (see later).

Table 12-1 depicts some of the atypical combinations of Q, R, and S waves and possible underlying cardiac pathologic processes.

12-1 • SELECTED VARIANTS OF THE QRS COMPLEX

Complex	Location (Leads)	Possible Significance
QS complex	Any contiguous leads	MI
		Premature ventricular contraction *(singlets or couplets, and wide complex)*
	V_1, V_2	Septal MI
		Left bundle branch block *(wide complex)*
	V_1–V_4	Anteroseptal MI
		Amyloidosis
	III, aVF, aVL, or V_1	Normal variant
	V_6	Ventricular tachycardia *(wide complex)*
		Ventricular paced rhythm *(wide complex)*
QR complex	V_1, V_2	qR variant of RBBB
	V_1, V_2	Septal MI
	V_1	qR variant of RVH
	V_1	Ventricular tachycardia *(wide complex)*
	III, aVF, or aVL	Normal variant
RSR′ complex	V_1, V_2	Complete RBBB *(if QRS >0.12 sec)*
		Ventricular tachycardia—especially if RSr′ pattern *(wide complex)*
		Brugada syndrome (with associated ST segment elevation—may be V_1–V_3)
		Incomplete RBBB *(if QRS <0.12 sec)*
		Right ventricular hypertrophy
		Acute right ventricular dilation—as in pulmonary embolism
		Tricyclic antidepressant toxicity *(wide complex)*
		Pectus excavatum; straight back syndrome *(if QRS <0.12 sec)*
		Normal variant *(if QRS <0.12 sec)*
		Superior misplacement of V_1, V_2 electrodes

MI, myocardial infarction; RBBB, right bundle branch block; RVH, right ventricular hypertrophy.

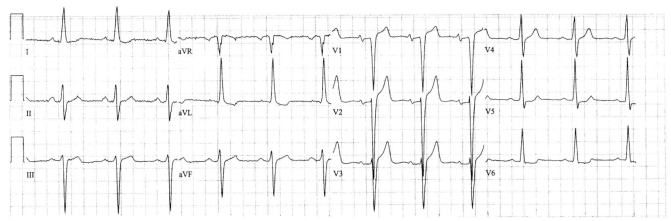

FIGURE 12-5 · **Large amplitude QRS complexes.** This patient meets multiple ECG criteria for left ventricular hypertrophy, including QRS complex voltage in lead aVL >11 mm; S wave in lead V_1 + R wave in lead V_5 or V_6 >35 mm; R wave in lead aVL + S wave in lead V_3 >28 mm in men; QRS complex duration >0.09 sec; and repolarization "strain" abnormality seen in leads I, aVL, and V_6 (see Chapter 35, Ventricular Hypertrophy).

Normal QRS complex duration

Large Amplitude.   Increased amplitude is suggestive of *ventricular enlargement* (Fig. 12-5). Left ventricular hypertrophy (LVH) has many voltage criteria with varying sensitivities and specificities (see Chapter 35, Ventricular Hypertrophy), some of which involve the precordial leads, others the limb leads, and still others a combination of both. Right ventricular hypertrophy similarly has a variety of voltage-related criteria (see Chapter 35, Ventricular Hypertrophy). Abnormally large QRS complexes are sometimes seen in athletes and as normal variants; they may be seen in *benign early repolarization* (BER), but QRS amplitude per se is not a defining component of BER. QRS complex amplitude may mimic ventricular hypertrophy in *hyperthyroidism.*

Diminished Amplitude.   Decreased amplitude, or "low voltage," is usually considered to be present when the total QRS complex voltage in each of the limb leads is less than 5 mm (0.5 mV), or less than 10 mm (1.0 mV) in each of the precordial leads. This is seen with *pericardial effusion, amyloidosis, myxedematous hypothyroidism, nephrotic syndrome, anasarca, pneumothorax, left pleural effusion, restrictive cardiomyopathy, hemochromatosis, scleroderma* (with cardiac involvement), *starvation,* and chest conditions featuring increased anteroposterior diameter, such as *chronic obstructive pulmonary disease.* QRS complex amplitude usually decreases with age and with weight gain.

Prolonged QRS complex duration

Large Amplitude.   Increased QRS complex amplitude with prolonged duration (>0.12 sec) is seen with a variety of disorders. *Ventricular enlargement* may feature increased voltage and a widened QRS (see Chapter 35, Ventricular Hypertrophy; Fig. 12-5). *Left bundle branch block* features prominent QRS complex amplitude, although amplitude is not part of the defining characteristics (see Chapter 21, Intraventricular Conduction Abnormalities; Fig. 12-6). *Ectopic ventricular complexes* (e.g., premature ventricular complexes, couplets, ventricular tachycardia) will, by definition, be wider than normal, and may be increased in amplitude (Fig. 12-7). *Ventricular paced rhythms,* which are essentially artificially induced ventricular complexes, are also by definition widened,

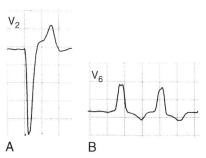

FIGURE 12-6 · **Left bundle branch block (LBBB).** LBBB is demonstrated in lead V_2 (*A*; note the large amplitude), and lead V_6 (*B*).

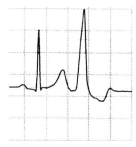

FIGURE 12-7 · **Ectopic ventricular complex.** Note the relatively larger amplitude and longer duration of the second complex in the figure; this is a premature ventricular beat.

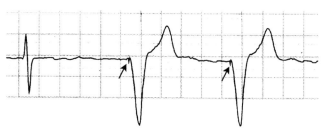

FIGURE 12-8 · **Ventricular paced beats.** Note that the second and third beats, generated by an artificial ventricular pacemaker, are larger in amplitude, and wider, than the native beat that precedes them. Note also the small pacemaker spikes (*arrows*).

and may be of increased amplitude—although pacemaker spikes are the key to detecting this condition (Fig. 12-8).

Normal Amplitude.   The QRS complex may be widened, yet of normal amplitude, in a variety of conditions. QRS complex widening may signify LVH (see Chapter 35, Ventricular Hypertrophy). Any cardiac condition that causes delay in conduction through ventricular tissue (e.g., *cardiomyopathy, myocarditis, preexcitation,* primary conduction system disease) results in widening of the QRS complex. Impulses originating in the ventricle (*ectopic ventricular complexes, ventricular tachycardia, ventricular paced rhythms*) are widened by definition. Various *drugs,* in toxic amounts, may cause widening of the QRS (see Chapters 49 through 57, on toxicology). *Hyperkalemia* may also widen the QRS complex; this usually occurs after the T waves have become abnormally tall and peaked (Fig. 12-9; see Chapter 58, Electrolyte Abnormalities).

Diminished Amplitude.   Decreased amplitude, or "low voltage," may occur with *pericardial effusion, amyloidosis, myxedematous hypothyroidism, nephrotic syndrome, anasarca, obesity, pneumothorax, left pleural effusion, restrictive cardiomyopathy, hemochromatosis, scleroderma* (with cardiac involvement), *starvation,* and chest conditions featuring increased anteroposterior diameter, such as *chronic obstructive pulmonary*

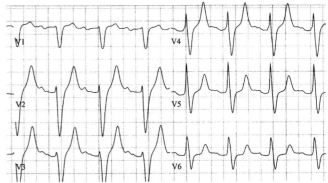

FIGURE 12-9 · Hyperkalemia. Note the widened QRS complex in the precordial leads. In leads V_5 and V_6, normal amplitude is found in the setting of a widened QRS complex. Conversely, leads V_2, V_3, and V_4 demonstrate both large amplitude and widened QRS complexes. Also note the prominent T waves in the right to mid-precordial leads. This ECG suggests hyperkalemia; the clinician must also consider left bundle branch block and left ventricular hypertrophy in the ECG differential diagnosis.

disease. All entities discussed previously in the sections on large and normal amplitude may manifest as widened QRS complexes of diminished amplitude in these conditions.

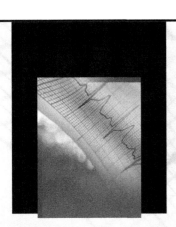

Chapter 13

ST Segment

William J. Brady

The ST segment of the cardiac electrical cycle represents the period between depolarization and repolarization of the left ventricle. In the normal state, the ST segment is isoelectric, meaning that it is neither elevated nor depressed relative to the TP segment. ST segment elevation or depression results from a number of clinical syndromes, including acute coronary syndrome (ACS) and non-ACS presentations.

ELECTROCARDIOGRAPHIC DIAGNOSIS

ST segment elevation

Magnitude.   Greater total amounts of ST segment elevation (STE) are associated with acute myocardial infarction (AMI) compared with other, noninfarction syndromes.

Morphology.   The contour of the STE may be of assistance in diagnostic considerations: Concave morphology is generally associated with a non-AMI causes (Fig. 13-1A) and convex morphology is usually seen seen in patients with AMI (Fig. 13-1B).

Distribution.   The anatomic location of the STE can suggest the diagnosis. More widespread STE is associated with non-AMI causes, whereas localized changes occur more frequently with AMI.

Prominent Electrical Forces.   Large QRS complexes are a possible indication of electrocardiographic (ECG) left ventricular hypertrophy (LVH), which, if present, may explain ST segment/T wave changes.

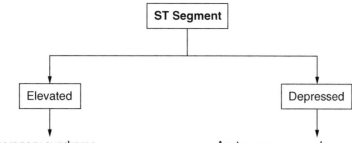

```
                    ST Segment

        Elevated                Depressed
```

Elevated

- Acute coronary syndrome
- Prinzmetal's angina (vasospastic)
- Myocardial infarction
  - ST segment elevation AMI
- Acute pericarditis
- Benign early repolarization
- Left ventricular aneurysm
- Bundle branch block (left and right)
- Left ventricular hypertrophy
- Ventricular paced rhythm
- Cardiomyopathy
- Acute myocarditis
- Hypothermia
- Hyperkalemia
- Post-electrical cardioversion
- Non-ACS myocardial injury (e.g., contusion)
- CNS injury
- Brugada syndrome
- Preexcitation syndromes

Depressed

- Acute coronary syndrome
- Myocardial ischemia
- Myocardial infarction
  - Non-ST segment elevation AMI
  - Posterior AMI (leads V_1–V_3)
- Bundle branch block
- Left ventricular hypertrophy
- Ventricular paced rhythm
- Digitalis effect
- Tachycardia/rate-related
- Metabolic syndromes
- Post-electrical cardioversion
- Non-ACS myocardial injury (e.g., contusion)

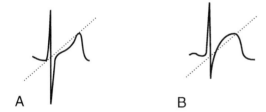

FIGURE 13-1 · **Morphology of the elevated ST segment.** A line is drawn from the J point to the apex of the T wave. The morphology is termed concave if the ECG waveform falls below the line and convex if the ECG waveform is above the line: *A*, Non–acute myocardial infarction (AMI) presentation with a concave morphology. *B*, AMI presentation with convex morphology.

QRS Complex Width. A widened QRS complex is one criterion for bundle branch block (BBB) or ventricular-paced rhythm, which may cause ST segment/T wave abnormalities.

Other Features. The presence of ST segment depression distant from the elevated ST segments suggests AMI. PR segment depression is highly associated with acute pericarditis.

ST segment elevated syndromes

Acute Coronary Syndrome/Prinzmetal (Variant) Angina. The elevated ST segment is usually obliquely straight or convex and is difficult to distinguish from that associated with AMI.

Acute Coronary Syndrome/Myocardial Infarction (ST Segment Elevation Acute Myocardial Infarction). STE related to AMI is present in at least two anatomically contiguous ECG leads. The STE itself may assume one of three morphologies: concave, obliquely straight, or convex. The initial upsloping portion of the ST segment usually is either convex or flat in AMI; concave contours are most often associated with non-AMI syndromes (Fig. 13-2).

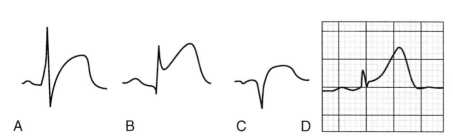

FIGURE 13-2 · **The ST segment elevation morphology in acute myocardial infarction.** *A*, Convex. *B*, Obliquely straight. *C*, Convex. *D*, Concave.

Benign Early Repolarization. The ECG definition of benign early repolarization includes the following characteristics: (1) STE; (2) upward concavity of the initial portion of the ST segment; (3) notching or slurring of the terminal QRS complex; (4) symmetric, concordant T waves of large amplitude; (5) widespread or diffuse distribution of STE on the ECG; and (6) relative temporal stability (Fig. 13-3).

Acute Pericarditis. STE, usually with a concave morphology, can be seen in the early stages of acute pericarditis. This finding may be seen in association with PR segment depression in certain individuals (Fig. 13-4).

Bundle Branch Block. STE is usually concave and, if present, most often associated with prominently negative QRS complexes. The correct configurations are predicted by the rule of appropriate discordance, which states that the ST segment/ T wave structure is directed opposite the terminal portion of the QRS complex. In right BBB (RBBB), STE is seen in the lateral leads. In left BBB, STE is seen in the right to mid-precordial leads as well as the inferior leads (Fig. 13-5).

Left Ventricular Hypertrophy. STE is usually concave and associated with prominently negative QRS complexes. STE is usually seen in the right to mid-precordial leads (Fig. 13-6).

Ventricular Paced Rhythm. STE is usually concave and associated with prominently negative QRS complexes. The correct configurations are predicted by the rule of appropriate discordance, which states that the ST segment/T wave structure is directed opposite the terminal portion of the QRS complex. STE is usually seen in the inferior and precordial leads (Fig. 13-7).

Left Ventricular Aneurysm. Left ventricular aneurysm is characterized electrocardiographically by persistent STE seen several weeks after AMI. The actual ST segment abnormality due to the left ventricular aneurysm may present with varying morphologies, ranging from obvious, convex STE to minimal, concave elevations. The distinction from STE in the patient with AMI may be difficult. In most cases of left ventricular aneurysm, a fully developed Q wave is noted, but this can also be seen in the early evolution of AMI (Fig. 13-8).

Central Nervous System Injury. Certain intracranial disasters may produce significant ST segment/T wave changes, including varying degrees of STE (Fig. 13-9).

Hypothermia. This hypothermia-related ECG change involves the juncture between the terminal portion of the QRS complex and the initial ST segment—the J point. The J point itself and the immediately adjacent ST segment appear to have lifted off the isoelectric baseline. The resultant configuration

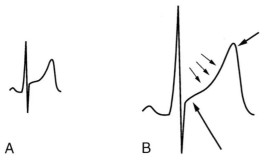

FIGURE 13-3 · **ST segment elevation in benign early repolarization.** *A,* Elevated ST segment at the J point with preservation of the normal concavity of the ST segment. *B,* Accentuation of the elevated ST segment at the J point (*large arrow*) with preservation of the normal concavity (*small arrows*) of the ST segment and prominent T waves (*intermediate arrow*).

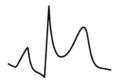

FIGURE 13-4 · **Acute pericarditis.** Note concave ST segment elevation, PR segment depression, and prominent T wave.

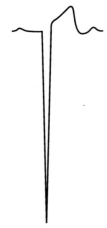

FIGURE 13-6 · **Left ventricular hypertrophy (LVH).** LVH-related ST segment elevation is seen in lead V_2 in this patient.

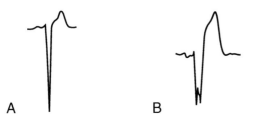

FIGURE 13-5 · **Bundle branch block (BBB).** *A,* BBB-related ST segment elevation (STE) is seen in this patient. The magnitude of STE in this example is considered appropriate for the BBB. *B,* "Excessive" STE is seen in this BBB presentation; this patient was diagnosed with an acute anterior wall myocardial infarction.

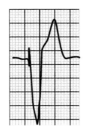
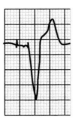
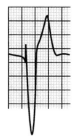

FIGURE 13-7 · **ST segment elevation related to ventricular paced rhythms.**

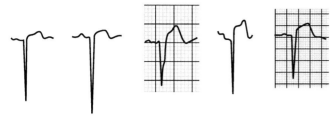

FIGURE 13-8 · **Left ventricular aneurysm–related ST segment elevation.** Note the varying magnitudes, ranging from minimal to maximal, and morphologies, including concave and convex varieties, of the ST segment elevation.

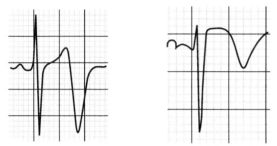

FIGURE 13-9 · **ST segment elevation in intracranial hemorrhage.** These tracings are from two patients with intracranial hemorrhage and marked ST segment/T wave abnormality. Note the ST segment elevation.

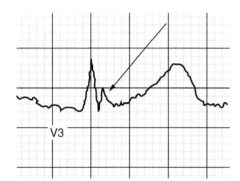

FIGURE 13-10 · **ST segment elevation in hypothermia.** This ECG is from a patient "found down" on a city street with an ambient environmental temperature of 45°F. The ST segment is minimally elevated with a J, or Osborn, wave (*arrow*).

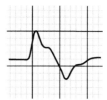

FIGURE 13-11 · **ST segment elevation in hyperkalemia.** Hyperkalemia-related ST segment elevation is seen in a patient with a serum potassium of 8.1 mEq/dL.

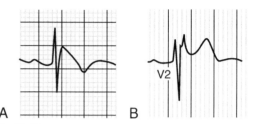

FIGURE 13-12 · **ST segment elevation morphology types in the Brugada syndrome.** *A,* Convex. *B,* Concave ("saddle-type").

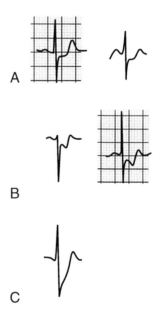

FIGURE 13-13 · **Examples of ST segment depression.** *A,* Horizontal or flat. *B,* Downsloping. *C,* Upsloping.

produces the J wave, also known as the *Osborn wave* and *Osborn J wave* (Fig. 13-10).

Hyperkalemia. The QRS complex may become widened, ultimately forming the sine wave configuration in hyperkalemia. In earlier forms of this QRS complex widening, the ST segment may appear elevated. In general, this pseudo-STE associated with hyperkalemia is characterized by J point elevation and prominent, hyperacute T waves. The initial, upsloping portion of the ST segment is concave, rather than the flat or convex patterns seen in the patient with AMI with STE (Fig. 13-11).

Brugada Syndrome. The Brugada syndrome, encountered in patients with syncope or cardiac arrest, presents electrocardiographically with RBBB and STE in right precordial leads. The STE may take one of two forms, convex or concave

"saddle-type" (Fig. 13-12; see Chapter 26, Ventricular Tachycardia).

Other Causes of ST Segment Elevation. Other causes of nonspecific STE include cardiomyopathy, acute myocarditis, post-electrical cardioversion, and non-ACS myocardial injury (e.g., trauma, contusion).

ST segment depression

Morphology. Horizontal (flat) or downsloping ST segment depression is more often associated with ACS-related forms, although nonischemic causes of ST segment depression may also present with similar morphologies (Fig. 13-13).

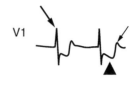

FIGURE 13-14 · Acute coronary syndrome–related ST segment depression. *A*, Horizontal. *B*, Downsloping.

Distribution.   A specific anatomic distribution is not helpful in the diagnosis of ACS. An anatomic distribution, however, is significant in the LVH, BBB, and ventricular paced patterns, as suggested by the rule of appropriate discordance.

Prominent Electrical Forces (QRS Complex Amplitude). The presence of prominent QRS complex forces suggests the possibility of LVH and related repolarization abnormality.

QRS Complex Width.   The presence of a widened QRS complex suggests the presence of either BBB, ventricular paced rhythm, or LVH pattern, with the possibility of ST segment depression related to a nonischemic etiology.

ST segment depressed syndromes

Acute Coronary Syndrome (Myocardial Ischemia and Non–ST Segment Elevation Acute Myocardial Infarction). A combination of two diagnostic criteria have typically been required in at least one ECG lead to diagnose ACS: (1) at least 1 mm (0.1 mV) depression at the J point, and (2) either horizontal or downsloping ST segment depression. ST segment depression due to ACS is usually diffuse. ST segment depression may be located in either anterior or inferior leads; alternatively, it is not necessarily localizing. The specificity of this finding must be discussed relative to its morphology, with a downsloping segment more specific for the diagnosis of ischemia than horizontal depression; a depressed but upsloping ST segment lacks adequate specificity for ACS (Fig. 13-14).

Acute Coronary Syndrome (Posterior Acute Myocardial Infarction).   ECG abnormalities suggestive of a posterior wall AMI include the following (in leads V_1, V_2, or V_3): (1) horizontal ST segment depression with tall, upright T waves; (2) a tall, wide R wave; and (3) an R/S wave ratio greater than 1 in lead V_2 (Fig. 13-15).

Reciprocal ST Segment Depression.   Reciprocal segment depression—also known as *reciprocal change*—is

FIGURE 13-15 · Acute posterior wall myocardial infarction in an adult male with chest pain. Note the prominent R wave (*large arrow*), ST segment depression (*arrowhead*), and upright T wave (*small arrow*).

defined as horizontal or downsloping ST segment depression in leads that are separate and distinct from leads manifesting STE. The presence of reciprocal change increases the positive predictive value for a diagnosis of AMI to greater than 90%— in other words, ST segment depression on the ECG in the setting of anatomically arrayed STE greatly increases the chance that the STE results from AMI. ST segment depression seen in ECG situations involving LVH, BBB, or ventricular paced patterns is not considered reciprocal ST segment depression (Fig. 13-16).

Bundle Branch Block (Left and Right).   Intraventricular conduction delays such as left and right BBB demonstrate ST segment changes as a consequence of the altered conduction. The rule of appropriate discordance states that in BBB, ST segment/T wave configurations are directed opposite from the major, terminal portion of the QRS complex. As such, leads with either QS or rS complexes should have significantly elevated ST segments, whereas leads with a large monophasic R wave demonstrate ST segment depression (Fig. 13-17).

Ventricular Paced Rhythm.   As with the BBB pattern, the ventricular paced pattern has associated ST segment changes,

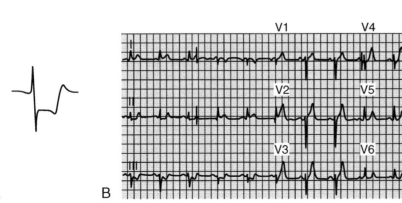

FIGURE 13-16 · Reciprocal ST segment depression. *A*, Reciprocal ST segment depression in lead V_3 in a patient with anterior ST segment elevation, consistent with anterior wall acute myocardial infarction (AMI). *B*, Early anterolateral AMI with minimal ST segment elevation in leads I and aVL and prominent, hyperacute T waves in leads V_2 to V_4. The presence of ST segment depression in leads II, III, and aVF, in this case reciprocal change due to the coexisting ST segment elevation in the inferior leads, reinforces the diagnosis of ST segment elevation AMI of the anterolateral walls.

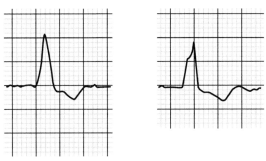

FIGURE 13-17 · **Bundle branch block–related ST segment depression.** Note the downsloping morphology of the depression with a gradual initial limb and a more rapid, abrupt return to the baseline of the terminal limb.

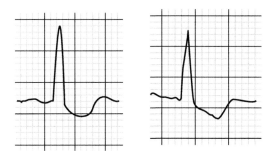

FIGURE 13-19 · Digitalis-related ST segment depression. Note the "scooped" appearance of the depressed ST segment, with a gradual initial limb and a more rapid, abrupt return to the baseline of the terminal limb.

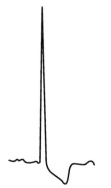

FIGURE 13-18 · Left ventricular hypertrophy–related ST segment depression.

including depression, which is predicted by the rule of appropriate discordance.

Left Ventricular Hypertrophy. Significant ST segment T waves are encountered in approximately 70% of ECG LVH cases. This pattern is characterized by downsloping ST segment depression with abnormal T waves in leads with prominent R waves (I, aVL, V_5, and V_6) and is also referred to as a "strain" pattern. The downsloping ST segment depression—usually without J point depression—is greater than 1 mm and is followed by an inverted T wave (Fig. 13-18).

Digitalis Effect. The ECG manifestations of digitalis—the digoxin effect—includes a "scooped" form of ST segment depression, most prominent in the inferior and anterior leads and usually absent in the rightward leads. The J point is usually found at the isoelectric baseline; occasionally, the J point is depressed. The ST segment morphology is characterized by a gradual, downsloping initial limb and an abrupt return to the baseline. Note that this form of ST segment depression is not indicative of digoxin toxicity (Fig. 13-19).

Tachycardia. Downsloping ST segment depression may be seen in patients with supraventricular tachycardias, including sinus tachycardia. The rate-related depression may not represent acute coronary ischemia.

Other Causes. Other causes of ST segment depression include non-ACS myocardial injury (e.g., contusion), metabolic disturbances (e.g., hypokalemia, hyperkalemia), and post-electrical cardioversion.

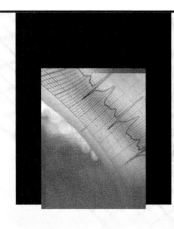

Chapter 14

T Wave

William J. Brady

The T wave of the cardiac electrical cycle represents the period of ventricular repolarization. In the normal state, the T wave is positive (upright) in most electrocardiographic leads (leads I, II, and V_3 to V_6); it is negative (inverted) in lead aVR; and it is variably situated in leads III, aVL, aVF, V_1, and V_2. In the pathologic state, the T wave can assume one of several morphologies, including the prominent, inverted, biphasic, or flattened presentations.

ELECTROCARDIOGRAPHIC DIAGNOSIS

Features to consider in the electrocardiographic differential diagnosis include morphology, magnitude, nature of the QRS complex, temporal nature, and other features.

Prominent T wave

Acute Coronary Syndrome (Early ST Segment Elevation Acute Myocardial Infarction). The initial electrocardiographic finding resulting from the ST segment elevation acute myocardial infarction (AMI) is the prominent T wave—termed *hyperacute* in the context of AMI—which is noted as early as 30 minutes after the onset of infarction. The hyperacute T waves of AMI are asymmetric with a broad base. The R wave also increases in amplitude at this stage. In addition, the "J" (or junction) point may also be elevated, indicative of impending ST segment elevation (Fig. 14-1).

Acute Coronary Syndrome (Posterior Acute Myocardial Infarction [Leads V_1 to V_3]). Posterior wall AMI may present with tall T waves in leads V_1 to V_3. The tall T waves of posterior wall AMI are analogous to the T wave inversions characteristic of anterior and inferior wall AMIs. In contrast to the transient nature of hyperacute T waves of anterior wall AMI, the tall T waves representing posterior wall AMI tend to persist many days and may even be permanent.

Hyperkalemia. The T waves associated with hyperkalemia tend to be tall, narrow, and peaked with a prominent or sharp apex—these T waves resemble the tall, vaulting appearance of a church steeple. Also, these T waves tend to be symmetric in morphology. As the serum potassium level increases, the T waves tend to become taller, peaked, and narrowed in a

symmetric fashion in the anterior distribution (Fig. 14-2).

Benign Early Repolarization. Prominent T waves of large amplitude and slightly asymmetric morphology are encountered; the T waves may appear "peaked," suggestive of the hyperacute T wave encountered in patients with AMI. The T waves are concordant with the QRS complex and are usually found in the precordial leads (Fig. 14-3).

Acute Myopericarditis. Prominent T waves may be seen in association with concave ST segment elevation and PR segment depression.

Bundle Branch Block. Large, positive T waves may be seen in leads with entirely negative QRS complexes, as predicted by the rule of appropriate discordance. Such a presentation is seen in left bundle branch block pattern in leads V_1 to V_3 and, less commonly, in right bundle branch block in the left precordial leads.

Left Ventricular Hypertrophy. Large, positive T waves may be seen in leads with entirely negative QRS complexes, as predicted by the rule of appropriate discordance, in leads V_1 to V_3.

Inverted T wave

Acute Coronary Syndrome. Inverted T waves produced by myocardial ischemia or infarction are classically narrow and symmetric. T wave inversion associated with acute coronary syndrome (ACS) is morphologically characterized by an isoelectric ST segment that is usually bowed upward and followed by a sharp, symmetric downstroke. These findings can occur in all stages of ACS, including myocardial ischemia and non–ST segment elevation and ST segment elevation AMI. These inversions may be seen post-AMI. T wave inversions may also occur with reperfusions (Fig. 14-4).

Wellen's Syndrome. An important subgroup of patients with noninfarction ACS present with significantly abnormal T wave inversions (symmetric, deeply inverted T waves) of the precordial leads (particularly leads V_2 and V_3). Refer to Figure 14-2 for an example. These electrocardiographic patterns frequently occur in the pain-free state (Fig. 14-5).

Bundle Branch Block. Bundle branch block may produce significant T wave changes. Inverted T waves are seen in leads

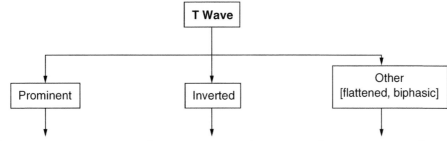

```
                        ┌──────────┐
                        │  T Wave  │
                        └──────────┘
        ┌───────────────────┼───────────────────┐
        ▼                   ▼                   ▼
 ┌────────────┐      ┌────────────┐      ┌──────────────────┐
 │  Prominent │      │  Inverted  │      │       Other      │
 └────────────┘      └────────────┘      │[flattened, biphasic]│
        │                   │            └──────────────────┘
        ▼                   ▼                   ▼
```

• Acute coronary
  syndrome
   – AMI
   – Posterior AMI
     (leads V_1–V_3)
• Hyperkalemia
• Benign early
  repolarization
• Acute myopericarditis
• Bundle branch block
• Left ventricular
  hypertrophy

• Acute coronary syndrome
   – Myocardial ischemia
   – Non-STE AMI
   – Wellen's syndrome
• Past myocardial infarction
• Bundle branch block
• Pericarditis
• Pulmonary embolism
• Left ventricular
  hypertrophy
• Digitalis effect
• CNS injury
• Ventricular paced rhythm
• Intra-abdominal disorders
• Metabolic syndromes
• Toxic syndromes
• Preexcitation syndrome
• Juvenile T wave pattern

• Acute coronary syndrome
• Myocardial ischemia
• Myocardial infarction
   – Non-STE AMI
• Metabolic syndromes
• Post-electrical cardioversion

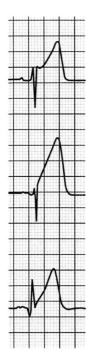

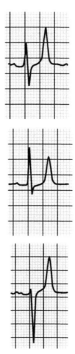

FIGURE 14-1 · Prominent T waves of early acute myocardial infarction.

FIGURE 14-2 · Prominent T waves associated with hyperkalemia.

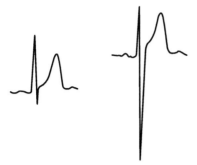

FIGURE 14-3 · Prominent T waves of benign early repolarization.

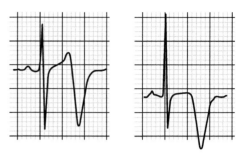

FIGURE 14-5 · T wave inversions characteristic of Wellen's syndrome.

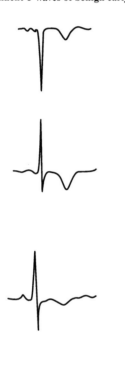

FIGURE 14-4 · T wave inversions associated with acute coronary syndrome.

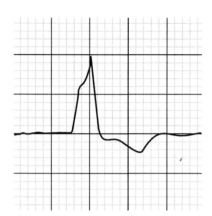

FIGURE 14-6 · T wave inversion in bundle branch block pattern.

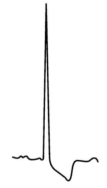

FIGURE 14-7 · T wave inversion associated with left ventricular hypertrophy.

with either entirely or predominantly positive QRS complexes, as predicted by the rule of appropriate discordance. These T waves are widely splayed and asymmetric with the initial portion gradually downsloping and the terminal limb rapidly, abruptly returning to the baseline; the amplitude ranges from minimal to significant (Fig. 14-6).

Left Ventricular Hypertrophy. The "strain" pattern, electrocardiographic changes resulting from repolarization abnormality in the patient with left ventricular hypertrophy, is characterized by ST segment depression with asymmetric, biphasic, or

inverted T waves in leads with prominent R waves (the lateral lead I). The ST segment/T wave is initially bowed upward, followed by a gradual downward sloping into an inverted, asymmetric T wave with an abrupt return to the baseline. The T wave may be minimally or deeply inverted (Fig. 14-7).

Digitalis Effect. The T wave is usually inverted and a component of the depressed ST segment (Fig. 14-8).

Central Nervous System Injury. Inverted T waves due to a central nervous system event are symmetric, deeply inverted, and variable in width. T wave inversions range from small in structure to very prominent; the most prominent inversions, termed *wellenoid* in appearance, are symmetric, very deep, rather prominent inverted T waves (Fig. 14-9).

Acute Myopericarditis. These T wave inversions are frequently small in size and symmetric in morphology. These changes are a late-stage finding in acute myopericarditis.

Pulmonary Embolism. T wave inversions of varying magnitude may be seen in the precordial leads.

Ventricular Paced Rhythm. T wave inversions are seen in leads with prominent, positive QRS complexes, as predicted by the rule of appropriate discordance. Morphologically, they are asymmetric with a gradual downward slope and a more rapid, abrupt return to the baseline.

Preexcitation Syndrome. T wave inversions may be seen in leads with prominent R waves. These inversions are frequently small in size and symmetric in morphology.

Persistent Juvenile T Wave Pattern. Juvenile T wave inversions may appear in the precordial leads (e.g. V_1, V_2, and V_3).

Such a finding is considered normal in the child and young adolescent; this finding, however, should evolve into the upright T wave of adulthood as the child ages (usually in the early to mid-teen years). The T wave inversion is usually small in amplitude and symmetric in structure (Fig. 14-10).

Other Causes. T wave inversions may be seen in intra-abdominal disorders, metabolic and toxic etiologies, or as a normal variant.

Other T wave abnormalities

Acute Coronary Syndrome. In early non-AMI ACS presentations, the T wave may become either diminished or flattened. In the non–ST segment elevation AMI, similar T wave changes may be seen.

Wellen's Syndrome. An important subgroup of patients with unstable angina present with significantly abnormal T wave inversions (biphasic T waves) of the precordial leads (particularly leads V_2 and V_3).

Other Causes. T wave abnormalities may be seen in intra-abdominal disorders, metabolic and toxic etiologies, post-electrical cardioversion, or as a normal variant.

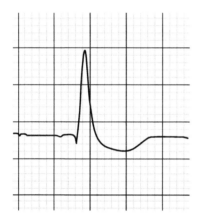

FIGURE 14-8 · **T wave inversion seen in digoxin-treated patient.**

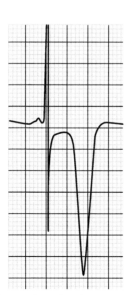

FIGURE 14-9 · **T wave inversion in a patient with subarachnoid hemorrhage.**

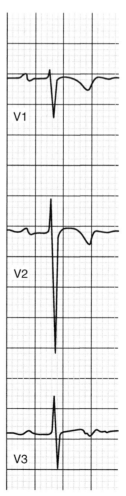

V1

V2

V3

FIGURE 14-10 · **T wave inversions seen in the adult patient with persistent juvenile T wave pattern.**

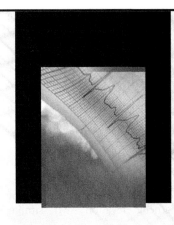

Chapter 15

QT Interval

Richard A. Harrigan

The QT interval reflects the systolic phase for the ventricles, and includes ventricular activation (QRS complex) as well as recovery. It is measured from the beginning of the QRS complex until the end of the T wave. Within any 12-lead tracing, there is lead-to-lead variation in QT interval duration (see Chapter 73, QT Dispersion); in general, the longest measurable QT interval is regarded as determining the overall QT interval for a given tracing. QT interval varies with age (increases slightly with age), sex (slightly longer in women than men), and heart rate (the higher the rate, the shorter the QT interval). The QT interval is also usually longer during the night. A correction factor for rate is automatically included on most tracings with computer printouts across the top of the tracing; this *corrected QT interval* (QT$_C$) is determined by dividing the QT interval by the square root of the R-R interval.

$$QTc = QT/\sqrt{RR}$$

Estimating the QT interval is difficult at times. If U waves occur, T-U wave fusion may make determination of the cessation of the T wave difficult. Similarly, T-P wave fusion may occur at higher heart rates, creating a similar dilemma. In such cases, the onset (of the U wave) or termination (of the P wave) should serve as markers of the terminus of the QT interval.

ELECTROCARDIOGRAPHIC DIAGNOSIS

Short QT interval

It is difficult to find universal agreement on what constitutes a short QT interval, especially in light of the coincident effects of age, sex, rate, and diurnal variation, as well as the lack of pathologic processes associated with short QT intervals. A short QT interval for normal sinus rates would be

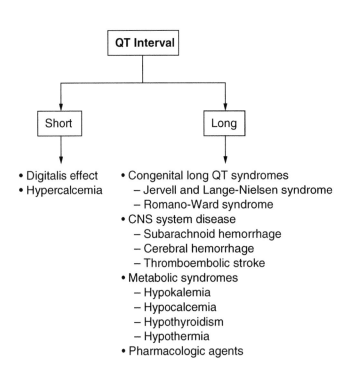

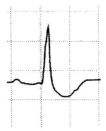

FIGURE 15-1 · **Digitalis effect.** Shown here in lead V_6, scooped ST segment depression includes the T wave and demonstrates a short QT interval.

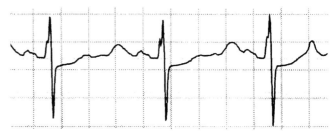

FIGURE 15-3 · **Long QT interval.** The QT interval seen here in lead V_3 exceeds 0.70 sec; the T wave nearly merges with the P wave from the following complex. ST segment depression is also evident. Serum potassium was 1.6 mEq/L.

roughly in the range of 0.28 to 0.33 sec. A very short QT interval may appear to encroach on the ST segment.

Digitalis Effect. Among the earliest findings seen on the electrocardiogram exhibiting digitalis effect is a shortening of the QT interval, due to earlier repolarization of myocardial cells. QT interval shortening may or may not be seen with digitalis therapy (not related to toxicity), as well as PR interval prolongation, "scooped" ST segment depression, and diminished T wave amplitude (Fig. 15-1).

Hypercalcemia. Serum calcium levels are inversely related to QT interval. The T wave in hypercalcemia may abruptly rise out of the ST segment, which itself may or may not be evident (Fig. 15-2).

Long QT interval

A long QT interval at normal sinus rates is, conservatively, greater than 0.44 sec, whereas others have advanced 0.46 sec in men and 0.47 sec in women as sex-specific upper limits of normal. QT interval differences due to sex have not been observed in infants and children younger than 14 years of age. A rule of thumb for individuals with heart rates within normal limits (60 to 100 bpm) is that the QT interval should be less than half the preceding R-R interval. QT interval prolongation is seen in a variety of metabolic, toxicologic, and noncardiac diseases, as well as in primary cardiac diseases (see Chapter 47, Long QT Syndromes).

Congenital Long QT Syndromes. Familial QT interval prolongation associated with syncope, sudden death, and congenital deafness, and transmitted through an autosomal

recessive pattern, is referred to as the *Jervell and Lange-Nielsen syndrome.* A similar syndrome lacking the hearing loss and transmitted in an autosomal dominant fashion is the *Romano-Ward syndrome.* These syndromes can show marked variability in QT interval within an individual at different points in time, and thus present randomly and unpredictably.

Mitral Valve Prolapse. The relationship between mitral valve prolapse and QT interval prolongation is not clear; however, QT interval prolongation may occur in this population, and has been suggested as a marker of ventricular dysrhythmia.

Central Nervous System Disease. A number of disorders of the central nervous system can present with QT interval prolongation, including *subarachnoid hemorrhage, intracerebral hemorrhage,* and *thromboembolic cerebrovascular stroke.* A marked increase in T wave amplitude, frequently with deep, symmetric T wave inversion (so-called roller coaster T waves), is another characteristic of these syndromes.

Metabolic Syndromes. *Hypokalemia* and *hypocalcemia* are known to cause QT prolongation. Hypomagnesemia is not known directly to prolong the QT interval; however, effects on the QT interval seen in its presence may be mediated by associated low levels of potassium or calcium. Whereas hypokalemia also can cause ST segment depression (Fig. 15-3), T wave flattening, and U waves, hypocalcemia does not displace the ST segment or affect the T wave.

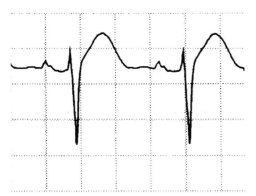

FIGURE 15-2 · **Short QT interval.** These complexes from lead V_3 in a man with bladder cancer and an elevated serum calcium of 14.8 mEq/L demonstrate a short QT interval and the virtual disappearance of a distinct ST segment before the T wave.

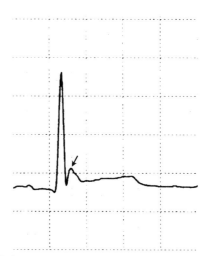

FIGURE 15-4 · **Long QT interval.** The slightly prolonged QT interval (0.49 sec) shown here in lead V_5 is secondary to hypothermia (rectal temperature was 26.5°C [81°F]); note the Osborn wave (*arrow*).

Hypothyroidism may cause QT interval prolongation, as well as bradycardia, low voltage, and T wave changes. *Hypothermia* may cause prolongation of all intervals in the cardiac cycle; the characteristic notched J waves (Osborn waves) after the QRS complexes should be sought (Fig.15-4), as well as bradydysrhythmias (e.g., sinus bradycardia, atrial fibrillation with slow ventricular response).

Drug Effects. An increasing number of pharmaceutical agents have been linked with varying degrees of certitude to QT interval prolongation. Some general rules are helpful in remembering drugs with a propensity to prolong the QT interval. *Potassium channel blocking agents* prolong the QT interval, but are not a class of drugs readily familiar to most physicians for that effect. Some *antidysrhythmics* are classically linked to QT interval prolongation, including Vaughan Williams class Ia, Ic, and III agents, and as such may prolong the QT interval with or without widening the QRS complex, depending on the drug. Various *psychotropic* medications may prolong the QT interval. Several *antibiotics* (e.g., sparfloxacin, erythromycin, clarithromycin, pentamidine) also can lengthen the QT interval (see Chapters 49 through 57, on toxicology).

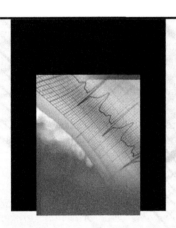

Chapter 16
U Wave

Theodore C. Chan

The U wave follows the T wave and is the last deflection seen in the normal cardiac cycle. The U wave is the most inconspicuous deflection and is often not well visualized or is misinterpreted as part of the T wave on the electrocardiogram (ECG). The exact mechanism of the U wave is unclear. Theories as to the source of the U wave include repolarization of Purkinje fibers or some other portion of the ventricular myocardium, afterpotentials generated by mechanicoelectrical coupling during ventricular relaxation, longer duration of the action potential of conduction myocytes, and repolarization of the papillary muscle cells.

ELECTROCARDIOGRAPHIC DIAGNOSIS

Normal U wave

The normal U wave is a small, rounded deflection occurring just after the T wave. The ascent of the wave is usually shorter than the descent, although the U wave can appear symmetric in morphology. The amplitude is usually less than 1 mm. At normal heart rates, the duration from the apex of the T wave to the apex of the U wave is approximately 0.1 sec.

The normal U wave axis is directed anteriorly and to the left at approximately +60 degrees, and is similar to that of the T wave. That is, for a given lead, the U wave is directed similar to the T wave. The amplitude of the U wave varies, but is no more than 25% of the T wave amplitude. The U wave is usually monophasic (positive or negative), but rarely can be biphasic. The upright U wave is best seen in leads II and V_2 to V_4. The U wave can have a negative deflection in lead aVR, and occasionally in leads III and aVF.

The U wave can appear inconspicuous, particularly at higher heart rates. In addition, it can be mistaken as part of the T wave, erroneously suggesting a prolonged QT interval on ECG.

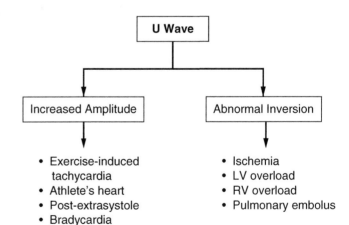

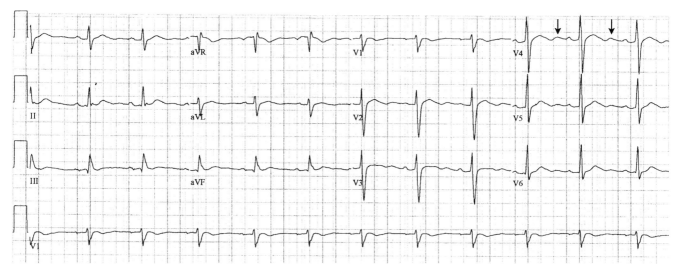

FIGURE 16-1 · U wave with increased amplitude in a healthy, young athlete.

Abnormal U waves include those that have increased amplitude and those that are inverted (i.e., are directed in the opposite direction of the T wave for a given lead).

Increased U wave amplitude

Exercise. Increased U wave amplitude can be seen with exercise, but may be masked by the superimposed P wave from a shortened R-R interval tachycardia.

Athlete's Heart. Young athletic individuals may have a normal U wave with amplitude as great as 2 mm, most prominently seen in the mid-precordial leads (Fig. 16-1).

Post-Extrasystole. Larger U waves can be seen after the next beat following a long pause, as occurs with extrasystole beats.

Bradycardias. With bradycardias, U waves can become more prominent.

Hypokalemia. The U wave increases in magnitude with decreasing serum potassium levels. This large U wave can be mistaken for the T wave because the latter diminishes with hypokalemia. The uncommon giant U waves are seen with hypokalemia associated with hypochloremic metabolic alkalosis (Fig. 16-2). In addition, a U wave electrical alternans (alternation of amplitude) can be seen with hypokalemia.

Central Nervous System Events. Increased U wave amplitude greater than 1.5 mm can be seen in central nervous system events (such as cerebrovascular accident), particularly in leads V_2 to V_4. However, this finding can be obscured by the increase in T wave amplitude and QT interval duration.

Hypertension. Chronic hypertension has been associated with increased U wave amplitude. Large U waves have also been associated with pheochromocytomas.

Medications. Increased U wave amplitude has been associated with catecholamine agents, digoxin, as well as quinidine and amiodarone.

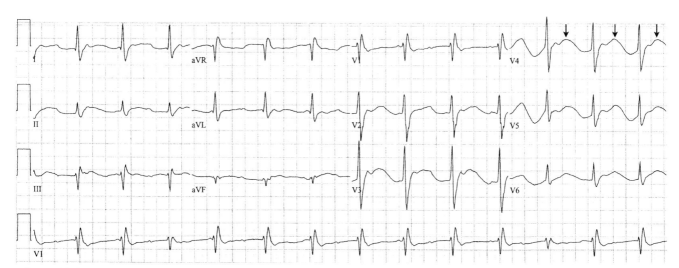

FIGURE 16-2 · **Examples of giant U waves from hypokalemia.** The U waves merge into the T waves in this patient with a serum potassium level of 1.6 mEq/L.

Inverted U waves

Ischemia. Inverted U waves can be seen with cardiac ischemia. The change in the U wave occurs progressively from decreased amplitude, to biphasic morphology, to inversion. These changes are often best seen in leads I, II, III, aVL, and V_4 to V_6. Similar U wave inversions can be seen with vasospastic or Prinzmetal angina.

Left Ventricular Overload. Inverted U waves in leads V_4 to V_6 are often associated with left ventricular overload due to left ventricular hypertrophy or valvular disease, including mitral regurgitation, aortic regurgitation, and aortic stenosis.

Right Ventricular Overload. Inverted U waves in leads II and III and the right precordial leads are associated with right ventricular overload, which in turn is often associated with valvular disease, including atrial septal defect with large left-to-right shunt, pulmonic stenosis, and mitral stenosis. This finding occurs less commonly in right ventricular overload due to pulmonary disease.

Pulmonary Embolus. Patients with pulmonary embolism can have transient U wave inversions seen in the right precordial leads, likely related to right ventricular pressure changes and overload.

Section III

Electrocardiographic Manifestations of Disease

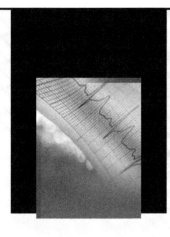

Chapter 17

Bradycardia and Escape Rhythms

Christopher J. Ware and Jacob W. Ufberg

Clinical Features

Bradycardia describes a number of separate clinical and electrocardiographic (ECG) entities, ranging from benign to life-threatening, all with the common end point of a slow heart (ventricular) rate. In the adult patient, bradycardia is defined as a ventricular rate less than 60 bpm; pediatric bradycardia is an age-dependent phenomenon (see Chapter 5, The Pediatric Electrocardiogram). Patients may be asymptomatic or present with generalized weakness, dizziness, syncope, dyspnea, or chest pain. The heart rate in asymptomatic individuals may drop to 35 to 40 bpm during sleep[1] or in endurance athletes, and symptoms may be absent at even lower rates, as long as the stroke volume is able to rise sufficiently to compensate and maintain cardiac output.

The various portions of the cardiac conduction system share the ability to generate impulses independently of the sinoatrial (SA) node. The rate of spontaneous depolarization varies along the conduction system such that those tissues closer to the SA node generate impulses faster than those further away.[2] The area with the highest intrinsic rate (usually the SA node), under normal circumstances, suppresses the ability of other pacemaker sites, a concept known as *overdrive suppression*. Conversely, should a higher pacemaker site fail, a focus below that site will assume the responsibility of impulse generation, a concept known as *escape rhythm*. Such rhythm disturbances may be divided into primary (defect intrinsic to the conduction system) and secondary (defect extrinsic to the conduction system) causes.

Primary etiologies are less often encountered clinically; these abnormalities most often result from damage to the conduction system that occurs slowly, usually associated with aging. Examples of primary conduction system disorders include sick sinus syndrome (see Chapter 29, Sick Sinus Syndrome), Lenegre's syndrome (fibrotic degenerative disease of the His-Purkinje system), Lev's syndrome (fibrotic and calcific degeneration of the fibrous skeleton of the heart with involvement of the conduction system), and congenital atrioventricular (AV) block.

Secondary causes are due to factors extrinsic to the cardiac conduction system and represent the most frequently encountered form of bradydysrhythmia. A wide spectrum of etiologies are seen in the secondary category, including cardiovascular syndromes (both ischemic and nonischemic) as well as pharmacologic, toxicologic, reflex-mediated, neurologic, infectious, rheumatologic, and metabolic disease states.

Concerning ischemic-mediated bradydysrhythmia, the right coronary artery supplies the SA node and the AV node in most patients,[3] so diligence in examining the inferior and posterior ECG leads is essential with new or evolving bradycardia. Pharmacologic agents may produce bradycardia because of either therapeutic or toxic effect. Parasympathetic nervous system activity causes a slowing of impulse generation as well as

---

ELECTROCARDIOGRAPHIC HIGHLIGHTS

Sinus bradycardia

- QRS complex rate is less than 60 bpm and regular.
- Each P wave is followed directly by a QRS complex, so the P-P interval should closely match the R-R interval.
- Each P wave should be identical in morphology in any single lead.

Junctional escape rhythm

- QRS complex rate is usually 40 to 60 bpm and regular.
- QRS complex duration is usually less than 120 msec.
- If P waves are present, they will occur immediately adjacent to the QRS complex (before or after), and may be inverted.

Idioventricular escape rhythm

- Rate is usually 20 to 40 bpm and regular.
- QRS complex duration is greater than 120 msec.
- If P waves are present, there should be no correlation between the P wave and the wide-complex QRS.

ELECTROCARDIOGRAPHIC PEARLS

- In a new or evolving bradycardia, look closely for evidence of inferior or posterior ischemia because the right coronary artery is the common blood supply to these areas in most patients.
- When P waves are present with a narrow-complex bradycardia, be sure that each P wave is followed directly by a subsequent complex to differentiate sinus bradycardia from normal sinus rhythm with third degree atrioventricular (AV) block and a junctional escape rhythm.
- Supraventricular activity with high-degree AV block may produce junctional or idioventricular escape rhythms.
- In the diagnosis of idioventricular escape rhythm, be sure to rule out the firing of a mechanical pacemaker or a supraventricular rhythm with bundle branch block.

conduction. The bradycardic effect of parasympathetic influence may be transient, as in episodes of vasovagal syncope. Prolonged effects are seen in trained athletes, who may have bradycardia at rest, in part because of increased baseline parasympathetic tone. Infectious causes such as Lyme disease may produce a transient disruption of the conduction system, leading to bradycardia. Furthermore, systemic diseases may change the composition of the tissue itself, as with deposition from infiltrative diseases or collagen vascular disorders. Endocrinologic abnormalities such as hypothyroidism or environmental insults such as hypothermia may cause bradycardia in the setting of otherwise normal conduction tissue. Electrolyte abnormalities may also produce bradycardia by interfering with the normal ionic milieu necessary for impulse generation and propagation to occur. Finally, surgical or iatrogenic trauma disrupts or destroys conduction tissue.

Electrocardiographic Manifestations

The diagnosis of bradycardia on the ECG is made when the ventricular rate is less than 60 bpm. Characteristic ranges of rate, QRS morphologies, and the presence or absence of atrial depolarization as displayed by the P wave differentiate the rhythms that give rise to bradycardia. Some abnormalities lead to bradycardia by way of blocks in the conduction system.

Sinus Bradycardia. Sinus bradycardia exists when each P wave is followed by an accompanying QRS complex occurring at a rate consistent with bradycardia (<60 bpm). In general, the QRS complex is narrow, but there are instances when a sinus bradycardia may present with a prolonged QRS duration. In cases of intraventricular conduction delay or

bundle branch block, sinus beats are present, and the PR interval is typically constant, but the QRS duration is prolonged. The underlying rhythm is sinus bradycardia as long as each QRS complex is preceded by a P wave. Sinus bradycardia may be difficult to differentiate from second degree, 2:1 SA block, in which every other impulse generated in the SA node fails to reach the atrial myocardium. The difference may become evident only if the onset or termination of block is witnessed by a sudden halving (onset) or doubling (termination) of the heart rate (Fig. 17-1).

Junctional Rhythm. Junctional rhythm, a supraventricular escape rhythm, is characterized by the presence of regular, narrow QRS complexes, not associated with preceding P waves or aberrant atrial rhythms (atrial fibrillation or flutter, or wandering atrial pacemaker). A junctional escape rhythm typically has a rate of 40 to 60 bpm (Fig. 17-2). Junctional rhythms at rates less than 40 bpm are known as *junctional bradycardias*; those at rates greater than 60 bpm are termed *accelerated junctional rhythms*. Retrograde P′ waves may be seen immediately adjacent to the QRS complex, occurring before or after. These P waves may be either upright or inverted.

Lack of overdrive suppression causes the automaticity of the AV node to "escape." This process illustrates the origin of the term *escape rhythm*, which is sometimes used to describe regular depolarizations from foci below the SA node, often seen in cases of bradycardia. A typical narrow QRS complex is therefore generated, independent of the P waves. Wide QRS complexes may be seen with a junctional rhythm in the setting of bundle branch block and aberrant conduction.

Idioventricular Escape Rhythms. Idioventricular escape rhythms typically display rates between 20 and

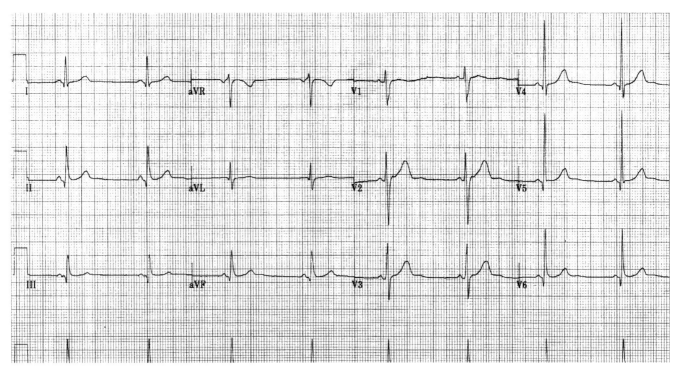

FIGURE 17-1 · Sinus bradycardia. Twelve-lead ECG demonstrating a sinus bradycardia, in a patient with a history of myocardial infarction. The rate is 49 bpm. There are P waves preceding each QRS complex, and the QRS duration is less than 0.12 sec.

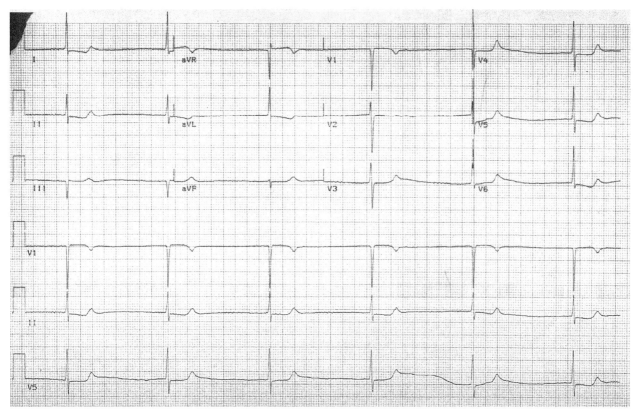

FIGURE 17-2 · Junctional escape rhythm. Twelve-lead ECG demonstrating a junctional escape rhythm in a patient with a past history of atrial fibrillation and digoxin use. Each QRS complex is narrow and is not preceded by a P wave. The rate is 35 bpm, slightly lower than the typical 40 to 60 bpm of junctional escape rhythm. Therefore, the interpretation of this ECG is junctional bradycardia.

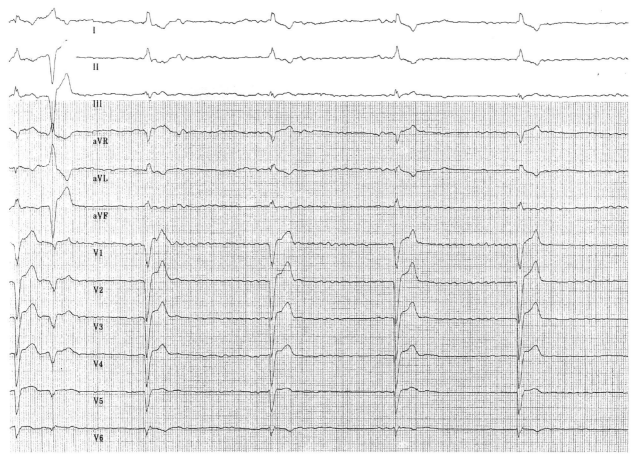

FIGURE 17-3 · Idioventricular escape rhythm. Twelve-lead ECG demonstrating an idioventricular rhythm due to inadvertent beta-adrenergic blocking agent ingestion. The QRS complex is wide, with a rate of 27 bpm. There are no P waves noted on this rhythm strip.

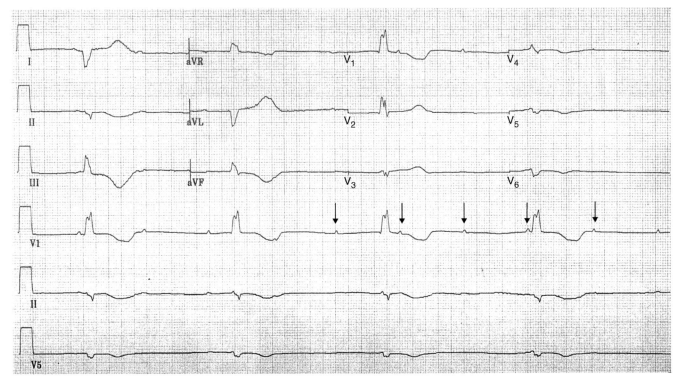

FIGURE 17-4 • **Idioventricular escape rhythm.** Twelve-lead ECG demonstrating an idioventricular rhythm in a patient status post-cardiorespiratory arrest. The QRS complex is wide and each complex is not preceded by a P wave. There are P waves (*arrows*) present on this ECG, however, with a sinus rate of slightly less than 60 bpm. The interpretation of this ECG would therefore be third degree atrioventricular block and idioventricular escape rhythm.

40 bpm, but can be higher in the case of accelerated idioventricular rhythms. Their wide QRS morphology, similar to that seen in other ventricular beats, such as premature ventricular contractions and ventricular tachycardia, makes their origin clear (Figs. 17-3 and 17-4).

References

1. Olgin JE, Zipes DP: Specific arrhythmias: Diagnosis and treatment. In Braunwald E, Zipes DP, Libby P (eds): Heart Disease: A Textbook of Cardiovascular Medicine, 6th ed. Philadelphia, WB Saunders, 2001, p 822.
2. Netter FH: A Compilation of Paintings on the Normal and Pathologic Anatomy and Physiology, Embryology, and Diseases of the Heart. The Ciba Collection of Medical Illustrations, Volume 5. Cincinnati, Ohio, The Hennegan Co., 1992, pp 48–49.
3. Mangrum JM, DiMarco JP: The evaluation and management of bradycardia. N Engl J Med 2000;342:703.

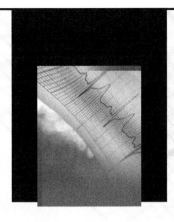

Chapter 18

Sinus Pause/Sinus Arrest

Jacob W. Ufberg

Clinical Features

Sinus pause and sinus arrest refer to the failure of impulse formation in the sinus node. Because no electrical impulse emerges from the node, no deflections appear on the electrocardiogram (ECG), which shows an isoelectric line. A brief failure is termed *sinus pause*, whereas a more prolonged failure is termed *sinus arrest*. No universally accepted definition exists regarding the time at which sinus pause becomes sinus arrest, so the terms are often used interchangeably. Pauses of up to 2.5 sec have been noted in healthy young people on ambulatory ECG monitoring.[1] Recurrent pauses of greater than 2.5 sec are considered abnormal and likely indicate sinoatrial (SA) dysfunction.[2] Brief sinus pauses are often asymptomatic and not indicative of an underlying pathologic process. Patients with more pronounced pause or arrest may also be asymptomatic; conversely, such patients may experience lightheadedness, dizziness, syncope, or, in the extreme, death. The degree of symptomatic expression depends on the timeliness of the appearance of an escape rhythm.

The precise mechanism causing sinus pause/arrest frequently cannot be determined. Sinus pause/arrest may be physiologic or may occur in patients with increased vagal tone or carotid sinus hypersensitivity. Various factors may produce sinus pause or arrest, including medications such as digoxin, metabolic derangements, including hyperkalemia, or heightened parasympathetic activity. In addition, cardiac disease such as acute myocardial infarction, acute myocarditis, and other heart diseases may cause sinus arrest, particularly when the sinus node is involved.

Electrocardiographic Manifestations

Because no sinus impulse occurs, no atrial depolarization is seen on the ECG, leading to an absence of the P wave and the resultant QRS complex and T wave. Thus, an isoelectric "pause" of indefinite duration appears on the ECG (Fig. 18-1). The P-P interval of the pause should *not* be a multiple of the basic underlying rhythm. Sinus pause/arrest may occur during normal sinus rhythm or may follow ectopic beats (Fig. 18-2) or runs of ectopic tachycardia that suppress the sinus node's usual automaticity. The sinus node may also be suppressed by

---

ELECTROCARDIOGRAPHIC HIGHLIGHTS

- Sinus pause/arrest is of indefinite duration with absent PQRST complex.
- P-P interval of pause/arrest is not a multiple of the basic P-P interval.
- In a tracing with multiple pauses, they will likely vary in duration.

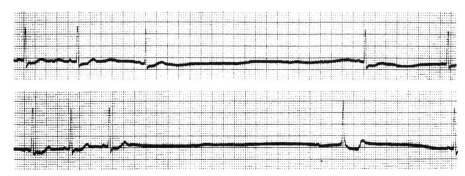

FIGURE 18-1 · Sinus arrest. Sinus arrest in an elderly man with recurrent syncope. (From Chou TC, Knilans TK: Electrocardiography in Clinical Practice: Adult and Pediatric, 4th ed. Philadelphia, WB Saunders, 1996, Fig. 15-10.)

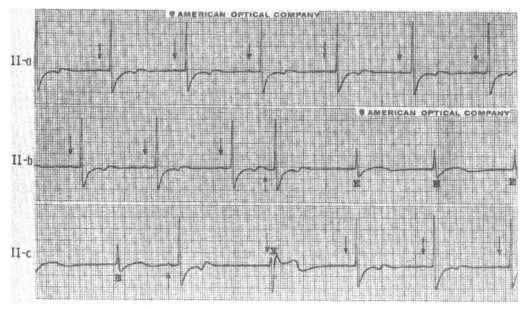

FIGURE 18-2 · **Sinus pause/ arrest.** Leads IIa through IIc are continuous. Sinus P waves are indicated by *downward arrows*. The rhythm is sinus bradycardia with first degree atrioventricular block and infrequent premature atrial contractions (*upward arrows*), followed by sinus pause/arrest. The first episode is interrupted by a ventricular escape rhythm (E) and the second is interrupted by a ventricular escape beat (X) from a separate focus. (From Chung EK: Principles of Cardiac Arrhythmias, 3rd ed. Baltimore, Williams & Wilkins, 1983, Fig. 4-18.)

ELECTROCARDIOGRAPHIC PEARLS

- Sinus pause/arrest may be preceded by an ectopic beat, ectopic tachycardia, or junctional escape rhythm.
- Sinus pause/arrest can be terminated by sinus rhythm, junctional escape, or idioventricular escape.
- Sinus pause/arrest is difficult to distinguish from sinoatrial exit block, particularly with underlying sinus arrhythmia.

---

ectopic discharge from the atrioventricular (AV) node during junctional escape rhythms, leading to sinus arrest.[3]

Frequently, sinus rhythm returns after sinus pause/arrest before the emergence of any escape beats or rhythm. If sinus rhythm does not return, AV junctional escape beats appear in order to control ventricular contraction. When the AV node fails to emerge as the escape pacemaker, ventricular beats will likely appear (see Fig. 18-2). In the absence of any sinus or escape pacemaker activity, asystole results.

It is often difficult to distinguish sinus pause/arrest from SA exit block because they both lead to absence of the entire PQRST complex. The major distinction can often be made by measuring the P-P interval involving the pause and comparing it with the P-P interval of the basic rhythm. The P-P interval during sinus pause is unrelated to the basic P-P interval, and subsequent pauses should vary in duration. The P-P interval during SA exit block should always be a multiple of the basic P-P interval. Such a distinction, however, may be impossible to make with marked underlying sinus arrhythmia.

References

1. Vitasalo MT, Kala R, Eisalo A: Ambulatory electrocardiographic recording in endurance athletes. Br Heart J 1982;47:213.
2. Shaw DB, Southall DP: Sinus node arrest and sinoatrial block. Eur Heart J 1984;5(Suppl A):83.
3. Chung EK: Principles of Cardiac Arrhythmias, 3rd ed. Baltimore, Williams & Wilkins, 1983.

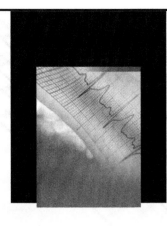

Chapter 19

Sinoatrial Exit Block

Jacob W. Ufberg

Clinical Features

Sinoatrial (SA) exit block, also known as SA block, refers to a dysfunction in the conduction of electrical impulses from the SA node (the heart's normal pacemaker) to the surrounding atrial myocardium. The degree of dysfunction ranges from slight conduction delays to complete block of the impulses from the SA node with the need for an alternate (escape) pacemaker to sustain life. Electrocardiographic (ECG) findings associated with SA exit blocks range from a normal ECG to various changes in the P-P interval to a complete lack of P waves, depending on the type of block involved.

SA exit blocks, like atrioventricular blocks, are classified into first, second, and third degree blocks, with second degree blocks subclassified into type I (Wenckebach), type II, and 2:1 blocks. The symptoms related to SA exit blocks are usually transient[1] and depend on the degree of block involved. Most patients with first degree and type I second degree blocks are asymptomatic, and these blocks are of little clinical significance.[2] Patients with other types of second degree block may notice an "uneasy" feeling with the onset and termination of the block. Third degree block with the slow emergence of an escape rhythm may cause dizziness, light-headedness, and syncope.

The causes of SA exit block are many and varied. Children, young adults, and well-conditioned athletes[3] may have asymptomatic SA exit block. Increased vagal activity may induce SA exit block during esophagoscopy or bronchoscopy, or during episodes of great pain or fear.

SA exit block may occur in patients with several types of cardiac pathologic processes, including myocarditis, cardiomyopathy, sick sinus syndrome, Prinzmetal angina, and early on in an acute inferior myocardial infarction. Drugs such as digoxin, calcium channel antagonists, beta-adrenergic blocking agents, procainamide, quinidine, amiodarone, and other antidysrhythmic medications (especially in supratherapeutic doses) may also cause SA exit block.

Electrocardiographic Manifestations

First Degree Sinoatrial Exit Block. First degree SA exit block is manifested by an increased time for the impulse generated by the SA node to reach and cause contraction of the atrial myocardium. Because SA node depolarization produces no deflection on the surface ECG, these blocks can be

---

ELECTROCARDIOGRAPHIC HIGHLIGHTS

First degree SA exit block
- Normal-appearing ECG

Second degree SA exit block/type I
- Progressive shortening of the P-P interval, followed by a dropped P-QRS-T complex
- Grouped beating

Second degree SA exit block/type II
- Normal sinus rhythm with an intermittent dropped P-QRS-T complex
- Length of P-P interval that includes dropped beat is twice the normal P-P interval

Second degree SA exit block/2:1 block
- Appears identical to sinus bradycardia
- Can be diagnosed only if tracing catches onset (rate halves) or termination (rate doubles)

Third degree SA exit block
- Complete absence of P waves
- May see long sinus pause/sinus arrest at onset
- Usually junctional escape rhythm

ELECTROCARDIOGRAPHIC PEARLS

- First degree sinoatrial (SA) exit block is not manifested in any way on the ECG.
- Grouped beating is a useful clue in diagnosing second degree type I SA exit block.
- In high degree SA exit blocks, the P-P interval of the dropped beat(s) is a multiple of the normal P-P interval.
- Often, third degree SA exit block cannot be distinguished from sinus arrest.

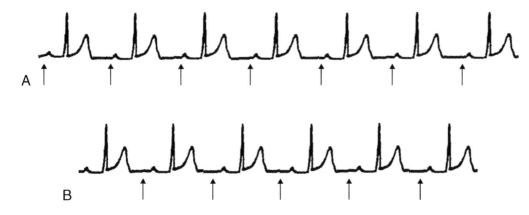

FIGURE 19-1 · **Sinus rhythm compared with first degree sinoatrial (SA) exit block.** *Arrows* represent the sinus node impulses that are not seen on the surface ECG. *A,* Normal sinus rhythm. *B,* First degree SA exit block leads to a prolonged interval between the sinus node impulse and the P wave, which cannot be detected by the surface ECG.

diagnosed only by specialized sinus node recordings. Thus, the ECG demonstrates normal sinus rhythm (Fig. 19-1).

Second Degree Sinoatrial Exit Block/Type I. This type of block occurs when the time from the SA impulse to the P wave gradually lengthens until an SA impulse is not conducted. This appears on the ECG as a gradually shortening P-P interval followed by a pause in which no P-QRS-T complex appears. This may appear on the ECG as Wenckebach, or "grouped" beating, or simply as a very irregular sinus rhythm (Fig. 19-2).

Second Degree Sinoatrial Exit Block/Type II. This block is characterized by a constant time from SA impulse to atrial depolarization with an intermittent SA impulse that is not conducted to the atria, resulting in an occasional missed P-QRS-T complex. The resultant P-P interval that includes the missed P-QRS-T is twice the length of the normal P-P interval (Fig. 19-2).

Second Degree Sinoatrial Exit Block with 2:1 Conduction. This is a second degree block in which SA impulses are only alternately conducted to the atria. Thus, every other P-QRS-T complex is missing. This appears on the ECG as sinus bradycardia. The only way to differentiate this block from sinus bradycardia on ECG is if the recording shows either the onset of the block when the heart rate is suddenly halved or the termination of the block when the heart rate suddenly doubles (Fig. 19-2).

Third Degree Sinoatrial Exit Block. This block occurs when none of the SA node impulses reaches or activates the atria. This results in a prolonged pause in which the ECG recording is isoelectric until an escape rhythm, usually a junctional rhythm, begins or until normal sinus rhythm is restored (Fig. 19-3). If normal sinus rhythm is restored, the pause should be a multiple of the normal P-P interval.

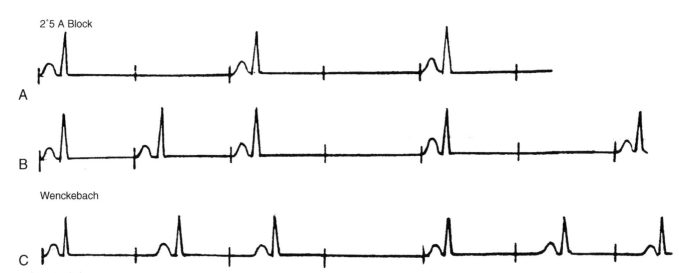

FIGURE 19-2 · **Second degree sinoatrial (SA) exit blocks.** Vertical hash marks represent the sinus node impulses; these do not appear on the ECG. In second degree SA block with 2:1 conduction (*A*), every other sinus impulse is non-conducted, making the rhythm indistinguishable from sinus bradycardia. In second degree SA block, the pause resulting from the non-conducted sinus impulse is a multiple of the basic P-P interval (*B*), and thus can be differentiated from a sinus pause. The Wenckebach phenomenon in second degree SA block (*C*) results in a progressive shortening of the P-P interval before the pause due to the dropped P-QRS-T. (From: Surawicz B, Knilans TK: *Chou's Electrocardiography in Clinical Practice.* 5th ed. W.B. Saunders, Philadelphia, 2001, p 321.)

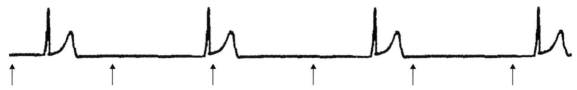

FIGURE 19-3 · Third degree sinoatrial exit block. *Arrows* represent the sinus node impulses that are not seen on the surface ECG. Only the escape rhythm is visible on the ECG.

References

1. Olgin JE, Zipes DP: Specific arrhythmias: Diagnosis and treatment. In Braunwald E, Zipes DP, Libby P (eds): Braunwald's Heart Disease: A Textbook of Cardiovascular Medicine, 6th ed. Philadelphia, WB Saunders, 2001, pp 815–889.

2. Sandoe E, Sigurd B: Arrhythmia: A Guide to Clinical Electrocardiology. Bingen, Germany, Publishing Partners Verlags GmbH, 1991.

3. Bjornstad H, Storstein L, Meen HD, et al: Ambulatory electrocardiographic findings in top athletes, athletic students, and control subjects. Cardiology 1994;84:42.

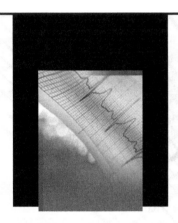

Chapter 20

Atrioventricular Block

William J. Brady and Richard A. Harrigan

Clinical Features

Atrioventricular (AV) block involves a dysfunction in the transmission of electrical impulses from the supraventricular portion of the cardiac conduction system to the ventricles. The degree of dysfunction varies from minimal, with essentially normal conduction, to maximal, with both a complete cessation of impulse transmission and total independent activity of the atria and ventricles. On the electrocardiogram (ECG), AV block is manifested by a prolongation of the PR interval or an altered relationship of the P wave to the QRS complex. AV block results from any of a wide range of syndromes, with clinical impacts varying from none to life-threatening.

AV conduction system dysfunction, which includes first, second (types I and II), and third degree AV block, is etiologically divided into primary and secondary causes. Primary causes are due to an intrinsic defect in the generation or conduction of an impulse in the conduction system itself[1]; primary etiologies are less often encountered in patients, accounting for only 15% of cases in the emergency department setting.[2,3] Secondary causes are due to factors extrinsic to the cardiac conduction system,[1] including both ischemic and nonischemic cardiovascular syndromes as well as pharmacologic, toxicologic, reflex-mediated, neurologic, infectious, rheumatologic, endocrinologic, and metabolic disease states. Approximately 55% of secondary causes result directly from acute coronary ischemic events, most of which are acute myocardial infarction (AMI); the remaining causative syndromes are encountered at the following frequencies: pharmacologic/toxicologic, 20%; metabolic, 5%; neurologic, 5%; electronic pacemaker failure, 2%—among other miscellaneous etiologies.[2,3]

The most frequently encountered cause of AV block is acute ischemic heart disease, particularly AMI. The rhythm disturbances that may complicate AMI include first degree and second degree type I AV block; they are found in 15% and 10% of patients, respectively. Second degree type II AV block is rare, and complete heart block (third degree AV block) complicates 10% of infarctions and represents the most frequent unstable bradyarrhythmia encountered in the patient with AMI.[2,3] The pathophysiologic mechanisms underlying most of the AV blocks in patients with AMI involve either reversible ischemic injury to, or irreversible necrosis of, the

---

ELECTROCARDIOGRAPHIC HIGHLIGHTS

First degree atrioventricular (AV) block

- PR interval prolonged greater than 0.20 sec
- Constant PR interval without progressive change

Second degree AV block/Mobitz type I (Wenckebach)

- Progressive lengthening of PR interval, followed by dropped beat
- Progressive shortening of the R-R interval
- R-R interval length of the dropped beat less than twice the shortest R-R cycle
- Grouped beating

Second degree AV block/Mobitz type II

- Dropped beat occurs with either normal or prolonged PR interval
- PR interval constant
- QRS complex usually wide
- Magnitude of AV block expressed as a ratio of P waves to QRS complexes

Third degree AV block (complete heart block)

- No relation of P waves to QRS complexes
- Complete independent activity of atria and ventricles
- Atrial rate greater than ventricular rate
- QRS complex usually wide

---

conduction system; altered autonomic function frequently is also a significant factor, particularly in the inferior AMI scenario, with its increased parasympathetic supply.

Electrocardiographic Manifestations

First Degree Atrioventricular Block. In first degree AV block, the PR interval is prolonged, with a duration greater than 0.20 sec, and is constant without progressive change (Fig. 20-1). The P wave has normal morphology and precedes every QRS complex. The QRS complex usually has a normal morphology and axis for the given patient and clinical situation. Every atrial impulse is conducted to the ventricles. First degree AV block may be associated with other conduction abnormalities as well.

Second Degree Mobitz Type I Atrioventricular Block. In second degree Mobitz type I AV block, also known as Wenckebach AV block, a specific pattern to the P wave–QRS complex relationship is encountered. The PR interval is often normal in the first beat of the series. Progressive PR interval lengthening with subsequent beats is observed until an impulse is unable to reach the ventricles, resulting in a nonconducted P wave. After the dropped beat, the PR interval returns to normal and the cycle repeats itself. A pattern to the R-R interval is also seen. As the PR interval lengthens with subsequent beats, the R-R interval becomes shorter. After the

dropped beat, the R-R interval in the subsequent beats tends to shorten. The site of the block is usually at or above the AV node; as such, the QRS complex is narrow and normal in terms of morphology. The longest R-R interval containing the dropped beat is shorter than twice the shortest R-R interval (which is the preceding interval). Successive R-R interval shortening with PR interval lengthening may appear counterintuitive. With second degree type I AV block, as the PR interval increases with each successive beat, the degree of increase is smaller with each beat. Therefore, the greatest increase in PR interval is associated with the first beat featuring a prolonged PR interval, and each subsequent PR interval increase is incrementally shorter until the dropped QRS-T occurs (Fig. 20-2). The clinician also will notice on the rhythm strip a grouping of beats that is especially noticeable with tachycardia. Such a finding is referred to as *grouped beating of Wenckebach.*

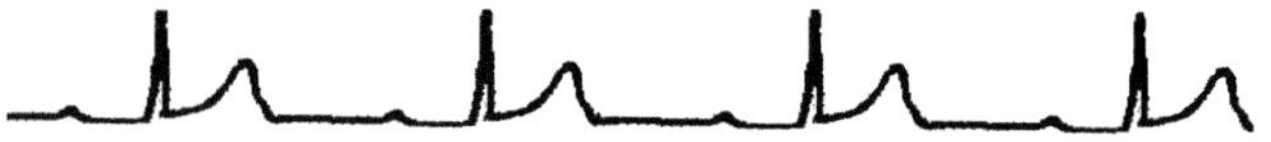

Evidence on the ECG for Mobitz type I AV block includes the following: (1) progressive lengthening of the PR interval, then dropped beat; (2) progressive shortening of the R-R interval; (3) the R-R interval length of the dropped beat is less than twice the shortest cycle; and (4) grouped beating.

Second Degree Mobitz Type II Atrioventricular Block. The PR interval in type II second degree AV block is constant (Fig. 20-3). However, the PR interval may either be normal or prolonged, but is always constant without progressive PR interval lengthening. The QRS complex, conversely, is widened in most instances of type II second degree AV block (Fig. 20-3*B*), although a narrow complex may be seen (Fig. 20-3*A*). The magnitude of the AV block is expressed as a ratio of P waves to QRS complexes. For example, if there are three P waves for two QRS complexes, then it is a 3:2 conduction ratio, as in Figure 20-3.

Second Degree Atrioventricular Block with 2:1 Conduction. Distinguishing type I from type II block is relatively straightforward unless there is 2:1 conduction, as seen in Figure 20-4. In this situation, there is no way to compare the PR intervals for the conducted beats and hence make the distinction between Mobitz type I and type II AV blocks. The width of the QRS complex in Mobitz type II block is usually characterized by a widened QRS complex, although a narrow QRS complex rhythm may be seen (Fig. 20-4). Nonetheless, the physician should initially "assume the worst" in situations of 2:1 conduction; that is, the block is a Mobitz II unless proven otherwise.

Second Degree Type II Atrioventricular Block with High-Grade Block. In Mobitz type II AV block, high-grade block occurs when two or more P waves are not conducted (Fig. 20-5). This pattern implies advanced conduction disease and high risk for sudden development of complete heart block. These patients tend to have widened QRS complexes with ventricular rates of 20 to 40 bpm and a higher risk of progression to complete heart block.

Third Degree Atrioventricular Block. In third-degree heart block, also known as complete heart block, no atrial impulses reach the ventricle through the AV conduction system. Therefore, the atria and ventricle are controlled by different pacemaker sites and hence are functioning independently. The atrial pacemaker can be either sinus or ectopic. The ventricular escape rhythm can also have varying pacemaker sites, resulting in differing rates. Rarely, there is no ventricular

FIGURE 20-1 · First degree atrioventricular block.

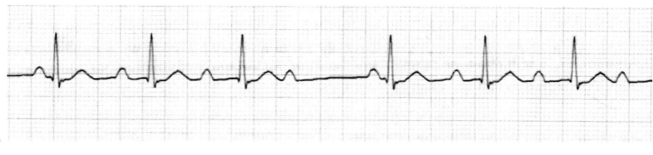

A

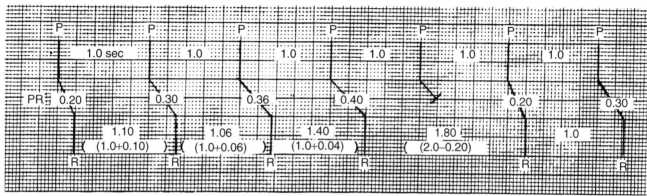

B

FIGURE 20-2 • **Second degree type I atrioventricular block.** *A*, Rhythm strip reveals progressive PR interval prolongation until the 4th P wave is non-conducted. *B*, Ladder diagrammatic depiction of Wenckebach phenomenon in second degree atrioventricular (AV) block, Mobitz type I. This variation of AV block features progressive lengthening of the PR interval–along with the counterintuitive progressive shortening of the R-R interval–prior to the dropped beat (a P wave followed by a dropped QRS-T; here occurring in the fifth beat). This seeming paradox can be explained by noting that, given a constant P-P interval (1.0 sec), the PR intervals are getting longer (0.20 sec, 0.30 sec, 0.36 sec, 0.40 sec), yet the beat-to-beat incremental increase in the R-R intervals (1.0 + 0.10 sec, 1.0 + 0.06 sec, 1.0 + 0.04 sec) is decreasing. This is because, with each beat, the PR interval lengthens by a progressively shorter *increment*; from the first to second beat, it increased by 0.10 sec, yet between the second and third beats, it increased by only 0.06 sec, etc. (From Surawicz B, Knilans TK: Chou's Electrocardiography in Clinical Practice, 5th ed. W. B. Saunders, Philadelphia, 2001, p 442.)

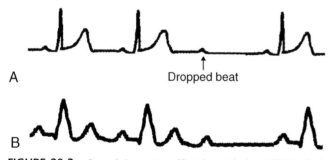

A

↑ Dropped beat

B

FIGURE 20-3 • **Second degree type II atrioventricular (AV) block.** *A*, Second degree type II AV block with a narrow QRS complex. *B*, Second degree type II AV block with a wide QRS complex.

ELECTROCARDIOGRAPHIC PEARLS

- In patients with second degree atrioventricular (AV) block and 2:1 conduction, beware of diagnosing type I block.
- Narrow QRS complex rhythms do not guarantee a more benign form of AV block.
- Alterations in the ECG machine chart speed and amplitude may assist in the diagnosis of AV block by more clearly delineating the ECG waveforms.
- Grouped beating is a useful ECG clue for the diagnosis of second degree type I AV block.

FIGURE 20-4 • *A*, Second degree unknown type AV block (AVB) with 2:1 conduction pattern and a narrow QRS complex escape. This patient ultimately progressed to a second degree type II AVB with 3:2 conduction. *B*, Second degree unknown type AVB with 2:1 conduction. The 2:1 conduction pattern makes the differentiation of type I from type II AVB. A wide QRS complex escape, as seen here, is most often associated with type II physiology. This patient ultimately manifested a typical second degree type II AVB.

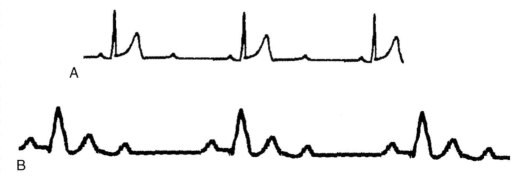

A

B

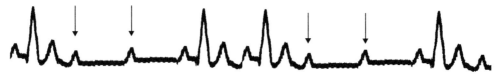

FIGURE 20-5 · **Second degree type II atrioventricular block with high-grade block.** *Arrows* denote P waves with consecutive dropped QRS complexes.

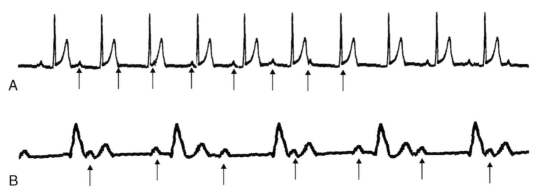

FIGURE 20-6 · **Third degree atrioventricular (AV) block.** *A,* Third degree AV block with a narrow QRS complex. *Arrows* denote P wave activity. *B,* Third degree AV block with a wide QRS complex. *Arrows* denote P wave activity.

escape rhythm and the patient presents in asystolic arrest. More often, the site of escape is just below the level of the block. The atrial rate is always greater than the ventricular rate in patients with third degree AV block. There is no meaningful relationship between the P waves and the QRS complexes. The P waves appear in a regular rhythm and "march" through the rhythm strip at a specific atrial rate. The QRS complexes should appear in a regular fashion and also "march" through the rhythm strip. The duration of the QRS complex and the ventricular rate depends on the site of the block. When the ventricular escape rhythm is located near the His bundle, the rate is greater than 40 bpm and the QRS complexes tend to be narrow (Fig. 20-6*A*). When the site of escape is distal to the His bundle, the rate tends to be less than 40 bpm and the QRS complexes tend to be wide (Fig. 20-6*B*).

References

1. Ornato JP, Peberdy MA: The mystery of bradyasystole during cardiac arrest. Ann Emerg Med 1996;27:576–587.
2. Brady WJ, Swart G, DeBehnke DJ, et al: The efficacy of atropine in the treatment of hemodynamically unstable bradycardia and atrioventricular block: Prehospital and emergency department considerations. Resuscitation 1999;41:47–55.
3. Swart G, Brady WJ, DeBehnke DJ, et al: Acute myocardial infarction complicated by hemodynamically unstable bradyarrhythmia: Prehospital and emergency department treatment with atropine. Am J Emerg Med 1999;17:647–652.

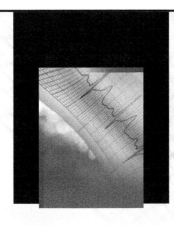

Chapter 21

Intraventricular Conduction Abnormalities

Amal Mattu and Robert L. Rogers

Clinical Features

Intraventricular conduction abnormalities (IVCA) are common electrocardiographic (ECG) entities. These abnormalities include unifascicular blocks (right bundle branch block [RBBB], left anterior fascicular block [LAFB], and left posterior fascicular block [LPFB]), bifascicular blocks (RBBB + LAFB, RBBB + LPFB, and left bundle branch block [LBBB]), trifascicular blocks, and nonspecific intraventricular conduction delays (NSIVCD).

The potential causes of IVCA are extensive. Any process that affects the intrinsic ventricular conduction system or slows intraventricular conduction can lead to the development of an intraventricular block or conduction delay. Overall, the most common cause of IVCA is atherosclerotic heart disease, resulting in ischemic damage to the conduction system. Paradoxically, these abnormalities can also simulate or even mask the expected findings of acute cardiac ischemia. Another common cause is underlying structural heart disease, such as infiltrative cardiomyopathy (e.g., sarcoidosis, hemochromatosis). Progressive fibrosis of the Purkinje fibers, termed Lenegre's disease or Lev's disease, may develop in some patients, resulting in IVCA.[1–3] Patients undergoing right heart catheterization may experience transient conduction blocks, most commonly RBBB, as the catheter enters the right heart. Hyperkalemia is well known to cause IVCAs that may simulate any of the unifascicular or bifascicular blocks.[4] In Central and South America, one of the most common causes of IVCA is Chagas disease. An RBBB can also be caused by other miscellaneous conditions such as congenital heart disease (e.g., Ebstein's anomaly), pulmonary embolism, cyclic antidepressant poisoning, scleroderma, and myocarditis.[5] Finally, both RBBB and LBBB may occasionally be seen in normal healthy individuals.[6]

A normal cardiac conduction impulse begins in the sinoatrial node and is propagated to the atrioventricular (AV) node through right and left atrial tissue. The impulse is then conducted through the His bundle, into the right and left bundle branches. The left bundle branch is further subdivided into the anterior and posterior fascicles. When there is a pathologic process involving the normal ventricular conduction system, a "block" in conduction may result. If the block completely involves the right or left bundle branches, the ECG will show evidence of QRS complex prolongation owing to the slower conduction from the remaining intact bundle branch through ventricular tissue.

Electrocardiographic Manifestations

Unifascicular blocks

Right Bundle Branch Block. With complete RBBB, the QRS complex duration must be at least 0.12 sec. The initial portion of the QRS complex is normal. The classic morphology of the QRS complex in V_1 is an M-shaped rSR′ pattern (Fig. 21-1), but other patterns are commonly seen, including a wide monophasic, notched R wave, or qR morphology. The onset of the R′ wave (the time to peak deflection, termed the *intrinsicoid deflection*) is delayed 0.08 sec or more. There is a broad, shallow S wave in lateral leads I or V_6. When these morphologic criteria are met but the QRS complex duration is less than 0.12 sec (usually 0.08 to 0.11 sec), the diagnosis of incomplete RBBB is made[5] (Fig. 21-2). RBBB is associated with secondary ST and T wave changes, especially in leads V_1 to V_3. The ECG often demonstrates mild ST segment depression with inverted T waves in some or all of these leads.

Left Anterior Fascicular Block. In LAFB, also termed *left anterior hemiblock*, there is a leftward axis shift in the frontal plane QRS complex (Fig. 21-3). The degree of left axis deviation has been debated, and ranges from a minimum of −30 to −45 degrees. Although there are many causes of left axis deviation, LAFB can be distinguished from the rest by a qR pattern or an isolated R wave in lead I. Lead aVL usually has a qR pattern as well. The inferior leads (II, III, aVF) have an rS pattern. The QRS complex duration is normal unless there is another cause of IVCA present. Patients with LAFB often have low-amplitude R waves in leads V_1 to V_3 (i.e., delayed transition zone), often leading to the erroneous diagnosis of anteroseptal myocardial infarction. In the absence of other

ELECTROCARDIOGRAPHIC HIGHLIGHTS

Right bundle branch block

- Lead V₁: M-shaped QRS complex (rSR′); sometimes single wide or notched R wave or qR
- Lead V₆: wide S wave
- Lead I: wide S wave
- QRS complex duration ≥0.12 sec (if preceding criteria are met but duration is <0.12 sec, "incomplete right bundle branch block" is evident)
- A unifascicular block

Left anterior fascicular block

- Left axis deviation (between −30 (or −45) and −90 degrees; usually ≥−60 degrees)
- Small q wave and prominent R wave or isolated prominent R wave in lead I
- Small q wave and prominent R wave in lead aVL
- Small r wave and prominent S wave in leads II, III, and aVF
- Usually normal QRS complex duration (unless associated with another cause of intraventricular conduction abnormality)
- A unifascicular block

Left posterior fascicular block

- Right axis deviation (usually ≥+120 degrees)
- Small r wave and prominent S wave in leads I and aVL
- Small q wave and prominent R wave in lead III (often in leads II and aVF as well)
- No evidence for right ventricular hypertrophy or other causes of right axis deviation
- Usually normal QRS complex duration (unless associated with another cause of intraventricular conduction abnormality)
- A unifascicular block

Left bundle branch block

- Right precordial leads: QS or rS complex
- Leads V₅ and V₆: no q waves, monophasic prominent R wave
- Lead I: no q wave, monophasic prominent R wave
- QRS complex duration ≥0.12 sec (if preceding criteria are met but duration is <0.12 sec, "incomplete left bundle branch block" is evident)
- A bifascicular block

Trifascicular blocks

- Evidence of permanent block in one fascicle and an intermittent/alternating block in the other two fascicles
- Definitive diagnosis requires His bundle recording; however, it is strongly suggested by the following:
  - Incomplete trifascicular block: bifascicular block with first or second degree atrioventricular block
- Complete trifascicular block: bifascicular block with complete heart block

Nonspecific intraventricular conduction delay

- QRS complex duration of ≥0.11 sec
- Does not satisfy criteria for specific bundle branch or fascicular block

ELECTROCARDIOGRAPHIC PEARLS

- Consider hyperkalemia as the cause of a new unifascicular or bifascicular block.
- ST segment elevation or upright T waves in leads V₁ to V₃ in the presence of right bundle branch block could suggest an acute coronary syndrome or Brugada syndrome.
- Left anterior fascicular block is often mistaken for past anteroseptal myocardial infarction.
- Other causes of right axis deviation should be ruled out before the diagnosis of left posterior fascicular block is made.
- Left bundle branch block (LBBB) is associated with significant secondary ST segment and T wave abnormalities that are discordant to the major vector of the QRS complexes across the precordium. Therefore, the presence of concordant ST segment elevation or concordant T wave orientation suggests myocardial ischemia.
- LBBB can be distinguished from left ventricular hypertrophy by the presence of prominent monophasic R waves and the absence of q waves in leads I and V₆.

characterized by a rightward axis shift and an rS pattern in leads I and aVL (Fig. 21-4). A qR pattern is present in lead III and often in leads II and aVF as well (see Box 21-2). LPFB should not be diagnosed in the presence of right ventricular hypertrophy (see Chapter 35, Ventricular Hypertrophy). The QRS complex duration is normal unless there is another cause of IVCA present. In a sense, LPFB manifests as the "opposite" of LAFB; the axes are opposite (left in LAFB, right in LPFB), and the morphologic findings seen in the lateral leads (I, aVL) of each are seen in the inferior leads (II, III, aVF) in the other.

Bifascicular blocks

Right Bundle Branch Block Plus Left Anterior Fascicular Block. The combination of RBBB and LPFB is the most common form of bifascicular block.[5] This combination has the ECG manifestations of both RBBB and LAFB noted previously (Fig. 21-5). The leftward axis persists and the QRS complex duration is greater than 0.12 sec.

Right Bundle Branch Block Plus Left Posterior Fascicular Block. The combination of RBBB and LAFB is an uncommon form of bifascicular block. The ECG demonstrates the key features of both RBBB and LPFB (Fig. 21-6). The rightward axis persists and the QRS complex duration is greater than 0.12 sec.

Left Bundle Branch Block. Because the left bundle branch is subdivided into anterior and posterior fascicles, complete LBBB can be considered a form of bifascicular block. The ECG in patients with LBBB (Fig. 21-7) demonstrates a QRS complex duration greater than 0.12 sec with a delayed intrinsicoid deflection in lead V₆ of at least 0.08 sec.[5] If the QRS complex duration is less than 0.12 sec but other criteria for LBBB are met, the diagnosis of incomplete LBBB is made. The right precordial leads in LBBB demonstrate QS or rS complexes. Leftward axis deviation may be present. Leads I and V₆ should manifest prominent monophasic R waves; the presence of even small q waves in these leads rules out the diagnosis. The ST segments and T waves should be oriented

types of repolarization abnormalities (e.g., left ventricular hypertrophy [LVH]), there are usually no significant differences in the ST segments and T waves compared with normal individuals.[1]

Left Posterior Fascicular Block. LPFB, also termed *left posterior hemiblock*, is rare in contrast to LAFB. It is

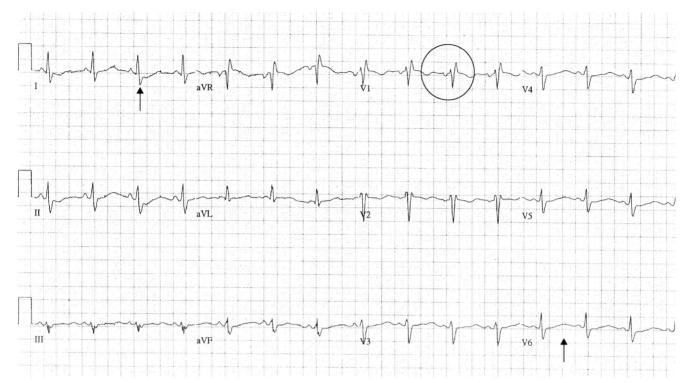

FIGURE 21-1 · **Right bundle branch block.** Note the rSR′ pattern of the wide QRS complex in lead V_1 (*circle*), and the wide S wave in leads I and V_6 (*arrows*).

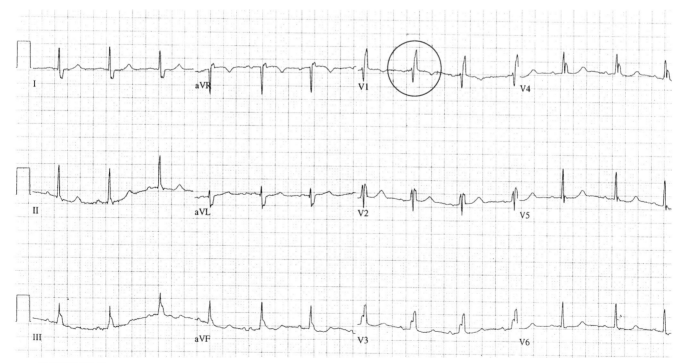

FIGURE 21-2 · **Incomplete right bundle branch block.** Note the QRS complex of intermediate width with an rSR′ pattern in lead V_1 (*circle*).

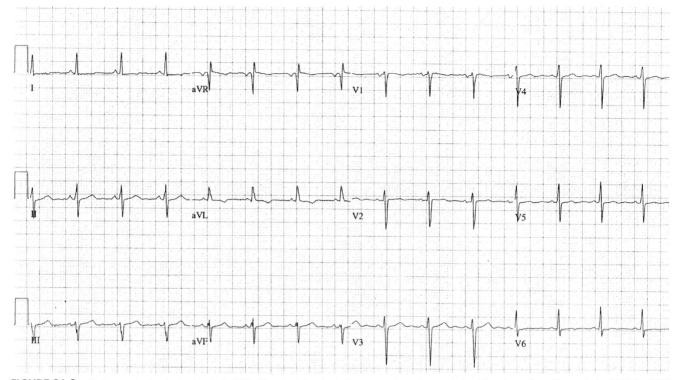

FIGURE 21-3 · Left anterior fascicular block (LAFB). Note the left axis deviation, prominent R wave in lead I, and prominent S wave in lead III. The QRS complex is of normal duration. Also typical of LAFB is the delayed transition zone in the precordial leads.

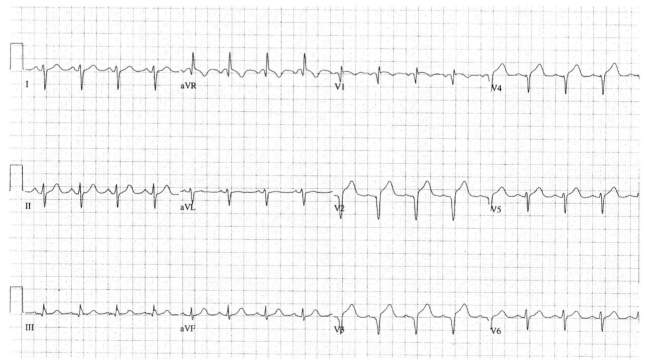

FIGURE 21-4 · Left posterior fascicular block. The tracing demonstrates an evolving anteroseptal MI with Q waves and ST segment elevation in leads V_1 through V_4, along with left posterior fascicular block (LPFB). LPFB is diagnosed by right axis deviation, prominent S wave in lead I, and prominent R wave in lead III. The QRS complex is of normal duration.

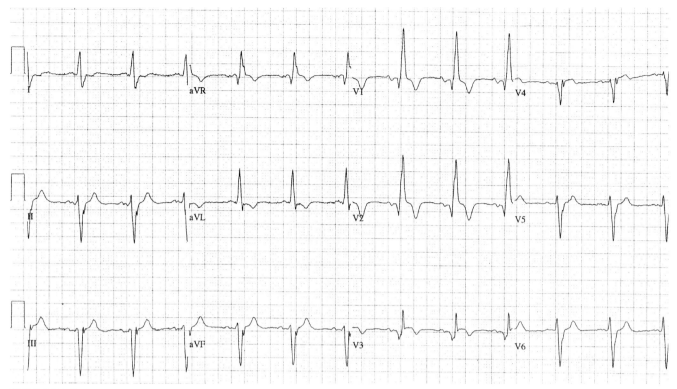

FIGURE 21-5 • **Bifascicular block (right bundle branch block [RBBB] + left anterior fascicular block [LAFB]).** Although somewhat atypical, this ECG meets the criteria for RBBB and LAFB.

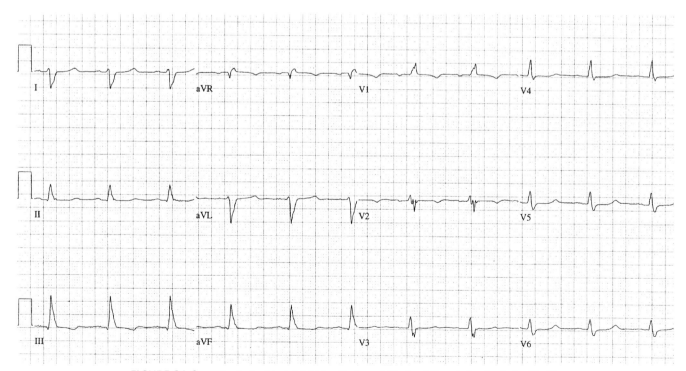

FIGURE 21-6 • **Bifascicular block (right bundle branch block + left posterior fascicular block).**

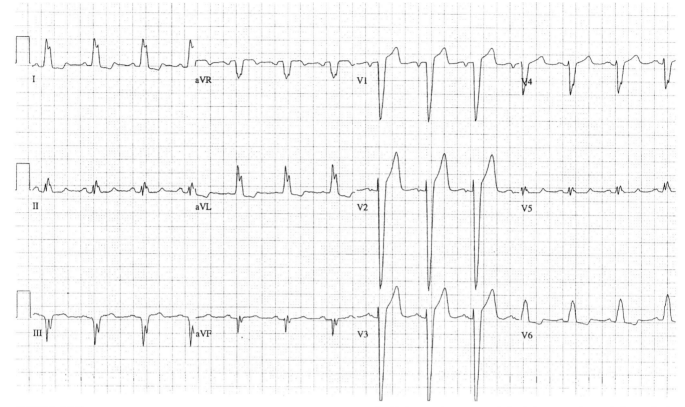

FIGURE 21-7 · **Left bundle branch block.** Note the wide QRS complex associated with the prominent R wave in leads I, aVL, and V_6 and qS complex in lead V_1. The ST segment/T wave changes are appropriately discordant to the QRS complex in the right and left precordial leads, as well as leads I and aVL.

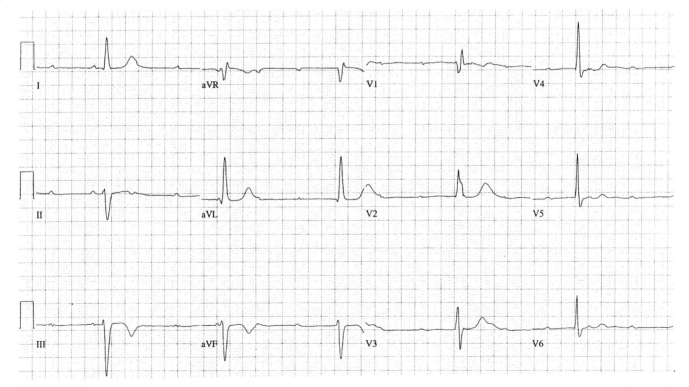

FIGURE 21-8 · **Trifascicular block (third degree heart block + right bundle branch block [RBBB] + left anterior fascicular block [LAFB]).** A prior ECG demonstrated preexisting RBBB and LAFB, a bifascicular block. With the development of third degree heart block, a trifascicular block was diagnosed. In this ECG, the atrial rate is 100 bpm, whereas the ventricular rate is 35 bpm.

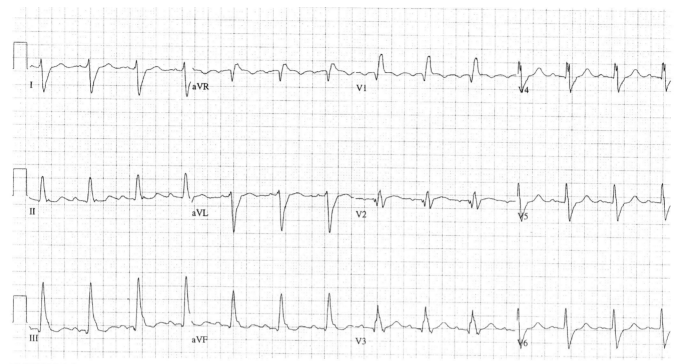

FIGURE 21-9 · **Incomplete trifascicular block.** This ECG shows suspected incomplete trifascicular block (first degree atrioventricular block + right bundle branch block + left posterior fascicular block [LPFB]), in a setting of previous anteroseptal myocardial infarction. Right ventricular hypertrophy (as a cause of the prominent R wave and qR pattern in lead V_1, as well as for the right axis deviation) should be excluded by echocardiography before this pattern can be definitively concluded to represent LPFB.

in a direction opposite (discordant) to the main deflection of the QRS complex in these leads. For this reason, the expected abnormalities of acute myocardial ischemia and infarction are not reliable (see Chapter 34, Acute Myocardial Infarction: Confounding Patterns).

Trifascicular blocks

Trifascicular block is suspected when there is a permanent block in one fascicle and an intermittent block in the other two fascicles. For example, if the patient has a chronic RBBB and alternating LAFB and LPFB develop, trifascicular block is diagnosed. When a complete trifascicular block occurs, the ECG shows evidence of a bifascicular block with third degree AV block (Fig. 21-8). If the block in one of the fascicles is incomplete, the ECG demonstrates a bifascicular block with first or second degree AV block[1] (Fig. 21-9). However, this pattern of AV block does not always guarantee that the conduction disturbance is due to fascicular disease; the conduction delay may be at the level of the AV node or the His bundle.[1] Definitive diagnosis of trifascicular block requires His bundle recording.[1,7] It is safer to assume that first or second degree AV block in the presence of bifascicular block heralds impending complete trifascicular block because there is no way to discern the cause of the AV block (fascicle versus AV nodal) at the bedside.

Nonspecific intraventricular conduction delay

In NSIVCD, the QRS complex duration is greater than 0.12 sec, but the ventricular conduction delay does not meet strict criteria for a specific bundle branch or fascicular block. In many cases, the delay is explained by the presence of drugs (e.g., cyclic antidepressants) or other conditions (e.g., hyperkalemia, hypothermia) that slow ventricular conduction. LVH is often associated with conduction delay as well, and may produce significant prolongation of the QRS complex. This is not necessarily a pathologic condition. LVH with a widened QRS complex can sometimes be mistaken for LBBB, but the presence of small q waves and absence of a prominent monophasic R wave in leads I and V_6 rules out LBBB.

References

1. Surawicz BS, Knilans TK: Chou's Electrocardiography in Clinical Practice, 5th ed. Philadelphia, WB Saunders, 2001.
2. Lenegre J: Etiology and pathology of bilateral bundle branch block in relation to complete heart block. Prog Cardiovasc Dis 1964;6:409.
3. Lev M: Anatomic basis for atrioventricular block. Am J Med 1964;37:742.
4. Mattu A, Brady WJ, Robinson DA: Electrocardiographic manifestations of hyperkalemia. Am J Emerg Med 2000;18:721.
5. Fowler NO: Clinical Electrocardiographic Diagnosis: A Problem Based Approach. Philadelphia, Lippincott Williams & Wilkins, 2000.
6. Wagner GS: Marriott's Practical Electrocardiography, 10th ed. Philadelphia, Lippincott Williams & Wilkins, 2001.
7. Levitas R, Haft JL: Significance of first degree heart block (prolonged PR interval) in bifascicular block. Am J Cardiol 1975;34:259.

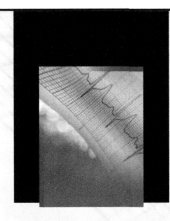

Chapter 22

Atrial Fibrillation and Atrial Flutter

Keith Wrenn

Clinical Features

Atrial Fibrillation. The prevalence of atrial fibrillation is increasing and its incidence doubles with each decade of adult life, with 5% of persons aged 65 years and older affected. Atrial fibrillation complicates 5% to 10% of acute myocardial infarctions and 40% of cardiac surgeries.[1] Presentations range from palpitations to pulmonary edema and stroke. Nonspecific symptoms such as fatigue and altered mentation are common in the elderly.[2] In patients with paroxysmal atrial fibrillation, asymptomatic episodes are more common than symptomatic episodes.

There are many causes for atrial fibrillation, including pericarditis, chronic hypertension, pulmonary embolism, coronary artery disease, alcohol abuse (holiday heart), rheumatic valvular disease (particularly mitral and tricuspid), thyrotoxicosis, and cardiac surgery. It is very rare for ischemic heart disease to present as atrial fibrillation in the absence of other signs and symptoms of ischemia.[2] Up to 30% of cases are not associated with hypertension or other demonstrable underlying cardiopulmonary disease (known as "lone" atrial fibrillation).[3]

The common pathophysiologic process is atrial enlargement (especially the left atrium), atrial inflammation, and fibrosis. Triggering events include altered sympathetic or parasympathetic tone, acute or chronic changes in atrial wall tension, ischemia, bradycardia, atrial premature contractions, and conduction through accessory atrioventricular (AV) pathways.[1] These triggers are prodysrhythmic because they accelerate repolarization and shorten the refractory state of atrial tissue. Currently, the preeminent theory of the genesis of atrial fibrillation is the multiple wavelet hypothesis.[1,2] After a triggering event, multiple, random atrial micro-reentrant waves are generated, collide, and extinguish one another, and arise again. Another recently discovered mechanism for the initiation of atrial fibrillation involves a rapidly firing focus in or near the atrial sleeves of the pulmonary veins.[1]

There are four classifications of atrial fibrillation based on the duration of the dysrhythmia: (1) acute—lasting less than 48 hours; (2) paroxysmal—more than one acute self-terminating

episode; (3) persistent—lasting longer than 48 hours without spontaneous termination; and (4) permanent—resistant to pharmacologic or electrical cardioversion.[4]

Atrial Flutter. Atrial flutter is second only to atrial fibrillation in frequency of atrial dysrhythmias, and shares many of the same predisposing causes (with the addition of chronic obstructive pulmonary disease). It is also closely associated with atrial fibrillation; atrial fibrillation often precedes or follows atrial flutter and may actually coexist in the same patient at the same time. Unlike atrial fibrillation, which is often chronic, atrial flutter is typically paroxysmal, rarely lasting more than a few hours, usually reverting to either sinus rhythm or atrial fibrillation. In most cases, atrial flutter is thought to be caused by a macro-reentrant circuit in the right atrium, involving a zone of slowed conduction between the tricuspid annulus and the crista terminalis, usually in a counterclockwise direction.

ELECTROCARDIOGRAPHIC HIGHLIGHTS

Atrial fibrillation

- Irregularly irregular ventricular response (presence of QRS complexes)
- Narrow QRS complex unless preexisting intraventricular conduction abnormality or rate-related bundle malfunction
- Chaotic baseline
- No evidence of organized atrial activity (i.e., no P waves)
- Ventricular rate varies from very slow (30 bpm) to very fast (>150 bpm), with typical rate of 110 to 130 bpm

Atrial flutter

- Ventricular response regular in most cases
- Narrow QRS complex unless preexisting intraventricular conduction abnormality or rate-related bundle malfunction
- Atrial activity present with obvious flutter waves in a sawtooth pattern in most leads
- Atrial rate of 250 to 350/minute
- Ventricular rate most often 150 bpm (2:1 conduction)

Atrial flutter usually causes symptoms related to rate.[5] The ventricular response to atrial flutter at rest is usually faster than in atrial fibrillation because of the typical 2:1 AV conduction in untreated patients.

Electrocardiographic Manifestations

Atrial Fibrillation. Atrial fibrillation usually presents as an irregularly irregular rhythm. The baseline oscillates rather than being isolectric. There are fibrillatory waves of different amplitude, duration, and morphology (Fig. 22-1) that do not appear as distinct P waves or flutter waves. Small fibrillatory waves (<0.5 mm in amplitude) are called fine atrial fibrillation (Fig. 22-2), whereas larger fibrillatory waves (>0.5 to 1.0 mm) are called coarse atrial fibrillation (Fig. 22-3). Fine atrial fibrillation is seen more often in chronic ischemic heart disease, whereas coarse atrial fibrillation is encountered more commonly in rheumatic heart disease.[6] Occasionally, fibrillatory waves may be so fine as to be undetectable in any lead, with the baseline appearing isoelectric.

The mean rate in untreated patients is usually in the range of 110 to 130 bpm. The atrial fibrillatory rate is typically in excess of 400 bpm. Fibrillatory impulses may partially penetrate the AV node, making it refractory, which accounts for the typically slower ventricular response rates commonly observed. The QRS complexes are usually narrow unless preexisting (see Figs. 22-1 and 22-2) or rate-related intraventricular conduction abnormalities are present.

Occasionally, when there is associated AV block, the rate may be slower and the ventricular response more regular because of a subsidiary pacemaker focus in the AV node or His-Purkinje system (Fig. 22-3). Another cause of regularization

is medication, heightened vagal tone, and digitalis toxicity. Resting ventricular response rates above 150 bpm may be due to fever, volume depletion, thyrotoxicosis, or other hyperadrenergic states such as alcohol withdrawal.[2,7] When the ventricular response rates exceed 200 to 220 bpm, the presence of an accessory AV pathway is likely. In this setting, the QRS complexes often are wide with bizarre configurations because of antegrade conduction through the bypass tract.

Another cause of wide QRS complexes in atrial fibrillation is a coexisting bundle branch block (see Figs. 22-1 and 22-2). When a right bundle branch block (RBBB) and left anterior fascicular block (bifascicular block) accompany atrial fibrillation in a child, an ostium primum septal defect should be suspected (Fig. 22-2). When a right ventricular conduction delay (sometimes called incomplete RBBB) occurs with atrial fibrillation in a young person, an ostium secundum defect should be suspected.[7]

One last important electrocardiographic aspect of atrial fibrillation or any irregular rhythm like multifocal atrial tachycardia or atrial flutter with variable block is *Ashman's phenomenon* (Fig. 22-4). The length of the refractory period after a particular beat is determined by the preceding R-R interval. If the preceding R-R interval is long, then the following refractory period will also be long. If, by chance, another QRS complex falls in this longer refractory period (often called a "long-short" R-R cycle), then it may be conducted aberrantly, usually with an RBBB pattern (see Fig. 22-4). These wide QRS complexes are often misinterpreted as premature ventricular contractions.

Atrial Flutter. Atrial flutter is usually a regular rhythm. Again, like atrial fibrillation, the baseline is not isoelectric. Flutter waves, both more distinct and uniform than atrial

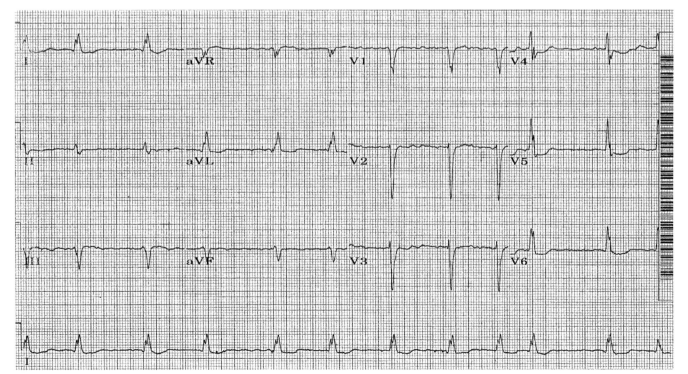

FIGURE 22-1 · Atrial fibrillation with slow ventricular response and left bundle branch block. Note the irregularly irregular rhythm and oscillatory baseline, seen best in lead V₁.

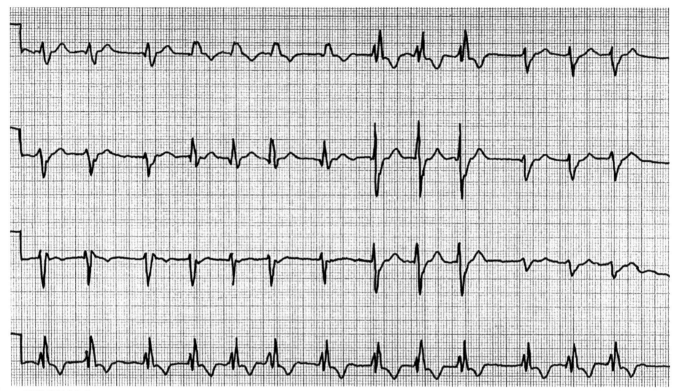

FIGURE 22-2 • **Atrial fibrillation with slow response and left anterior fascicular block.** Note the fine fibrillatory waves (<0.5 mm in amplitude).

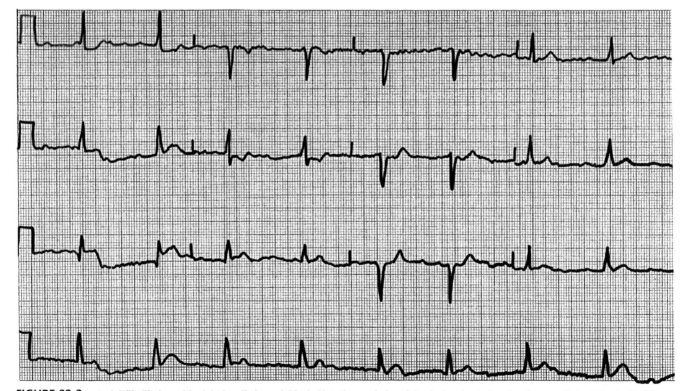

FIGURE 22-3 • **Atrial fibrillation with right bundle branch block.** Note the regularity of the rhythm due to junctional escape. In lead V_1, the fibrillatory waves are coarse (0.5 mm in amplitude).

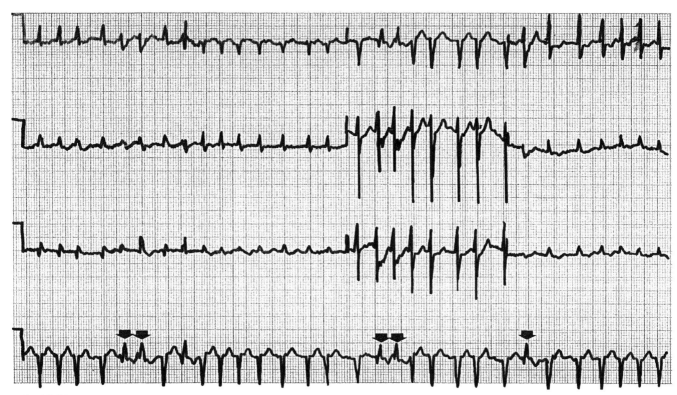

FIGURE 22-4 · Atrial fibrillation with rapid ventricular response and Ashman's phenomenon. Note the aberrantly conducted beats in the rhythm strip (*arrows*) with right bundle branch block pattern following a longer R-R interval.

activity observed in atrial fibrillation, are seen between QRS complexes (the so-called sawtooth pattern), most prominently in the inferior leads (II, III, aVF) and lead V_6 (Fig. 22-5).[5] Flutter waves that are positively deflected in lead V_1 imply the typical counterclockwise reentrant circuit, whereas negatively deflected flutter waves in V_1 imply the atypical clockwise current.

The atrial rate is typically between 250 and 350 bpm. The most common ventricular response rate is approximately 150 bpm owing to physiologic 2:1 AV conduction. High degree AV block greater than 2:1 usually results from treatment with AV nodal blocking drugs. Furthermore, 1:1 conduction is rare, but may be precipitated by hyperadrenergic states or medications (type 1A antidysrhythmics), or in Wolff-Parkinson-White syndrome (WPW) when conduction to the ventricles occurs through the bypass tract.

Less commonly, atrial flutter results in an irregular rate because of variable AV conduction. This irregularity may occur because of conducting system disease or medications used for rate control or conversion. Slower atrial flutter wave rates (below 250 bpm) occur in the presence of medical therapy or can be associated with the marked right atrial enlargement accompanying certain congenital heart defects (possibly due to an increased reentrant circuit length).

The QRS is usually normal in length. The QRS complexes can be wide in the setting of a coexisting intraventricular conduction delay or in WPW with bypass tract conduction. Occasionally, in the inferior distribution, the flutter waves merge, making the QRS complex appear wide and forming a pseudo-S wave.

Differentiating Atrial Fibrillation and Flutter from Other Supraventricular Tachydysrhythmias. Atrial flutter is usually regular whereas atrial fibrillation is most often irregular. When atrial flutter is irregular because of varying degrees of AV block, the more regular oscillation of the baseline due to flutter waves should help differentiate flutter from fibrillation. Atrial fibrillation and flutter often coexist in the same patient. There is also an entity called atrial fibrillation–flutter in which it is very hard to differentiate the two because the atrial rates are a bit faster than typical flutter, the flutter waves a little more morphologically indistinct, and the ventricular rhythm irregular. It is believed that in this setting there is often atrial fibrillation in the left atrium coexisting with atrial flutter in the right atrium.[8]

Unlike atrial fibrillation or flutter, multifocal atrial tachycardia should have an isoelectric baseline and distinct, although morphologically different P waves before each QRS complex. Tremor artifact, as in Parkinson's disease or shivering, may mimic fibrillatory waves in the baseline, particularly in the limb leads.[6] The ventricular response should be regular, however, if tremor is the only issue (Fig. 22-6).

Sinus tachycardia can be confused with atrial flutter because of the regular rate, but tends to be a more variable rate over time. Vagal maneuvers may help differentiate the two because sinus tachycardia tends to slow gradually, whereas in atrial flutter there is either no response or an increase in AV block causing abrupt slowing, at which time the flutter waves can usually be seen more easily.

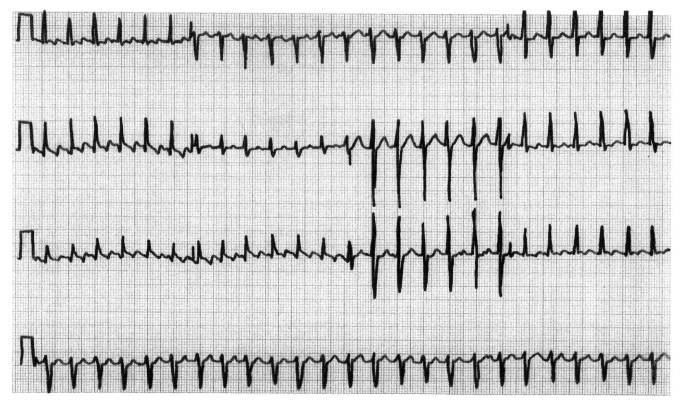

FIGURE 22-5 · **Atrial flutter.** Note the classic sawtooth pattern, seen best in leads II, III, aVF.

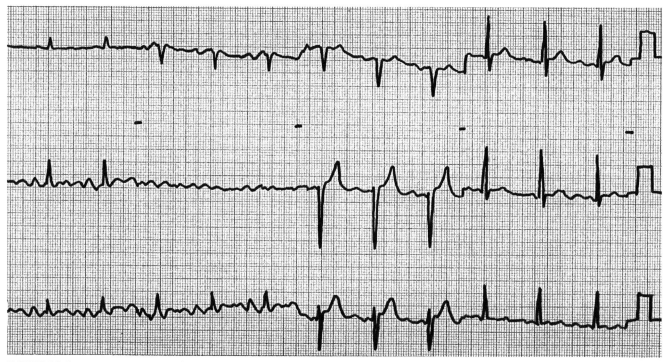

FIGURE 22-6 · **Tremor artifact in limb leads mimicking atrial fibrillation.** Note the regularity of the rhythm and the presence of P waves in the precordial leads.

<table>
<tr><td colspan="2">

</td></tr>
</table>

Atrial flutter is probably misdiagnosed as paroxysmal supraventricular tachycardia (PSVT) more often than any other rhythm. If the rate is right around 150 bpm, flutter should be suspected. In PSVT, the rates are usually in excess of 160 bpm. With PSVT, vagal maneuvers cause either a conversion to sinus rhythm or nothing. Adenosine has similar effects, but may cause prolonged episodes of ventricular asystole in atrial flutter (10 seconds or longer), during which flutter waves can be seen more easily.

Paroxysmal atrial tachycardia (PAT) with block usually results in a slower atrial rate than atrial flutter (<200 bpm). In PAT with block, there is an isoelectric baseline and the P waves are more distinctly P wave–like than in atrial flutter.

References

1. Allessie MA, Boyden PA, Camm AJ, et al: Pathophysiology and prevention of atrial fibrillation. Circulation 2001;103:769.
2. Falk RH: Medical progress: Atrial fibrillation. N Engl J Med 2001;344:1067.
3. Toft AD, Boon NA: Thyroid disease and the heart. Heart 2000;84:455.
4. Davies W: The management of atrial fibrillation. Clin Med 2001;1:190.
5. Waldo AL: Treatment of atrial flutter. Heart 2000;84:227.
6. Thurmann M, Janney JG Jr: The diagnostic importance of fibrillatory wave size. Circulation 1962;25:991.
7. Hurst JW: Ventricular Electrocardiography. New York: Gower Medical Publishing, 1991:1.2–13.36.
8. Waldo AL: Pathogenesis of atrial flutter. J Cardiovasc Electrophysiol 1998;9(8 Suppl):s18.

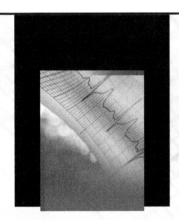

Chapter 23

Wandering Atrial Pacemaker and Multifocal Atrial Tachycardia

Keith Wrenn

Clinical Features

Wandering Atrial Pacemaker. Wandering atrial pacemaker (WAP) is a variant of sinus arrhythmia usually of no pathologic significance. Although occasionally seen with other cardiopulmonary problems such as sick sinus syndrome or congenital heart disease in children, it is most often associated with individuals who have well-developed vagal reflexes—for example, athletes and wind instrument musicians.[1] WAP is postulated to result from an imbalance in the sympathetic and parasympathetic tone in the heart. In situations where the resting rate is naturally slow or repetitive respiratory strain activates vagal stretch receptors and the cardioinhibitory center in the medulla, the resultant inhibition of the sinoatrial (SA) node allows latent subsidiary atrial pacemaker sites to become active. Conversely, it is possible that sympathetic stimulation could directly stimulate these subsidiary pacemaker sites, causing WAP.

Multifocal Atrial Tachycardia. Multifocal atrial tachycardia (MAT), also called *chaotic atrial rhythm*, is almost always associated with significant underlying cardiopulmonary disease such as chronic obstructive pulmonary disease (COPD), congestive heart failure (CHF), or the cardiothoracic postoperative setting.[2,3] The average age of patients with MAT is in

---

ELECTROCARDIOGRAPHIC HIGHLIGHTS

Wandering atrial pacemaker

- Slight irregularity
- Normal to slow rate
- Three or more P waves of different morphology in a single lead
- PR intervals vary minimally from beat to beat
- QRS complexes of normal duration

Multifocal atrial tachycardia

- Rate greater than 100 bpm
- Three morphologically distinct P waves in a single lead (best seen in leads II, III, and V_1)
- Irregularity of the P-P, PR, and R-R intervals
- Isoelectric baseline between P waves

---

the range of 70 to 75 years. Many of these patients have coexisting coronary artery disease. In-hospital mortality rates are reportedly as high as 60% in patients in whom MAT develops, and the mean survival after diagnosis is just over a year.[2,3]

Importantly, it is not the dysrhythmia itself, but rather the underlying disease process that accounts for this high mortality rate. Occasionally, MAT at higher rates may directly cause hemodynamic compromise or myocardial ischemia, resulting in death. Overt pulmonary disease is seen in at least 60% of patients with MAT, although up to a third may have CHF, which often coexists with COPD.[2–4] Other important associations with MAT include theophylline toxicity and metabolic disorders such as hypokalemia or hypomagnesemia.[2–4]

In children, MAT is associated with a coexisting disease only approximately half the time, and is often asymptomatic. When associated with myocarditis or congenital heart disease, the mortality rate is significantly higher.[5]

MAT represents a state in which there is the absence of a single dominant pacemaker. Right atrial abnormality, hypoxia, hypercarbia, acidosis, and excess catecholamines, either alone or more commonly in combination, lead to increased atrial automaticity due to triggered electrical activity from late or delayed after depolarizations. MAT is frequently a self-limited dysrhythmia that resolves with correction or improvement of the underlying problem. However, recurrence is common.[4]

Electrocardiographic Manifestations

Wandering Atrial Pacemaker. WAP is manifested on the surface electrocardiogram as a rhythm with slight irregularity, normal to slow rate, and three or more P waves of different morphology, all occurring in a single lead. The PR intervals vary slightly from beat to beat. The QRS complexes are typically of normal duration or at least have the same morphology from beat to beat. WAP might be considered when there are frequent atrial extrasystoles. Occasionally, the varied P waves may come from within the SA node itself (Fig. 23-1).

Differentiating WAP from sinus dysrhythmia relies primarily on being able to recognize different P wave morphologies in WAP. Both rhythms show slight irregularity, are benign, and are associated with heightened vagal tone. In sinus dysrhythmia, the PR interval should also be constant, unlike in WAP.

Multifocal Atrial Tachycardia. MAT is electrocardiographically manifested as (1) a rate greater than 100 bpm;

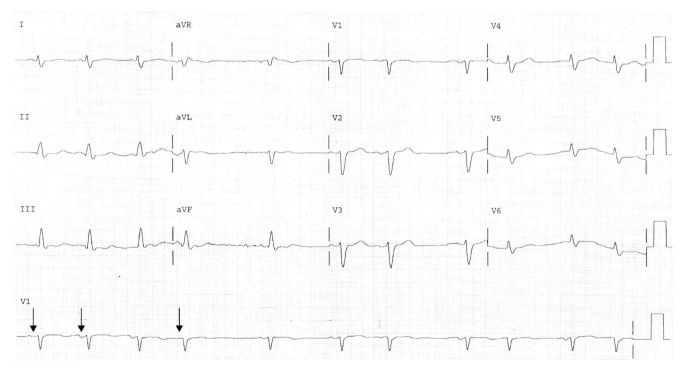

FIGURE 23-1 · **Wandering atrial pacemaker.** Note in the lead V_1 rhythm strip there are at least three different P wave morphologies (*arrows*) at a rate less than 100 bpm. Subsequent pauses may represent sinus node dysfunction.

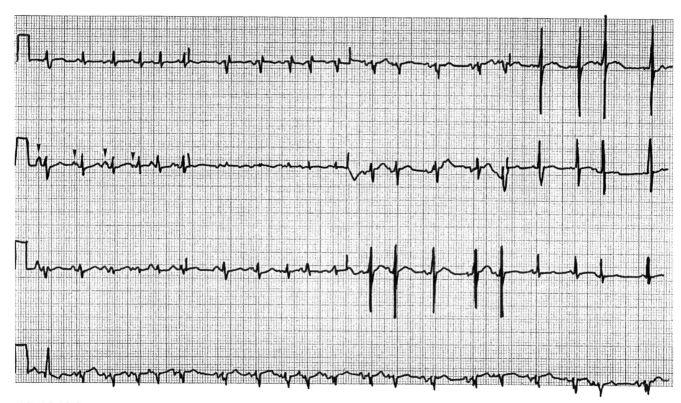

FIGURE 23-2 • **Multifocal atrial tachycardia.** Note four different P wave morphologies in lead II (*arrowheads*), with an average ventricular response 100 to 120 bpm, in a patient with chronic obstructive pulmonary disease.

(2) at least three morphologically different (but discrete) non-sinus P waves in a single lead; (3) irregularity of the P-P, PR, and R-R intervals; and, importantly, (4) an isoelectric baseline between P waves. The variable P wave morphology is usually seen best in leads II, III, and V_1 (Fig. 23-2). There is some disagreement about whether the three different P wave morphologies must be "nonsinus."

Because it is sometimes difficult to tell which P wave morphology is from the SA node, many investigators believe that any three morphologically distinct P waves should qualify as MAT. There is also disagreement about the requirement that the rate be greater than 100 bpm because there are often patients who fulfill the other requirements and fit the clinical picture but have heart rates below 100 bpm.

MAT is often mistaken for atrial fibrillation, another very common, chaotic, irregular atrial dysrhythmia. MAT has a true isoelectric baseline, whereas atrial fibrillation and flutter do not. When rates are especially fast, it is more difficult to see the irregularity and to assess the shorter baseline. In addition, atrial fibrillation and flutter often occur in the same clinical settings as MAT. Atrial fibrillation may precede or follow MAT. Atrial flutter is usually regular, unlike MAT, and because 2:1 block is usually present, the ventricular rate is often 150 bpm, although it can be irregular with coexisting variable atrioventricular block. In situations where it is truly

unclear whether the patient has MAT, atrial fibrillation, or atrial flutter, esophageal or intra-arterial leads may show the distinct P waves of MAT versus the fibrillatory or flutter waves. Perhaps more practically, pharmacologic slowing of the rate often allows this differentiation.

Sinus tachycardia and paroxysmal supraventricular tachycardia (PSVT), like MAT, are characterized by an isoelectric baseline, but can be differentiated from MAT primarily by their regularity. In sinus tachycardia at rest, the rate rarely exceeds 140 bpm; a single P wave morphology is seen. In PSVT, P waves are not usually observed and, when present, have an abnormal orientation. The rates usually exceed 160 bpm.

References

1. Borgia JF, Nizet PM, Gliner JA, Horvath SM: Wandering atrial pacemaker associated with repetitive respiratory strain. Cardiology 1982;69:70.
2. Schwartz M, Rodman D, Lowenstein SR: Recognition and treatment of multifocal atrial tachycardia: A critical review. J Emerg Med 1994; 12:353.
3. Kastor JA: Multifocal atrial tachycardia. N Engl J Med 1990;322:1713.
4. Scher DL, Arsura EL: Multifocal atrial tachycardia: Mechanisms, clinical correlates, and treatment. Am Heart J 1989;118:574.
5. Bradley DJ, Fischbach PS, Law IH, et al: The clinical course of multifocal atrial tachycardia in infants and children. J Am Coll Cardiol 2001;38:401.

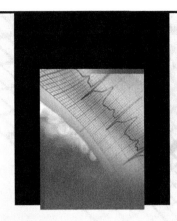

Chapter 24

Other Supraventricular Tachydysrhythmias

A. Antoine Kazzi and Hubert Wong

Clinical Features

The supraventricular tachycardias (SVT) are defined as any tachycardic rhythms that rely on the atrium or atrioventricular (AV) node to be triggered or sustained.[1] Although sinus tachycardia (ST) is included in this chapter, in general, SVTs involve an abnormal impulse generation or conduction in atrial or AV nodal tissue.

SVTs are some of the most common cardiac dysrhythmias seen in the emergency department.[2] They can occur in all age groups and have an increasing incidence with age (with the exception of SVTs associated with preexcitation). Although most patients complain of palpitations (as high as 90%), the clinical presentation is variable and includes asymptomatic presentations as well as any manifestations of cardiac failure, end-organ ischemia, or shock.[3]

Clinicians frequently use the term *paroxysmal supraventricular tachycardia* (PSVT). This term refers to SVTs that manifest a pattern of episodic sudden onset and termination. Factors that contribute to the onset of PSVT include any increase in sympathetic stimulation, such as anxiety, caffeine intake, and illicit drug use (e.g., cocaine, amphetamines, and methamphetamines).

SVTs are broadly categorized as *atrial tachydysrhythmias* or *atrioventricular tachydysrhythmias*. Atrial tachydysrhythmias result from impulses generated in atrial tissue due to abnormal automaticity or triggered activity. These tachydysrhythmias include ST, inappropriate ST (IST), sinus nodal reentrant tachycardia (SNRT), and atrial tachycardia (AT). Multifocal AT (MAT), atrial flutter, and atrial fibrillation are also atrial tachydysrhythmias, but are covered elsewhere in this text.

AV tachydysrhythmias result from an abnormal impulse generated in or dependent on the AV node (usually as part of the reentry circuit). These tachydysrhythmias include the following: AV nodal reentrant tachycardia (AVNRT), AV reentrant tachycardia (AVRT), junctional ectopic tachycardia, and nonparoxysmal junctional tachycardia. Because the AV node is a part of the reentry circuit or source of abnormal impulse generation, AV node blocking measures (such as vagal or

Valsalva maneuvers, carotid sinus massage, or medications) often result in termination of the tachydysrhythmia.[4]

Electrocardiographic Manifestations

Typically, SVT manifests electrocardiographically as a narrow-complex tachycardia with a regular rate. Exceptions are atrial fibrillation, atrial flutter with variable block, AT with variable block, and MAT, which usually have an irregular rate and rhythm. SVTs can occasionally result in wide-complex QRS morphologies in the setting of aberrant conduction (SVT with aberrancy) or AVRT with antidromic conduction (see later).

PSVT is defined generally by the sudden onset of a minimum of three premature supraventricular beats. PSVTs are often initiated by an atrial premature beat followed by a prolonged PR interval. The heart rate usually ranges between 140 and 250 bpm.

ELECTROCARDIOGRAPHIC HIGHLIGHTS

- Supraventricular tachycardias (SVTs) result in a regular tachycardia at rates of 100 to 250 bpm.
- SVTs produce a narrow QRS complex tachycardia with the exception of SVT with aberrancy and antidromic atrioventricular reentrant tachycardia (AVRT).
- Sinus tachycardia has a gradual onset and resolution as opposed to other SVTs, which have a more paroxysmal presentation.
- Atrial tachycardias are usually due to a single atrial focus producing the same recurrent ectopic P wave (unlike multifocal atrial tachycardia).
- With atrioventricular nodal reentrant tachycardia (AVNRT; the most common type of SVT other than sinus tachycardia), the P wave is often not seen or is buried in the QRS complex, producing distortion of the terminal portion (pseudo-S or R′ wave).
- AVNRT cannot be differentiated from orthodromic AVRT on the 12-lead ECG.

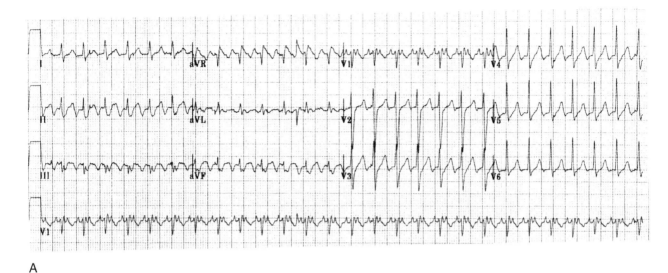

A

B

FIGURE 24-1 • Tachycardia of unclear etiology. *A,* ECG reveals tachycardia of unclear etiology. *B,* Doubling the paper speed artificially slows the tracing down, allowing easier detection of atrial activity (*arrows*). The diagnosis of atrial flutter with 2:1 block becomes clear.

In the setting of rapid heart rates, native atrial P wave activity can often be difficult to detect on a standard 12-lead electrocardiogram (ECG) because of overlying QRS complexes, ST segments, and T waves. Diagnosis can be enhanced by increasing the ECG machine paper speed (usually by doubling it, to 50 mm/sec). Doing so artificially slows the rhythm on the 12-lead ECG and may allow underlying atrial activity to be seen[5] (Fig. 24-1).

Atrial Tachydysrhythmias. Atrial tachydysrhythmias (including ST) are generated in atrial tissue above the AV node. As a result, these rhythms are also termed *AV node independent.* These tachydysrhythmias may be present in the setting of AV block, and treatment aimed at AV blockade (which may decrease the ventricular response rate) will not necessarily terminate the atrial dysrhythmia.

Sinus Tachycardia. ST is essentially a physiologic response to a stress such as hypoxia, fever, hypovolemia, pain, hyperthyroidism, anxiety, exercise, or drugs (e.g., caffeine, stimulants, or sympathomimetics). ST is usually regular and consists of an accelerated baseline sinus rhythm. The threshold rate is age dependent (with higher rates in children) and always exceeds 100 bpm. The rate of the tachycardia varies during presentation and usually has a gradual, rather than sudden, onset and resolution (Fig. 24-2).

Inappropriate Sinus Tachycardia. IST is typically found in healthy adults, most commonly young women, who manifest an elevated resting heart rate and an exaggerated rate increase during minimal exercise. IST has not been related to structural heart disease. It is attributed to autonomic hypersensitivity or to an abnormality of the sinus node. IST resembles ST, except that clinicians cannot identify a responsible stressor.

Sinus Node Reentrant Tachycardia. SNRT consists of an acceleration of the underlying rhythm caused by a reentry circuit, in or close to the sinus node. SNRT represents up to 10% of PSVTs. Often misdiagnosed as IST, SNRT starts and ends abruptly. The ECG shows a normal P wave morphology with a rate of 100 to 150 bpm.

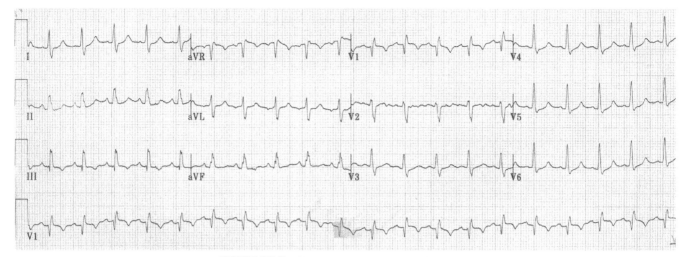

FIGURE 24-2 · Sinus tachycardia at a rate of 119 bpm.

Atrial Tachycardia. AT is typically due to a single ectopic atrial pacer, and attributed to either a trigger such as digoxin toxicity or to increased automaticity or reentry of the atrial tissue. Also known as *paroxysmal AT*, AT makes up fewer than 10% of PSVTs. The atrial rhythm is regular and the rate ranges between 100 and 250 bpm—slower than atrial flutter, with which it can be confused. AV block can be present with AT, leading to a lower ventricular rate. In addition, whereas AV blockade may slow the ventricular response, it will not terminate the tachydysrhythmia. In fact, an ensuing AV block may limit conduction of the tachycardia to the ventricles and cause an atrial flutter–like state.

Because the origin is a single ectopic atrial pacer, the shape of the ectopic P wave is usually different from the baseline sinus node P wave. A minimum of three consecutive atrial premature beats with the same ectopic P wave is required to make the diagnosis of AT (Fig. 24-3). The location of the ectopic atrial focus can often be determined by analysis of the P wave in leads aVL and V_1. A P wave with positive deflection in lead V_1 suggests a left atrial focus, whereas a positive deflection in lead aVL suggests a right atrial focus.[6]

Atrial fibrillation and atrial flutter are discussed in Chapter 22, and multifocal atrial tachycardia in Chapter 23.

Atrioventricular Tachydysrhythmias. AV tachydysrhythmias are generated at the AV node either by abnormal impulse generation or a reentry circuit. As a result, these tachycardias are termed *AV node dependent*, do not coexist with AV blockade, and can be terminated with appropriate AV blocking treatment.

Atrioventricular Nodal Reentrant Tachycardia. AVNRT affects all ages in the general population, although it has been associated with myocardial ischemia, rheumatic heart disease, pericarditis, mitral valve prolapse, and the preexcitation syndromes. AVNRT is the most common (50% to 60%) of the PSVTs.

AVNRT results from a reentrant circuit loop, formed by the presence of two pathways, slow and fast, in the AV node. The tachydysrhythmia is essentially triggered when a premature atrial impulse succeeds in conducting antegrade to the ventricles through either pathway, and then subsequently retrograde back to the atria through the other pathway as a result of different refractory periods. This AV nodal reentry causes a rapid, nearly simultaneous depolarization of both the ventricles and atria. The retrograde impulse then causes depolarization again down the antegrade pathway, completing the circuit and establishing the tachydysrhythmia.

With AVNRT, the QRS complex is typically narrow and regular, and the heart rate ranges between 120 and 250 bpm (Figs. 24-4 and 24-5). The ventricles are not part of the impulse circuit and the QRS complex morphology is therefore not affected by the reentry mechanism of AVNRT. However, because atrial depolarization may occur simultaneously with ventricular depolarization, the P wave may be "buried" in the QRS complex. The location of the P wave relative to the QRS complex depends on the type of reentrant circuit in the AV node and the duration of the anterograde PR interval relative to that of the retrograde RP interval. Most of the time (66%), the P wave is hidden in the QRS and is therefore not visible. This buried P wave can cause a deformity of the QRS complex, most commonly a distortion of the terminal portion (the so-called pseudo-S wave in the inferior leads, or pseudo-R' wave in lead V_1).[7]

When visible, the P wave is located *just after* (in 30% of AVNRT) or *immediately before* (in only 4%) the QRS complex. When visible, the P wave is usually inverted in the inferior leads II, III, and aVF as a result of the retrograde direction of atrial depolarization from the AV node.

Atrioventricular Reentrant Tachycardia. AVRT is the second most common form of PSVT and tends to present at an earlier age than AVNRT. The incidence of AVRT in male patients is twice that in female patients, and is associated with congenital Ebstein's anomaly.

This dysrhythmia is attributed to a large reentry circuit caused by the presence of aberrant myocardial accessory pathways, or bypass tracts, connecting atria to ventricles. The reentry circuit occurs when impulses travel through these accessory pathways in addition to the AV node, resulting in recurrent activation of the atria and ventricles. Accessory pathway conduction can be either anterograde or retrograde. In some patients, the direction taken by atrial impulses can also alternate through the same fibers. During sinus rhythm, these accessory pathways often transmit impulses in addition to the AV node, resulting in preexcitation of the ventricles (see Chapter 25, Preexcitation Syndromes). However, some

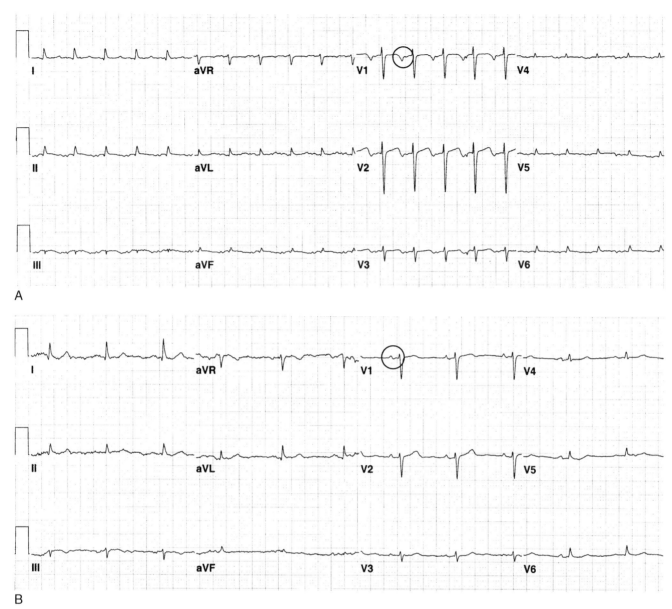

FIGURE 24-3 · Atrial tachycardia. *A*, Atrial tachycardia at a rate of 126 bpm originating from an ectopic atrial focus. Note the abnormal P wave axis and morphology, particularly in lead V₁ (*circle*). *B*, Same patient with a return to sinus rhythm. Note the change in P wave morphology in lead V₁ (*circle*).

accessory tracts cannot be detected in an ECG during sinus rhythm transmission. These pathways are capable only of retrograde conduction and are therefore "concealed." They are apparent only during an AVRT rhythm.

With an AVRT rhythm, *orthodromic* conduction is more common, occurring when anterograde conduction proceeds down the normal His-Purkinje pathway, followed by retrograde conduction up the accessory pathway. Because ventricular depolarization occurs along the normal conduction pathway, orthodromic AVRT results in a narrow QRS complex (Fig. 24-6). Because the atria are depolarized late by conduction retrograde up the accessory pathway, the P wave follows a normal QRS complex during the episode of AVRT. Depending on the location of the accessory pathway, the P wave may be upright, inverted, or flat. AVRT due to orthodromic conduction may be difficult to distinguish from some forms of AVNRT.

ELECTROCARDIOGRAPHIC PEARLS

- Patients with atrioventricular (AV) reentrant tachycardia (AVRT) often have evidence of ECG preexcitation at baseline sinus rhythm.
- AV blockade slows the ventricular response for most SVTs, but does not terminate atrial tachydysrhythmias (AV nodal independent).
- AV blockade can terminate AV tachydysrhythmias (AV nodal dependent), but must be used cautiously, particularly with AVRT, because it may accelerate conduction down the accessory pathway.
- Differentiating among supraventricular tachycardia with aberrancy, AVRT with antidromic conduction, and ventricular tachycardia (VT) can be difficult. When in doubt, initial management should focus on treating VT.

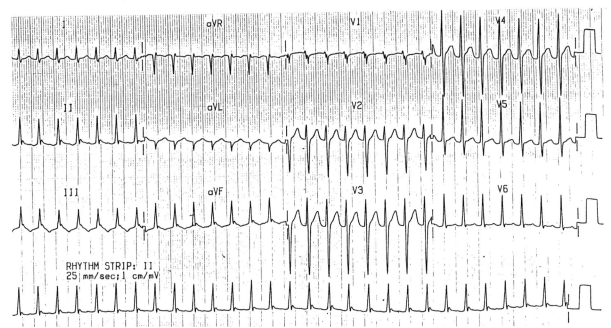

FIGURE 24-4 · Atrioventricular nodal reentrant tachycardia (AVNRT). Supraventricular tachycardia was detected in a 36-year-old man presenting with palpitations, ultimately diagnosed with AVNRT on electrophysiologic study. Note the regular, narrow QRS complex tachycardia at a rate of 180 bpm. In most cases, AVNRT cannot be distinguished from orthodromic AV reentrant tachycardia on the 12-lead ECG.

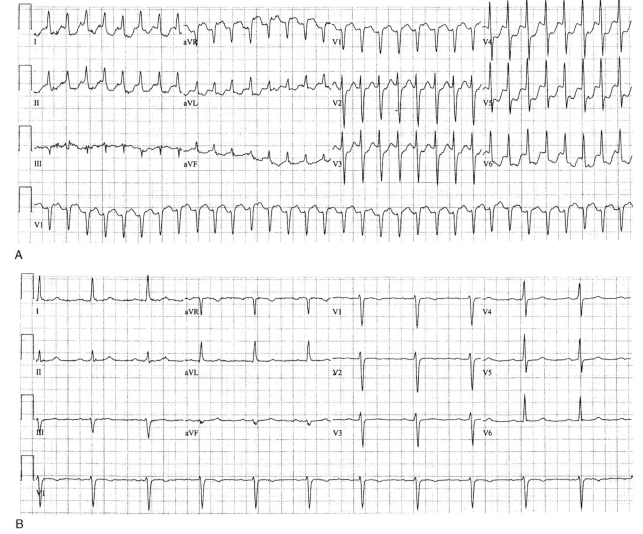

FIGURE 24-5 · Atrioventricular nodal reentrant tachycardia (AVNRT). *A,* Supraventricular tachycardia was detected in a 97-year-old woman with chest pain, later diagnosed with AVNRT. Note the regular, narrow QRS complex tachycardia at a rate of 195 bpm with ST segment depression in the anterolateral leads. *B,* After converting to sinus rhythm, the rate-related ischemic ST segment findings have resolved.

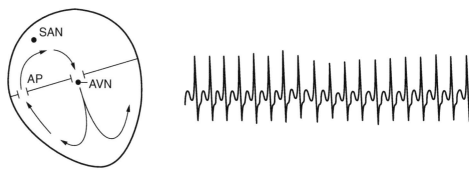

FIGURE 24-6 • Atrioventricular (AV) reentrant tachycardia with orthodromic conduction. Ventricular depolarization occurs down along the normal conduction pathway through the AV node, resulting in a narrow QRS complex tachycardia.

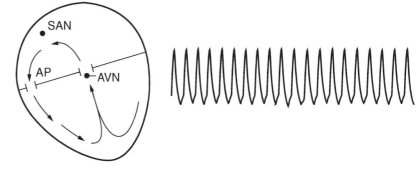

FIGURE 24-7 • Atrioventricular reentrant tachycardia with antidromic conduction. Ventricular depolarization occurs down the accessory pathway, resulting in a wide QRS complex tachycardia.

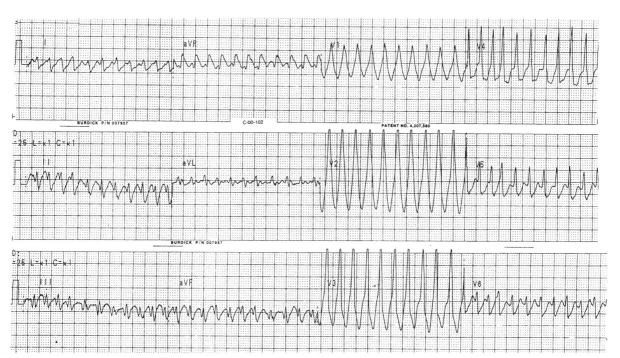

FIGURE 24-8 • Wide QRS complex tachycardia. A 20-year-old woman presented with palpitations and a regular, wide QRS complex tachycardia consistent with atrioventricular reentrant tachycardia with antidromic conduction as a result of a previously undiagnosed accessory pathway.

Antidromic conduction occurs when anterograde conduction proceeds down the accessory pathway followed by retrograde conduction back up the normal pathway (Fig. 24-7). Because the ventricles are aberrantly depolarized through the accessory pathway, a bizarre wide QRS complex tachycardia results and may be difficult to distinguish from ventricular tachycardia (VT) or AVNRT with aberrancy.

The rapid unblocked ventricular depolarization is nondecremental and presents with extremely rapid rates (Figs. 24-7 and 24-8).

Nonparoxysmal Junctional Tachycardia and Junctional Ectopic Tachycardia. These two types of AV tachydysrhythmias are very rare and have been attributed to triggers such as ischemia and digoxin toxicity or to enhanced

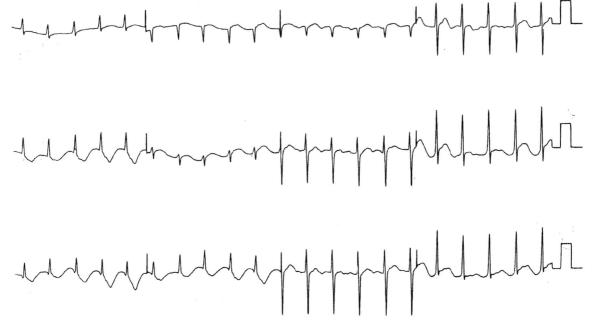

FIGURE 24-9 · Junctional tachycardia. Junctional tachycardia (or accelerated junctional rhythm) is seen in a patient presenting with acute digoxin toxicity. Note the regular, narrow QRS complex tachycardia with no discernible atrial activity.

automaticity after cardiac surgery or infarction. These two dysrhythmias are typically regular in rhythm and feature a narrow QRS complex with no visible P waves, even though AV dissociation may rarely be seen (Fig. 24-9).

Supraventricular Tachycardia with Wide QRS Complex Morphology. SVT rhythms can result in a wide QRS complex morphology in the setting of aberrancy or AVRT. This typically occurs when the supraventricular impulse must be

conducted through a preexisting or rate-dependent ventricular conduction delay. As noted earlier, a wide QRS complex morphology also occurs with AVRT with antidromic conduction (Fig. 24-10).

SVT with aberrancy may be difficult to distinguish from VT or AVRT with antidromic conduction.

The differentiation between SVT and VT in young children can be especially difficult because of the age-dependent

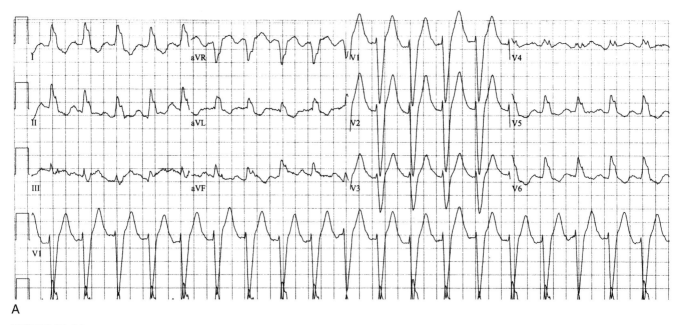

A

FIGURE 24-10 · A, Wide QRS complex tachycardia. In this wide QRS complex tachycardia, note the widened QRS complex with a regular ventricular rate of 117 bpm and left bundle branch block pattern.

Figure continues

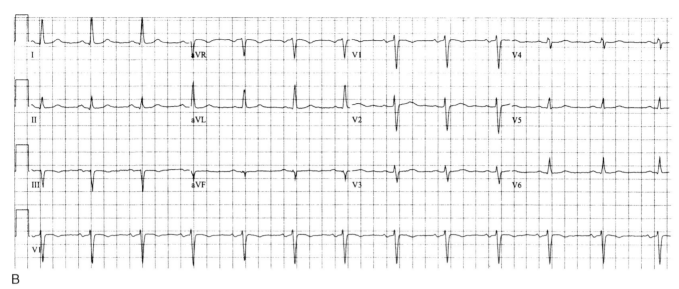

FIGURE 24-10 · *B*, Wide QRS complex tachycardia. The patient converted to normal sinus rhythm with a narrow QRS complex morphology. This presentation is consistent with supraventricular tachycardia with aberrant ventricular conduction due to rate-dependent bundle branch block.

variation in QRS complex width. For both adults and children, when the diagnosis is unclear, initial management should assume VT is present. (See Chapter 26, Ventricular Tachycardia and Ventricular Fibrillation.)

References

1. Chauhan VS, Krahn AD, Klein GJ, et al: Supraventricular tachycardia. Med Clin North Am 2001;85:193.
2. Orejarena LA, Vidaillet H, DeStevano F, et al: Paroxysmal supraventricular tachycardia in the general population. J Am Coll Cardiol 1998;31:150.
3. Pollack ML, Brady WJ, Chan TC: Electrocardiographic manifestations: Narrow QRS complex tachycardias. J Emerg Med 2003;24:35.
4. Ornato JP, Rees WA, Clark RF, et al: Treatment of paroxysmal supraventricular tachycardia in the ED by clinical decision analysis. Am J Emerg Med 1988;8:555.
5. Accardi AJ, Holmes JF: Enhanced diagnosis of narrow complex tachycardias with increased electrocardiograph speed. J Emerg Med 2002;22:123.
6. Tang CW, Van Hare GF, et al: Use of P wave configuration during atrial tachycardia to predict site of origin. J Am Coll Cardiol 1995;26:1315.
7. Kalbfleisch SJ, el-Atassi R, Calkins H, et al: Differentiation of paroxysmal narrow QRS complex tachycardias using the 12-lead electrocardiogram. J Am Coll Cardiol 1993;21:85.
8. Meldon SW, Brady WJ, Berger S, Mannebach M: Pediatric ventricular tachycardia: A report of three cases with a review of the acute diagnosis and management. Pediatr Emerg Care 1994;110:294.

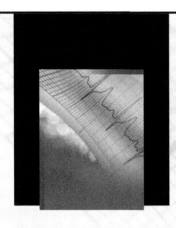

Chapter 25

Preexcitation Syndromes

John R. Lindbergh and William J. Brady

Clinical Features

Preexcitation is a phenomenon by which the ventricle is activated earlier than would be expected, had the electrical impulse traveled through the normal atrioventricular (AV) node. Preexcitation in and of itself is not a harmful condition; however, its presence allows the possibility for malignant tachycardic rhythms to emerge. There are essentially two different mechanisms for tachycardia in the presence of preexcitation. The first is a reentrant circuit, which allows reactivation of the atria earlier than would have occurred by the sinus node. The second occurs when very rapid atrial rates (as in atrial fibrillation or flutter) are transmitted to the ventricles by way of an accessory pathway (AP). The rapid activation of the ventricles by either of these mechanisms puts the patient at risk of ventricular fibrillation in the worst of cases, but in most cases it causes only transient paroxysms of tachycardia.

Wolff-Parkinson-White syndrome (WPW) is relatively uncommon, occurring in 0.1 to 3.0 per 1000 persons, more commonly in men than in women.[1,2] It is caused by the presence of accessory pathways, known as bundles of Kent, which effectively short-circuit the time-delay feature of the AV node and the slower automaticity of the sinoatrial node. Induction of a tachycardic rhythm is usually due to a premature beat of either ventricular or atrial origin, which then causes the normal pathways to be refractory to their usual direction of conduction. This allows for the possibility of abnormal reentrant circuits to emerge, resulting in a sustained tachycardia.[3] There are a multitude of tachycardia-inciting events that patients report, such as fright, anger, alcohol, belching, bending over, infection, or exercise.

Only approximately half of the patients with electrocardiographically diagnosed preexcitation have symptoms at the time of diagnosis, which can include palpitations, dizziness, shortness of breath, chest pain, and syncope. The most frequently reported type of dysrhythmia is a form of paroxysmal or reentry supraventricular tachycardia (AV reentrant tachycardia).[4]

Other Types of Preexcitation. Traditionally, patients with a shortened PR interval but a normal QRS complex duration and no delta wave, who have paroxysms of tachycardia are labeled with Lown-Ganong-Levine (LGL) syndrome. The LGL syndrome is currently thought to be an anachronism. Its existence remains unconfirmed with the advent of modern electrophysiologic studies, and no referable anatomic analog has been identified. Another variant of preexcitation, termed *Mahaim type*, typically features a normal PR interval with a delta wave.

Electrocardiographic Manifestations

Preexcitation syndromes either can be obvious, when the conventional electrocardiographic features are present, or may be quite puzzling to diagnose when more subtle manifestations occur. It is common for preexcitation to be confused with supraventricular tachycardias, myocardial infarction patterns, bundle branch blocks, and ventricular tachycardias. The electrocardiographic morphologies when the patient is in a normal sinus rhythm differ from those during the tachycardic rhythm.

ELECTROCARDIOGRAPHIC HIGHLIGHTS

Sinus rhythm ECG

- The P wave is usually normal in its morphology and axis.
- The PR interval is shortened to less than 0.12 sec.
- The QRS complex has an initial slurring (the delta wave), and is prolonged at greater than 0.12 sec.
- The T waves are frequently inverted.
- Q waves in an infarction territory pattern may occur.

Tachycardic ECG

- The rate is usually 200 to 350 bpm.
- The P wave occurs shortly after the QRS complex or is hidden in the QRS complex.
- The QRS complex looks like a normal, non-preexcited supraventricular beat in orthodromic conduction, and a wide-complex tachycardia in antidromic conduction or rapid conduction of atrial flutter and atrial fibrillation.
- The T waves are inverted.

The electrocardiogram during sinus rhythm

Rapid conduction through an AP, which bypasses the AV node, accounts for the shortened PR interval of less than 0.12 sec. This abnormally early ventricular activation is responsible for slurring of the initial portion of the QRS complex, known as the delta wave, and widening of the QRS complex to more than 0.12 sec. These three phenomena are the often-cited classic findings in WPW (Figs. 25-1, 25-2B, and 25-3). When AP conduction predominates, the PR interval is short and the delta wave is large. Conversely, when AV node conduction predominates, the PR interval is more normal and the delta wave is smaller.

Approximately 70% of patients with WPW manifest Q waves simulating a myocardial infarction pattern in an anterior, inferior, or posterior pattern (the latter as an R wave in the right precordial leads), depending on the sequence of ventricular depolarization.[4,5] This pseudoinfarction pattern due to

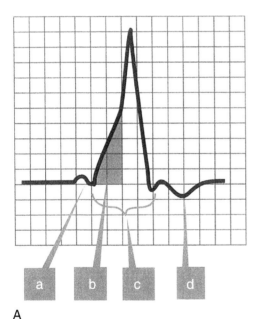

A

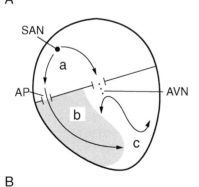

B

FIGURE 25-1 · Preexcitation during normal sinus rhythm. *A,* Classic manifestations of preexcitation during normal sinus rhythm. a, shortened PR interval (<0.12 sec); b, delta wave slurring of initial portion of QRS complex; c, QRS complex widening (>0.12 sec); d, T wave inversion due to repolarization abnormalities secondary to abnormal myocardial activation sequence. *B,* Anatomic depiction of classic manifestations of preexcitation during normal sinus rhythm. AP, accessory pathway; AVN, atrioventricular node; SAN, sinoatrial node.

a negatively deflected delta wave is seen in the inferior or anterior precordial leads (downward deflection; Fig. 25-4), or as a prominent R wave in the anterior leads (simulating posterior infarction, right bundle branch block, or right ventricular hypertrophy) (Fig. 25-3).

Rate. The heart rate is normal during nontachycardic periods.

P Wave. The P wave usually is normal in its morphology and axis.

PR Interval. The PR interval often is shortened to less than 0.12 sec; its duration is inversely related to the width of the QRS complex.

QRS Complex. The QRS complex is characterized by initial slurring, or delta wave, and is prolonged at greater than 0.12 sec. The delta wave can be subtle. In cases of unclear preexcitation, maneuvers to increase vagal tone, such as Valsalva maneuver or carotid sinus massage, have been shown to enhance conduction over the accessory pathway by decreasing AV nodal conduction, and can thus make the syndrome more electrocardiographically obvious. Adenosine has also been shown to enhance preexcitation in unclear cases.[6]

ST Segment and T Wave. The ST segment and T wave frequently demonstrate repolarization abnormalities that are thought to be secondary to the abnormal ventricular activation sequence. This usually manifests as T waves that are discordant with the QRS complex (see Fig. 25-3).

Concealed Conduction. Concealed conduction occurs when an AP is present that is refractory to antegrade conduction and therefore preexcitation, but is able to conduct in a retrograde fashion and therefore able to sustain a tachycardia. The electrocardiogram in these patients, in a normal rhythm, does not show the characteristic shortened PR interval or delta wave that is seen in most patients with WPW, hence the term *concealed* (Fig. 25-2F).

The electrocardiogram during tachycardia

Tachycardia resulting from preexcitation occurs as a result of one of two mechanisms: (1) reentrant tachycardia using the normal AV conduction system and the AP as a reentry circuit loop; or (2) rapid conduction of an atrial tachycardic rhythm through the AP to activate the ventricles.

Reentrant Tachycardias (Atrioventricular Reentrant Tachycardia). It is frequently a source of confusion that the electrocardiographic features of WPW change during the tachycardic phase, often with loss of the defining characteristics of the delta wave and the shortened PR interval, particularly with reentrant tachycardias. This occurs because there is no longer any ventricular preexcitation, and the AP now serves as one of the loops of the reentrant circuit.

Orthodromic Conduction. Orthodromic reciprocating (or reentrant) tachycardia is a reentrant rhythm that uses the AV node for antegrade conduction (hence the term *orthodromic*) to activate the ventricles, and the AP for retrograde conduction to reactivate the atria, thus completing the circuit loop (Fig. 25-2C). This type of circuit usually results in a narrow-complex tachycardia (Figs. 25-5 and 25-6).

Rate. The heart rate is quite fast, usually from 200 to more than 300 bpm.

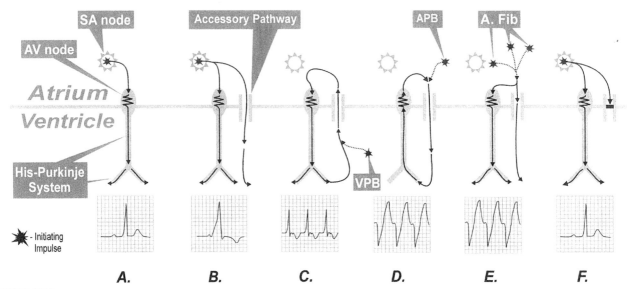

FIGURE 25-2 · **Schematic representation of preexcitation pathways and mechanisms of tachycardia.** *A,* Normal conduction through the AV node with normal ECG manifestations. *B,* Preexcitation without tachycardia with an ECG showing the classic manifestations of Wolff-Parkinson-White syndrome. *C,* Orthodromic reentrant tachycardia usually initiated by a ventricular premature beat and sustained by retrograde conduction through the accessory pathway (AP). *D,* Antidromic reentrant tachycardia using the atrioventricular node as the reentry circuit and the AP as the antegrade conduction pathway, resulting in a wide-complex tachycardia. *E,* Atrial tachycardia with rapid AP conduction, resulting in a wide-complex tachycardia. *F,* Concealed conduction in which an AP is present, but refractory to antegrade conduction, resulting in a normal resting ECG. A. Fib, atrial fibrillation; APB, atrial premature beat; VPB, ventricular premature beat.

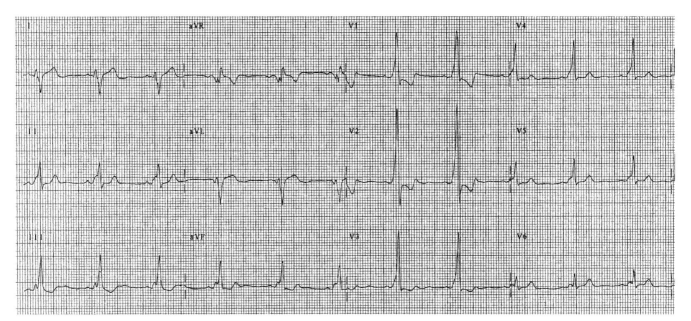

FIGURE 25-3 · **Preexcitation on sinus rhythm electrocardiogram.** Classic manifestations of preexcitation are shown in the resting ECG of a 36-year-old man with paroxysms of tachycardia. Note the shortened PR interval, prominent delta waves in the anterior and inferior leads, and T wave inversion in leads V₁ and V₃.

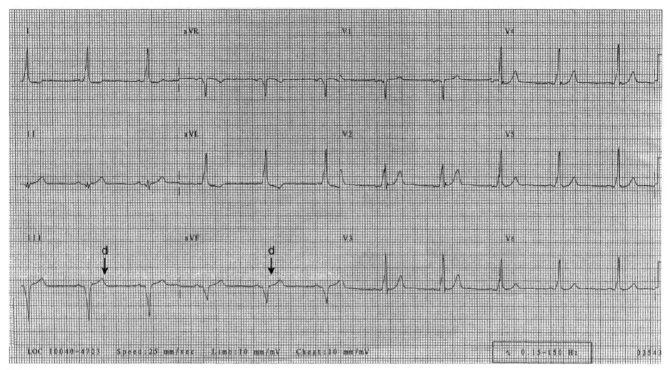

FIGURE 25-4 · **Pseudoinfarction pattern of Wolff-Parkinson-White syndrome (WPW).** The pseudoinfarction pattern of WPW mimics an inferior myocardial infarction with Q waves in leads II, III, and aVF. These Q waves are caused by negatively deflected delta waves (d).

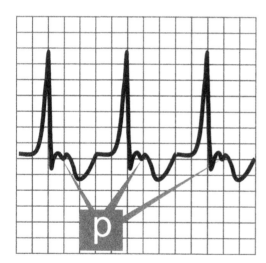

FIGURE 25-5 · **Orthodromic reentry tachycardia.** Orthodromic reentry tachycardia is the most common of the paroxysmal tachycardias seen in Wolff-Parkinson-White syndrome. Note that the delta wave is no longer present, and that the P wave appears shortly after the QRS complex in a retrograde fashion (p).

P Wave.   The P wave usually appears shortly after the QRS complex or may be hidden in it.

QRS Complex.   The QRS complex resembles a normal, non-preexcited supraventricular beat. The characteristic delta wave is absent because the preexcitation pathway is now being occupied by the reentrant circuit. If there is no pre-existing bundle branch block, the QRS complex should appear narrow.

ST Segment and T Wave.   T waves are usually inverted, and the ST segments may be depressed.

Antidromic Conduction.   Antidromic reciprocating (or reentrant) tachycardia is much less common than orthodromic conduction and occurs in approximately 5% of patients with WPW. In antidromic conduction, the AP provides the antegrade impulse pathway for the activation of the ventricles (hence the term *antidromic*), and the AV node provides the reentrant pathway to reactivate the atria (Fig. 25-2D). Ventricular activation through the AP rather than the normal conduction system results in a wide QRS complex tachycardia (Fig. 25-7).

Atrial Tachycardias with Accessory Pathway Conduction.   Tachycardia can also result when atrial tachycardic rhythms are conducted through the AP, resulting in rapid activation of the ventricles. This can occur when atrial fibrillation or flutter emerges in the presence of an AP. These rapid atrial rates can then be rapidly conducted to the ventricle by way of the AP, bypassing the inherent time delay feature of the AV node (Fig. 25-2E). This type of conduction also results in a

---

ELECTROCARDIOGRAPHIC PEARLS

- The ECG morphology differs in normal sinus rhythm and tachycardic rhythms. Preexcitation may be intermittent, either beat-to-beat or some other period of time (Fig. 25-9).
- Narrow-complex tachycardias usually result from orthodromic conduction.
- Wide-complex tachycardias usually result from antidromic conduction, or from the rapid conduction of atrial tachycardias through the accessory pathway.
- In concealed conduction, patients may have preexcitation and have a perfectly normal resting ECG.

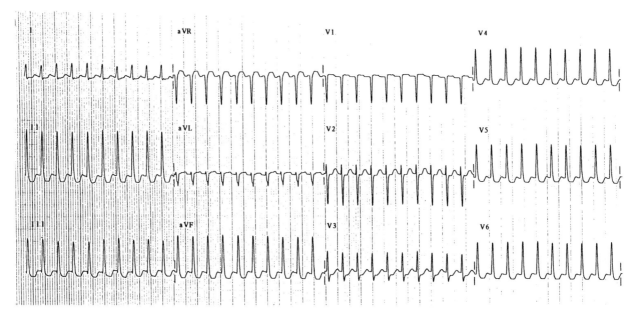

FIGURE 25-6 · **Orthodromic reentry tachycardia.** This electrocardiogram shows orthodromic reentry tachycardia with a rate of approximately 250 bpm. This rhythm exhibits regular, narrow complexes and the absence of discernible P waves.

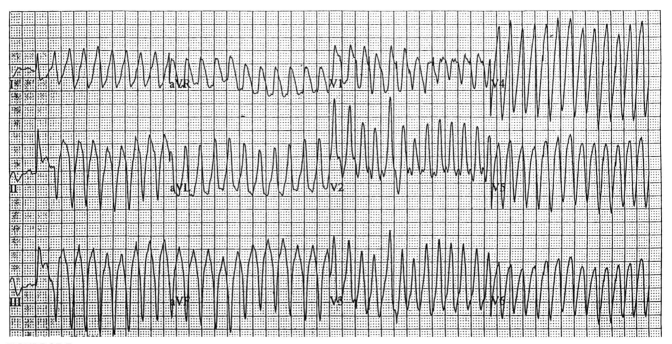

FIGURE 25-7 · **Antidromic reentry tachycardia.** This electrocardiogram shows antidromic reentry tachycardia with a rate of approximately 300 bpm. Note the wide-complex regular tachycardia.

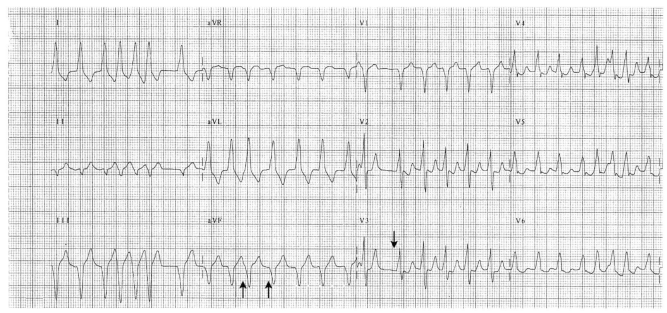

FIGURE 25-8 • Atrial fibrillation. Atrial fibrillation is demonstrated in this ECG from a 47-year-old patient with known Wolff-Parkinson-White syndrome, who presented with a rapid, wide QRS complex irregular tachycardia. *Arrows* denote delta waves.

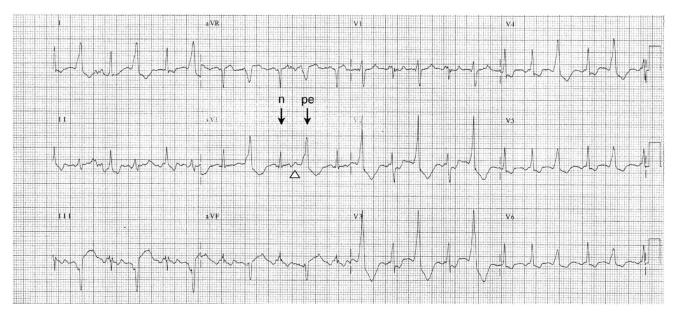

FIGURE 25-9 • Bigeminal rhythm. This ECG is from a 74-year-old man with known Wolff-Parkinson-White syndrome who developed this bigeminal rhythm with alternating normal beats (n) and preexcited beats (pe). *Open arrowhead* denotes the P wave preceding the preexcited beat.

wide-complex tachycardia because normal activation of the ventricles is bypassed (Fig. 25-8). Atrioventricular node blocking agents should be avoided in patients with known or suspected preexcitation and wide QRS complex tachycardia because of the risk of increasing AV conduction block and precipitating or increasing conduction through the AP.

References

1. Rosner MH, Brady WJ, Kefer MP, Martin ML: Electrocardiography in the patient with the Wolff-Parkinson-White syndrome: Diagnostic and initial therapeutic issues. Am J Emerg Med 1999;17:705.

2. Herbert M, Tully G: Wolff-Parkinson-White Syndrome. eMed J 2001;2:8.

3. Wellens HJJ: Paroxysmal supraventricular tachycardia, including Wolff-Parkinson-White syndrome. In Kastor JA (ed): Arrhythmias. Philadelphia, WB Saunders, 2000, p 198.

4. Al-Khatib SM, Pritchett LC: Clinical features of Wolff-Parkinson-White syndrome. Am Heart J 1999;138:403.

5. Vukmir RB: Cardiac arrhythmia diagnosis. Am J Emerg Med 1995;13:2.

6. Xie B, Thakur RK, Shah CP, Hoon VK: Emergency management of cardiac arrhythmias: Clinical differentiation of narrow QRS complex tachycardia. Emerg Med Clin North Am 1998;16:295.

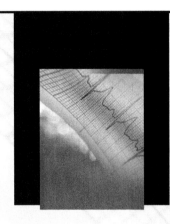

Chapter 26

Ventricular Tachycardia and Ventricular Fibrillation

Sharone Jensen and Sarah A. Stahmer

Clinical Features

Eight of 10 patients presenting with a wide-complex tachycardia (QRS complex >120 msec with a ventricular rate >100 bpm) are diagnosed with ventricular tachycardia (VT). If the patient has a history of coronary artery disease, the incidence increases to 95%.[1-3] Careful inspection of the 12-lead electrocardiogram (ECG) allows correct determination of the diagnosis in approximately 90% of patients.[4,5] Despite this fact, VT is frequently misinterpreted as being supraventricular tachycardia (SVT) with aberrancy. Common errors include the assumption that VT cannot be "narrow" or occur in an awake or stable patient as well as lack of familiarity with ECG criteria for VT.[4,6,7] Both SVT and VT can cause hemodynamic instability, and a common mistake is to assume a stable rhythm is SVT with aberrancy and an unstable rhythm is VT.[5-7]

VT is frequently encountered as a complication of coronary artery disease because of active ischemia or presence of chronic scar tissue, both of which can create substrates for ventricular dysrhythmias. Patients with cardiomyopathies, particularly the idiopathic dilated type, are the second largest group of patients at risk. Rarely, VT can also occur in healthy individuals or may be the first indication of organic heart disease, such as right ventricular dysplasia. Medications, particularly some antidysrhythmic therapies, can be proarrhythmic under certain clinical conditions, and give rise to ventricular dysrhythmias. These include digoxin, type I antidysrhythmics, phenothiazines, tricyclic antidysrhythmics, and sympathomimetics. Medications that cause prolongation of the QT interval can generate a specific polymorphic form of VT known as *torsades de pointes*. Finally, severe or acute electrolyte imbalances, particularly hypokalemia and hyperkalemia, can give rise to VT.

The mechanisms responsible for initiation and maintenance of VT are reentry, enhanced automaticity, and triggered activity. Reentry is the most common mechanism, consisting of the following characteristics: (1) two functionally distinct conduction pathways with different conduction velocities and refractory periods; (2) a unidirectional block in one pathway; and (3) slower conduction down the other pathway. Reentry circuits can develop as a result of ischemia, myocardial scarring,

infiltrative disease, metabolic derangements, or adverse affects of medications.[1,3]

Electrocardiographic Manifestations

The 12-lead ECG is critical to determining the etiology of a wide-complex tachycardia. A number of decision rules have been proposed attempting to aid in the diagnosis of VT. The criteria vary in their reliability when applied individually and must be interpreted in conjunction with the other criteria, the patient's clinical presentation, medical history, and old ECGs when available.[4,5,8-10]

Atrioventricular Dissociation. Dissociation between atrial and ventricular activity during a wide-complex tachycardia is the hallmark of VT. During VT, the sinus node continues

---

ELECTROCARDIOGRAPHIC HIGHLIGHTS

- QRS width >0.14 sec in right bundle branch block (RBBB) and >0.16 sec in left bundle branch block (LBBB)
- Atrioventricular dissociation
- Capture or fusion beats
- Precordial QRS complex concordance
- Axis: −90 degrees to +180 degrees
- QRS configuration
  - No RS in any lead
  - Lead V_1 positive (RBBB type):
    V_1: Monophasic or biphasic
        Triphasic with taller left peak (RSr')
        QR or RS complex
    V_6: R:S ratio <1 in lead V_6
  - Lead V_1 negative (LBBB type):
    Right axis deviation
    V_1: r wave in lead V_1 >0.03 sec in duration
        Duration from the start of the r wave to nadir of
          S wave = 0.06 sec
        Slurred downstroke to nadir of S wave
    V_6: QR or QS pattern
        S wave or QS amplitude >15 mm deep

---

to create impulses, which are usually blocked at the level of the atrioventricular (AV) node by retrograde ventricular activation from the ectopic ventricular pacemaker. The sinus rate is usually slower than the ventricular rate, which explains why few beats that originate in the atrium are conducted into the ventricle—the ectopic foci keep the AV node or infranodal tissue electrically "busy" and therefore unable to conduct. The atrial and ventricular pacemakers are independent of one another, and clear evidence of this on the ECG is diagnostic of VT. AV dissociation (Fig. 26-1) is more readily appreciated when the rate of ventricular tachycardia is slow. Although highly specific, AV dissociation is seen too infrequently (<25% of patients with confirmed VT) to be helpful in the majority of undifferentiated wide-complex tachycardias.[4,5,9]

When P waves are clearly seen, the lack of relationship between atrial and ventricular beats must be demonstrated before true AV dissociation can be diagnosed. Ventricular beats can be conducted retrograde into the atria, and has been observed in up to 50% of patients with confirmed VT.[4,8] The retrograde beats give rise to P waves, which may be matched in a one-to-one fashion to the QRS complexes, or intermittent because of retrograde AV nodal block.

Capture and Fusion Beats. The key to interpretation of wide-complex dysrhythmias may be found when a break occurs in the rhythm pattern. One example is the appearance of a narrow complex in the midst of a run of wide-complex tachycardia. This interruption is usually due to a supraventricular beat that is successfully conducted, *capturing* the ventricle. Although rare, capture beats are extremely helpful in confirming the presence of VT (Fig. 26-2).

Fusion beats represent partial capture of the ventricles at the same time a ventricular ectopic beat fires. The resultant QRS complex is intermediate, or *fused*, in appearance between the ectopic ventricular beat and the "normal" QRS complex (Fig. 26-3). Both capture and fusion beats are more likely to be seen in slower VT rhythms.

QRS Complex Width. The duration of the QRS complexes is usually 0.12 sec or longer owing to the abnormal pattern of ventricular activation. The further the focus is from the normal pathways of activation, the more bizarre and wide the complexes. In general, the combination of QRS complex width and morphology can provide clues to the diagnosis of VT. A QRS complex width greater than 0.14 sec with a right bundle branch block (RBBB) morphology (lead V_1 positive), or greater than 0.16 sec with a left bundle branch block (LBBB) morphology (lead V_1 negative) suggests VT.

There is significant overlap in QRS complex widths among patients with SVT and VT, particularly those on antidysrhythmic medications or with underlying BBB.[4,8] In addition, if the focus is high in the septum, the resultant QRS complex may be relatively narrow, leading to erroneous diagnosis of SVT. The QRS complex width alone cannot be used reliably to exclude the diagnosis of VT, and must be interpreted in the context of other findings.

Regularity. The rhythm in monomorphic VT is generally regular. There may be some initial irregularity, with the average difference in cycle lengths being 127 ± 72 msec.[11] This degree of variability usually persists for the first few beats and then resolves. Gross, sustained irregularity suggests the source of the rhythm is supraventricular, likely atrial fibrillation.

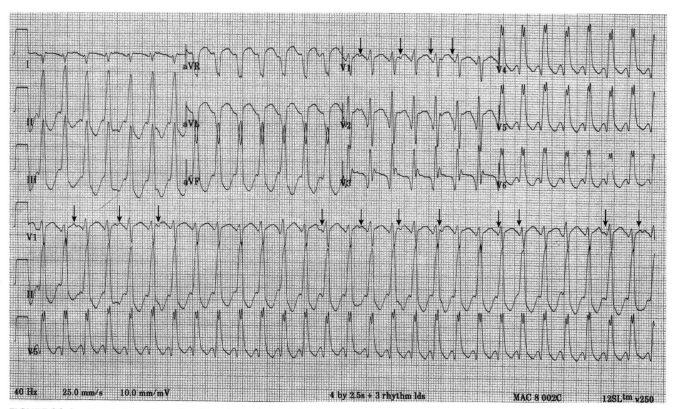

FIGURE 26-1 • **Ventricular tachycardia with atrioventricular (AV) dissociation.** *Arrows* indicate P wave activity unrelated to the QRS complex consistent with AV dissociation.

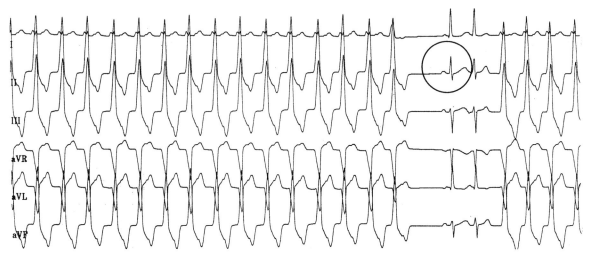

FIGURE 26-2 · Ventricular tachycardia with capture beats (*circle*).

Frequent capture or fusion beats can also make the rhythm appear irregular, particularly in slow ventricular dysrhythmias.

Ventricular Rate. The ventricular rate in VT is usually between 140 and 200 bpm. Slower VT may be seen in patients taking various cardioactive medications, particularly amiodarone (Fig. 26-4). Slower rates, less than 110 bpm, are referred to as *accelerated idioventricular rhythms*. These rhythms are typically associated with reperfusion in acute myocardial infarction (MI). Rates greater than 200 bpm may resemble a sine wave, and are referred to as *ventricular flutter* (Fig. 26-5). Ventricular rate alone does not differentiate VT from SVT with aberrancy.

QRS Axis. The axis of the ventricular depolarization reflects the site of abnormal activation. Any portion of the ventricle can be the site of an ectopic pacemaker; as such, the axis in

VT is subsequently highly variable. The more "abnormal" the axis, the more likely the dysrhythmia focus is ventricular. Left axis deviation is the most common axis deviation seen in VT, but is clearly not unique to VT.[8,12] The only axis that is specific for VT is the extreme or superior axis (−90 degrees to +180 degrees), which is more commonly seen in patients who have had a previous MI.[13] A negative QRS complex in leads I and aVF easily identifies a QRS axis in this quadrant, which indicates an ectopic site located at or near the apex of the heart conducting toward the base of the heart. Patients with idiopathic (nonischemic) VT are more likely to have a normal QRS complex axis.[12,14]

Concordance. This term refers to the precordial QRS complex axes and describes the interlead relationship of the axes across the precordial leads. During normal sinus rhythm, the QRS complex axis varies in direction from lead V_1 through lead V_6 (from predominantly negative to predominantly positive). Concordance is defined as the QRS axis in the precordial leads V_1 through V_6 being either all negative (negative concordance) or all positive (positive concordance). Concordance is highly suggestive of VT. Positive concordance results from ventricular activation originating in the posterobasal region of the left ventricle. This pattern can be seen in patients with VT, but can also be seen in patients conducting anterograde down an accessory pathway, which inserts into the posterobasal portion of the left ventricle. Negative concordance results from ventricular activation originating in the anteroapical portion of the left ventricle. In rare cases, LBBB with a marked left axis deviation may result in negative concordance. In one study of patients with wide-complex tachycardias, 22% of patients with VT had either positive (12%) (Fig. 26-6A) or negative (10%) concordance[4] (Fig. 26-6B).

QRS Complex Morphology. The appearance of the QRS complex in VT depends on the origin of the ectopic beat. If the ectopic pacemaker site is in the right ventricle, the QRS complex resembles an LBBB because the left ventricle is initially activated from the right. Left-sided activation has an RBBB appearance. The activation sites are usually distant from the His bundle, so the resultant patterns vary from the usual LBBB or RBBB patterns seen in supraventricular rhythms.

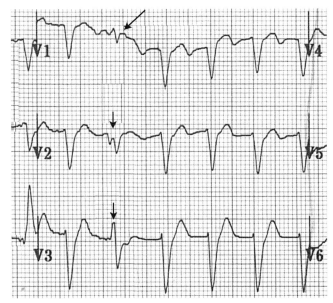

FIGURE 26-3 · **A 57-year-old man with chest pain and lightheadedness.** The QRS complex width is greater than 0.14 sec with fairly typical left bundle branch block pattern. The key to identification of ventricular tachycardia in this ECG is the presence of fusion beat (*arrows*).

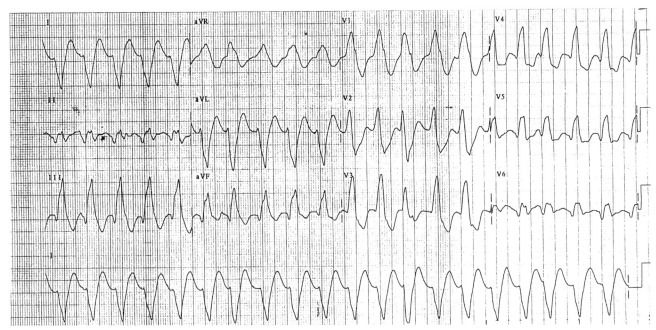

FIGURE 26-4 · **A 62-year-old woman with recent myocardial infarction on amiodarone.** Note the rate of 123 bpm, a relatively slow rate resulting from amiodarone therapy. The QRS width is greater than 0.14 sec. Right axis deviation and positive QRS complex concordance are noted. A monophasic QRS complex is seen in lead V_1.

QRS complexes originating from the apex of the heart look unlike either BBB pattern, have a superior axis, and give rise to mostly negative forces in the precordial leads. In general, the more peripheral the site of activation, the more aberrant and atypical the complex. For the sake of simplicity, QRS morphology is discussed in terms of lead V_1–positive VT and lead V_1–negative VT. QRS complexes that have an indeterminate axis in lead V_1 are more likely to be VT.

A positive QRS complex in lead V_1 implies a left-sided ectopic focus and the morphology can provide important clues to the diagnosis of VT. A monophasic or biphasic RBBB-type QRS complex in lead V_1 is highly suggestive of VT (Fig. 26-4). Patients with a triphasic complex in lead V_1 (rSR′) are more likely to have an SVT with RBBB aberrancy, but reversal of the pattern (RSr′, the "reversed rabbit ears") is seen only in patients with VT[1,5,8,15,16] (Fig. 26-7). It must be emphasized that a "normal"-appearing RBBB pattern does not exclude the diagnosis of VT. When confronted by a triphasic QRS complex morphology, inspection of lead V_6 is often

helpful. Typically in aberrancy, the complex in lead V_6 starts with a Q wave followed by a tall R wave and a wide S wave, reflecting delayed activation of the right side of the heart. An R/S ratio of less than one or a QS complex in lead V_6 is not seen in RBBB aberrancy and supports the diagnosis of VT[1,5,8,15,16] (Fig. 26-8).

Lead V_1–negative QRS complexes and LBBB morphologies are common in wide-complex tachycardias and VT. Close inspection of the QRS morphology and frontal lead axis is helpful in identifying those patients with VT. The presence of an R wave in lead V_1 or V_2 greater than 0.03 sec in duration is highly suggestive of VT and not normally not seen in SVT with LBBB aberrancy.[10,15] The presence of any Q wave in lead V_6 also suggests VT.[5,8,12] In SVT with aberrancy with LBBB morphology, the downstroke of the S wave in lead V_1 is usually rapid and smooth. In VT, the duration from the onset of the QRS complex to the nadir of the S wave in leads V_1 or V_2 is often greater than 0.06 sec. The longer the measured duration, the more likely is the diagnosis of VT. Further inspection of the S wave may also reveal notching on the downstroke in lead V_1 or V_2, which is also highly suggestive of VT[4,5,10,12] (Figs. 26-9 and 26-10).

Absence of RS complexes in any of the precordial leads has been proposed by some to be virtually diagnostic of VT[5,9] (Fig. 26-11). Brugada and colleagues proposed a four-step algorithm using the ability to identify RS complexes as the initial decision point. If RS complexes are present, then the R-to-S interval is measured; if the time from onset of the R wave to the nadir of the S wave is greater than 0.10 sec, then VT is the likely diagnosis. If none of the preceding criteria is met, the ECG is examined for two other features: evidence of AV dissociation and morphologic criteria in leads V_1 and V_6 (as noted previously). Although this algorithm has reported sensitivity and specificity of 99% and 97%, respectively, when applied retrospectively by emergency physicians, it has performed less favorably.[5,6,17]

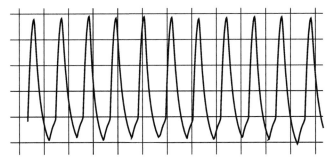

FIGURE 26-5 · **Ventricular flutter.** Rhythm strip demonstrates continuous sine wave configuration at a rate of approximately 300 bpm with no distinction between QRS complex, ST segment, and T wave.

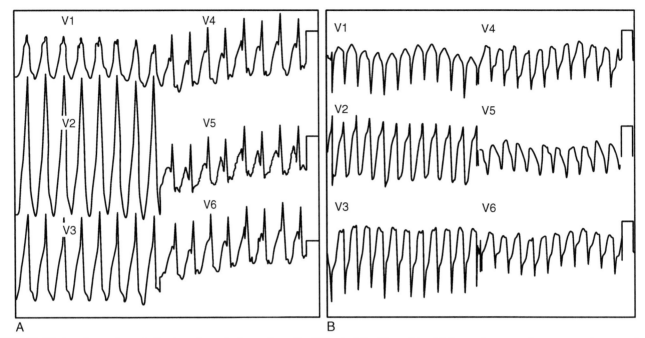

FIGURE 26-6 · **Concordance indicative of ventricular tachycardia (VT).** *A,* VT with positive QRS complex concordance across the precordium. *B,* VT with negative QRS complex concordance across the precordium.

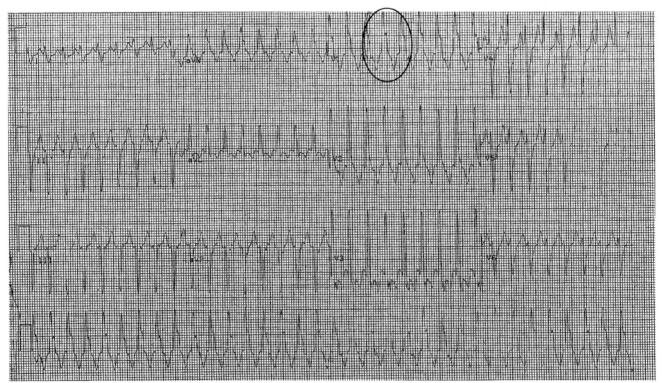

FIGURE 26-7 · **A 53-year-old man involved in a motor vehicle accident after experiencing a syncopal event.** The QRS complex width is greater than 160 msec in a lead V₁–positive pattern. There is reversal of the "rabbit ears" in lead V₁, with the first ear larger (RSr′; *circle*). The R/S ratio in lead V₆ is less than 1.

Specific Types of Ventricular Tachycardia

Right Ventricular Outflow Tract Ventricular Tachycardia. This form of VT is seen in patients without underlying heart disease. Impulses originate from or near the right ventricular outflow tract, and typically result in an LBBB morphology and right inferior axis (Fig. 26-12).

Ventricular Tachycardia in the Setting of a Preexisting Bundle Branch Block. Many of the various morphologic criteria for VT are present in patients with preexisting BBB. This scenario may confound the use of the ECG in diagnosing VT—unless an old ECG is available. One study examined patients with BBB in sinus rhythm, and identified five criteria for VT that were not present in the patients

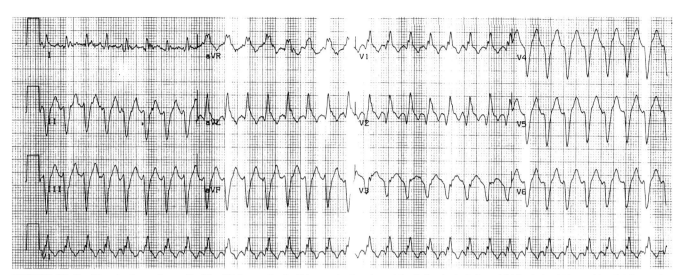

FIGURE 26-8 • **Ventricular tachycardia.** The QRS complex is 124 msec in duration with a left axis deviation. A biphasic lead V$_1$–positive QRS complex with "typical" right bundle branch block pattern is seen.

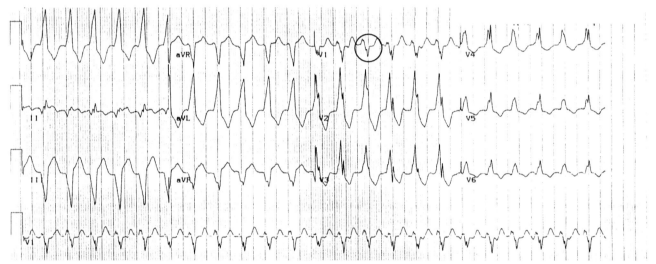

FIGURE 26-9 • **Ventricular tachycardia with notching of the downstroke of the S wave in lead V$_1$** (*circle*).

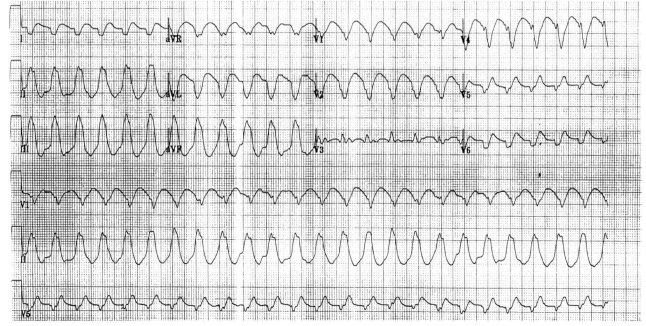

FIGURE 26-10 • **Ventricular tachycardia.** The QRS complex width is greater than 160 msec with right axis deviation. Notching of the downstroke of the S wave is clearly seen in leads V$_1$ and V$_2$, as is the delay from onset of R to S nadir.

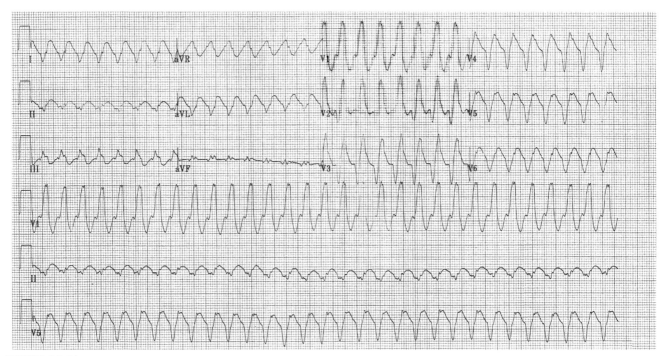

FIGURE 26-11 • **Ventricular tachycardia.** The QRS complex width is greater than 140 msec in lead V$_1$, which is positive. The axis is superior with no RS complexes seen in the precordial leads.

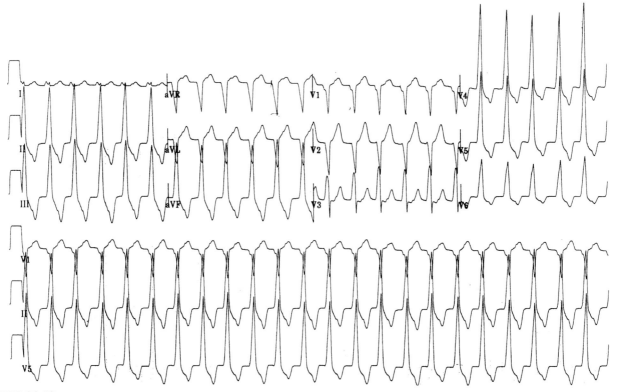

FIGURE 26-12 • **Right ventricular outflow tract ventricular tachycardia (VT).** This rhythm strip demonstrates right ventricular outflow tract VT with typical left bundle branch block morphology and right inferior axis.

with supraventricular rhythm and BBB, including:[18]

1. RSr′ or Rr′ pattern in lead V_1 in setting of RBBB
2. QS, QR, or R pattern in lead V_6 in the presence of an RBBB
3. Any Q wave in lead V_6 in the presence of an LBBB
4. Concordance in precordial leads
5. Absence of RS complex in all precordial leads

Torsades de Pointes.   Torsades de pointes (TdP) is a rapid form of polymorphic VT that is characterized by beat-to-beat variability in the QRS complexes, which vary in both amplitude and polarity. The resultant QRS complexes appear to "twist" around the isoelectric line. A prerequisite for the rhythm is baseline prolongation of the QT interval, which may be congenital or acquired, such as can occur with medications (type Ia antidysrhythmics) and electrolyte imbalances (hypokalemia, hypomagnesemia). TdP is initiated by a series of ectopic beats that begin with a premature ventricular beat

or salvo of ventricular beats, followed by a pause, and then a supraventricular beat. Another premature ventricular beat arrives at a relatively short coupling interval and falls on the preceding T wave, precipitating the rhythm.

TdP is usually paroxysmal in nature and the underlying rhythm and intervals can be identified during "breaks" in the rhythm. Typically, 5 to 20 complexes are seen in each cycle; the rhythm may either self-terminate or degenerate into ventricular fibrillation. The ventricular rate is usually between 200 and 250 bpm, and the amplitude of the QRS complexes varies in a sinusoidal pattern (Fig. 26-13). The baseline ECG usually provides important clues to diagnosis, including corrected QT interval prolongation and ST segment and T wave changes related to the underlying metabolic abnormality (Fig. 26-14).

Polymorphic Ventricular Tachycardia (Normal QRS).   This form of VT often appears similar to TdP, with the important difference being the absence of QT prolongation. Patients with

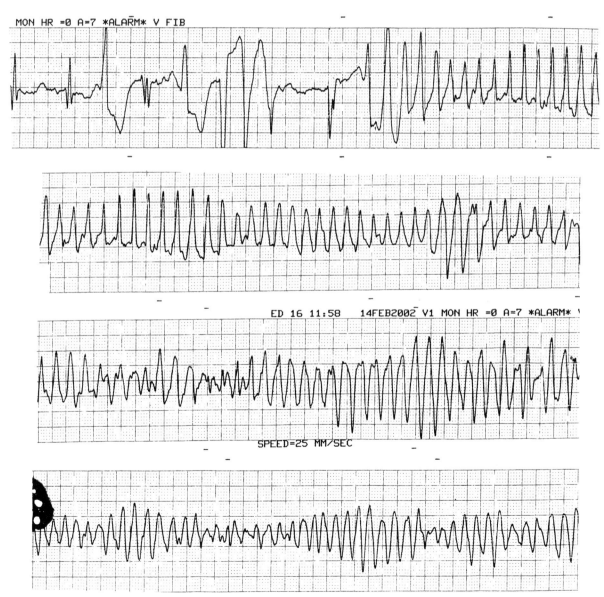

FIGURE 26-13 • Torsades des pointes. This rhythm strip demonstrates the initiation of torsades des pointes by a series of ectopic beats that begin with a premature ventricular beat or salvo of ventricular beats, followed by a pause, and then a supraventricular beat. Another premature ventricular beat arrives at a relatively short coupling interval and falls on the preceding T wave, precipitating the rhythm. The baseline corrected QT interval was 0.64 sec.

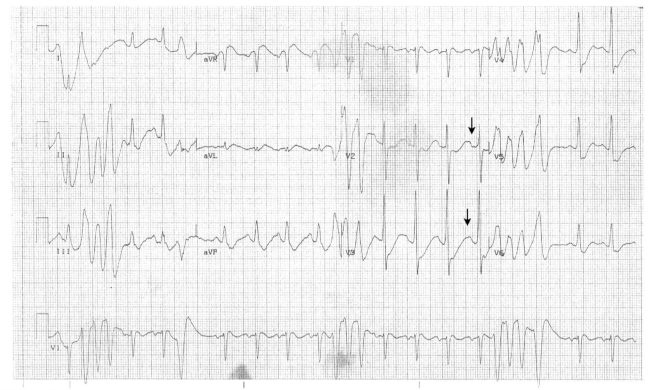

FIGURE 26-14 • **Polymorphic ventricular tachycardias with hypokalemia.** Paroxysms of multifocal ventricular ectopy are seen in this ECG from a patient with a serum potassium of 1.9 mEq/dL. Note the ST segment depression and "giant" U waves (*arrows*).

this rhythm are often found to have unstable coronary artery disease, and acute coronary ischemia is thought to be an important prerequisite for this dysrhythmia[1,19] (see Fig. 26-14).

Ventricular Flutter/Fibrillation. Both ventricular flutter and fibrillation are fatal unless terminated abruptly. The ECG in flutter appears as a continuous sine wave, with no distinction between the QRS complex, ST segment, and T waves (see Fig. 26-5). Ventricular fibrillation is unmistakable—the complexes are chaotic and irregular, without discrete QRS complexes (Fig. 26-15). The patient is always unconscious because this rhythm is unable to generate synchronous ventricular contractions.

Digoxin-Toxic Fascicular Tachycardia. This unusual form of ventricular tachycardia is usually a monomorphic VT that has a relatively narrow QRS and can be mistaken for SVT. It can also present as a bidirectional tachycardia, where the QRS usually has a baseline RBBB morphology and alternates its electrical axis with alternating beats. This VT subtype is thought to be due to alternating block in anterior and posterior fascicles of the left bundle branch.

Brugada Syndrome. Brugada and Brugada described a syndrome that was associated with sudden death in individuals with a structurally normal heart and no evidence of atherosclerotic coronary disease.[20] Patients with this syndrome,

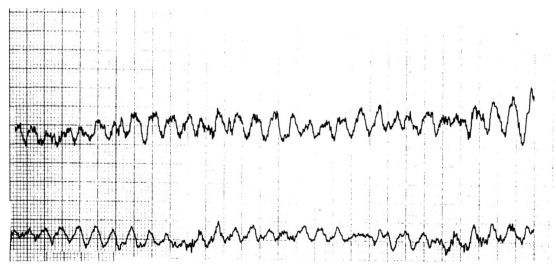

FIGURE 26-15 • **Ventricular fibrillation.** Ventricular fibrillation is characterized by chaotic, irregular complexes without discrete QRS complex morphology.

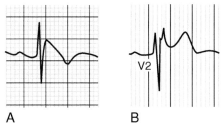

FIGURE 26-16 · **Brugada syndrome.** *A,* The convex-type ST segment elevation. *B,* The saddle-type ST segment elevation with concave morphology.

known as the Brugada syndrome, were noted to have a distinct set of ECG abnormalities, characterized by an incomplete or complete RBBB pattern with ST segment elevation in the right precordial leads[21] (Fig. 26-16*A* and *B*). Patients with the Brugada syndrome have unpredictable episodes of ventricular tachycardia (most commonly polymorphic).[21] These patients may present with self-terminating episodes of ventricular tachycardia manifested as syncope or near-syncope. Alternatively, patients with persistent dysrhythmia present with ventricular fibrillation. Untreated, the natural history of the syndrome is ominous, with an associated mortality rate of 20% at 2 years.[21]

ECG abnormalities that suggest the diagnosis were first described by Brugada and Brugada,[21] when it was noted that patients with sudden death or aborted sudden death had ECGs with RBBB and ST segment elevation in leads V_1 to V_3.[20] The RBBB pattern may be complete or incomplete.[22–24] Two types of ST segment elevation morphologies have been described in the right precordial leads: convex (see Fig. 26-16*A*) and concave[22,23,25] (saddle type; see Fig. 26-16*B*).

Differentiating Ventricular Tachycardia from Other Causes of Wide QRS Complex Tachycardia

Distinguishing the cause of a wide QRS complex tachycardia may be problematic. Potential causes include:

- Supraventricular tachycardia with preexisting bundle branch block
- Supraventricular tachycardia with aberrant ventricular conduction
- Preexcited (Wolff-Parkinson-White syndrome–related) supraventricular tachycardia

- Metabolic derangement–related wide QRS complex tachycardia
- Toxin-related wide QRS complex tachycardia
- Pacemaker-mediated tachycardia

Clues to the presence of an SVT with preexisting BBB are the "typical" appearance of the QRS complex with duration less than 0.14 sec and an axis within the normal range. Triphasic complexes in lead V_1–positive rhythms are highly suggestive of SVT with aberrancy, although *reversal* of the rSR′ (left "rabbit ear" greater than right "rabbit ear," i.e., RSr′) is seen only in VT. SVTs with LBBB patterns are more likely to have a rapid downstroke from the onset of the QRS complex to the nadir of the S wave (<0.06 sec). The most useful finding is the presence of a BBB with identical appearance on an old ECG.

The likelihood that a beat will be conducted aberrantly depends on the proceeding cycle length and underlying rhythm. SVT with aberrant ventricular conduction is often seen in irregular rhythms such as atrial fibrillation, where a beat with a short R-R interval is aberrantly conducted if it follows a beat with a longer R-R interval (Ashman's phenomenon). This finding is due to the fact that the ventricular refractory period is set on a beat-to-beat basis, with longer cycle lengths having longer refractory periods. Most aberrantly conducted beats have an RBBB appearance because the right bundle is both longer and more slowly conducting.[5,26] The appearance of the aberrantly conducted beat

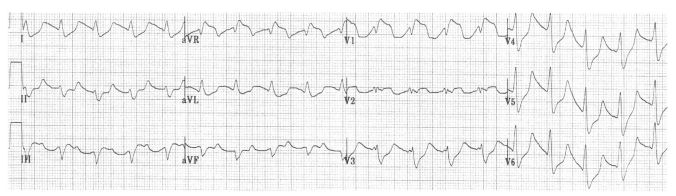

FIGURE 26-17 · **Hyperkalemia.** In this rhythm strip, hyperkalemia is causing marked prolongation of the QRS complex greater than 0.14 sec. The relatively "slow" ventricular rates and peaked T waves in leads V_4 to V_6 are clues to the correct diagnosis.

is similar to a fixed BBB, the axis is within normal range, and the rate is determined by the underlying supraventricular rhythm. Rate-related aberrancy depends on demonstration of the "widest" beat occurring at the shortest cycle length.

The ECG appearance of tachycardias conducting anterograde down a bypass track can be readily confused with VT. These tachycardias are often rapid and wide and may demonstrate concordance, which is almost always positive because of the basal-to-apical direction of ventricular conduction. Monophasic and biphasic QRS complexes are common in both RBBB and LBBB patterns, making differentiation from VT based on QRS morphology alone difficult. Prior history of tachyarrhythmias in a younger patient, response to vagal maneuvers, and an old ECG showing shortened PR intervals and delta waves are all helpful. Bypass tracts in the setting of atrial fibrillation can be readily identified by the irregular rhythm, extremely rapid ventricular rate, varying beat-to-beat QRS complex appearance, and often the narrowest QRS complex at the shortest R-R interval.

Electrolyte abnormalities that prolong conduction in the ventricles can give rise to rhythms that can be mistaken for VT. Hyperkalemia, in particular, can create significant prolongations in the QRS complex, which give the appearance of a ventricular origin of the rhythm. Clues to the diagnosis include a slower ventricular rate because the rhythm is still sinus, diffuse QRS complex widening, and prominent S waves in lead I and the left precordial leads[16] (Fig. 26-17).

References

1. Akhtar M: Clinical spectrum of ventricular tachycardia. Circulation 1990;82:1561.
2. Munger TM: Ventricular tachycardia electrocardiographic diagnosis (including aberration) and management. In Murphy JG (ed): Mayo Clinic Cardiology Review. Armonk, NY, Futura, 1997, pp 457–466.
3. Gupta AK, Thakur RK: Wide QRS complex tachycardias. Med Clin North Am 2001;85:245.
4. Akhtar M, Shenasa M, Jazayeri M, et al: Wide QRS complex tachycardia: Reappraisal of a common clinical problem. Ann Intern Med 1988;109:905.
5. Drew BJ, Scheinman MM: ECG criteria to distinguish between aberrantly conducted supraventricular tachycardia and ventricular tachycardia: Practical aspects for the immediate care setting. Pacing Clin Electrophysiol 1995;18:2194.
6. Herbert ME, Votey SR, Mortan MT, et al: Failure to agree on the electrocardiographic diagnosis of ventricular tachycardia. Ann Emerg Med 1996;27:35.
7. Stewart RB, Bardy GH, Greene HL: Wide complex tachycardia: Misdiagnosis and outcome after emergent therapy. Ann Intern Med 1986;104:766.
8. Wellens HJJ, Bar FWHM, Lie KI: The value of the electrocardiogram in the differential diagnosis of a tachycardia with a widened QRS complex. Am J Med 1978;64:27.
9. Brugada P, Brugada J, Mont L, et al: A new approach to the differential diagnosis of a regular tachycardia with a wide QRS complex. Circulation 1991;83:1649.
10. Kindwall KE, Brown J, Josephson ME: Electrocardiographic criteria for ventricular tachycardia in wide complex left bundle branch block morphology tachycardias. Am J Cardiol 1988;61:1279.
11. Volosin KJ, Beauregard LM, Fabiszewski R, et al: Spontaneous changes in ventricular cycle length. J Am Coll Cardiol 1991;17:409.
12. Wellens HJJ, Brugada P: Diagnosis of ventricular tachycardia from the 12-lead electrocardiogram. Cardiol Clin 1987;5:511.
13. Coumel P, Leclercq JF, Attuel P, et al: The QRS morphology in post-myocardial infarction ventricular tachycardia: A study of 100 tracings compared with 70 cases of idiopathic ventricular. Eur Heart J 1984;5:792.
14. Morady F, Baerman JM, DiCarlo LA, et al: A prevalent misconception regarding wide complex tachycardias. JAMA 1985;254:2790.
15. Mattu A, Brady WJ, Perron AD, et al: Prominent R wave in lead V1: Electrocardiographic differential diagnosis. Am J Emerg Med 2001;19:504.
16. Chou T, Knilans TK: Electrolyte imbalance. In Chou T, Knilans TK (eds): Electrocardiography in Clinical Practice: Adult and Pediatric, 4th ed. Philadelphia, WB Saunders, 1996, p 532.
17. Brady WJ, Skiles J: Wide QRS complex tachycardia: ECG differential diagnosis. Am J Emerg Med 1999;17:376.
18. Alberca T, Almendral J, Sanz P, et al: Evaluation of the specificity of morphological electrocardiographic criteria for the differential diagnosis of wide QRS complex tachycardia in patients with intraventricular conduction defects. Circulation 1997;96:3257.
19. Passman R, Kadish A: Polymorphic ventricular tachycardia, long Q-T syndrome, and torsades de pointes. Med Clin North Am 2001;85:321.
20. Brugada P, Brugada J: Right bundle branch block, persistent ST segment elevation and sudden cardiac death: A distinct clinical and electrocardiographic syndrome. J Am Coll Cardiol 1992;20:1391.
21. Brugada P, Brugada R, Brugada J: The Brugada syndrome. Curr Cardiol Rep 2000;2:507.
22. Alings M, Wilde A: "Brugada" syndrome: Clinical data and suggested pathophysiological mechanism. Circulation 1999;99:666.
23. Monroe MH, Littmann L: Two-year case collection of the Brugada syndrome electrocardiogram pattern at a large teaching hospital. Clin Cardiol 2000;23:849.
24. Gussak I, Antzelevitch C, Bjerregaard P, et al: The Brugada syndrome: Clinical, electrophysiologic and genetic aspects. J Am Coll Cardiol 1999;33:5.
25. Furuhashi M, Uno K, Tsuchihashi K, et al: Prevalence of asymptomatic ST segment elevation in right precordial leads with right bundle branch block (Brugada-type ST shift) among the general Japanese population. Heart 2001;86:161.
26. Pollack ML, Chan TC, Brady WJ: Electrocardiographic manifestations: Aberrant ventricular conduction. J Emerg Med 2000;19:363.

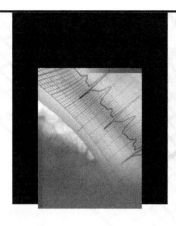

Chapter 27

Pacemakers: Normal Function

Taylor Y. Cardall and Theodore C. Chan

Clinical Features

This chapter summarizes the electrocardiographic (ECG) manifestations of the normally functioning implantable cardiac pacemaker. Cardiac pacemakers were first used in the 1950s to prevent Stokes-Adams attacks. Since then, the technology behind implantable cardiac pacemakers has advanced steadily; similarly, the number of patients receiving them has increased. In 1998, the American College of Cardiology and the American Heart Association published updated recommendations concerning "Guidelines for Permanent Cardiac Pacemaker Implantation," listing indications, including atrioventricular (AV) node dysfunction, sinus node dysfunction, hypersensitive carotid sinus syndrome and neurally mediated syncope (vasovagal syncope), prevention of tachycardia with long QT syndrome, and hypertrophic cardiomyopathy.[1] Recent literature expands these indications to include selected patients with congestive heart failure and for the prevention of atrial fibrillation. Advances in technology, expanding indications, and the aging of the population ensure that clinicians will encounter patients with cardiac pacemakers on a regular basis.

Pacing Modes. As pacemakers have evolved and assumed more functions and capabilities, a five-position code has been developed by the North American Society of Pacing and Electrophysiology (NASPE) and the British Pacing and Electrophysiology Group (BPEG).[2] Position I indicates the chambers being paced: atrium (A), ventricle (V), both (D, dual), or none (O). Position II gives the location where the pacemaker senses native cardiac electrical activity (A, V, D, or O). Position III indicates the pacemaker's response to sensing: triggering (T), inhibition (I), both (D), or none (O). Older versions of the code only designated these three positions, and pacemakers are still commonly referred to in terms of these three codes. Position IV indicates two things: the programmability of the pacemaker, and the capability to control rate adaptively (R). The code in this position is hierarchical with no programmability (O), simple programmability (P), multiprogrammable capability (M), and ability to communicate with external equipment (i.e., telemetry; C). Position V identifies the presence of antitachydysrhythmia functions, including the antitachydysrhythmia pacing (P) or shocking (S), both (D), or none (O). From a practical standpoint, most pacemakers encountered in the emergency department or clinic setting will be AAIR, VVIR, DDD, DDDR, or "back-up" pacing modes for cardioverter–defibrillator devices (Table 27-1).

AAI Pacing. An AAI pacemaker is one that paces the atrium, senses the atrium, and inhibits the pacing activity if it

27-1 • THE NASPE/BPEG GENERIC (NBG) PACEMAKER CODE				
Position				
I	**II**	**III**	**IV**	**V**
Chamber(s) paced	Chamber(s) sensed	Response to sensing	Programmability, rate modulation	Antitachydysrhythmia functions
O = none	O = none	O = none	O = none	O = none
A = atrium	A = atrium	T = triggered	P = simple programmable	P = pacing (antitachydysrhythmia)
V = ventricle	V = ventricle	I = inhibited	M = multiprogrammable	S = shock
D = dual (atrium and ventricle)	D = dual (atrium and ventricle)	D = dual (atrial triggered and atrial and ventricular inhibited)	C = communicating	D = dual (pacing + shock)
			R = rate modulation	

NASPE/BPEG, North American Society of Pacing and Electrophysiology/British Pacing and Electrophysiology Group.

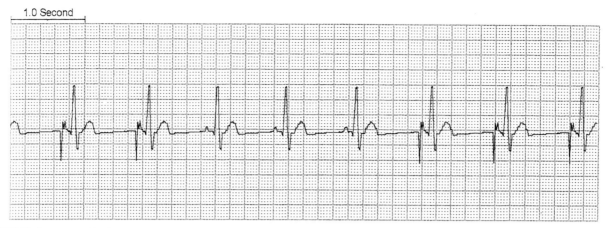

FIGURE 27-1 · **AAI pacing in a patient with sinus node dysfunction.** The first two P waves are paced, whereas the following three P waves are native, so atrial pacing is inhibited. The next three P waves are again paced. (Courtesy of St. Jude Medical, St. Paul, Minnesota.)

senses spontaneous atrial activity (Fig. 27-1). If, at the end of a preset interval, no atrial activity is sensed, it generates an atrial pacing stimulus. Thus, it is termed an *atrial demand mode* of pacing. This mode of pacing prevents the atrial rate from decreasing below a preset level, and is useful for patients with sinus node dysfunction and intact AV node conduction.

VVI Pacing. VVI pacing is useful in those with chronically ineffective atria, such as chronic atrial fibrillation or atrial flutter (Fig. 27-2). This mode is similar to AAI in that it is a demand mode, except that the ventricle is sensed and the ventricle is paced rather than the atrium.

DDD Pacing. DDD pacing is a form of dual-chambered pacing, where both the atria and the ventricles are paced. In DDD pacing, both the atrium and the ventricle are sensed, and either paced or inhibited depending on the native cardiac activity sensed (Figs. 27-3 and 27-4). In DDD pacing, if the pacer does not sense any native atrial activity after a preset interval, it generates an atrial stimulus (Fig. 27-5). An atrial stimulus, whether native or paced, initiates a period known as the AV interval. During the AV interval, the atrial channel of

---

ELECTROCARDIOGRAPHIC HIGHLIGHTS

Atrial paced rhythm

- Pacer spike just before the P wave
- P wave with normal morphology

Ventricular paced rhythm

- Pacer spike just before the QRS complex
- QRS morphology similar to left bundle branch block
- QRS complex and T waves discordant
- Wide, mainly negative QS or rS complexes with poor R wave progression in leads V_1 to V_6
- QS complexes in leads II, III, and aVF
- Large R wave in leads I and aVL
- Usually left axis deviation

Dual-chambered pacing

- As in the above categories, plus
- Pacing spikes may be present before P waves, QRS complexes, or both

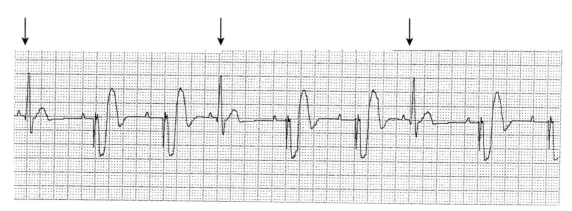

FIGURE 27-2 · **VVI pacing in a patient with second degree atrioventricular (AV) block.** The first, fourth, and seventh QRS complexes are native (*arrows*), whereas the others are paced. Note that in VVI pacing there is no AV synchrony. (Courtesy of St. Jude Medical, St. Paul, Minnesota.)

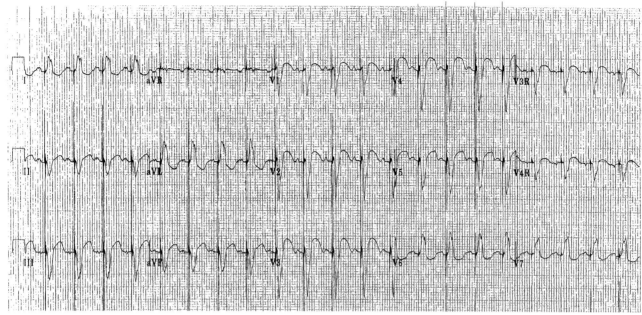

FIGURE 27-3 · ECG of normal DDD pacemaker. In this case, the sinus node is functioning properly, so there is no atrial pacing occurring. The tracing demonstrates the widened QRS complexes typical in ventricular paced rhythm. Note the resemblance to a left bundle branch block pattern with left axis deviation, as well as the T wave/QRS complex discordance and ST segment elevation. These are expected findings in a patient with a ventricular paced rhythm.

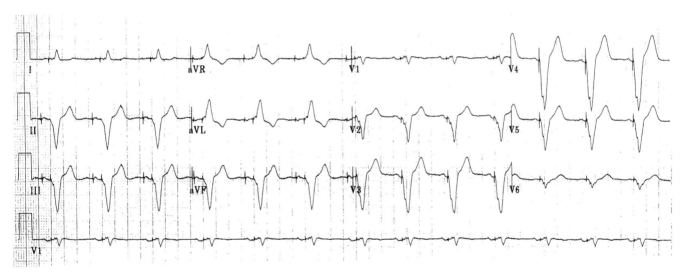

FIGURE 27-4 · ECG of normal DDD pacemaker. In this case, both atrial and ventricular pacing are evident by evaluating different leads.

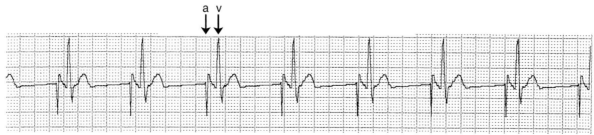

FIGURE 27-5 · DDD pacing in a patient with sinus node dysfunction and intact atrioventricular (AV) node conduction. In this case, there is atrial pacing (a) with ventricular sensing, but no ventricular pacing because intact AV node conduction allows for native ventricular stimulation (v). (Courtesy of St. Jude Medical, St. Paul, Minnesota.)

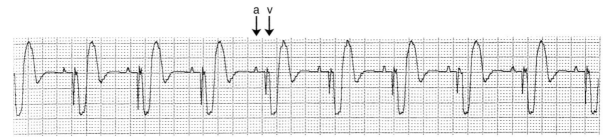

FIGURE 27-6 · **DDD pacing in a patient with intact sinus node and complete atrioventricular block.** In this case, there is atrial sensing (a) with ventricular pacing (v). (Courtesy of St. Jude Medical, St. Paul, Minnesota.)

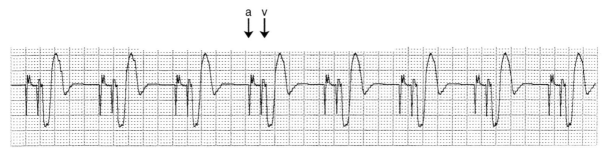

FIGURE 27-7 · **DDD pacing with sinus node dysfunction and complete heart block.** Both atrial (a) and ventricular pacing (v) occur. (Courtesy of St. Jude Medical, St. Paul, Minnesota.)

the pacer is inactive, or refractory. At the end of the present AV interval, if no native ventricular activity is sensed by the ventricular channel, the pacer generates a ventricular stimulus (Fig. 27-6). The atrial refractory period, begun at the onset of the AV interval, continues so as to prevent sensing the ventricular stimulus or resulting retrograde P waves as native atrial activity. Figure 27-7 shows DDD pacing in a patient with both sick sinus syndrome and complete heart block, yielding pacing of both the atria and the ventricles.

As one might imagine, if supraventricular tachycardia were to develop in a patient with a DDD pacemaker, the pacemaker might pace the ventricles at the rapid rate (up to the preprogrammed upper rate limit, of course). To prevent this, most DDD pacemakers now use algorithms whereby if an atrial tachydysrhythmia develops, the pacer switches to a pacing mode where there is no atrial tracking, such as VVI. On cessation of the dysrhythmia, the pacer reverts to DDD mode, thus restoring AV synchrony without being complicit in the transmission of paroxysmal atrial tachydysrhythmias. This is termed *mode switching.*

Electrocardiographic Manifestations

The Paced Electrocardiogram. When a pacemaker is active and pacing, small spikes signify that the electrical signal emanating from the pacemaker leads are usually evident on the ECG. Low-amplitude pacemaker artifacts may not be visible in all leads. Pacing artifacts are much smaller with bipolar electrode systems than with unipolar leads, and consequently may be difficult to visualize.

Typically, atrial pacing appears as a small pacer spike just before the P wave. Because atrial pacing leads are implanted in the appendage of the right atrium, the P wave is usually of

a normal morphology. In contrast, the ventricular paced rhythm (VPR) is quite abnormal. Because the ventricular pacing lead is placed in the right ventricle, the ventricles depolarize from right to left by slow-conducting myocytes, rather than by the regular conduction system. Thus, the overall QRS complex morphology is similar to that of a left bundle branch block (LBBB), with prolongation of the QRS complex interval (occasionally, patients have epicardial, rather than intracardiac pacemaker leads that may be placed over the left ventricle, resulting in a right bundle branch block ventricular paced pattern).

With this LBBB pattern, the altered ventricular conduction is manifested by wide, mainly negative QS or rS complexes with poor R wave progression in leads V_1 to V_6. QS complexes are commonly seen in leads II, III, and aVF, whereas a large R wave is typically seen in leads I and aVL (see Fig. 27-3). Leads V_5 and V_6 sometimes have deep S waves because the depolarization may be traveling away from the plane of those leads (see Fig. 27-4).

Usually, the ventricular lead is placed near the apex, causing the ventricles to contract from apex to base, yielding frontal plane QRS complex left axis deviation on the ECG. If the lead is implanted toward the right ventricular outflow tract, depolarization forces travel from base to apex, yielding a right axis deviation.

Because of the abnormal ventricular depolarization, repolarization also occurs abnormally. ST segments and T waves should typically be *discordant* with the QRS complex, unlike the usual ECG pattern. Thus, T wave inversions with VPR are the rule, not the exception. This is known as the *rule of appropriate discordance* or *QRS complex/T wave axis discordance* for ventricular pacing. This becomes important when trying to interpret the ECG with VPR in the context of

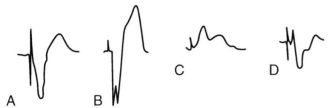

FIGURE 27-8 · ECG changes in patients with ventricular paced rhythm associated with acute myocardial infarction.[3] *A,* Normal, expected QRS complex/ST segment/T wave discordance. *B,* Discordant ST segment elevation ≥5 mm. *C,* Concordant ST segment elevation ≥1 mm. *D,* ST segment depression ≥1 mm in leads V_1, V_2, or V_3. (From Kozlowski FH, Brady WJ, Aufderheide TP, Buckley RS: The electrocardiographic diagnosis of acute myocardial infarction in patients with ventricularly paced rhythms. Acad Emerg Med 1998;5:52–57; copyright 1998 by Hanley & Belfus Inc. Reproduced with permission from Hanley & Belfus Inc. in the format Textbook via Copyright Clearance Center.)

possible cardiac ischemia[3,4] (Fig. 27-8; see Chapter 34, Acute Myocardial Infarction: Confounding Patterns).

Application of the Magnet and Other Maneuvers. Often patients may present with native heart rates above the pacing threshold, so pacer activity cannot be evaluated on a baseline ECG. Placing a magnet over the generator of most pacemakers typically eliminates sensing and initiates an asynchronous mode of pacing, most commonly AOO, VOO, or DOO (Fig. 27-9; a small minority of pacemakers exhibit a different preprogrammed effect or no effect when a magnet is applied). This procedure is useful for assessing pacemaker capture, evaluating battery life, and treating pacemaker-mediated tachycardia (see Chapter 28, Electronic Pacemakers: Abnormal Function). In addition, in some pacemakers, the pace rate with the magnet changes as the battery approaches the end of its life.

Vagal maneuvers such as carotid sinus massage may also help in some circumstances by slowing the patient's spontaneous heart rate and allowing pacemaker function to be evaluated. Short-acting drugs such as adenosine or edrophonium can be similarly used.[5] These maneuvers should be used only with extreme caution in a pacemaker-dependent patient where one suspects pacer malfunction.

Electrocardiographic Differentiation of Ventricular Paced Rhythm, Bundle Branch Block, and Ventricular Hypertrophy. As discussed previously, the VPR is typically very similar in appearance to LBBB. For this reason, a 12-lead

---

ELECTROCARDIOGRAPHIC PEARLS

- Usually left bundle branch block can be differentiated from ventricular paced rhythm (VPR) by inspection of the major QRS vector in lead V_6.
- Application of a magnet should convert pacing mode to asynchronous pacing and allow for assessment of capture (beware of pacemaker-dependent patients).
- Check for pacemaker spikes in multiple leads; rhythm strip is not sufficient.

Acute Myocardial Infarction Difficult in the Setting of VPR

- Serial ECGs as well as comparison of current ECG to prior study may be helpful in evaluating acute myocardial infarction as well as other pacing functions.
- Exaggerated discordance or inappropriate concordance of QRS complex and T waves may indicate myocardial ischemia or injury.

ECG should be obtained and all leads scrutinized, because on a monitor strip pacing spikes may not be evident. Distinguishing between VPR and LBBB is easier in most cases by looking at lead V_6. In LBBB, the QRS complex is upright, whereas in VPR the QRS complex is principally below the isoelectric line—because of pacemaker impulse generation from apex to base being oriented superiorly, or in the opposite direction of the V_6 individual lead axis (which is leftward and somewhat inferior).

Left ventricular hypertrophy (LVH) can cause left axis deviation and interventricular conduction delays, as well as QRS complex/T wave discordance, causing an appearance similar to that of VPR. However, with LVH, the ECG should also meet other criteria for LVH (see Chapter 35, Ventricular Hypertrophy, for details). Finally, signal artifacts, from motion, short circuit, poor lead connection, and the like, may produce artifacts that can mimic pacer spikes. However, these should be random in appearance, and not consistently correlated with cardiac activity.

Electrocardiographic Diagnosis of Acute Myocardial Infarction in the Ventricular Paced Patient. The ECG diagnosis of myocardial ischemia or infarct in the patient with a VPR is complicated because of pacing artifacts and changes in depolarization vectors that obscure the classic ECG

m

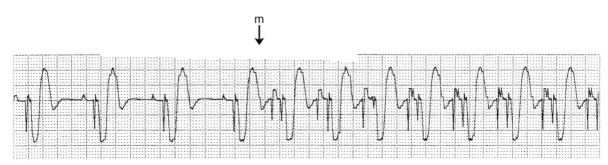

FIGURE 27-9 · Effect of magnet application on pacemaker function. This ECG shows DDD pacing in a patient with third degree atrioventricular block. Initially, atrial sensing and ventricular pacing occur. After the third beat, the magnet is applied (m), which converts the pacing mode to DOO. In this mode there is no sensing and both atria and ventricles are paced. (Courtesy of St. Jude Medical, St. Paul, Minnesota.)

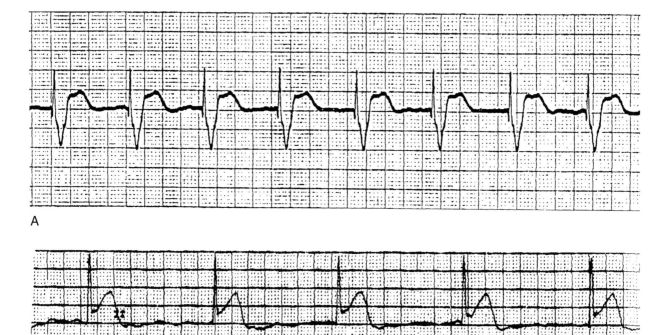

A

B

FIGURE 27-10 · **Effects of ventricular pacing on ST segments and T waves.** The effects of ventricular pacing on ST segments and T waves can make the diagnosis of acute myocardial infarction (AMI) difficult. *A,* This rhythm strip from a patient with ventricular paced rhythm (VPR) in the emergency department (ED) demonstrates the normal QRS morphology for VPR. *B,* In this rhythm strip obtained by the paramedics before arriving at the ED, the patient's native rhythm is fast enough to suppress pacing, so native QRS complexes can be seen. When not paced, it is apparent that the patient has ST segment elevations consistent with the diagnosis of AMI. (Courtesy of William J. Brady, MD, University of Virginia Health System, Charlottesville, Virginia.)

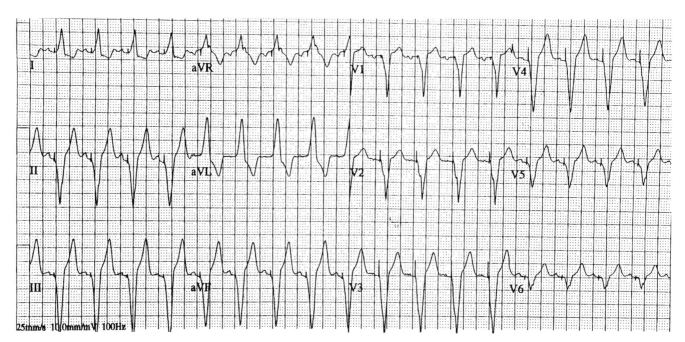

FIGURE 27-11 · **Baseline ECG with ventricular paced rhythm (VPR).** The tracing demonstrates the widened QRS complexes typical in VPR, as well as the expected QRS complex/T wave discordance. (From Kozlowski FH, Brady WJ, Aufderheide TP, Buckley RS: The electrocardiographic diagnosis of acute myocardial infarction in patients with ventricularly paced rhythms. Acad Emerg Med 1998;5:52–57; copyright 1998 by Hanley & Belfus Inc. Reproduced with permission from Hanley & Belfus Inc. in the format Textbook via Copyright Clearance Center.)

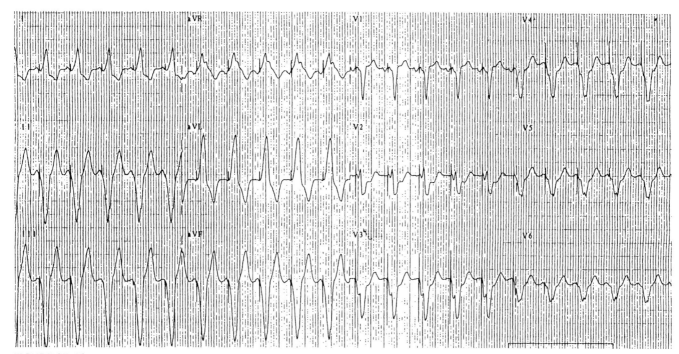

FIGURE 27-12 • Acute cardiac ischemia. This ECG, from the same patient in Figure 27-11, now shows findings of acute cardiac ischemia. Instead of the expected discordance between the QRS complex and the ST segment, there is concordant depression of the ST segment by >1 mm in the precordial leads, most prominently V_2. (From Kozlowski FH, Brady WJ, Aufderheide TP, Buckley RS: The electrocardiographic diagnosis of acute myocardial infarction in patients with ventricularly paced rhythms. Acad Emerg Med 1998;5:52–57; copyright 1998 by Hanley & Belfus Inc. Reproduced with permission from Hanley & Belfus Inc. in the format Textbook via Copyright Clearance Center.)

findings of acute injury.[3,4] In addition to the paced LBBB-like pattern and discordant T waves, ventricular paced patients may demonstrate large ST segment elevation (STE) without experiencing any myocardial ischemia or injury. Conversely, the paced repolarization ST segment/T wave abnormalities can obscure ischemia or injury patterns. Finally, the T waves themselves in VPR often appear hyper-acute or inverted, which can imitate cardiac ischemia (Figs. 27-10, 27-11, and 27-12).

As in the nonpaced patient, comparison with an old ECG may reveal changes. Serial ECGs can also be helpful by illustrating dynamic changes. Inhibition of ventricular pacing in patients who are not pacemaker dependent (by methods such as chest wall stimulation in rate-modulated patients) allows evaluation of the native QRS complex, ST segment, and T waves (see Fig. 27-10). However, caution should be used when interpreting these because ST segment and T wave abnormalities produced by the pacemaker may persist beyond the cessation of pacing.

Several investigators have sought to find ECG changes in the patient with VPR that are characteristic of acute myocardial infarction (AMI). Only three of these traditional criteria have been shown to have independent value in the diagnosis of AMI in patients with VPRs.[3,6] These are:

1. STE ≥5 mm discordant with the QRS complex—or an exaggerated discordance (normally discordant STE in patients with VPR should be less than 3 mm)
2. STE ≥1 mm concordant with the QRS complex—a violation of the rule of appropriate discordance

3. ST depression ≥1 mm in leads V_1, V_2, or V_3—a violation of the rule of appropriate discordance

Figures 27-8, 27-11, and 27-12 illustrate how these criteria can be used to diagnose AMI in a patient with VPR. However, the sensitivity and specificity of these criteria remain controversial.

References

1. Gregoratos G, Cheitlin MD, Conill A, et al: ACC/AHA guidelines for implantation of cardiac pacemakers and antiarrhythmia devices: Executive summary—A report of the American College of Cardiology/American Heart Association Task Force on Practice Guidelines (Committee on Pacemaker Implantation). Circulation 1998;97:1325.
2. Bernstein AD, Camm AJ, Fisher JD, et al: North American Society of Pacing and Electrophysiology policy statement: The NASPE/BPEG Defibrillator Code. Pacing Clin Electrophysiol 1993;16:1776.
3. Sgarbossa EB, Pinski SL, Gates KB, et al: Early electrocardiographic diagnosis of acute myocardial infarction in the presence of ventricular paced rhythm. Am J Cardiol 1996;77:423.
4. Kozlowski FH, Brady WJ, Aufderheide TP, Buckley RS: The electrocardiographic diagnosis of acute myocardial infarction in patients with ventricular paced rhythms. Acad Emerg Med 1998;5:52.
5. Atlee JL: Management of patients with pacemakers or ICD devices. In: Atlee JL (ed): Arrhythmias and Pacemakers: Practical Management for Anesthesia and Critical Care Medicine. Philadelphia, WB Saunders, 1996, p 295.
6. Sgarbossa EB, Pinski SL, Barbagelata A, et al: Electrocardiographic diagnosis of evolving acute myocardial infarction in the presence of left bundle branch block. GUSTO-I Investigators. N Engl J Med 1996; 334:481.

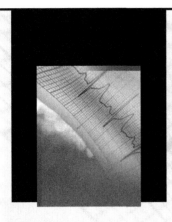

Chapter 28

Pacemakers: Abnormal Function

Taylor Y. Cardall and Theodore C. Chan

Clinical Features

Malfunctions of artificial pacemakers are disorders of sensing, capture, or rate. Patients with pacemaker malfunction often have vague and nonspecific symptoms. Therefore, complaints such as palpitations, irregular heartbeat, syncope, presyncope, dizziness, chest pain, dyspnea, orthopnea, paroxysmal nocturnal dyspnea, or fatigue should prompt an evaluation, which must include a 12-lead electrocardiogram (ECG). If there is no pacemaker activity on the ECG, the clinician should attempt to obtain a paced ECG by applying a magnet, which typically switches the pacemaker to asynchronous

pacing and allows for assessment of capture, but not sensing. If the patient's native cardiac rhythm is above the lower-rate threshold for pacing, cautious attempts to slow the rate with carotid massage, adenosine, or edrophonium may be useful.[1] However, these should be performed with extreme caution in the pacemaker-dependent patient.

If routine evaluation yields no pacemaker abnormalities, the pacemaker should be interrogated. Most patients have a card in their wallet identifying the make and model of pacemaker. Manufacturers also place an identification number in the generator that is visible at times on the chest radiograph and can be referenced to provide detailed information on the pacemaker.

Clinically significant abnormal pacemaker function includes the following: failure to pace, failure to capture, undersensing, pacemaker-mediated tachycardia, and the pacemaker syndrome.

Failure to Pace. Pacemaker output failure occurs when the pacemaker fails to fire in a situation where pacing should occur. Failure to pace has many causes, including oversensing, pacing lead problems (dislodgement or fracture), battery or component failure, and electromagnetic interference. Oversensing, the most common cause, occurs when inappropriate sensing of electrical signals inhibits firing.[2,3] These signals may occur with native cardiac activity, skeletal muscle myopotentials, or "make–break" signals from metal-to-metal contact.

Failure to Capture. Failure to capture occurs when a pacing stimulus is generated but fails to trigger myocardial depolarization (Table 28-1). The most common cause is exit block—elevations in the threshold voltage required for depolarization. Exit block can be caused by maturation of tissues at the electrode–myocardium interface after implantation (postimplantation failure) or tissue damage from defibrillation.

Undersensing. Undersensing occurs when a pacemaker that is programmed to sense cardiac signals of a certain amplitude and frequency fails to sense or detect native cardiac activity. Anything that changes the amplitude, vector, or frequency of these electrical signals can result in undersensing. These include all causes of failure to capture, as well as the

---

ELECTROCARDIOGRAPHIC HIGHLIGHTS

Failure to pace
- Absence of pacing where it is expected
- No visible pacing spikes
- Application of magnet yields no pacing spikes

Failure to capture
- Pacing spikes seen but no depolarization follows
- May be intermittent
- May be atrial or ventricular
- Application of magnet shows regular pacing spikes, but without 100% capture

Undersensing
- Difficult to diagnose by ECG
- May be inferred from the behavior of the surface ECG coupled with knowledge of expected pacemaker behavior

Pacemaker-mediated tachycardia
- Tachycardic paced rhythm
- Stops with magnet placement

Pacemaker syndrome
- Loss of atrioventricular synchrony
- Retrograde P waves

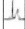
28-1 • SOME CAUSES OF FAILURE TO CAPTURE

- Pacing voltage programmed too low
- Lead dislodgement
- Lead fracture or insulation defect
- Exit block
- Post-lead implantation
- After external cardiac defibrillation
- Low battery life
- Elevated pacing thresholds
- Acute myocardial infarction
- Electrolyte abnormalities (especially hyperkalemia)
- Metabolic derangements (acidemia, hypothyroidism, hypoxemia)

development of new native cardiac bundle branch blocks (BBBs), premature ventricular contractions (PVCs), or atrial or ventricular tachydysrhythmias.

Pacemaker-Mediated Dysrhythmias. Pacemakers can be useful to treat or prevent dysrhythmias, but can themselves become a source of dysrhythmias. Examples include pacemaker-mediated tachycardia (PMT), runaway pacemaker, dysrhythmias due to lead dislodgement, and sensor-induced tachycardias.

Pacemaker-Mediated Tachycardia. PMT, also known as *endless-loop tachycardia*, is a reentry dysrhythmia occurring in dual-chamber pacemakers with atrial sensing where the pacemaker itself acts as part of the reentry circuit. PMT occurs when a retrograde P wave (most commonly as a result of a PVC occurring after the pacemaker's postventricular atrial refractory period [PVARP]) is interpreted as a native atrial stimulus, which in turn triggers ventricular pacing, and another retrograde P wave, ad infinitum. The pacemaker acts as the anterograde conductor for the reentrant rhythm, while retrograde conduction occurs through the intact atrioventricular (AV) node. PMT can also occur as a result of oversensing or the removal of the pacing magnet.[4]

Runaway Pacemaker. The runaway pacemaker is an exceedingly rare primary component failure in older-generation pacemakers in which there are inappropriately rapid discharges (up to 400 pulses per minute), potentially inducing ventricular tachycardia or fibrillation. This phenomenon is usually limited to older pacemakers without preprogrammed upper rate limits.

Dysrhythmias Due to Lead Dislodgement. A lead that has become dislodged may bounce against the ventricular wall and provoke ectopic beats and dysrhythmias.

Sensor-Induced Tachycardias. Many modern pacemakers are equipped with rate-modulation features that attempt to raise the heart rate appropriately to meet physiologic needs (designated by an "R" in IV position of the pacemaker code). These sensors respond to vibration, respiratory changes, hemodynamic parameters, or acid–base status. Pacemaker rates may be inappropriate if the sensors are stimulated by nonphysiologic parameters, such as loud noises, vibrations from heavy equipment (e.g., aeromedical helicopter transport), sleeping on the side of the implant, fever, hyperventilation, arm movement, or electrocautery.[5–12]

Pacemaker Syndrome. Pacemaker syndrome is a constellation of signs and symptoms in patients with suboptimal

pacing modes or programming in an otherwise normally functioning pacemaker. The pathophysiologic process of pacemaker syndrome is complex and multifactorial, but the major factor appears to be suboptimal AV synchrony.[13,14] This AV dyssynchrony leads to unfavorable hemodynamics and decreased perfusion, resulting in variable nonspecific symptoms.

Pseudomalfunction. Pseudomalfunction occurs when pacing is actually occurring, but pacing spikes are not seen or result in "abnormal" rhythms on the ECG despite normal pacemaker function. Pseudomalfunction also occurs when the clinician mistakenly expects the pacer to be triggering when it is appropriately inactive (Table 28-2).

Electrocardiographic Manifestations

Failure to Pace. Failure to pace manifests itself on the ECG by an absence of pacer spikes at a point where pacer spikes would be expected based on the rate of native cardiac activity. In dual-chambered pacing systems, isolated atrial or ventricular failure to pace may be evident.

Oversensing. Abnormal electrical signals that result in oversensing may or may not be seen on the ECG. For example, oversensing from skeletal muscle myopotentials, particularly from the pectoralis and rectus abdominis muscles as well as the diaphragm, may be reproduced by running a 12-lead rhythm strip while having the patient stimulate the rectus and pectoralis muscles. The 12-lead ECG will demonstrate the results of oversensing, most commonly failure to pace. Oversensing, however, can cause PMT in patients where oversensing of atrial activity results in recurrent ventricular pacing.

Failure to Capture. On the ECG, failure to capture is identified by the presence of pacing spikes without associated myocardial depolarization, or capture. Failure to capture can

28-2 • TROUBLESHOOTING PACEMAKER MALFUNCTION

No Pacing Seen on ECG
- Appropriate pacemaker function; no pacing needed
- Failure to pace
- Failure to capture
- Lead dislodgement or exit block
- Pacing occurring but spikes not visible on ECG (may occur with bipolar pacing systems and analog ECG recorders)

Irregularly Paced Beats
- Appropriate pacing behavior; pacing inhibited when native cardiac activity sensed
- Intermittent left bundle branch block masquerading as paced rhythm
- Failure to capture
- Pseudomalfunction (i.e., pacemaker Wenckebach rhythm)
- Oversensing of extracardiac signals

Tachycardiac Paced Rhythm
- Appropriate pacing function
- Pacemaker-mediated tachycardia
- Tachydysrhythmia due to lead dislodgement
- Sensor-induced tachycardia
- Runaway pacemaker
- Native ventricular tachycardia

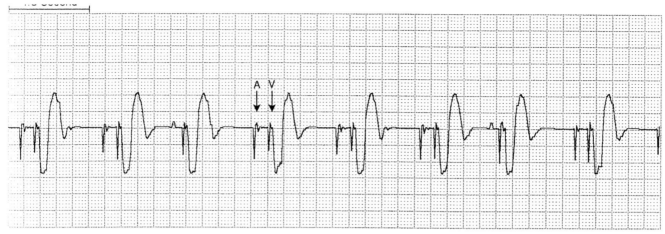

FIGURE 28-1 · Loss of atrial capture. Both atrial (A) and ventricular pacing spikes (V) are visible, but only the ventricular stimuli are capturing. There are no P waves after the atrial spikes. (Courtesy of St. Jude Medical, St. Paul, Minnesota.)

occur with atrial pacing, ventricular pacing, or both (Figs. 28-1 and 28-2). Native cardiac electrical activity, including escape rhythms, is seen and may occur simultaneously with pacemaker spikes, resulting in fusion beats or other unique ECG findings (Fig. 28-2). Many pacemakers are programmed for "safety pacing" to prevent a paced stimulus from falling on the T wave of a paced or native ventricular beat if there is failure to capture (Fig. 28-3). Capture can be assessed by applying a pacer magnet over the generator, switching the pacemaker to asynchronous pacing (Fig. 28-4).

Undersensing. Unlike failure to capture, there is often no obvious finding on ECG to suggest undersensing because pacing artifacts may or may not be easily detectable. Instead, the clinician must infer from the ECG whether the pacemaker is sensing properly and responding with an appropriate output based on its program. Figure 28-5 shows an example of atrial undersensing. Native P waves are not being sensed, and the pacemaker responds by triggering atrial and ventricular pacing spikes. In this case the appropriate pacer activity would be to sense the native atrial activity and inhibit atrial pacing, but pace the ventricle in response to the native atrial activity. Figure 28-6 demonstrates ventricular undersensing with the presence of both a native QRS complex and ventricular paced rhythms.

Pacemaker-mediated dysrhythmias

Pacemaker-Mediated Tachycardia. On the ECG, PMT appears as a regular, ventricular paced tachycardia at a rate

at or less than the maximum upper rate of the pacemaker. PMT cannot exceed the maximum programmed rate of the pacemaker, usually 160 to 180 bpm.

Rarely, the inciting event (PVC with retrograde P wave, oversensing, magnet removal) may be captured on a rhythm strip (Fig. 28-7). Treatment consists in the application of the magnet to initiate asynchronous pacing and break the reentry circuit. PMT can also be terminated by achieving AV conduction block with adenosine or vagal maneuvers.[15–17] Modern pacemakers also feature programming to terminate PMT automatically by temporarily prolonging the PVARP or omitting a single ventricular stimulus (Fig. 28-8).

Runaway Pacemaker. On the ECG the runaway pacemaker appears as a paced ventricular tachycardia, with a rate often exceeding the expected maximum upper limit of a pacemaker.

The runaway pacemaker is a true medical emergency. Application of a magnet may induce a slower pacing rate. If emergency interrogation and reprogramming are not successful, emergent surgical intervention to disconnect the leads may be necessary.[18]

Dysrhythmias Due to Lead Dislodgement. A dislodged lead may provoke ventricular extrasystoles or ventricular dysrhythmias. On the ECG, a change from the characteristic left BBB morphology to a right BBB morphology in a patient with a right ventricular transvenous electrode is suggestive of myocardial perforation.

Sensor-Induced Tachycardias. Sensor-induced tachycardias appear on the ECG as paced tachycardias. Unlike the

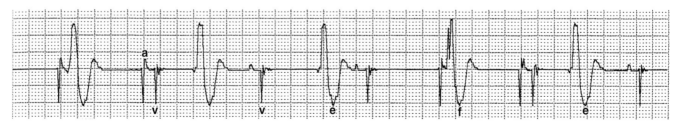

FIGURE 28-2 · Loss of ventricular capture. In this tracing there is DDD pacing in a patient with sick sinus syndrome and complete heart block. Atrial sensing and pacing is occurring; when no native P waves are detected, atrial pacing occurs (a). However, no QRS complexes follow ventricular pacing spikes (v) and ventricular stimulation fails to capture. The QRS complexes on this tracing are slow ventricular escape beats (e). In the fourth QRS complex, the pacemaker generates a stimulus at the same time a ventricular escape beat occurs, yielding a type of fusion beat (f). (Courtesy of St. Jude Medical, St. Paul, Minnesota.)

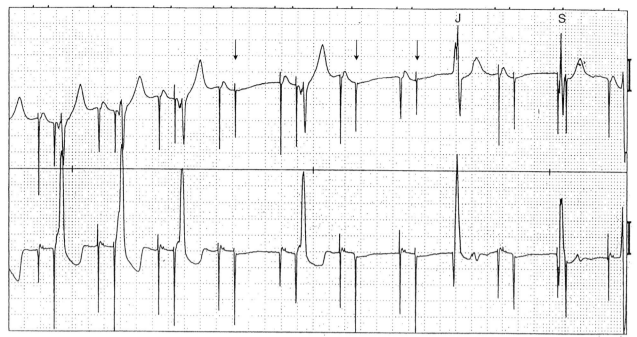

FIGURE 28-3 · **DDD pacing with intermittent loss of ventricular capture (*arrows*).** After the third loss of capture event there is a junctional escape beat (J). In the next-to-last beat, a junctional escape beat is bracketed by two pacing spikes (S). This is an example of "safety pacing." The pacing spikes in this complex have a shorter atrioventricular (AV) interval because a ventricular event was sensed. Rather than inhibiting ventricular pacing (and risk having no ventricular output if the sensed event were not truly a native ventricular depolarization), the AV interval is shortened by the pacemaker and a paced output occurs. This safety pacing preserves ventricular output and also prevents a paced stimulus from falling on the T wave. (Modified from Cardall TY, Brady WJ, Chan TC, et al: Permanent cardiac pacemakers: Issues relevant to the emergency physician, part II. J Emerg Med 1999;17:697–709; used with permission.)

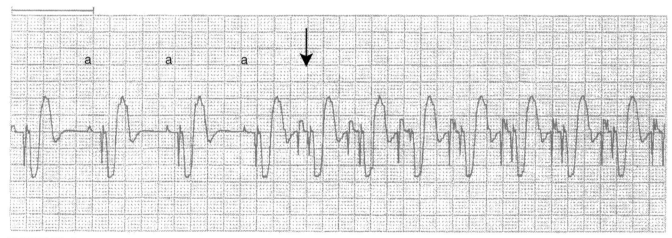

FIGURE 28-4 · **Placement of magnet inhibits sensing and reverts the pacemaker to asynchronous pacing.** The magnet allows for assessment of capture (but not sensing), as well as termination of certain types of pacemaker-mediated dysrhythmias. In this case, native atrial beats (a) are triggering ventricular pacing spikes and depolarization. The native atrial activity inhibits atrial pacing. When the magnet is placed *(arrow),* atrial sensing is halted, and asynchronous atrial and ventricular pacing occurs.

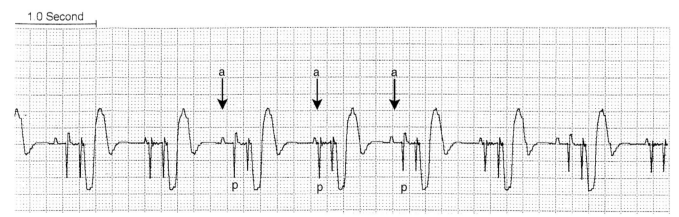

FIGURE 28-5 · **Atrial undersensing.** In this patient with a DDD pacemaker and complete heart block, the native atrial events are not sensed (a). If atrial sensing were occurring, atrial pacing (p) would be inhibited. (Courtesy of St. Jude Medical, St. Paul, Minnesota.)

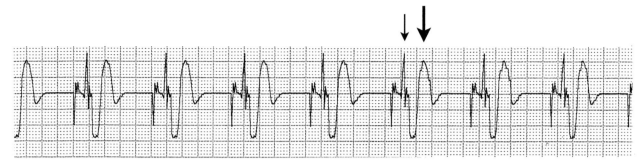

FIGURE 28-6 · Ventricular undersensing. In this patient with a DDD pacemaker and sinus node dysfunction, but intact AV conduction, the intrinsic ventricular events are not sensed. Note a native, upright, narrow QRS complex (*thin arrow*) after each atrial stimulus. These complexes are not sensed, and before ventricular repolarization has a chance to get started, ventricular pacing occurs, triggering the wider QRS complexes (*thick arrow*) evident on the tracing. (Courtesy of St. Jude Medical, St. Paul, Minnesota.)

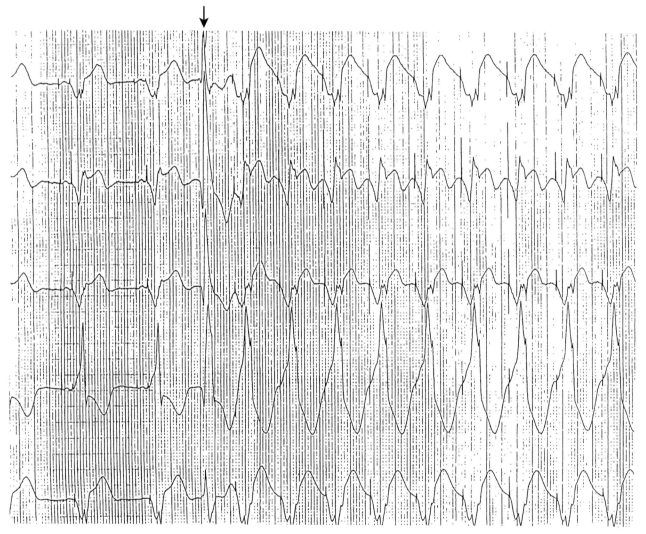

FIGURE 28-7 · Pacemaker-mediated or endless-loop tachycardia. In this patient with a DDD pacing system, a premature ventricular contraction occurs after the second QRS complex (*arrow*), triggering a run of pacemaker-mediated tachycardia. The pacemaker senses the resultant retrograde P wave (buried in the T wave), interprets it as native atrial activity, and paces the ventricle. This sets up the reentry rhythm as the pacemaker senses the retrograde P wave yet again. (Modified from Cardall TY, Brady WJ, Chan TC, et al: Permanent cardiac pacemakers: Issues relevant to the emergency physician, part II. J Emerg Med 1999;17:697–709; used with permission.)

runaway pacemaker, these tachycardias are typically benign and cannot exceed the pacemaker's upper rate limit. If necessary, they can always be broken with application of the magnet.

Pseudomalfunction.   Proper pacer functioning may appear to be abnormal on the ECG (Fig. 28-9). For example, fixed heart blocks mediated by the pacemaker may occur, particularly with marked tachycardias. The total atrial refractory period (TARP) is the period during which the atrium is refractory to depolarization after an atrial beat (essentially, the AV interval plus the PVARP). In DDD pacers, if the TARP is programmed longer than the upper rate interval (the cardiac cycle duration at the pacemaker's maximum ventricular rate), the cardiac cycle length may actually decrease with rapid atrial tachycardias to the point that it is shorter than the TARP. If this occurs, some native P waves will occur during the TARP and go undetected, resulting in AV block (most commonly seen as a 2:1 AV block) on ECG. This may be uncomfortable, particularly in active patients, because they may experience a sudden reduction in ventricular rate with exercise.

To avoid this sudden reduction in ventricular pacing, the TARP is often programmed to be shorter than the upper rate interval. However, this programming can lead to an alternate Wenckebach AV block rhythm in DDD pacing with atrial tachycardias. In this case, as the atrial rate rises, the P-P interval approaches the TARP, which is less than the upper rate interval. Ventricular pacing, however, cannot exceed the upper rate interval. Thus, when a sensed atrial event occurs faster than the upper rate interval, the pacemaker will wait to trigger the accompanying ventricular stimulus until the end of the upper rate interval. This AV delay increases with successive cycles until a dropped beat occurs, creating a pacemaker-mediated Wenckebach AV block. If the atrial rate continues to rise, the P-P interval will become less than the TARP and a fixed block like that described previously will occur.

The Pacemaker Syndrome.   Although the diagnosis cannot be made solely from the ECG, the lack of AV synchrony in the appropriate clinical situation suggests the diagnosis. Retrograde P waves suggest ventriculoatrial conduction, which in the context of AV dyssynchrony may cause atrial

---

ELECTROCARDIOGRAPHIC PEARLS

- Application of a magnet should convert pacing mode to asynchronous pacing and yields useful information.
- Interrogation of the pacemaker also yields useful information about pacemaker programming and function.
- Fixed 2:1 atrioventricular block or paced Wenckebach rhythm may be normal in DDD pacing at atrial rates near maximum upper limit of pacer.

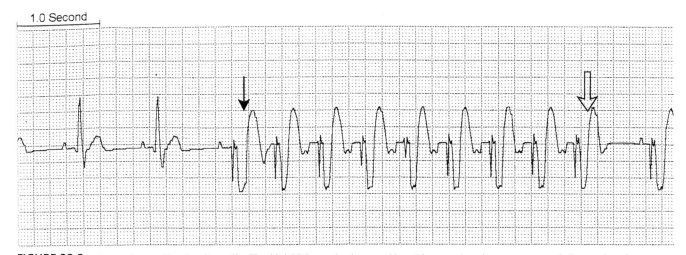

1.0 Second

FIGURE 28-8 · Pacemaker-mediated tachycardia. The third QRS complex is a paced beat (*thin arrow*), and causes a retrograde P wave that triggers a run of pacemaker-mediated tachycardia (PMT). In this case, the pacemaker detects the PMT and, in the penultimate beat (*thick arrow*), temporarily lengthens the postventricular atrial refractory period, preventing atrial sensing of the retrograde P wave and breaking the reentrant loop. (Courtesy of St. Jude Medical, St. Paul, Minnesota.)

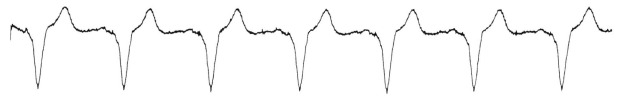

FIGURE 28-9 · Pseudomalfunction of a DDD pacemaker. In this tracing of lead II of a DDD pacer, the pacemaker is functioning properly, and pacing is occurring, but pacer spikes are not visible. This is common in bipolar pacing systems and represents normal pacemaker function. For this reason, a 12-lead ECG should be used where possible to evaluate pacemaker function because pacing spikes may be visible on some leads but not others.

overload, part of the pacemaker syndrome. In addition, the systolic blood pressure may drop 20 mm Hg or more when the patient goes from a spontaneous native rhythm to a paced rhythm. Treatment consists in upgrading to dual-chambered pacing to restore AV synchrony when pacemaker syndrome occurs in ventricular pacemakers.

References

1. Atlee JL: Management of patients with pacemakers or ICD devices. In Atlee JL (ed): Arrhythmias and Pacemakers: Practical Management for Anesthesia and Critical Care Medicine. Philadelphia, WB Saunders, 1996, p 295.
2. Love CJ, Hayes DL: Evaluation of pacemaker malfunction. In Ellenbogen KA, Kay GN, Wilkoff BL (eds): Clinical Cardiac Pacing. Philadelphia, WB Saunders, 1995, p 656.
3. Barold SS, Falkoff MD, Ong LS, Heinle RA: Oversensing by single-chamber pacemakers: Mechanisms, diagnosis, and treatment. Cardiol Clin 1985;3:565.
4. Oseran D, Ausubel K, Klementowicz PT, Furman S: Spontaneous endless loop tachycardia. Pacing Clin Electrophysiol 1986;9:379.
5. Lau CP, Tai YT, Fong PC, et al: Pacemaker mediated tachycardias in single chamber rate responsive pacing. Pacing Clin Electrophysiol 1990;13:1575.
6. Snoeck J, Berkhof M, Claeys M, et al: External vibration interference of activity-based rate-responsive pacemakers. Pacing Clin Electrophysiol 1992;15:1841.
7. Gordon RS, O'Dell KB, Low RB, Blumen IJ: Activity-sensing permanent internal pacemaker dysfunction during helicopter aero-medical transport. Ann Emerg Med 1990;19:1260.
8. French RS, Tillman JG: Pacemaker function during helicopter transport. Ann Emerg Med 1989;18:305.
9. Fromm RE Jr, Taylor DH, Cronin L, et al: The incidence of pacemaker dysfunction during helicopter air medical transport. Am J Emerg Med 1992;10:333.
10. Volosin KJ, O'Connor WH, Fabiszewski R, et al: Pacemaker-mediated tachycardia from a single chamber temperature sensitive pacemaker. Pacing Clin Electrophysiol 1989;12:1596.
11. Vanderheyden M, Timmermans W, Goethals M: Inappropriate rate response in a VVI-R pacemaker. Acta Cardiol 1996;51:545.
12. Seeger W, Kleinert M: An unexpected rate response of a minute-ventilation dependent pacemaker [letter]. Pacing Clin Electrophysiol 1989;12:1707.
13. Ellenbogen KA, Stambler BS: Pacemaker syndrome. In Ellenbogen KA, Kay GN, Wilkoff BL (eds): Clinical Cardiac Pacing. Philadelphia, WB Saunders, 1995, p 419.
14. Ellenbogen KA, Gilligan DM, Wood MA, et al: The pacemaker syndrome: A matter of definition [editorial]. Am J Cardiol 1997;79:1226.
15. Conti JB, Curtis AB, Hill JA, Raymenants ER: Termination of pacemaker-mediated tachycardia by adenosine. Clin Cardiol 1994;17:47.
16. Barold SS, Falkoff MD, Ong LS, Heinle RA: Pacemaker endless loop tachycardia: Termination by simple techniques other than magnet application. Am J Med 1988;85:817.
17. Friart A: Termination of magnet-unresponsive pacemaker endless loop tachycardia by carotid sinus massage [letter]. Am J Med 1989;87:1.
18. Mickley H, Andersen C, Nielsen LH: Runaway pacemaker: A still-existing complication and therapeutic guidelines. Clin Cardiol 1989;12:412.

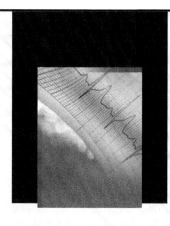

Chapter 29

Sick Sinus Syndrome

Wendy M. Curulla and Ioliene Boenau

Clinical Features

Sick sinus syndrome is a term originally used by Lown in 1967 to describe a prolonged recovery of normal sinus node function with "chaotic atrial activity" after cardioversion of an atrial tachydysrhythmia.[1] Since that time, the term has been used to describe a range of sinoatrial (SA) node dysfunction that can present with various electrocardiographic (ECG) findings. These presentations include sinus bradycardia, sinus arrhythmia, sinus pauses/arrest, SA exit block, atrioventricular (AV) junctional escape rhythm, and the bradycardia-tachycardia syndrome. Patients may exhibit one or more of these manifestations. Episodes of sick sinus syndrome may be intermittent. The incidence of sick sinus syndrome has been estimated to be as high as 1 in 600 in individuals over the age of 65 years.[2]

Clinical manifestations of sick sinus syndrome are due to severe or inappropriate bradycardia, which leads to a decrease in cardiac output and resultant organ hypoperfusion. Neurologic symptoms predominate owing to cerebral hypoperfusion and include lethargy and fatigue when bradycardia is persistent. Dizzy spells, lightheadedness, near-syncope, and syncope are common during abrupt episodes of bradycardia or cardiac standstill. In addition to the symptoms of bradycardia, patients with the bradycardia-tachycardia syndrome may also experience palpitations during episodes of tachycardia. Syncope often follows an episode of tachycardia when long pauses occur at the termination of the tachycardia, before recovery of normal SA node function.

There are multiple causes of sick sinus syndrome, including both intrinsic and extrinsic etiologies. Intrinsic sinus node disease is most commonly due to idiopathic degeneration and fibrosis of nodal tissue due to aging. Fibrosis of the node can also be due to ischemia, surgical trauma, and inflammatory or systemic diseases. Physical destruction of the node can occur during surgery. Infiltrative and connective tissue diseases such as sarcoidosis, amyloidosis, hemochromatosis, systemic lupus erythematosus, and scleroderma can also damage the SA node.[2,3]

Extrinsic causes of SA node dysfunction include pharmacologic therapy and noncardiac disease such as hypothyroidism, hypothermia, increased intracranial pressure, and states of increased vagal tone, including gastrointestinal disorders.[2,3] Many of the medications implicated are antihypertensive and antidysrhythmic agents such as beta-adrenergic blocking agents, calcium channel antagonists, digoxin, quinidine, procainamide, and clonidine. Although many causes have been identified, most cases are idiopathic in origin.

ELECTROCARDIOGRAPHIC HIGHLIGHTS

Sinus bradycardia

- Rate 60 bpm or less
- Identical upright P waves followed by a narrow QRS complex in a 1:1 ratio

Sinus arrhythmia

- Cyclical variation in sinus length
- Identical upright P waves followed by a narrow QRS complex in a 1:1 ratio
- Longest P-P interval >0.16 sec longer than shortest P-P interval

Sinoatrial exit block

- Pause is due to dropped P-QRS-T, whereas in atrioventricular block, pause is due to dropped QRS-T
- P-P interval of the pause is a multiple of the basic P-P interval
- Second degree sinoatrial block is the only type seen on 12-lead ECG

Sinus pause or arrest

- P-P interval of the pause is not a multiple of the basic P-P interval

Bradycardia-tachycardia syndrome

- Sinus bradycardia or junctional bradycardia interrupted by paroxysms of tachycardia, most often of a supraventricular type
- The termination of tachycardia is often followed by a slow recovery of the sinus rhythm, which may manifest with pauses
- Documentation of both the bradycardia and tachycardia are necessary

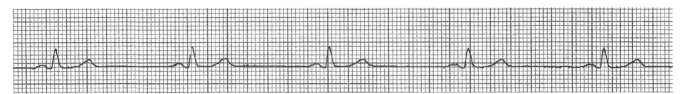

FIGURE 29-1 · **Sinus bradycardia.** Sinus bradycardia at 45 bpm in lead II rhythm strip.

Electrocardiographic Manifestations

Multiple ECG presentations are possible with sick sinus syndrome.

Sinus Bradycardia. Sinus bradycardia may be pathologic when due to depressed automaticity in the SA node and when appropriate increases in heart rate cannot occur. Electrocardiographically in the adult, sinus bradycardia is present when the heart rate is less than 60 bpm, a normal P wave axis is observed, and every P wave is usually associated with a narrow QRS complex[3] (Fig. 29-1). Sinus bradycardia may be a manifestation of sick sinus syndrome when the patient experiences symptoms (see Chapter 17, Bradycardia and Escape Rhythms).

Sinus Arrhythmia. Like sinus bradycardia, sinus arrhythmia is often seen in normal individuals, particularly children. It is usually asymptomatic and correlates with the respiratory cycle. The sinus rate increases with inspiration and decreases during expiration. When not associated with normal respiratory variation, it can be an early sign of sinus node disease, particularly in the elderly. Electrocardiographically, a gradual, cyclic variation is seen in the sinus beats, with the longest P-P interval exceeding the shortest P-P interval by more than 0.16 sec (Fig. 29-2).[3]

Sinoatrial Exit Block. SA exit block (or SA block) occurs when impulses generated by the SA node are not conducted through to the atria. Similar to the better-known AV blocks, there are first, second, and third degree varieties of SA block. However, unlike their AV block counterparts, not all grades of SA block are evident on the 12-lead ECG—only second degree SA block is discernible on the surface ECG. First degree SA block refers to a delay in conduction from the SA node to the atria. This is apparent only in the electrophysiology laboratory with special SA tracings. Second degree SA block is further broken down into two types. Type I (Wenckebach variety) presents on surface ECG recordings as a progressive shortening of the P-P interval until a beat (P-QRS-T) is dropped. This appears as a pause. In type II second degree SA block, there is an intermittent lack of impulse conduction despite continued impulse formation. When this occurs, the pause is a multiple of the P-P interval because the pacing cells have continued firing at their basic rate. The P-P interval of the pause is typically approximately two to four times the length of the basic P-P interval (Fig. 29-3). Third degree SA block presents as an absence of P waves altogether and is indistinguishable from a prolonged sinus pause or arrest on the surface ECG (see Chapter 19, Sinoatrial Exit Block).

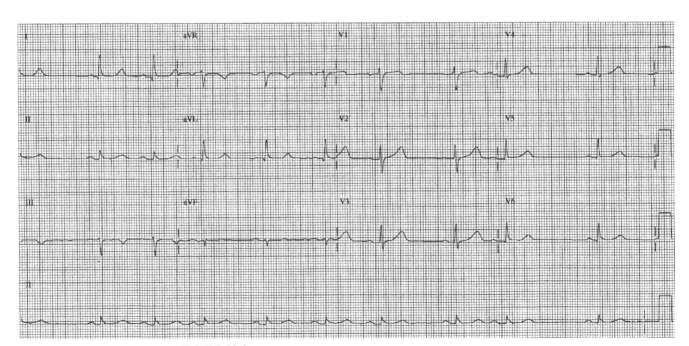

FIGURE 29-2 · **Sinus arrhythmia.** Sinus arrhythmia in an 82-year-old man.

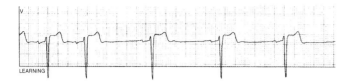

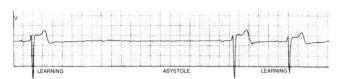

FIGURE 29-3 · **Type II sinoatrial exit block.** Note the P-P interval of the pause is three times the basic P-P interval established in the top rhythm strip.

ELECTROCARDIOGRAPHIC PEARLS

- Sinus bradycardia and sinus arrhythmia may be normal, but also may be an early indication of sinus node disease.
- If present for ECG acquisition, watch for variability in sinus complexes with respirations; if variability of complexes is independent of respiratory pattern, a pathologic process is more likely for sinus arrhythmia, particularly in the elderly.
- The determining ECG difference between sinus pause/arrest and sinoatrial exit block is whether the duration of the pause is a multiple of the basic P-P interval.
  - Sinoatrial exit block will be a multiple of the basic P-P interval.
  - Sinus pause/arrest will not be a multiple of the basic P-P interval.
- Sinoatrial and atrioventricular disease may be coexistent, making interpretation of ECG difficult.

Sinus Pause or Arrest. Sinus pause or sinus arrest (if the sinus pause is prolonged) occurs when the SA node fails to generate an impulse. Unlike SA block, dropped beats are random and not related to the regular P-P interval in any way (Fig. 29-4). A pause can be terminated by a sinus, junctional, or idioventricular escape beat.

Bradycardia-Tachycardia Syndrome. Bradycardia-tachycardia syndrome, alternatively known as the tachycardia-bradycardia

(or tachy-brady) syndrome, is a condition in which a bradycardic rhythm alternates with paroxysms of tachycardia, frequently of a supraventricular origin although accelerated junctional or ventricular rhythms can also be seen. A particularly notable ECG characteristic of the syndrome is the delayed recovery of the sinus mechanism after the abrupt spontaneous termination of the tachydysrhythmia. This may

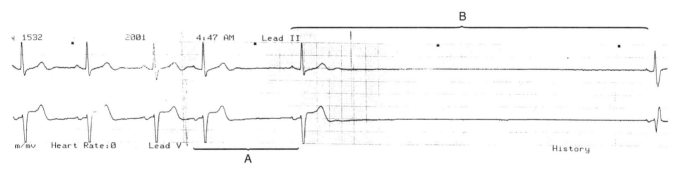

FIGURE 29-4 · **Sinus pause/sinus arrest.** This tracing reflects a rhythm strip simultaneously recorded in lead II (*top*) and a precordial lead (*bottom*). Note that neither pause (*A* or *B*) is a multiple of an underlying basic P-P interval.

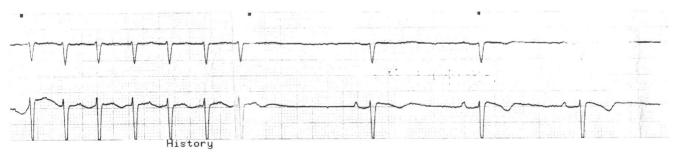

FIGURE 29-5 · **Bradycardia-tachycardia syndrome.** The rhythm strip is again recorded in two leads simultaneously. It demonstrates the alternation between the dysrhythmias, first tachycardic (probably atrial fibrillation), then bradycardic.

manifest as severe sinus bradycardia, sinus pauses, or SA block, or as a junctional rhythm. The transition from the tachydysrhythmia to the bradycardia is very difficult to capture on surface ECG, and therefore this diagnosis is often made based on clinical history and ambulatory monitoring of the patient's cardiac rhythm (Fig. 29-5).

References

1. Lown B: Electrical reversion of cardiac arrhythmias. Br Heart J 1967;29:469.
2. Mangrum JM, DiMarco JP: The evaluation and management of bradycardia. N Engl J Med 2000;342:703.
3. Applegate TE: Atrial arrhythmias. Prim Care 2000;27:677.

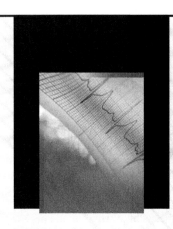

Chapter 30

Atrioventricular Dissociation

Lawrence Isaacs and Richard A. Harrigan

Clinical Features

Atrioventricular (AV) dissociation is a somewhat confusing, often misunderstood phenomenon. Simply defined, it is the independent beating of the atria and ventricles. In this condition, the atria and ventricles are controlled by different pacemakers, for either a single beat, multiple beats, or indefinitely. It is important to realize that AV dissociation is a description of a rhythm disturbance, not a type of dysrhythmia.[1,2] In general, there are three types of AV dissociation: *AV dissociation by default*, *AV dissociation by usurpation*, and *AV dissociation due to block*. Common etiologies for AV dissociation include ischemia, digitalis toxicity, electrolyte abnormalities, carotid sinus hypersensitivity, surgery, and normal variants.[1–5]

Clinically, the patient may present with syncope, chest pain, dyspnea, palpitations, dizziness, or weakness, or may be completely asymptomatic. Physical examination may reveal tachydysrhythmias or bradydysrhythmias, cannon *a* waves (due to simultaneous contraction of the atria and ventricles), increasing intensity of the first heart sound (*bruit de cannon*), or a paradoxical split of the second heart sound.[1] Management is based entirely on treating the underlying cause, not necessarily the rhythm—although there may be situations when medications or temporary cardiac pacing are required to maintain adequate perfusion while the underlying cause is being addressed.

Electrocardiographic Manifestations

By definition, the electrocardiogram (ECG) demonstrates independence of the P waves and QRS complexes. In other words, no evidence of P wave and QRS complex association is observed—these two ECG structures occur entirely independently of one another. AV dissociation may be transient or sustained. In the latter case, it is termed *complete* AV dissociation; the P-P and R-R intervals are uniform, but the PR intervals are variable. However, if the AV dissociation is "incomplete" (atrial beats occasionally capturing the ventricle), the R-R interval will occasionally be irregular. With regard to P wave morphology, the presence or shape of the P wave depends on the rhythm controlling the atria. For example, a normal P wave is seen in sinus rhythm, perhaps an inverted P wave in junctional rhythm, or flutter waves in atrial flutter.

Atrioventricular Dissociation by Default. *AV dissociation by default* occurs when the normally dominant pacemaker (usually the sinus node) slows to allow a normally subsidiary pacemaker (e.g., the AV node) to take control of the ventricles—for as little as one beat or for many beats. An example of this is a junctional escape beat occurring during significant sinus bradycardia. AV dissociation by default may emerge with other

---

ELECTROCARDIOGRAPHIC HIGHLIGHTS

- Independence of P waves and QRS complexes
- *Complete atrioventricular (AV) dissociation*: regularly spaced P waves and QRS complexes without temporal relationship to each other (P-P and R-R intervals are regular, PR interval variable)
- *Incomplete AV dissociation*: occasional narrow QRS complexes captured by P waves (R-R intervals are occasionally irregular)
- *P wave*: presence or shape depends on atrial rhythm

slow rhythms, such as sinus arrhythmia, sinus arrest, or sinoatrial exit block. It is not always reflective of a diseased heart.[5]

Atrioventricular Dissociation by Usurpation. *AV dissociation by usurpation* occurs when a normally slower, subsidiary pacemaker abnormally accelerates to take control of the ventricles. Examples of this include AV junctional tachycardia and ventricular tachycardia (Fig. 30-1).

Atrioventricular Dissociation Due to Block. The third classification is *AV dissociation due to block*, usually at the AV node. This block prevents the impulses from the dominant pacemaker from reaching the ventricles, allowing the ventricles to beat under the control of a normally subsidiary pacemaker (Fig. 30-2). Note that this differs from AV dissociation by default, where the normally dominant pacemaker slows,

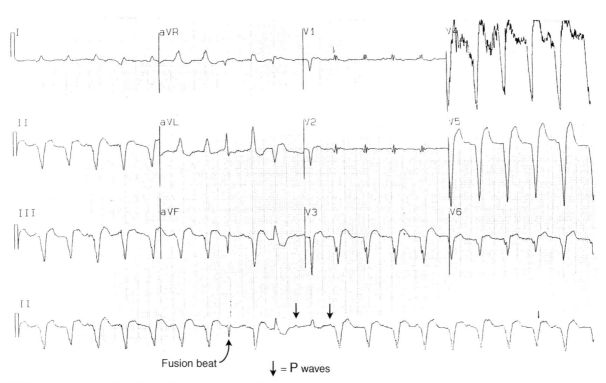

FIGURE 30-1 · **Atrioventricular dissociation by usurpation due to ventricular tachycardia.** Note the one fusion (eighth complex). Also note wide QRS complexes and P waves *(arrows)*, which have no relation to one another. (Reproduced from Harrigan RA, Perron A, Brady W: Atrioventricular dissociation. Am J Emerg Med 2001;19:218–222, with permission.)

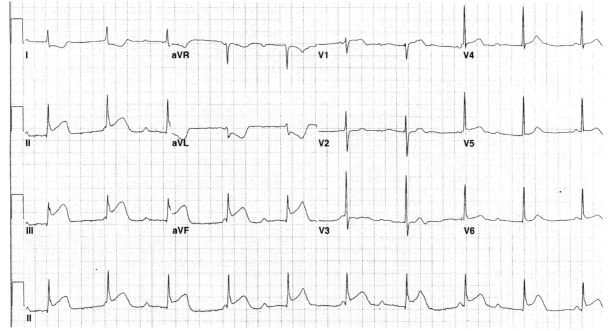

FIGURE 30-2 · **Inferior wall myocardial infarction with complete heart block due to block at the AV node.** This ECG demonstrates another type of atrioventricular dissociation resulting from a block at the AV node. The atrial rate is 80 bpm and the ventricular rate is 58 bpm, with variations in the PR interval.

ELECTROCARDIOGRAPHIC PEARLS

- Atrioventricular (AV) dissociation is a description of a rhythm, not a disease entity.
- The prognosis of AV dissociation depends on its cause; thus, the emergency physician should find and treat the underlying cause, if necessary.
- AV dissociation by default (slowing of the normal pacemaker) may be pathologic, but may also occur in normal hearts.
- AV dissociation by usurpation (quickening of a normally subsidiary pacemaker) reflects an abnormal, excitable state.
- Common etiologies include ischemia, electrolyte abnormalities, digitalis toxicity, and surgery.
- Third degree AV block (complete heart block) is a form of AV dissociation, but not all AV dissociation is due to third degree AV block.

---

and from AV dissociation by usurpation, where a secondary pacemaker has accelerated; here, the atrial rate continues as it would normally. It also differs in that, in both AV dissociation by default or by usurpation, the atrial rate is slower than that of the ventricles, whereas in AV dissociation due to AV block, the atrial rate is faster than the ventricular rate.[1–3]

AV dissociation and complete heart block (third degree AV block) are not synonymous. Complete heart block can be considered a type of AV dissociation, but not all AV dissociation is complete heart block.

Isorhythmic Atrioventricular Dissociation. In this special circumstance, the atria and ventricles are beating independently of each other, but the rates are very similar. The clinician must usually examine a long rhythm strip to observe the gradual, subtle variation in the PR interval. The etiology is unclear.[1,2,5,6]

References

1. Olgin JE, Zipes DP: Specific arrhythmias: Diagnosis and treatment. In Braunwald E, Zipes DP, Libby P (eds): Heart Disease: A Textbook of Cardiovascular Medicine, 6th ed. Philadelphia, WB Saunders, 2001, pp 815–889.
2. Surawicz B, Knilans TK: Chou's Electrocardiography in Clinical Practice: Adult and Pediatric, 5th ed. Philadelphia, WB Saunders, 2001.
3. Harrigan R, Perron A, Brady W: Atrioventricular dissociation. Am J Emerg Med 2001;19:218.
4. Kuner J, Enescu V, Utsu F, et al: Cardiac arrhythmias during anesthesia. Dis Chest 1967;52:580.
5. Marriott HJL, Menendez MM: AV dissociation revisited. Prog Cardiovasc Dis 1966;8:522.
6. Waldo AL, Vitikainen KJ, Harris PD, et al: The mechanism of synchronization in isorhythmic AV dissociation. Circulation 1968;38:880.

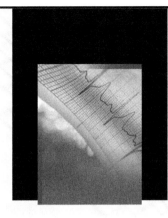

Chapter 31

Waveform Genesis in Acute Coronary Syndromes

Brian F. Ehrling and Andrew D. Perron

The electrocardiogram (ECG) demonstrates a dynamic spectrum of changes in the face of myocardial ischemia and infarction. Tissue ischemia potentially alters the morphology of the ST segment and the T wave, as well as the waves that comprise the QRS complex, leading to characteristic changes on the ECG (see Chapter 32, Acute Coronary Syndromes: Acute Myocardial Infarction and Ischemia). This usually occurs in a regional fashion because of impaired flow through one or more coronary arteries, and as such results in characteristic changes in ECG leads that represent the various anatomic regions of the heart (see Chapter 33, Acute Coronary Syndromes: Regional Issues).

Ischemic Conditions

With myocardial ischemia, there is a decrease in activity of the sodium-potassium–adenosine triphosphatase pump, and a consequent decrease in intracellular potassium. This pump is integral to maintaining the resting membrane potential as well

as generating the gradient necessary for phase 3 repolarization. Hence, there is a less negative resting membrane potential and a decrease in diastolic transmembrane potential. Phase 3 repolarization is also delayed. In addition, ischemic cells repolarize starting at the last point in the cell membrane to depolarize, which is opposite to that observed in normal cells. Therefore, the cellular repolarization vector in ischemic cells is opposite to that of normal cells, and is delayed, both of which are important in explaining pathologic ECG changes.

T Wave Changes

Subendocardial ischemia is the most common and earliest entity of acute coronary syndrome, and features delayed recovery of the ischemic zone. Repolarization proceeds from the epicardium to the endocardium in normal tissue, and therefore this delay does not change the direction of the repolarization vector. However, the prolonged repolarization does increase the amplitude of the vector, which generates a "hyperacute" T wave (Fig. 31-1).

FIGURE 31-1 · Repolarization in normal and ischemic cardiac tissue. The intrinsic delay of the endocardium to repolarize generates a positive T wave during normal repolarization. Subendocardial ischemia augments this delay and results in hyperacute T waves. Subepicardial ischemia results in a repolarization delay in the subepicardium, which reverses the repolarization vector and inverts the T wave. (Adapted with permission from Erling B, Brady W: Basic principles and electrophysiology. In Smith SW, Zvosec D, Henry TD, Sharkey SW [eds]: The ECG in Acute MI: An Evidence-based Manual of Reperfusion Therapy. Philadelphia, Lippincott Williams & Wilkins, 2002, pp 1-5.)

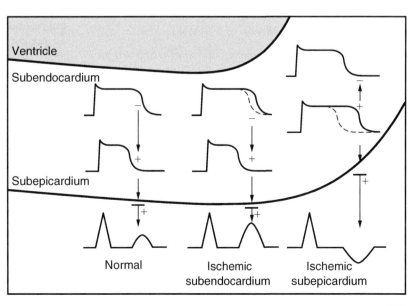

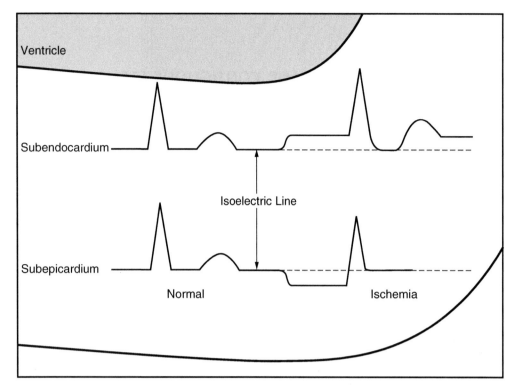

FIGURE 31-2 · The "current of injury" theory of ST segment depression and elevation. Injured tissue is less repolarized, and hence has a slightly less negative resting membrane potential. A positive reading electrode interprets this change during subendocardial ischemia as an upward shift of the isoelectric line because the electrode is distant from the tissue. During subepicardial ischemia, the electrode is adjacent to the tissue and interprets the less-negative resting membrane potential as a downward shift of the isoelectric line. The ST segment remains at the "baseline" isoelectric line because the tissue is still able to depolarize to the same degree. (Adapted with permission from Erling B, Brady W: Basic principles and electrophysiology. In Smith SW, Zvosec D, Henry TD, Sharkey SW [eds]: The ECG in Acute MI: An Evidence-based Manual of Reperfusion Therapy. Philadelphia, Lippincott Williams & Wilkins, 2002, pp 1-5.)

The repolarization delay in subepicardial ischemia carries greater electrical significance because it can completely reverse the direction of the repolarization vector. The result is the familiar and easily identified T wave inversion. In general, subepicardial ischemia is transmural, and only seldom occurs without involvement of the endocardium; however, because of its relatively larger mass as well as its closer proximity to the electrode, subepicardial ischemia dictates the electrical picture. This pattern holds true for lateral, inferior, and anterior ischemia on the standard 12-lead ECG.

The T wave inversions of transmural ischemia, theoretically, occur last during an infarction, after ST segment and Q wave changes. Realistically, each type of change can be seen at any given time during an infarction secondary to differing zones of ischemia around an infarct.

ST Segment Changes

The etiology of ST segment changes during myocardial injury is not entirely understood, although the "current of injury" theory has been proposed as a possible explanation. It is known that injured cells lose their membrane integrity, which produces a potassium leak out of the cell. Injured tissue is less repolarized, and hence has a slightly less negative resting membrane potential. The counter-charge on the outside of the cell is then slightly less positive. A distant, positive reading electrode interprets this change during subendocardial ischemia as an increase in the baseline vector. The result is an upward shift of the isoelectric line. During subepicardial ischemia, the electrode is adjacent to the tissue and interprets the less-positive charge as a decrease in the vector amplitude. The result is a downward shift of the isoelectric line. The ST segment, however, remains at the "baseline" isoelectric line because the tissue is still able to depolarize to the same degree (Fig. 31-2). In subepicardial/transmural ischemia, the baseline

isoelectric line, as demonstrated by the TP segment, decreases in voltage, and the ST segment is then relatively elevated. In subendocardial injury, the new isoelectric line increases and the ST segment appears depressed.

Another, quite opposite theory is that of "incomplete depolarization," which has its foundation in the belief that damaged cells do not completely depolarize. With this theory, there is no change to the isoelectric line. For example, in subepicardial/transmural injury, where the electrode is adjacent to these damaged cells, systole would be represented by a more positive ST segment. In subendocardial injury, electrodes over the normally depolarizing epicardium would interpret the distant partial depolarization as ST segment depression.

During transmural injury, ST segment elevations at adjacent electrodes may be accompanied by ST segment depressions at distant electrodes. These are known as *reciprocal changes*, and can be explained by either of the two aforementioned theories. There must be ST segment elevation at some recording electrode for ST segment depression to be termed a reciprocal change. Otherwise, the ST segment depression simply represents subendocardial injury, and not transmural infarction.

Q Waves

During normal ventricular activation, the septum is depolarized first during the initial 0.02 sec, and subsequently proceeds over the next 0.03 to 0.04 sec into the anterior, inferior, and lateral walls. Depolarization terminates in the posterior and high lateral walls. Either preexcitation or infarction can result in QRS changes in the first 0.04 sec of depolarization, the difference being that in the case of infarction, the dead tissue is electrically silent. A relatively large infarction (i.e., transmural) is necessary to generate pathologic Q waves. The pathologic Q wave is generated as the vector points away from this quiet tissue toward normal myocardium for the initial 40 msec.

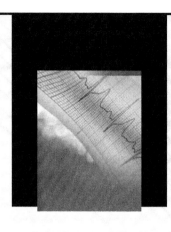

Chapter 32

Acute Coronary Syndromes: Acute Myocardial Infarction and Ischemia

Stephen W. Smith and Wayne Whitwam

Clinical Features

Acute coronary syndrome (ACS) encompasses the clinical presentation of those diseases most often associated with coronary artery disease (CAD) in which disruption of a vulnerable atherosclerotic plaque and subsequent exposure of the subendothelium stimulates platelet and fibrin activation, forming a thrombus that may occlude the coronary artery. The patient's symptoms are those associated with an imbalance between myocardial oxygen supply and demand, causing myocardial ischemia. By definition, this syndrome is characterized as either (1) acute myocardial infarction (AMI), defined as myocardial cell death due to prolonged ischemia and diagnosed by elevated levels of cardiac-specific serum markers; or as (2) unstable angina (UA), which implies fully reversible ischemia. Even though electrocardiographic (ECG) changes may indicate myocardial ischemia that has the potential to progress to myocardial infarction (MI), these changes are not sufficient by themselves to define AMI. The final diagnosis of myocardial necrosis depends on the detection of elevated cardiac biomarkers in the serum.

AMI may present initially with or without ST segment elevation (STE) on the ECG. ST segment elevation MI (STEMI) is a result of persistent complete occlusion of an artery supplying a significant area of myocardium without adequate collateral circulation. AMI without STE, although usually with ST segment depression or T wave changes, is referred to as non–ST segment elevation MI (NSTEMI), and its initial clinical and ECG presentation is frequently indistinguishable from UA. UA and NSTEMI result from non-occlusive thrombus, small risk area, brief occlusion, or an occlusion that maintains good collateral circulation (in addition, circumflex artery occlusion frequently manifests no STE). NSTEMI is differentiated from UA by cell death and the release of troponin in measurable amounts. However, both UA and, to a greater extent, NSTEMI confer a significant risk of subsequent death or MI that is significantly diminished by

aggressive medical therapy and, for those at highest risk, early revascularization.[1-3]

Approximately 45% of all AMIs manifest diagnostic STE.[4-6] However, a significant number of patients with AMI present with subtle STE and therefore are less easily recognized. Furthermore, most STE is a result of non-AMI etiologies.[7,8]

Electrocardiographic Manifestations

Primary and Secondary ST Segment and T Wave Abnormalities. Much of the ECG diagnosis of ACS depends on analysis of the ST segment and T wave. Such ST segment/T wave abnormalities may be *secondary* to QRS abnormalities, such as left ventricular hypertrophy (LVH) or left bundle branch block (LBBB), or they may be *primary* (i.e., not a result of an abnormal QRS). The ST segment/T wave abnormalities of ischemia are termed *primary*, although they may be superimposed on *secondary* abnormalities. Thus, with any ST segment/T wave abnormalities, one must not conclude hastily that they are due to ischemia/infarction, but rather consider the ST segment/T wave complex within the context of the entire QRST complex.

Traditionally, ST segment changes have been measured relative to the TP segment. Others have advanced the concept that ST segment changes should be viewed relative to the PR segment because of atrial repolarization[9-11] (Fig. 32-1).

Evolution of ST Segment Elevation Acute Myocardial Infarction on the Electrocardiogram. STEMI manifests as a developing sequence of transformations on serial ECGs (Fig. 32-2): An initial hyperacute T wave develops within the first minutes of an AMI; this is followed by STE; Q wave formation may begin within 1 hour and be completed by 8 to 12 hours; shallow T wave inversion is seen within 72 hours; and, finally, stabilization of the ST segment usually takes place within 12 hours, with or without STE resolution over the ensuing 72 hours.[12-14] STE resolves within 2 weeks after

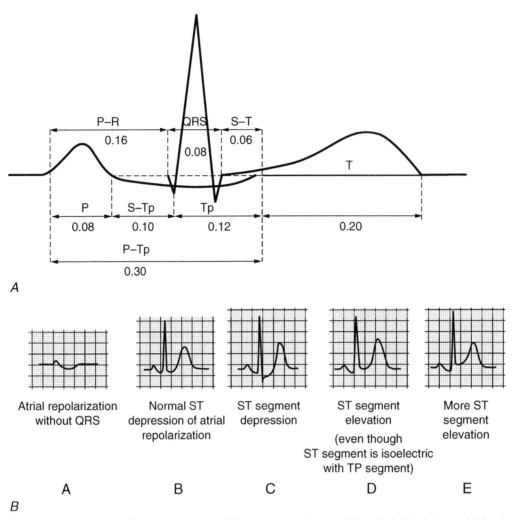

FIGURE 32-1 · Atrial repolarization as it affects measurement of ST segment elevation. *A,* Atrial repolarization follows atrial depolarization, producing a deflection called the T_p *(or T_a) wave*, not ordinarily seen because it is buried in the QRS complex. The T_p wave may falsely depress the ST segment at the junction between the QRS complex and the ST segment (called the *J point*). Therefore, ST segment elevation should be measured at the J point and relative to the PR segment. Alternatively, it may be measured at 0.06 to 0.08 sec after the J point and relative to the TP segment. (Reprinted from Tranchesi J, Adelardi V, de Oliverira JM: Atrial repolarization: Its importance in clinical electrocardiography. Circulation 1960;22:635. Used by permission of the American Heart Association, Inc.) *B,* "A" shows the P wave and atrial repolarization without a QRS complex superimposed; "B" shows the ST and PR segments are isoelectric (no ST segment depression); "C" shows the ST segment lower than the PR segment (true ST segment depression); "D" shows the ST segment at the level of the TP segment, but it should be depressed by the atrial repolarization and thus be at the level of the PR segment; therefore, there is ST segment elevation; "E" shows the ST segment above both the PR and TP segments (also ST segment elevation).

95% of inferior and 40% of anterior MI; persistence for more than 2 weeks after infarction is associated with greater morbidity.[14] Approximately 60% of patients with MI with persistent ST segment displacement have anatomic ventricular aneurysm (Fig. 32-3).

Most patients with completed, nonreperfused STEMI ultimately have Q waves, whereas a minority do not.[15] T waves may normalize over days, weeks, or months.[16] AMI has been classified as *Q wave* or *non–Q wave* MI, as well as the older *transmural* versus *subendocardial* MI; these terms were discovered to be both clinically and pathologically inaccurate, in part because there is little relationship between Q waves and transmural MI.[9–11,17] In STEMI, reperfusion of the infarct-related artery makes it significantly less likely that Q waves will develop.[13] Established Q waves disappear in days, weeks, or months in 15% to 30% of acute Q wave MIs.

Hyperacute T Wave. In the ECG evolution of AMI, alteration in T wave morphology or amplitude may be the first sign of coronary occlusion (Fig. 32-4). Experimentally, these

hyperacute T waves may form as early as 2 minutes after coronary ligation, but typically present within the first 30 minutes after a clinical event.[18–24] Even at this early phase, there is only subendocardial ischemia without cell death. The first change to the T wave may be an oblique straightening of the ST segment (Fig. 32-4), followed by a subtle enlargement of the T wave, with diminishing R wave amplitude. The T waves, often bulky and wide, without much upward concavity, are localized to the area of injury.[24–26] The J point is usually elevated, but may become depressed, with the T wave appearing to have its take-off below the isoelectric line[27,28] (see Fig. 32-4). The ratio of T wave amplitude to QRS amplitude is a better indicator of AMI than T wave amplitude alone, and that ratio correlates with the duration of coronary occlusion.[29] Reperfusion therapy begun while T waves are hyperacute has been demonstrated to correlate with a clinically better outcome because hyperacute T waves are a marker of early coronary occlusion.[29]

ST Segment Elevation. Although hyperacute T waves are the first sign of experimental AMI, this phase may be missed

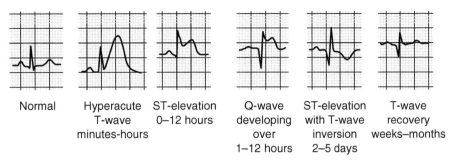

FIGURE 32-2 • **Progression of nonreperfused ST segment elevation myocardial infarction.** (Courtesy of K. Wang, Hennepin County Medical Center, Minneapolis, MN)

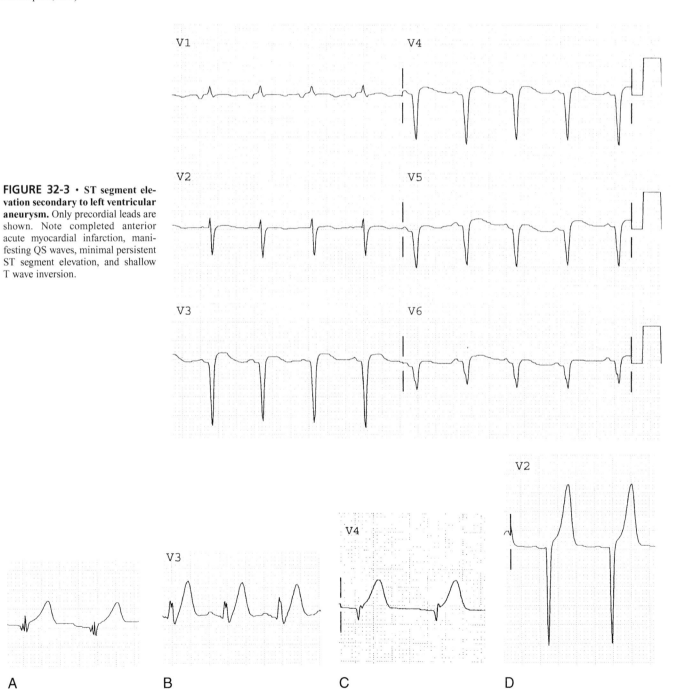

FIGURE 32-3 • **ST segment elevation secondary to left ventricular aneurysm.** Only precordial leads are shown. Note completed anterior acute myocardial infarction, manifesting QS waves, minimal persistent ST segment elevation, and shallow T wave inversion.

FIGURE 32-4 • **Four examples of hyperacute T waves.** *A,* In lead V_2, the T wave is massive compared with the QRS complex; there are also small Q waves present; *B,* Lead V_3 shows depressed ST segment take-off and straightening of the ST segment. *C,* Lead V_4 shows T waves that are wide and bulky, much larger than the QRS complex. *D,* This less common form of hyperacute T wave, seen here in lead V_2, is very peaked and tented, with an appearance of hyperkalemia.

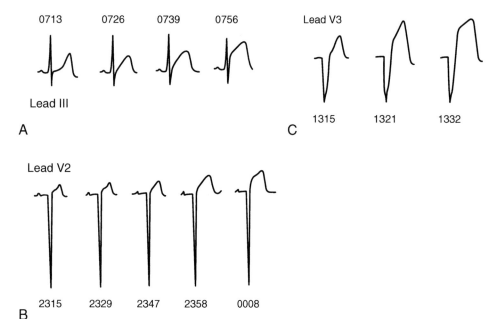

A

Lead III

0713   0726   0739   0756

B

Lead V2

2315   2329   2347   2358   0008

C

Lead V3

1315   1321   1332

FIGURE 32-5 • **Serial ECGs in three patients; time of tracing shown in parentheses.** *A,* This rhythm strip demonstrates the evolution of the ST segment from normal concave upward (0713) to straight (0726) to convex (0739) to still more ST segment elevation, confirming ST segment elevation myocardial infarction (0756). *B,* This tracing demonstrates the typical morphology of left ventricular hypertrophy (LVH) in lead V_2. Serial tracings reveal morphology evolution from straight and convex, with increased height of ST segments, suggesting acute myocardial infarction (AMI) superimposed on LVH. *C,* This tracing shows typical morphology of left bundle branch block in lead V_3, with subsequent increased ST segment elevation. The change is diagnostic of superimposed AMI.

in actual clinical situations. During prolonged ischemia, the ST segment often changes from a concave morphology to one that is straight, and then on to convex (Fig. 32-5). A concave ST segment morphology may persist with AMI, but is also common in nonischemic states. In anterior AMI, upward concavity is most common, but upwardly convex morphology is more specific for STEMI and is associated with greater infarct size and morbidity.[30,31] Coronary occlusion is often transient or dynamic, with "cyclic" reperfusion and reocclusion.[32] Indeed, transient STE appears in approximately 20% of STEMI, especially after aspirin therapy.[33]

Under the best of circumstances, the ECG has a sensitivity of 56% and specificity of 94% for AMI.[4-6,34] However, even STEMI is frequently not obvious, and ECG computer algorithms are especially insensitive for this diagnosis.[35] Various clinical trials of thrombolytic therapy have defined STE differently, using different criteria for amount of STE (1 or 2 mm [0.1 or 0.2 mV]), and for the number of leads required[36-44] (one or two leads; Fig. 32-6 and Table 32-1). A recent consensus document attempted to establish a better working definition. The authors define ST segment changes indicative of myocardial ischemia that may progress to infarction as new or presumed

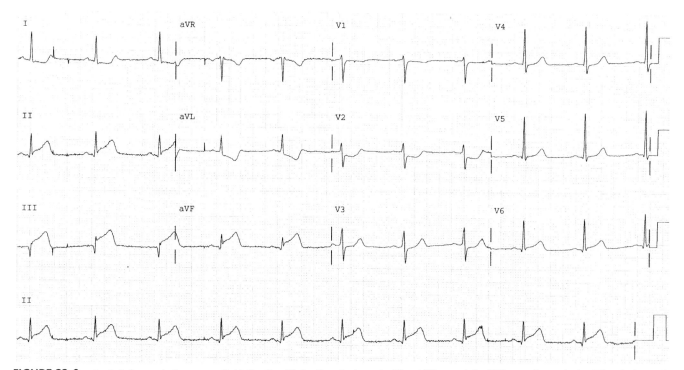

FIGURE 32-6 • **Acute inferoposterior myocardial infarction.** Notice there is also a significant QR wave in lead III soon after occlusion. There is the nearly obligatory reciprocal ST segment depression in lead aVL, but also reciprocal depression in leads V_2 and V_3 that is diagnostic of simultaneous posterior ST segment elevation myocardial infarction (right coronary artery occlusion with posterior branches).

32-1 • ST SEGMENT ELEVATION REQUIREMENTS: MAJOR THROMBOLYTIC TRIALS AND PRACTICE GUIDELINES*

Study or Practice Guidelines	Minimum Number, Consecutive Leads	Minimum ST Segment Elevation, Limb Leads (mm)	Minimum ST Segment Elevation, Precordial Leads (mm)
AHA/ACC	2	1	1
GISSI-1	1	1	2
GISSI-2	1	1	2
GUSTO	2	1	2
TIMI	2	1	1
TAMI	2	1	1
ISIS-2, ISIS-3	None, "suspected myocardial infarction" only		
Minnesota Code	1	1 mm: I, II, II, aVL, aVF, V_5, V_6	
		2 mm: V_1–V_4	

*Method and location of measurement of the ST segment are usually not stated.

ACC, American College of Cardiology; AHA, American Heart Association; GISSI, Gruppo Italiano per lo Studio della Sopravivenza Nell'Infarto Miocardio; GUSTO, Global Utilization of Streptokinase and Tissue Plasminogen Activator for Occluded Coronary Arteries; ISIS, International Study of Infarct Survival; TAMI, Thrombolysis and Angioplasty in Myocardial Infarction; TIMI, Thrombolysis in Myocardial Infarction.

Adapted with permission from Smith SW, Zvosec DL, Sharkey SW, Henry TD: The ECG in Acute MI: An Evidence-Based Manual of Reperfusion Therapy. Philadelphia, Lippincott Williams & Wilkins, 2002.

new STE at the J point in two or more contiguous leads with the cut-off points of 0.2 mV or more in leads V_1, V_2, or V_3 and 0.1 mV or more in other leads (contiguity in the frontal plane is defined by the lead sequence aVL, I, inverted aVR, II, aVF, III).[45] Whatever the clinical scenario, a well-informed subjective interpretation of the appearance of the ST segment is significantly more accurate than measured criteria.[35,46] Thus, always interpret ST segment deviation within the larger context of overall ECG morphology and clinical presentation.

Prognostic Features of ST Segment Elevation.   Anterior location of STE (anterior AMI), compared with inferior or lateral, correlates with much worse prognosis and greater benefit of reperfusion therapy.[47–51] Greater height of ST segments and greater number of leads involved correlate with higher mortality and greater benefit from reperfusion therapy (Fig. 32-7). A high *ST score* (the total millimeters of STE in

---

ELECTROCARDIOGRAPHIC HIGHLIGHTS

ST segment elevation

- Greater than 1 mm
- In at least two anatomically contiguous leads
- Typically straight or convex morphology, although may be concave

ST segment depression

- Downsloping or flat
- Greater than 1 mm

Hyperacute T wave

- Prominent
- Broad-based
- Asymmetrical
- Upright
- May be first sign of coronary occlusion

Nonspecific ST segment/T wave changes

- Less than 1 mm ST segment change
- T waves that are not hyperacute or inverted

Q wave

- At least 0.04 sec in duration or one-third the height of accompanying R wave

---

ELECTROCARDIOGRAPHIC PEARLS

- Aside from new left bundle branch block (LBBB), regional ST segment elevation (STE) is the only ECG indication for acute reperfusion therapy (STEMI); ST segment depression in leads V_1 to V_4 reflects a reciprocal view of posterior STE and is thus an exception.
- Non-STE acute events are not an indication for thrombolytics.
- Reciprocal ST segment depression on the ECG improves the specificity of STE for the diagnosis of acute myocardial infarction (AMI).
- With inferior AMI, look for reciprocal ST segment depression in lead aVL.
- ECG manifestations of high-risk STEMI are anterior location, multiple leads with STE, prominent STE, and reciprocal ST segment depression.
- Beware of missing subtle STE in inferior or lateral wall AMI.
- Because of *absence* of STE on the 12-lead ECG, posterior AMI is frequently overlooked.
- Right ventricular AMI increases the mortality risk of inferior AMI, and may be overlooked if a right-sided ECG is not recorded in inferior AMI.
- Anterior STE due to AMI may easily be misinterpreted as early repolarization.
- If the ECG is nondiagnostic and the symptoms are typical and persistent, record serial ECGs or use continuous ST segment monitoring
- LBBB may obscure the ECG diagnosis of AMI.
- Right bundle branch block (RBBB) does not obscure the ECG diagnosis of AMI.

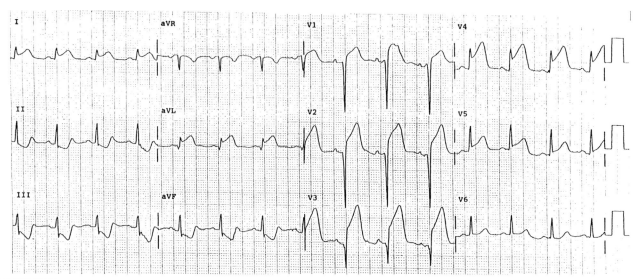

FIGURE 32-7 • **ST segment elevation (STE) myocardial infarction approximately 1 hour after occlusion but already manifesting Q waves.** These are QR waves, although the ST segment distorts the QRS complex to the point that the R wave is difficult to discern. The T waves are hyperacute and STE is very high. There is anterior and lateral STE, and inferior reciprocal ST segment depression, which correlates with an occlusion proximal to the first diagonal, and STE in lead V₁ correlates with septal infarction (occlusion proximal to the first septal perforator). Even with a history of 48 hours of chest pain, this ECG represents an acute occlusion, and is an indication for reperfusion therapy. (Reprinted with permission from Smith SW, Zvosec DL, Sharkey SW, Henry TD: The ECG in Acute MI: An Evidence-Based Manual of Reperfusion Therapy. Philadelphia, Lippincott Williams & Wilkins, 2002.)

all leads combined) correlates with higher mortality. Measured at the J point, a score greater than 12 to 13 mm for anterior AMI, and greater than 6 to 9 mm for inferior AMI, correlates with high risk of early complications.[50,52] Measured at 0.06 sec after the J point, risk is defined as relatively low, intermediate, or high based on ST score less than 12 mm, 12 to 20 mm, or greater than 20 mm, respectively (mean measurement at the J point [16 ± 9 mm] is significantly different from that at 0.06 sec after the J point [23 ± 11 mm]).[53] Total ST segment deviation, including reciprocal ST segment depression, may correlate with risk better than ST score alone.[53,54] Distortion of the terminal portion of the QRS (loss of

S wave in leads with RS configuration, or J point at least 50% the height of the R wave) is associated with a doubling of the mortality rate.[55] Nevertheless, although the correlations are real, there remains wide individual variation such that some patients without these features may have a very large AMI.[56]

Borderline ST Segment Elevation. Subtle STE (i.e., elevation <2 mm in the precordial leads, or ≤1 mm in other leads) may represent STEMI and easily be missed (Fig. 32-8). Such cases may be difficult to recognize, or difficult to differentiate from other etiologies, or both. Change from previous ECGs, changes over minutes to hours, the presence or absence of

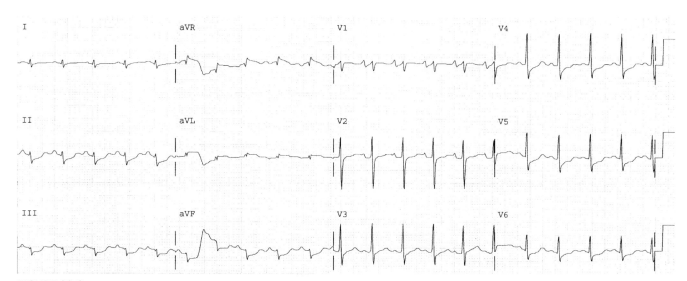

FIGURE 32-8 • **Subtle ST segment elevation.** In this case of circumflex artery occlusion, lateral ST segment elevation myocardial infarction is seen in one lead only (aVL). Reciprocal inferior ST segment depression is the most visible ECG sign. Inferior ST segment depression should prompt a search for ST segment elevation in lead aVL, which is there and is as high as it can be with such a low-voltage QRS complex.

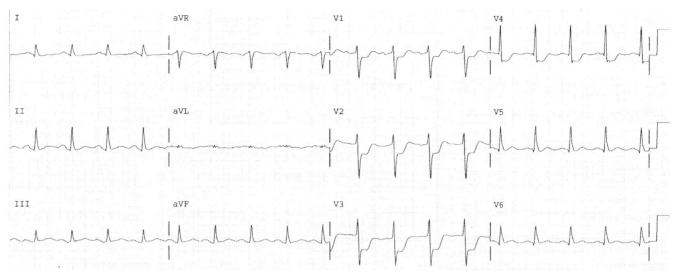

FIGURE 32-9 · Posterior AMI. There is no ST segment elevation (STE) on this ECG, yet this patient is a candidate for thrombolytics. The marked ST segment depression in leads V_1 to V_4 was a reciprocal view of a posterior wall STE myocardial infarction. Angiography revealed an occluded second obtuse marginal artery.

reciprocal ST segment depression, or presence of upward convexity, may help make the diagnosis. Circumflex or first diagonal artery occlusion may present with minimal or no STE because the lateral wall is in a more electrocardiographically silent area.[57–59] Nevertheless, the size of this myocardial risk area may be very large.[60,61] When R wave amplitude is low (frequently found in lead aVL), STE cannot possibly be any higher (see Fig. 32-8).

Reciprocal ST Segment Depression. Reciprocal ST segment depression improves the specificity for STEMI in the presence of normal conduction. Because reciprocal ST segment depression does not develop in a significant number of STEMIs, absence of reciprocal ST segment depression does not rule out STEMI.[8,62–66] In the presence of abnormal conduction (e.g., LVH, bundle branch block, or intraventricular conduction delay), ST segment depression is usually present as a result of the altered intraventricular conduction and therefore does not represent reciprocal ST segment depression[66] (see Chapter 34, Acute Myocardial Infarction: Confounding Patterns). Reciprocal ST segment depression presents as either (1) an opposing electrical view ("true" reciprocity) of the leads with STE (e.g., in inferior AMI, ST segment depression in lead aVL, which is 150 degrees opposite from lead III; see Fig. 32-6); (2) posterior STEMI (i.e., ST segment depression in leads V_1 to V_4, with or without STE in leads V_5 and V_6 or leads II, III, and aVF; see Figs. 32-6 and 32-9); or, much less commonly, (3) simultaneous UA/NSTEMI of another coronary distribution. The vast majority of inferior wall AMIs reveal reciprocal ST segment depression in lead aVL; many also manifest in precordial leads, indicating simultaneous posterior wall STEMI (see Fig. 32-6). Forty to 70% of anterior AMIs manifest reciprocal ST segment depression in at least one of leads II, III, and aVF; this ST segment depression correlates strongly with a proximal left anterior descending (LAD) coronary artery occlusion[67–70] (see Fig. 32-7). Reciprocal ST segment depression is associated with a higher mortality rate,[54] but also with greater benefit from thrombolytics.[53] This is especially true of precordial ST segment depression in

inferior AMI.[71] In some cases, reciprocal ST segment depression is the most visible sign of STEMI[28,72] (see Fig. 32-8).

T Wave Inversion. In the presence of normal conduction, the T wave is normally upright in the left-sided leads I, II, and V_3 to V_6; inverted in lead aVR; and variable in leads III, aVL, aVF, and V_1, with rare normal inversion in V_2. T wave inversion is associated with a number of conditions, and in the presence of symptoms suggesting ACS, T wave inversion is most likely a manifestation of ischemia. Isolated or minimally inverted nondynamic T waves (<1 mm) may be due to ACS but are not independently associated with adverse outcomes compared with patients with ACS and no ECG abnormalities.[3] However, T wave inversion due to ACS that is greater than 1 mm or seen in two or more leads is associated with higher-risk ACS.[73,74] T wave inversions without STE are never an indication for thrombolytics, but rather, in the appropriate clinical context, represent UA/NSTEMI.

During completed, nonreperfused AMI, as regional ST segments return to the isoelectric level, T waves invert in the same region, but not deeply (up to 3 mm).[75] Shallow T wave inversions in the presence of deep QS waves recorded at patient presentation usually represent AMI late in its course, with completed injury and necrosis.[75] Even with persistent STE, the opportunity for improvement with thrombolytic therapy may be lost (Fig. 32-10).

In the setting of reperfusion, whether spontaneous or as a result of therapy, there is often regional *terminal T wave inversion*.[76,77] This terminal inversion is identical to Wellens' pattern A and the *cove-plane T*.[73,78,79] The ST segments may retain some elevation, but the T waves invert, resulting in a biphasic appearance (Fig. 32-11). Later after reperfusion, the ST segments recover to the isoelectric level or slightly below, and are upwardly convex, sometimes with upward bowing, and the T wave inversion becomes more symmetrical and greater than 3 mm in depth.[75] This is identical to Wellens' pattern B (Fig. 32-12) or the *coronary T* or *Pardee T*[73,78,79] (Fig. 32-13). In both of these types of T wave inversion, the R wave is preserved; both are believed to be a result of

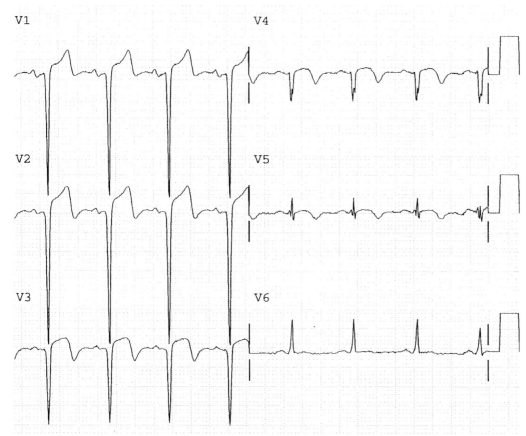

FIGURE 32-10 · **Simultaneous Q wave and ST segment elevation (STE).** This tracing shows anterior STE with QS waves and terminal T wave inversion. This is diagnostic of STE myocardial infarction, but suggests prolonged occlusion or spontaneous reperfusion. Indeed, this 37-year-old patient's symptoms had been constant for 32 hours. (Reprinted with permission from Smith SW, Zvosec DL, Sharkey SW, Henry TD: The ECG in Acute MI: An Evidence-Based Manual of Reperfusion Therapy. Philadelphia, Lippincott Williams & Wilkins, 2002.)

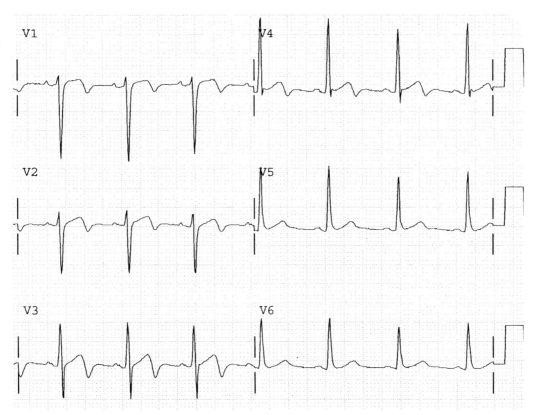

FIGURE 32-11 · **Wellens' syndrome.** Only precordial leads are shown. Wellens' syndrome, pattern A (analogous to "cove-plane T"), is demonstrated in a patient whose chest pain had recently resolved. The corrected QT interval is 0.45 sec, which helps to differentiate this from benign T wave inversion. Troponin, but not creatine kinase-MB, was minimally elevated, and there was a very tight left anterior descending artery stenosis. (Reprinted with permission from Smith SW, Zvosec DL, Sharkey SW, Henry TD: The ECG in Acute MI: An Evidence-Based Manual of Reperfusion Therapy. Philadelphia, Lippincott Williams & Wilkins, 2002.)

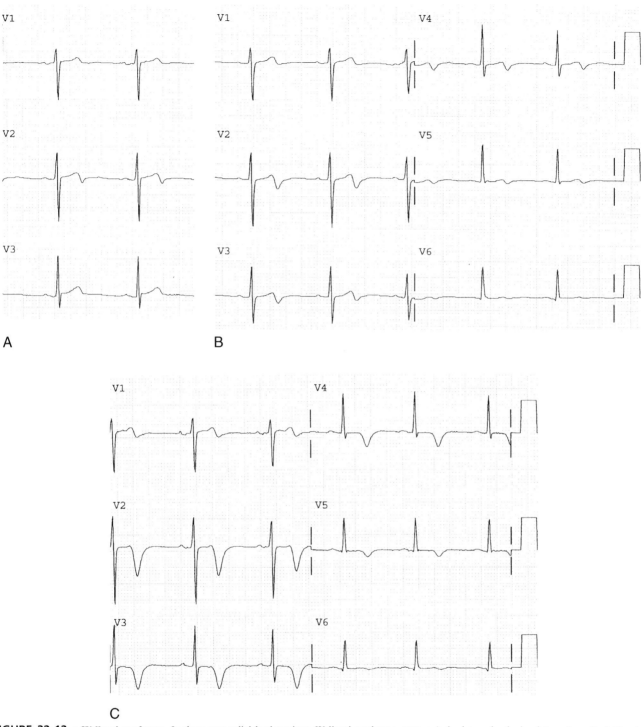

FIGURE 32-12 · Wellens' syndrome. In these precordial lead tracings, Wellens' syndrome, pattern A, is shown developing into pattern B. *A*, Terminal T wave inversion (Wellens' pattern A) in lead V_2 only, 1.5 hours after spontaneous resolution of chest pain with ST segment elevation. *B*, Terminal T wave inversion in leads V_2 to V_5 3 hours after chest pain resolution. *C*, Symmetrical T wave inversion the next morning (Wellens' pattern B; similar to *coronary T* or *Pardee T*). Troponin I, but not creatine kinase-MB, was elevated, and there was a very tight left anterior descending artery stenosis. (Fig. 32-12*C* is reprinted with permission from Smith SW, Zvosec DL, Sharkey SW, Henry TD: The ECG in Acute MI: An Evidence-Based Manual of Reperfusion Therapy. Philadelphia, Lippincott Williams & Wilkins, 2002.)

ischemia surrounding the infarct zone. If the T wave inversion is persistent, there will nearly always be troponin elevation, and this pattern is frequently termed *non–Q wave MI*. If no STE was recorded, this would be appropriately termed "NSTEMI," although frequently the transient STE simply went unrecorded.

Wellens' syndrome (see Figs. 32-11 and 32-12) refers to deep, prominent T wave inversion in leads V_2 to V_4 in the presence of persistent R waves, and represents probable transient STEMI due to occlusion of the LAD that, before the ECG recording, either spontaneously opened or received collateral flow.[28,73,74,80,81] This T wave inversion in the precordial leads is

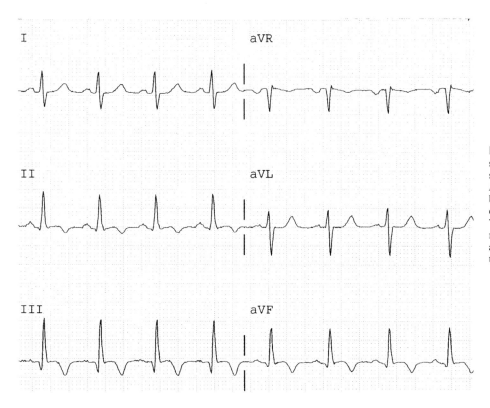

FIGURE 32-13 · Inferior Wellens' syndrome, pattern B. Only limb leads are shown. In this example, the *coronary T* or *Pardee T* morphology is evident (upward bowing of the ST segment and upward convexity before the symmetrically inverted T waves). Troponin was elevated and angiography revealed a very tight right coronary artery stenosis. (A qR wave in lead III at close to 0.04 sec may or may not be pathologic.)

associated with a high incidence of critical narrowing of the proximal LAD and indicates high risk for reocclusion with recurrent STEMI.[73,74] Identical T wave morphology is recorded after approximately 60% of cases of successful reperfusion therapy for anterior STEMI.[76,77] Similar patterns also occur in other coronary artery distributions (e.g., inferior [Figs. 32-13 and 32-14] or lateral [Fig. 32-14]), but the syndrome was originally described in the LAD. Reocclusion manifests as ST segment re-elevation and normalization of

terminal T wave inversion, called T wave *pseudonormalization* because the T wave flips upright (Fig. 32-15). Normalization of the T wave over weeks to months is part of the natural course of MI; true pseudonormalization—indicating reocclusion—is evident only if it occurs within days of the initial insult.

ST Segment Depression. Primary ST segment depression, if not reciprocal to STE or due to posterior STEMI, is an ECG sign of UA/NSTEMI (Figs. 32-16 and 32-17). ST segment

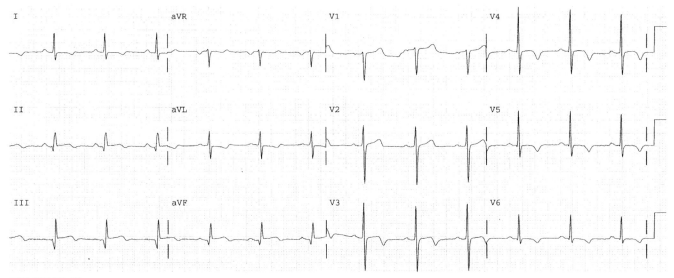

FIGURE 32-14 · Simultaneous inferior (pattern A) and lateral (pattern B) Wellens' syndrome. This tracing demonstrating simultaneous inferior (pattern A) and lateral (pattern B) Wellens' syndrome was recorded 10 hours after resolution of chest pain. The troponin I level was 20 ng/mL and there was an infero-posterior wall motion abnormality. A dominant right coronary artery was occluded, with collateral filling from two tightly stenotic obtuse marginals (off the circumflex artery). Pathologic qR waves are seen in the inferior leads.

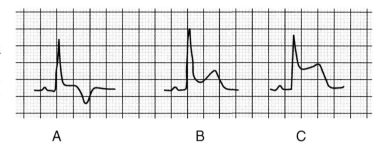

FIGURE 32-15 · **Schematic of reocclusion of a reperfused coronary artery.** *A,* T wave inversion is very suggestive of reperfused ST segment elevation myocardial infarction (Wellens' syndrome). *B,* The T wave has flipped upright ("pseudonormalization"), diagnostic of reocclusion. *C,* Persistent occlusion has elevated the ST segment still higher.

depression of only 0.5 mm, if changed from baseline, is associated with an increased mortality rate, but it is particularly significant when it is greater than 1 mm (0.10 mV) in two or more contiguous leads.[82] As with STE, it is measured at the J point. Although ST segment depression with or without T wave abnormality may be chronic, the ST segment depression associated with UA/NSTEMI is transient. Furthermore, it is usually flat or downsloping. Concurrent T wave inversion may or may not be present. ST segment depression of stable angina, due to coronary stenosis but not thrombosis, may be reproduced with exercise or activity. The proportionality of ST segment depression is important: 1 mm of ST segment depression after an R wave of less than 10 mm is more specific for ischemia, but less *sensitive*, than is 1 mm of ST depression after an R wave of greater than 20 mm.[83–86]

ST segment depression greater than 2 mm and present in three or more leads is associated with a high probability of serum marker–positive AMI, a 30-day mortality rate of up to 35%, and a 4-year mortality rate of 47%, regardless of whether there is complete coronary occlusion.[87] Lesser degrees of ST segment depression are associated with 30-day mortality rates from 10% to 26%. ST segment depression, with the exception of that which represents posterior STEMI, or that which is reciprocal to other STE, is not an indication for thrombolytic therapy.[1,54,88–90] ST segment depression (even as little as 0.5 mm), as well as positive troponin, remains a strong predictor of adverse outcome, and is one of the best indicators of benefit from an early invasive (within 48 hours) management strategy, in addition to intensive medical therapy with antiplatelet and antithrombotic agents as well as

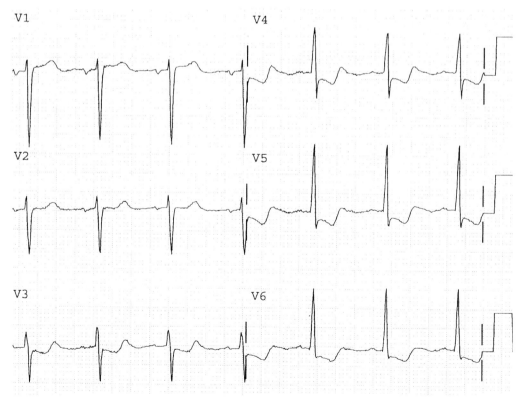

FIGURE 32-16 · **Downsloping ST segment depression of reversible anterior wall ischemia.** Only leads V_1 to V_6 are shown. Because the voltage meets left ventricular hypertrophy (LVH) criteria, one might erroneously attribute the ST segment depression in leads V_3 to V_6 to LVH, but it is, in fact, too deep and out of proportion to the R wave to be secondary to LVH alone. In lead V_3, ST segment depression is concordant with the majority of the QRS complex, whereas in LVH it should be discordant. Echocardiography revealed lateral and apical wall motion abnormality without LVH. After therapy, all ST segment depressions resolved. Angiography revealed nonocclusive 90% stenoses of the first diagonal and obtuse marginal arteries. (Reprinted with permission from Smith SW, Zvosec DL, Sharkey SW, Henry TD: The ECG in Acute MI: An Evidence-Based Manual of Reperfusion Therapy. Philadelphia, Lippincott Williams & Wilkins, 2002.)

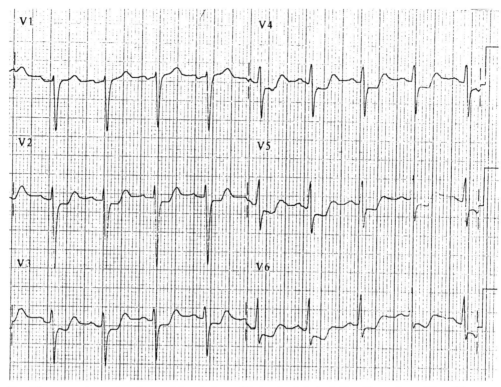

FIGURE 32-17 · **Flat ST segment depression of reversible anterior wall ischemia.** Only leads V_1 to V_6 are shown. When ST segment depression is most pronounced in lateral leads, circumflex occlusion is common, but left anterior descending artery unstable angina/ST segment elevation myocardial infarction (UA/NSTEMI) is probably more likely. Thus, thrombolytic therapy is not indicated. Furthermore, as in most UA/NSTEMI, the ST segment depression rapidly resolved with aspirin, sublingual nitroglycerin, and heparin. (Reprinted with permission from Smith SW, Zvosec DL, Sharkey SW, Henry TD: The ECG in Acute MI: An Evidence-Based Manual of Reperfusion Therapy. Philadelphia, Lippincott Williams & Wilkins, 2002.)

beta-adrenergic blocking agents.[2,3,82] Persistent ST segment depression in the setting of persistent angina, in spite of maximal medical therapy, is an indication for urgent angiography with possible percutaneous coronary intervention, but not for thrombolytic therapy.

Q Waves. A *normal* Q wave, representing the rapid depolarization of the thin septal wall between the two ventricles, may be found in most leads (Table 32-2). This initial negative deflection of the QRS complex is of very short duration and of low amplitude.

Pathologic Q waves, often a consequence of MI, are usually wider and deeper, and may be described as follows (Fig. 32-18): A *QR wave* denotes a Q wave followed by a substantial R wave; a *Qr wave* denotes a Q wave followed by a very small R wave; a *qR wave* denotes a small Q wave preceding a large R wave; and a *QS wave* denotes a single negative deflection without any R wave. After significant injury of the myocardium, electrically dead or necrotic tissue acts as an "electrical window," transmitting the depolarizing forces (R wave) as recorded from the opposite position of the heart. Thus, during or after a Q wave infarct of the left side of the heart, a left-positioned lead, such as lead I, does not record its own depolarizing positive vector, but instead records a depolarizing vector from the septum and from the right ventricle, moving away from lead I; this appears as a pathologic Q wave.[91]

Q waves may be transient markers of ischemia, not just of cell death, and frequently disappear after reperfusion.[92]

In fact, at 1 hour after LAD occlusion, up to 50% of anterior AMIs may manifest Q waves. These are apparently a result of ischemia of the conducting system, not necessarily of cellular necrosis.[12] Indeed, studies demonstrate that Q waves in AMI do not preclude aggressive reperfusion therapy[12] (see Figs. 32-6 and 32-7). Although patients with high STE and absence of Q waves have the greatest benefit from thrombolytic therapy, those with high STE and Q waves also receive significant benefit.[12] Q waves are usually completely developed within

---

32-2 · ABNORMAL Q WAVES

Lead V_2: Any Q wave
Lead V_3: Almost any Q wave
Lead V_4: >1 mm deep *or* at least 0.02 sec *or* larger than the Q wave in lead V_5
Any Q wave ≥0.03 sec (30 msec, 0.75 mm), except in leads III, aVR, or V_1 (see below)
Lead aVL: Q wave >0.04 sec or >50% of the amplitude of the QRS complex in the presence of an upright P wave
Lead III: Q wave ≥0.04 sec (a Q wave of depth >25% of R wave height is often quoted as diagnostic, but width is more important than depth)
Leads III, aVR, V_1: Normal subjects may have nonpathologic wide and deep Q waves

Adapted with permission from Smith SW, Zvosec DL, Sharkey SW, Henry TD: The ECG in Acute MI: An Evidence-Based Manual of Reperfusion Therapy. Philadelphia, Lippincott Williams & Wilkins, 2002.

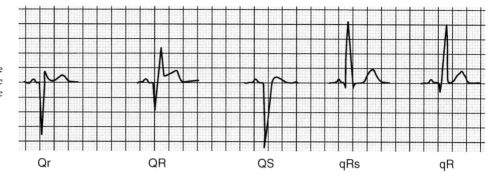

FIGURE 32-18 · Nomenclature of the QRS complexes. Capital letters denote large deflections, whereas lower-case letters indicate small deflections.

Qr   QR   QS   qRs   qR

8 to 12 hours of occlusion of a nonreperfused coronary artery.[12,13] However, in at least 10% of patients, Q waves do not develop until 3 to 11 days after an MI.[93] In most patients, these Q waves persist indefinitely, but in 15% to 30% of patients who do not receive any reperfusion therapy, the Q waves eventually disappear.[94] In contrast, when patients with Q waves receive early thrombolytic therapy, the Q waves disappear within a few days to weeks.[13,95]

There are a number of "Q wave equivalents," or electrical forces that are altered by the process of infarction.[9] The most notable examples include tall R waves in leads V_1 and V_2, representing "Q waves" of posterior infarction; localized R wave diminution (or "poor R wave progression"); and "reverse R wave progression," where R waves from leads V_1 to V_4 decrease in amplitude (they normally increase); in the latter case, precordial lead reversal should also be excluded.

Q wave analysis remains relevant to the reperfusion decision because (1) Q waves of a previous MI are evidence that a patient has CAD, and (2) QR waves in the presence of STE increase the probability that any STE is a direct result of AMI. Normal and abnormal Q waves may be distinguished by the following (see Table 32-2):

1. Any Q wave in leads V_2 and V_3, and Q waves of 0.03 sec or more in leads I, II, aVL, aVF, or V_4 to V_6, are associated with MI. The Q wave changes must be present in any two contiguous leads, and be greater than 1 mm in depth. A Q wave of depth greater than one fourth of the R wave height is often quoted as diagnostic, but width is more important than depth.[45]
2. Q waves on the right side of the standard 12-lead ECG (leads aVR, III, V_1) may be normal. Of healthy young men, 12% have Q waves in the inferior leads.[96] However, a Q wave in lead III greater than 0.04 sec (a single box), along with Q waves in the other inferior leads (II, aVF), is diagnostic of inferior MI.
3. Poor R wave progression, or reverse R wave progression, is equivalent to pathologic QR waves.
4. Pathologic QR waves (distinct from QS waves) are nearly always a sign of infarction, either old or acute.
5. QS waves in leads V_1 to V_3, which may occur with STE, may also be due to LBBB, LVH, cor pulmonale, or cardiomyopathy.

Normal or Nondiagnostic Electrocardiograms. A normal, initial ECG does not preclude the diagnosis of MI, and this is especially true for the initial ECG. Approximately 3.5% of patients with undifferentiated chest pain and a normal ECG experience AMI within the next 24 hours, and 9% of such patients with an abnormal but "nondiagnostic" or "nonspecific" ECG experience AMI.[5,97] However, a normal ECG recorded during an episode of chest pain makes significant ischemia less likely, and is associated with a better prognosis.[98]

Among patients diagnosed with AMI, 6% to 8% have normal ECGs and 22% to 35% have "nonspecific" ECGs. There is a significant associated relative mortality risk of AMI even with a "normal" ECG (0.59) or a "nonspecific" ECG (0.70) compared with a "diagnostic" ECG.[97,99,100]

Many additional patients with normal or nondiagnostic ECGs have UA (ACS without AMI). Those who are admitted for suspected ACS who have a "negative" ECG (no Q waves, LVH, or significant ST segment depression, T wave inversion, or STE, but may include T wave inversion in one lead or minor ST segment/T wave abnormalities) have significantly fewer in-hospital complications than those with a "positive" ECG, as long as subsequent ECGs remain negative.[101–103]

ST Segment Monitoring. There are several ECG methods that may help in the interpretation of equivocal or nondiagnostic ECGs; these are especially important in patients at high risk for ongoing coronary occlusion or reocclusion. The initial ECG should be compared with a *previous tracing*, particularly with those recorded during an asymptomatic period. *Continuous automated ST segment monitoring* may detect STE that would otherwise go unnoticed; it improves the sensitivity for STEMI from 46% on the initial ECG to 62%, while also enabling the exclusion of STEMI by *absence* of evolutionary changes[104,105] (Fig. 32-19). Continuous monitoring is also useful for diagnosing UA/NSTEMI by detection of dynamic ST segment depression.[106,107] Serial ECGs repeated every 15 to 20 minutes are a good substitute if continuous ST segment monitoring is unavailable (see Chapter 70, Serial Electrocardiography and ST Segment Trend Monitoring).

Reperfusion and Reocclusion. Reperfusion (whether spontaneous or therapy induced) of the infarct-related artery is measured angiographically by Thrombolysis in Myocardial Infarction (TIMI) trial flow classifications of 0 (no flow) to 3 (excellent flow).[38] Microvascular perfusion is assessed by TIMI myocardial perfusion (TMP) grading of 0 to 3. Although TIMI 3 flow is associated with excellent outcome, outcome is even more closely associated with TMP flow.[108] Along with angiographic evidence of microvascular perfusion, ST segment resolution is the best predictor of TMP flow and outcome from STEMI.[109]

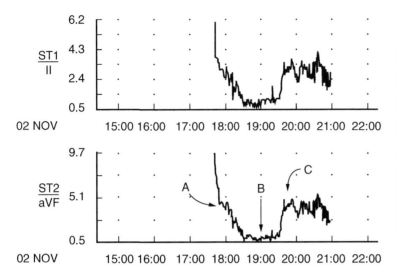

FIGURE 32-19 · ST segment trend monitoring after thrombolytic therapy. After the initial 12-lead ECG revealed inferior acute myocardial infarction with maximal ST segment elevation in leads II and aVF, these two leads were chosen for two-lead ST segment monitoring. Therapy to induce reperfusion was infused at approximately 17:30. At 17:42, ST segment elevation was 6.2 mm in lead II and 9.7 mm in lead aVF. By the time of admission to the cardiac care unit (A), ST segments had "recovered" to 2.4 and 5.0 mm (>50%, indicating successful reperfusion), respectively. By 19:00 (B), ST segments were nearly isoelectric. The alarm sounded at 19:30 (C), with the patient experiencing renewed chest pain (reocclusion). Angioplasty opened a 100% occluded right circumflex artery. (Reprinted with permission from Smith SW, Zvosec DL, Sharkey SW, Henry TD: The ECG in Acute MI: An Evidence-Based Manual of Reperfusion Therapy. Philadelphia, Lippincott Williams & Wilkins, 2002.)

On continuous ST segment monitoring after reperfusion therapy, a recovery of the ST segment to less than 50% of its maximal height by 60 minutes is strongly associated with TIMI 3 reperfusion,[110] and even more strongly associated with good microvascular perfusion (see Fig. 32-19).

A slightly less sensitive predictor of reperfusion, but highly specific, is terminal T wave inversion[76,77] (see Figs. 32-11 and 32-14). In patients with STEMI, the presence of negative T waves very early after presentation or very soon after therapy is associated with a very good prognosis.[111] Presence of negative T waves at time of discharge in patients with anterior STEMI is strongly correlated with both ST segment recovery to baseline and TIMI 3 flow.[112] Whether reperfusion is spontaneous or therapy induced, reocclusion can be detected by re-elevation of ST segments (see Fig. 32-19) or by "pseudo-normalization" of inverted T waves (see Fig. 32-15).

ELECTROCARDIOGRAPHIC DIFFERENTIAL DIAGNOSIS

Pseudoinfarction patterns (noninfarct ST segment elevation syndromes or ST segment elevation myocardial infarction lookalikes)

Pseudoinfarction patterns are ECG patterns that mimic or confound the diagnosis of acute coronary syndrome.

Hyperacute T waves (tall T waves)

- Benign early repolarization (BER; Fig. 32-20)
  Usually concave, steeper downward than upward slope, tall R waves
- Hyperkalemia (Fig. 32-21)

ST segment elevation

- BER (see Figs. 32-20 and 32-22)
  Tall R waves, elevated J point, young age, leads V_1 to V_4 primarily, no reciprocal ST segment depression
- Left ventricular hypertrophy (LVH; Figs. 32-5B and 32-23)
  ST segment elevation (STE) in leads V_1 to V_3 discordant and proportional to a high-voltage, mostly negative QRS complex
  ST segment depression in lateral leads proportional to positive QRS complex
  ST segment elevation or depression out of proportion to QRS complex should trigger suspicion of ischemia
- Left ventricular aneurysm (STE after previous myocardial infarction [MI]; Figs. 32-3 and 32-24)
  Mean ratio of T wave amplitude to QRS amplitude in leads V_1 to V_4 is low (<0.2)[49]
  QS waves or Qr waves, relatively low STE, some T wave inversion
- Acute myopericarditis (Fig. 32-25)
  Diffuse STE, easily confused with inferolateral MI, PR segment depression >0.5 to 0.8 mm
  Localized pericarditis may exactly mimic AMI on ECG
- Ventricular cardiac pacing
  Unlike LBBB, all precordial leads normally have negative QR complex
  Like LBBB, STE discordant to QRS, thus diffuse precordial STE, look for pacemaker spikes
- Left bundle branch block (LBBB; Fig. 32-26)
  STE and ST segment depression opposite (discordant) to most of QRS complex

ELECTROCARDIOGRAPHIC DIFFERENTIAL DIAGNOSIS—Cont'd

T wave inversion

Primary etiologies (QRS complex is normal)

NONPATHOLOGIC

- Benign T wave inversion (associated with BER, leads V_3 to V_5 biphasic T waves, corrected QT interval <0.40 to 0.425 sec)
- Persistent juvenile T waves (leads V_1 to V_3, up to age 30 years, especially in women)
- Physiologic changes (hyperventilation)
- Post-supraventricular tachycardia or ventricular tachycardia

PATHOLOGIC

- Myocardial stunning (associated with critical illness)
- Pulmonary embolism (especially in leads V_1 to V_3)
- Cerebrovascular accidents (subarachnoid hemorrhage)
- Pneumothorax (especially left sided)
- Acute myopericarditis
- Acute pancreatitis and gallbladder disease
- Electrolyte imbalance

Secondary etiologies (QRS complex is abnormal)

- Bundle branch block
- Right ventricular hypertrophy (RVH)
- LVH
- Wolff-Parkinson-White (WPW) syndrome (opposite to delta wave)
- Intraventricular conduction delay

ST segment depression

Primary etiologies (QRS complex is normal)

NONPATHOLOGIC

- Post-supraventricular tachycardia or ventricular tachycardia (very common)
- Hypokalemia
- Digoxin effect
- Baseline variant

PATHOLOGIC

- Acute pulmonary embolism
- Central nervous system events

- Pneumothorax
- Acute myocarditis (reciprocal depression)
- Inferior ventricular aneurysm (reciprocal depression in lead aVL)

Secondary etiologies (QRS complex is abnormal)

- Right bundle branch block (especially in right precordial leads with qR or RsR′)
- LBBB (discordant to positive QRS)
- RVH (right precordial leads V_1 to V_3)
- LVH (discordant to predominance of QRS)
- WPW syndrome (opposite to delta wave)
- Intraventricular conduction delay

Abnormal Q waves

Cardiac

MOST COMMON (QS WAVES IN LEADS V_1 TO V_3)

- LVH
- LBBB
- Dilated cardiomyopathy

LESS COMMON

- RVH
- Left anterior fascicular block
- Hypertrophic cardiomyopathy
- WPW syndrome
- Acute myocarditis
- Athlete's heart
- Dextrocardia

Noncardiac

- Misplacement of precordial electrode
- Chronic obstructive pulmonary disease
- Pulmonary embolism
- Pneumothorax
- Metabolic abnormalities
- Acute pancreatitis

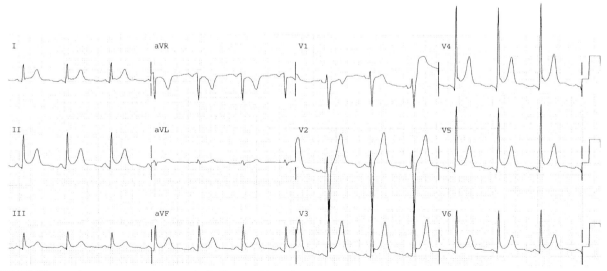

FIGURE 32-20 • Benign early repolarization. The findings on this tracing meet the criteria for left ventricular hypertrophy (LVH), but LVH was not present. ST segment elevation (STE) is 3 mm at the J point in lead V_2, and 7 mm at 80 msec after the J point. Notice that the large T waves do not tower over the R waves (as they often do in STE myocardial infarction) because the R waves are very prominent (as is generally true in this condition). Notice the typical J waves in leads V_3 and V_4, and the slurring of the J point in leads V_5 and V_6.

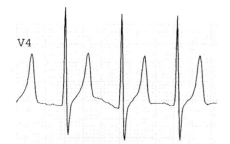

FIGURE 32-21 • **Hyperkalemia.** Lead V₄ only is shown. Note the typical peaked T wave of hyperkalemia, distinctly different from most hyperacute T waves.

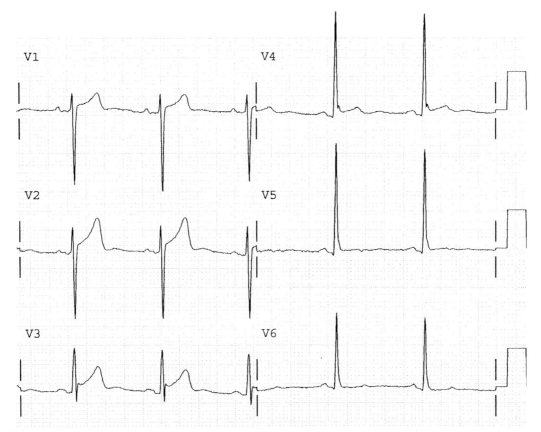

FIGURE 32-22 • **Benign early repolarization (BER) mimicking left ventricular hypertrophy (LVH).** Leads V₁ to V₆ only are shown. This ECG in an 83-year-old man with atypical chest pain has some features suggesting LVH with ST segment elevation. His ECG meets "criteria" for thrombolytics, but all previous ECGs were identical. Note the J waves in leads V₃ and V₄, with J point slurring in leads V₅ and V₆. This morphology is typical of BER, not of LVH, and is very unusual to see in an elderly patient. Serial ECGs were unchanged and troponins were negative.

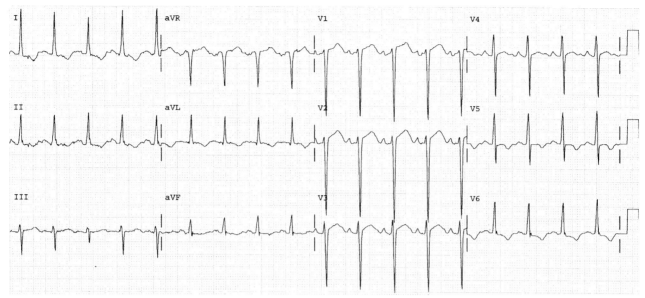

FIGURE 32-23 · Left ventricular hypertrophy (LVH) with secondary ST segment/T wave abnormalities. There is typical discordant ST segment elevation, up to 3 mm in lead V$_2$, which meets the "criteria" for thrombolytics, but is a result of LVH alone. Also note typical lateral ST segment depression and T wave inversion.

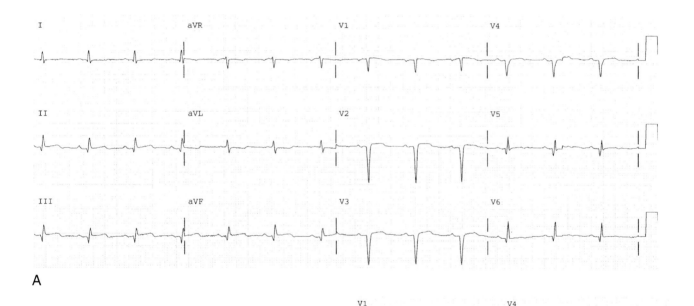

A

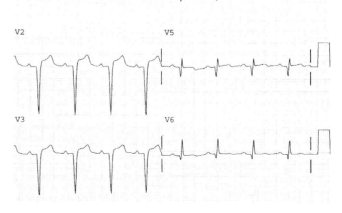

FIGURE 32-24 · Typical ventricular "aneurysm" morphology. *A,* In this baseline ECG, note that the anterior leads have a QS pattern, and inferior leads have a QR pattern. This is typical aneurysm morphology, and makes inferior aneurysm very difficult to distinguish from inferior acute myocardial infarction (AMI), whereas anterior aneurysm is usually not difficult to distinguish from AMI. *B,* Leads V$_1$ to V$_6$ only are shown. The same patient presented acutely ill, but without symptoms of acute coronary syndrome, and was subsequently diagnosed with acute pulmonary embolism. Note rise of anterior ST segments. There was a minimal troponin elevation, and subsequent ECGs showed ST segments back to baseline (*A*), but with shallow T wave inversion.

B

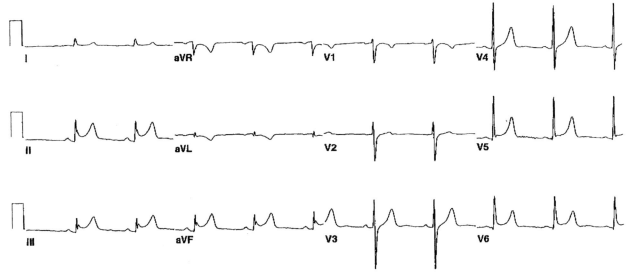

FIGURE 32-25 · Myopericarditis mimicking inferolateral acute myocardial infarction (AMI). A 77-year-old woman presented with sharp chest pain and a pericardial rub. ST segment elevation in leads II, III, and aVF, as well as V_5 and V_6, with reciprocal ST segment depression in lead aVL is "diagnostic" for inferolateral AMI. Angiography revealed no occlusion or stenosis, echocardiography was negative, and troponins were negative. Most myopericarditis is diffuse, with no reciprocal ST segment depression in lead aVL. When such ST segment depression is present, myopericarditis can exactly mimic inferolateral AMI. ST segment depression in lead aVR, a near-universal finding in myopericarditis, also occurs in inferior AMI. Marked PR segment depression, which frequently assists in the diagnosis of myopericarditis, is absent here. Most myopericarditis is not this difficult to distinguish from AMI.

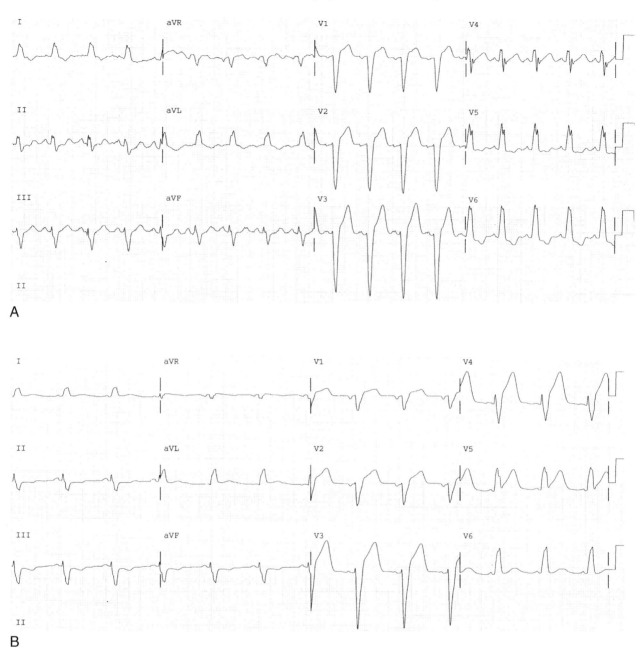

FIGURE 32-26 · Left bundle branch block (LBBB) with evolving acute myocardial infarction (AMI). A 60-year-old man presented with typical crushing chest pain. *A,* The previous ECG showed LBBB with typical discordant ST segments and T waves. *B,* The ECG recorded on presentation also manifests LBBB, but is distinctly different and diagnostic of ST segment elevation MI. There is increased width of the QRS complex; T waves are larger and bulkier, especially in lead V₄; there is concordant ST segment elevation and upright T waves in leads I, aVL, V₅, and V₆; and there is concordant reciprocal ST segment depression in inferior leads II, III, and aVF. The patient had immediate angiography and percutaneous coronary intervention for a 100% proximal left anterior descending artery occlusion.

References

1. Anderson HV, Cannon CP, Stone PH, et al: One-year results of the Thrombolysis in Myocardial Infarction (TIMI) IIIB clinical trial: A randomised comparison of tissue-type plasminogen activator versus placebo and early invasive versus early conservative strategies in unstable angina and non-Q wave myocardial infarction. J Am Coll Cardiol 1995;26:1643–1650.

2. Cannon CP, Weintraub WS, Demopoulos LA, et al: Comparison of early invasive and conservative strategies in patients with unstable coronary syndromes treated with the glycoprotein IIb/IIIa inhibitor tirofiban: (TACTICS)-TIMI 18. N Engl J Med 2001;344:1879–1887.

3. Diderholm E, Andren B, Frostfeldt G, et al: ST depression in ECG at entry indicates severe coronary lesions and large benefits of an early invasive treatment strategy in unstable coronary artery disease: The FRISC II ECG substudy. The Fast Revascularisation during InStability in Coronary artery disease. Eur Heart J 2002;23:41–49.

4. Rude RE, Poole WK, Muller J, et al: Electrocardiographic and clinical criteria for recognition of acute myocardial infarction based on analysis of 3,697 patients. Am J Cardiol 1983;52:936–942.

5. Rouan GW, Lee TH, Cook EF, et al: Clinical characteristics and outcome of acute myocardial infarction in patients with initially normal or nonspecific electrocardiograms (a report from the Multicenter Chest Pain Study). Am J Cardiol 1989;64:1087–1092.

6. Fesmire FM, Percy RF, Wears RL, MacMath TL: Initial ECG in Q wave and non-Q wave myocardial infarction. Ann Emerg Med 1989; 18:741–746.

7. Brady WJ: ST segment elevation in ED adult chest pain patients: Etiology and diagnostic accuracy for AMI. J Emerg Med 1998;16:797–798.

8. Otto LA, Aufderheide TP: Evaluation of ST segment elevation criteria for the prehospital electrocardiographic diagnosis of acute myocardial infarction. Ann Emerg Med 1994;23:17–24.

9. Phibbs B, Marcus F, Marriott HJ, et al: Q-wave versus non-Q wave myocardial infarction: A meaningless distinction. J Am Coll Cardiol 1999;33:576–582.

10. Fuster V, Badimon L, Badimon JJ, Chesebro JH: The pathogenesis of coronary artery disease and the acute coronary syndromes (1). N Engl J Med 1992;326:242–250.

11. Theroux P, Fuster V: Acute coronary syndromes: Unstable angina and non-Q-wave myocardial infarction. Circulation 1998;97:1195–1206.

12. Raitt MH, Maynard C, Wagner GS, et al: Appearance of abnormal Q waves early in the course of acute myocardial infarction: Implications for efficacy of thrombolytic therapy. J Am Coll Cardiol 1995;25:1084–1088.

13. Bar FW, Volders PG, Hoppener B, et al: Development of ST-segment elevation and Q- and R-wave changes in acute myocardial infarction and the influence of thrombolytic therapy. Am J Cardiol 1996;77:337–343.

14. Mills RM, Young E, Gorlin R, Lesch M: Natural history of S-T segment elevation after acute myocardial infarction. Am J Cardiol 1975;35:609–614.

15. Krone RJ, Greenberg H, Dwyer EMJ, et al: Long-term prognostic significance of ST segment depression during acute myocardial infarction: The Multicenter Diltiazem Postinfarction Trial Research Group. J Am Coll Cardiol 1993;22:361–367.

16. Chou TC, Knilans TK: Electrocardiography in Clinical Practice: Adult and Pediatric, 4th ed. Philadelphia, WB Saunders, 1996.

17. Phibbs B: "Transmural" versus "subendocardial" myocardial infarction: An electrocardiographic myth. J Am Coll Cardiol 1983;1:561–564.

18. Smith FM: The ligation of coronary arteries with electrocardiographic study. Arch Intern Med 1918;5:1–27.

19. Bayley RH, LaDue JS, York DJ: Electrocardiographic changes (local ventricular ischemia and injury) produced in the dog by temporary occlusion of a coronary artery, showing a new stage in the evolution of myocardial infarction. Am Heart J 1944;27:164–169.

20. Bohning A, Katz LN: Unusual changes in the electrocardiograms of patients with recent coronary occlusion. Am J Med Sci 1933;186:39–52.

21. Wood FC, Wolferth CC: Huge T-waves in precordial leads in cardiac infarction. Am Heart J 1934;9:706–721.

22. Graham GK, Laforet EG: An electrocardiographic and morphologic study of changes following ligation of the left coronary artery in human beings: A report of two cases. Am Heart J 1952;43:42–52.

23. Wachtel FW, Teich EM: Tall precordial T waves as the earliest sign in diaphragmatic wall infarction. Am Heart J 1956;51:917–920.

24. Pinto IJ, Nanda NC, Biswas AK, Parulkar VG: Tall upright T waves in the precordial leads. Circulation 1967;36:708–716.

25. Dressler W, Roesler H: High T waves in the earliest stage of myocardial infarction. Am Heart J 1947;34:627–645.

26. Freundlich J: The diagnostic significance of tall upright T waves in the chest leads. Am Heart J 1956;52:749–767.

27. Soo CS: Tall precordial T waves with depressed ST take-off: An early sign of acute myocardial infarction? Singapore Med J 1995;36:236–237.

28. Smith SW, Zvosec DL, Sharkey SW, Henry TD: The ECG in Acute MI: An Evidence-Based Manual of Reperfusion Therapy. Philadelphia, Lippincott Williams & Wilkins, 2002, p 320.

29. Hochrein J, Sun F, Pieper KS, et al: Higher T-wave amplitude associated with better prognosis in patients receiving thrombolytic therapy for acute myocardial infarction (a GUSTO-1 substudy): Global Utilization of Streptokinase and Tissue Plasminogen Activator for Occluded Coronary Arteries. Am J Cardiol 1998;81:1078–1084.

30. Smith SW: Upwardly concave ST segment morphology is common in acute left anterior descending coronary artery occlusion. Acad Emerg Med 2003;10:516.

31. Kosuge M, Kimura K, Ishikawa T, et al: Value of ST-segment elevation pattern in predicting infarct size and left ventricular function at discharge in patients with reperfused acute anterior myocardial infarction. Am Heart J 1999;137:522–527.

32. Clements IP: The Electrocardiogram in Acute Myocardial Infarction. Armonk, NY, Futura, 1998.

33. Adams J, Trent R, Rawles JM, on behalf of the GREAT Group: Earliest electrocardiographic evidence of myocardial infarction: Implication for thrombolytic treatment. BMJ 1993;307:409–413.

34. Menown IB, Mackenzie G, Adgey AA: Optimizing the initial 12-lead electrocardiographic diagnosis of acute myocardial infarction. Eur Heart J 2000;21:275–283.

35. Massel D, Dawdy JA, Melendez LJ: Strict reliance on a computer algorithm or measurable ST segment criteria may lead to errors in thrombolytic therapy eligibility. Am Heart J 2000;140:221–226.

36. ISIS-2 (Second International Study of Infarct Survival) Collaborative Group: Randomised trial of intravenous streptokinase, oral aspirin, both, or neither among 17,187 cases of suspected acute myocardial infarction: ISIS-2. Lancet 1988;2:349–360.

37. ISIS-3 (Third International Study of Infarct Survival) Collaborative Study Group: ISIS-3: A randomised comparison of streptokinase vs. tissue plasminogen activator vs anistreplase and of aspirin plus heparin vs aspirin alone among 41,299 cases of suspected acute myocardial infarction. Lancet 1992;339:753–770.

38. Chesebro JH, Knatterud G, Roberts R, et al: Thrombolysis in Myocardial Infarction (TIMI) Trial, Phase I: A comparison between intravenous tissue plasminogen activator and intravenous streptokinase: clinical findings through hospital discharge. Circulation 1987;76:142–154.

39. TIMI III A: Early effects of tissue-type plasminogen activator added to conventional therapy on the culprit coronary lesion in patients presenting with ischemic cardiac pain at rest: Results of the Thrombolysis in Myocardial Ischemia (TIMI IIIA) trial. Circulation 1993;87:38–52.

40. GISSI-2 (Gruppo Italiano per lo Studio della Sopravivenza Nell'Infarto Miocardio): GISSI-2: A factorial randomised trial of alteplase versus streptokinase and heparin versus no heparin among 12,490 patients with acute myocardial infarction. Lancet 1990;336:65–71.

41. Ryan TJ, Antman EM, Brooks NH, et al: 1999 Update: ACC/AHA guidelines for the management of patients with acute myocardial infarction. J Am Coll Cardiol 1999;34:890–911.

42. Topol EJ, Califf RM, Vandormael M, et al: A randomized trial of late reperfusion therapy for acute myocardial infarction: Thrombolysis and Angioplasty in Myocardial Infarction-6 (TAMI-6) Study Group. Circulation 1992;85:2090–2099.

43. GISSI (Gruppo Italiano per lo Studio della Sopravivenza Nell'Infarto Miocardio): Effectiveness of intravenous thrombolytic treatment in acute myocardial infarction. Lancet 1986;1:397–401.

44. Prineas J, Crow RS, Blackburn H: The Minnesota Code Manual of Electrocardiographic Findings: Standards and Procedures for Measurement and Classification. Littleton, Mass, John Wright, 1982.

45. Joint European Society of Cardiology/American College of Cardiology Committee: Myocardial infarction redefined: A consensus document of the Joint European Society of Cardiology/American College of Cardiology committee for the redefinition of myocardial infarction. J Am Coll Cardiol 2000;36:959–969.

46. Bell SJ, Leibrandt PN, Greenfield JC, et al: Comparison of an automated thrombolytic predictive instrument to both diagnostic software and an expert cardiologist for diagnosis of an ST elevation acute myocardial infarction. J Electrocardiol 2000;33(Suppl):259-262.

47. Hands ME, Lloyd BL, Robinson JS, et al: Prognostic significance of electrocardiographic site of infarction after correction for enzymatic size of infarction. Circulation 1986;73:885-891.

48. Stone PH, Raabe DS, Jaffe AS, et al: Prognostic significance of location and type of MI: Independent adverse outcome associated with anterior location. J Am Coll Cardiol 1988;11:453–463.

49. Mauri F, Gasparini M, Barbonaglia L, et al: Prognostic significance of the extent of myocardial injury in acute myocardial infarction treated by streptokinase (the GISSI trial). Am J Cardiol 1989;63:1291–1295.

50. Bar FW, Vermeer F, de Zwaan C, et al: Value of admission electrocardiogram in predicting outcome of thrombolytic therapy in acute myocardial infarction. Am J Cardiol 1987;59:6–13.

51. Lee KL, Woodlief LH, Topol EJ, et al: Predictors of 30-day mortality in the era of reperfusion for acute myocardial infarction: Results from an international trial of 41,021 patients. Circulation 1995;91:1659–1668.

52. Gwechenberger M, Schreiber W, Kittler H, et al: Prediction of early complications in patients with acute myocardial infarction by calculation of the ST score. Ann Emerg Med 1997;30:563–570.

53. Willems JL, Willems RJ, Willems GM, et al: Significance of initial ST segment elevation and depression for the management of thrombolytic therapy in acute myocardial infarction. Circulation 1990;82:1147–1158.

54. Savonitto S, Ardissino D, Granger CB, et al: Prognostic value of the admission electrocardiogram in acute coronary syndromes. JAMA 1999;281:707–713.

55. Birnbaum Y, Herz I, Sclarovsky S, et al: Prognostic significance of the admission electrocardiogram in acute myocardial infarction. J Am Coll Cardiol 1996;27:1128–1132.

56. Christian TF, Gibbons RJ, Clements IP, et al: Estimates of myocardium at risk and collateral flow in acute myocardial infarction using electrocardiographic indexes with comparison to radionuclide and angiographic measures. J Am Coll Cardiol 1995;26:388–393.

57. Huey BL, Beller GA, Kaiser D, Gibson RS: A comprehensive analysis of myocardial infarction due to left circumflex artery occlusion: Comparison with infarction due to right coronary artery and left anterior descending artery occlusion. J Am Coll Cardiol 1988;12:1156–1166.

58. Berry C, Zalewsky A, Kovach R, et al: Surface electrocardiogram in the detection of transmural myocardial ischemia during coronary artery occlusion. Am J Cardiol 1989;63:21–26.

59. Veldkamp RF, Sawchak S, Pope JE, et al: Performance of an automated real-time ST segment analysis program to detect coronary occlusion and reperfusion. J Electrocardiol 1996;29:257–263.

60. O'Keefe JHJ, Sayed-Taha K, Gibson W, et al: Do patients with left circumflex coronary artery-related acute myocardial infarction without ST-segment elevation benefit from reperfusion therapy? [See comments]. Am J Cardiol 1995;75:718–720.

61. Christian TF, Clements IP, Gibbons RJ: Noninvasive identification of myocardium at risk in patients with acute myocardial infarction and non-diagnostic electrocardiograms with technetium-99m-sestamibi. Circulation 1991;83:1615–1620.

62. Tighe M, Kellett J, Corry E, et al: The early diagnosis of acute myocardial infarction: Comparison of a simple algorithm with a computer program for electrocardiogram interpretation. Ir J Med Sci 1996;165: 159–163.

63. Rowlandson I, Kudenchuk PJ, Elko P: Computerized recognition of acute infarction: Criteria advances and test results. J Electrocardiol 1990; 23(Suppl):1–5.

64. Elko P, Weaver WD, Kudenchuk PJ, Rowlandson I: The dilemma of sensitivity versus specificity in computer-interpreted acute myocardial infarction. J Electrocardiol 1992;24(Suppl):2–7.

65. Elko P, Rowlandson I: A statistical analysis of the ECG measurements used in computerized interpretation of acute anterior myocardial infarction with applications to interpretive criteria development. J Electrocardiol 1993;25(Suppl):113–119.

66. Brady WJ, Perron AD, Syverud SA, et al: Reciprocal ST segment depression: Impact on the electrocardiographic diagnosis of ST segment elevation acute myocardial infarction. Am J Emerg Med 2002;20:35–38.

67. Birnbaum Y, Sclarovsky S, Solodky A, et al: Prediction of the level of left anterior descending coronary artery obstruction during anterior wall acute myocardial infarction by the admission electrocardiogram. Am J Cardiol 1993;72:823–826.

68. Engelen DJ, Gorgens AP, Cheriex EC, et al: Value of the electrocardiogram in localizing the occlusion site in the left anterior descending coronary artery in acute myocardial infarction. J Am Coll Cardiol 1999;34:389–395.

69. Tamura A, Kataoka H, Mikuriya Y, Nasu M: Inferior ST segment depression as a useful marker for identifying proximal left anterior descending artery occlusion during acute anterior myocardial infarction. Eur Heart J 1995;16:1795–1799.

70. Kosuge M, Kimura K, Toshiyuki I, et al: Electrocardiographic criteria for predicting total occlusion of the proximal left anterior descending coronary artery in anterior wall acute myocardial infarction. Clin Cardiol 2001;24:33–38.

71. Peterson ED, Hathaway WR, Zabel KM, et al: Prognostic significance of precordial ST segment depression during inferior myocardial infarction in the thrombolytic era: Results in 16,521 patients. J Am Coll Cardiol 1996;28:305–312.

72. Goldberger AL, Erickson R: Subtle ECG sign of acute infarction: Prominent reciprocal ST depression with minimal primary ST elevation. Pacing Clin Electrophysiol 1981;4:709–712.

73. de Zwaan C, Bar FW, Janssen JHA, et al: Angiographic and clinical characteristics of patients with unstable angina showing an ECG pattern indicating critical narrowing of the proximal LAD coronary artery. Am Heart J 1989;117:657–665.

74. de Zwaan C, Bar FW, Wellens HJJ: Characteristic electrocardiographic pattern indicating a critical stenosis high in left anterior descending coronary artery in patients admitted because of impending myocardial infarction. Am Heart J 1982;103:730–736.

75. Oliva PB, Hammill SC, Edwards WD: Electrocardiographic diagnosis of postinfarction regional pericarditis: Ancillary observations regarding the effect of reperfusion on the rapidity and amplitude of T wave inversion after acute myocardial infarction. Circulation 1993;88:896–904.

76. Doevendans PA, Gorgels AP, van der Zee R, et al: Electrocardiographic diagnosis of reperfusion during thrombolytic therapy in acute myocardial infarction. Am J Cardiol 1995;75:1206–1210.

77. Wehrens XH, Doevendans PA, Ophuis TJ, Wellens HJ: A comparison of electrocardiographic changes during reperfusion of acute myocardial infarction by thrombolysis or percutaneous transluminal coronary angioplasty. Am Heart J 2000;139:430–436.

78. Goldberger AL: Myocardial Infarction: Electrocardiographic Differential Diagnosis. St. Louis, Mosby, 1991.

79. Friedman HH: Diagnostic Electrocardiography and Vectorcardiography. New York, McGraw-Hill, 1985.

80. Tandy TK, Bottomy DP, Lewis J: Wellens' syndrome. Ann Emerg Med 1999;33:347–351.

81. Haines DE, Raabe DS, Gundel WD, Wackers FJ: Anatomic and prognostic significance of new T-wave inversion in unstable angina. Am J Cardiol 1983;52:14–18.

82. Hyde TA, French JK, Wong CK, et al: Four-year survival of patients with acute coronary syndromes without ST-segment elevation and prognostic significance of 0.5-mm ST-segment depression. Am J Cardiol 1999;84:379–385.

83. Ellestad MH, Crump R, Surbur M: The significance of lead strength on ST changes during treadmill stress tests. J Electrocardiol 1992; 25(Suppl):31–34.

84. Hollenberg M, Go JJ, Massie BM, et al: Influence of R-wave amplitude on exercise-induced ST depression: Need for a "gain factor" correlation when interpreting stress electrocardiograms. Am J Cardiol 1985;56:13.

85. Hakki AH, Iskandrian SD, Kutalek, et al: R-wave amplitude: A new determinant of failure of patients with coronary heart disease to manifest ST segment depression during exercise. J Am Coll Cardiol 1984;3:1155.

86. Santinga JT, Brymer JF, Smith F, Flora J: The influence of lead strength on the ST changes with exercise electrocardiography (correlative study with coronary arteriography). J Electrocardiol 1977;10:387.

87. Lee HS, Cross SJ, Rawles JM, Jennings KP: Patients with suspected myocardial infarction who present with ST depression. Lancet 1993;342:1204–1207.

88. Wong PS, el Gaylani N, Griffith K, et al: The clinical course of patients with acute myocardial infarction who are unsuitable for thrombolytic therapy because of the presenting electrocardiogram: UK Heart Attack Study Investigators. Coron Artery Dis 1998;9:747–752.

89. Fibrinolytic Therapy Trialists' (FTT) Collaborative Group: Indications for fibrinolytic therapy in suspected acute myocardial infarction: Collaborative overview of early mortality and major morbidity results from all randomised trials of more than 1000 patients. Lancet 1994;343:311–322.

90. Ryan TJ, Anderson JL, Antman EM, et al: ACC/AHA Guidelines for the management of patients with acute myocardial infarction: A report of the American College of Cardiology/American Heart Association Task

Force on Practice Guidelines (Committee on Management of Acute Myocardial Infarction). J Am Coll Cardiol 1996;28:1328–1428.

91. Wilson F, Johnston F, Hill I: The interpretation of the galvanometric curves obtained when one electrode is distant from the heart and the other near or in contact with the ventricular surface: II. Observations on the mammalian heart. Am Heart J 1934;10:176–183.

92. Barold SS, Falkoff MD, Ong LS, Heinle RA: Significance of transient electrocardiographic Q waves in coronary artery disease. Cardiol Clin 1987;5:367–380.

93. Kleiger RE, Boden WE, Schechtman KB, et al: Frequency and significance of late evolution of Q waves in patients with initial non-Q-wave acute myocardial infarction. Diltiazem Reinfarction Study Group. Am J Cardiol 1990;65:23–27.

94. Kaplan BM, Berkson DM: Serial electrocardiograms after myocardial infarction. Ann Intern Med 1964;60:430–435.

95. Blanke H, Scherff F, Karsch KR, et al: Electrocardiographic changes after streptokinase-induced recanalization in patients with acute left anterior descending artery obstruction. Circulation 1983;68: 406–412.

96. Fisch C: Abnormal ECG in clinically normal individuals. JAMA 1983;250:1321–1325.

97. Karlson BW, Herlitz J, Wiklund O, et al: Early prediction of acute myocardial infarction from clinical history, examination and electrocardiogram in the emergency room. Am J Cardiol 1991;68:171–175.

98. Braunwald E, Jones RH, Mark DB, et al: Diagnosing and managing unstable angina. Agency for Health Care Policy and Research. Circulation 1994;90:613–622.

99. McCarthy BD, Wong JB, Selker HP: Detecting acute cardiac ischemia in the emergency department: a review of the literature. J Gen Intern Med 1990;5:365–373.

100. Welch RD, Zalenski RJ, Frederick PD, et al: Prognostic value of a normal or nonspecific initial electrocardiogram in acute myocardial infarction. JAMA 2001;286:1977–1984.

101. Brush JE, Brand DA, Acampora D, et al: Use of the initial electrocardiogram to predict in-hospital complications of acute myocardial infarction. N Engl J Med 1985;312:1137–1141.

102. Zalenski RJ, Sloan EP, Chen EH, et al: The emergency department ECG and immediately life-threatening complications in initially uncomplicated suspected myocardial ischemia. Ann Emerg Med 1988;17:221–226.

103. Zalenski RJ, Rydman RJ, Sloan EP, et al: The emergency department electrocardiogram and hospital complications in myocardial infarction patients. Acad Emerg Med 1996;3:318–325.

104. Fesmire FM, Percy RF, Bardoner JB, et al: Usefulness of automated serial 12-lead ECG monitoring during the initial emergency department evaluation of patients with chest pain. Ann Emerg Med 1998; 31:3–11.

105. Fesmire FM: Which chest pain patients benefit from continuous ST-segment monitoring with automated serial ECG? Am J Emerg Med 2000;18:773–778.

106. Holmvang L, Andersen K, Dellbourg, et al: Relative contributions of a single-admission 12-lead electrocardiogram and early 24-hour continuous electrocardiographic monitoring for early risk stratification in patients with unstable coronary artery disease. Am J Cardiol 1999;83:667–674.

107. Jernberg T, Lindahl B, Wallentin L: ST-segment monitoring with continuous 12-lead ECG improves early risk stratification in patients with chest pain and ECG nondiagnostic of acute myocardial infarction. J Am Coll Cardiol 1999;34:1413–1419.

108. van't Hof AW, Liem A, Suryapranata H, et al: Angiographic assessment of myocardial reperfusion in patients treated with primary angioplasty for acute myocardial infarction: Myocardial blush grade. Zwolle Myocardial Infarction Study Group. Circulation 1998;97:2303–2306.

109. Claeys MJ, Bosmans J, Veenstra L, et al: Determinants and prognostic implications of persistent ST-segment elevation after primary angioplasty for acute myocardial infarction: Importance of microvascular reperfusion injury on clinical outcome. Circulation 1999;99: 1972–1977.

110. Krucoff MW, Croll MA, Pope JE, et al: Continuous 12-lead ST-segment recovery analysis in the TAMI 7 study: Performance of a non-invasive method for real-time detection of failed myocardial reperfusion. Circulation 1993;88:437–446.

111. Herz I, Birnbaum Y, Zlotikamien B, et al: The prognostic implications of negative T-waves in the leads with ST segment elevation on admission in acute myocardial infarction. Cardiology 1999;92:121–127.

112. Kusniec J, Slolodky A, Strasberg B, et al: The relationship between the electrocardiographic pattern with TIMI flow class and ejection fraction in patients with first acute anterior wall myocardial infarction. Eur Heart J 1997;18:420–425.

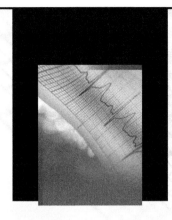

Chapter 33

Acute Coronary Syndromes: Regional Issues

Timothy G. Janz and Glenn C. Hamilton

Clinical Features

Myocardial ischemia and infarction can be localized to specific regions of the left ventricle (LV). The traditional regions include both the LV (anterior, inferior, lateral, septal, and posterior sections) and the right ventricle (RV). The amount of myocardium involved depends on the size of the artery involved and the location of obstruction in the artery. Although specific arteries correlate with regions of the LV, the electrocardiogram (ECG) is an imprecise instrument in identifying the involved vessel.[1,2] Underlying cardiac disease and anatomic variations alter the relationship between coronary arteries and the ECG regions of the left ventricle.

Disease in a large artery, such as the right coronary artery (RCA) or the left coronary artery (LCA), often affects more than one region of the left ventricle; therefore, isolated wall

involvement (i.e., inferior, anterior, lateral, septal, or posterior) is unusual. The more common occurrence is the involvement of more than one region (e.g., inferolateral or anteroseptal).

Electrocardiographic Manifestations

Anterior Wall. The anterior wall of the LV is perfused by the left anterior descending (LAD) coronary artery. Depending on reference source, the anterior wall is defined electrocardiographically by different leads of the 12-lead ECG.[3] The leads most commonly associated with acute coronary syndrome involving the anterior wall are precordial leads V_3 and V_4. Isolated involvement of the anterior wall is unusual (Fig. 33-1). Other anatomic regions of the LV also supplied by the LAD are commonly involved in infarctions and consist of the septum (anteroseptal) and the lateral wall (anterolateral).

The initial vector of the QRS complex typically deviates away from the area of a myocardial infarction (MI). This is classically represented on the ECG by the presence of an abnormal Q wave. In the absence of an abnormal Q wave, the deviation of the QRS complex may be represented by a diminished R wave. The loss of R wave progression (i.e., the absence of increasing R wave vector positivity from leads V_1 through V_6) in the precordial leads associated with an anterior wall MI is a classic example.[4]

Septum. The interventricular septum is supplied by the LAD and represented on the 12-lead ECG by precordial leads V_1 and V_2 (Fig. 33-2). Similar to the anterior wall, isolated involvement of the septum is unusual. The more common occurrence is disease of the LAD affecting both the interventricular septum and the anterior wall, which is referred to as the anteroseptal region. This area is represented by precordial leads V_1 through V_4 (Fig. 33-3). In patients presenting with an anteroseptal MI, ST segment elevation (STE) in lead aVR, complete right bundle branch block, and STE in lead V_1 greater than 2.5 mm strongly predict LAD artery occlusion proximal to the first septal perforator artery[5] (Fig. 33-4).

Reciprocal ST segment depression, also known as *reciprocal change*, associated with MI is located 180 degrees

ELECTROCARDIOGRAPHIC HIGHLIGHTS

Anatomic region	Coronary artery	Descriptive leads
Anterior wall	LAD	V_3 and V_4
Anteroseptal	LAD	V_1 to V_4
Anteroseptal–lateral	Proximal LAD	V_1 to V_6, I and aVL
Septal wall	LAD	V_1 and V_2
Inferior wall	RCA; LCX	II, III, and aVF
Inferior Right ventricle	Proximal RCA	II, III, aVF, V_1, V_2, and V_{3R} to V_{6R}
Inferoposterior	RCA; LCX	II, III, aVF, V_1, V_2, and V_7 to V_9
Posterior wall	RCA; LCX	V_1, V_2, and V_7 to V_9
Lateral wall	LAD	V_5, V_6, I, and aVL
Anterolateral	LAD; LCX	V_3 to V_6, I, and aVL
Inferolateral	LAD; LCX	II, III, aVF, I, aVL, V_5, and V_6
Posterolateral	LAD; LCX	V_1, V_2, V_7 to V_9, V_5, V_6, I, and aVL

LAD, left anterior descending coronary artery; LCX, left circumflex coronary artery; RCA, right coronary artery.

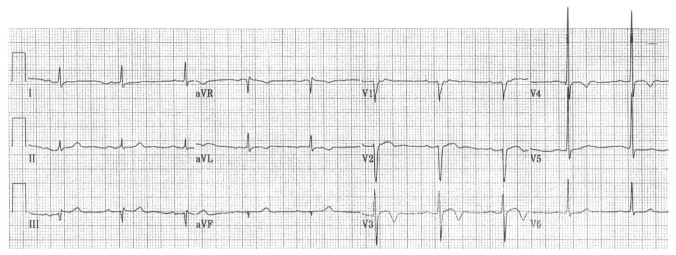

FIGURE 33-1 • **Acute anterior myocardial infarction.** This ECG from a 67-year-old man with chest pain demonstrates ST segment elevation with symmetrical T wave inversion in precordial leads V_2 through V_4.

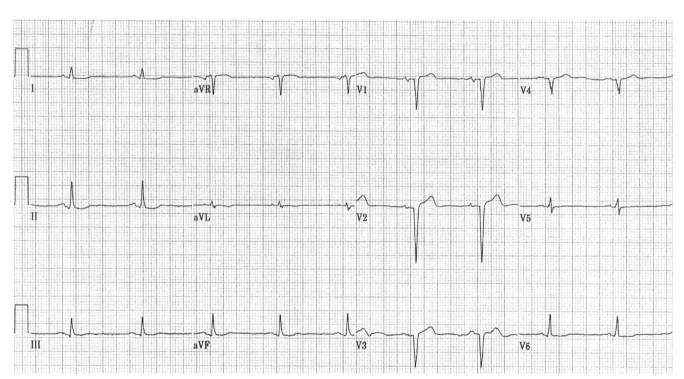

FIGURE 33-2 • **Anteroseptal myocardial infarction.** Note the Q waves in leads V_1 to V_4 and mild ST segment elevation in leads V_1 to V_3.

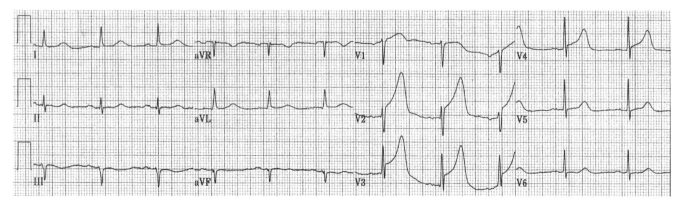

FIGURE 33-3 • **Anteroseptal myocardial infarction (MI).** The acute ST segment elevation in leads V_1 to V_4 of this 75-year-old man represents an anteroseptal MI. These ST segment changes resolved completely with the administration of a thrombolytic agent.

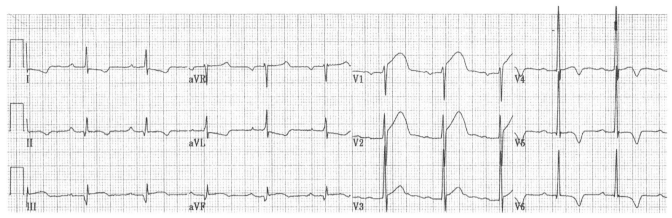

FIGURE 33-4 · Acute anteroseptal myocardial infarction (MI). The ST segment elevation (STE) in leads V_1 to V_4 of this 50-year-old man with chest pain is compatible with an acute anteroseptal MI. The STE in lead V_1 is greater than 2.5 mm, which is a strong prediction of a left anterior descending coronary artery occlusion that is proximal to the first septal perforator coronary artery.

from the involved region. Because no leads of the standard 12-lead ECG are located 180 degrees from the anterior or anteroseptal areas of the LV, acute MI (AMI) in these areas is not associated with reciprocal changes. Additional leads V_7 through V_9 (see section on Posterior Wall), however, would demonstrate reciprocal changes with these anteroseptal infarctions.

STE in lead aVR that is at least as great as STE in lead V_1 identifies left main coronary artery occlusion with 81% sensitivity, 80% specificity, and 81% accuracy (Fig. 33-5). The degree of STE in lead aVR is a quantitative measure of mortality in septal or anteroseptal MIs. STE in lead aVR of 1.5 mm has been found to predict death with 75% sensitivity, 75% specificity, and 75% accuracy.[6]

Lateral Wall. The lateral wall of the LV is commonly served by the LAD distal to the first septal perforator artery, but can also be supplied by the left circumflex artery (LCX). The lateral wall is represented by leads V_5 and V_6 in the precordial and leads I and aVL in the limb leads. Leads I and aVL represent the high lateral wall of the LV (Fig. 33-6).

Isolated lateral wall ischemia or infarction can occur. More commonly, however, the lateral wall is involved with other regions, such as inferolateral, anterolateral (Fig. 33-7), or anteroseptal with lateral extension. Acute coronary events of the lateral wall can also occur with involvement of the posterior wall (i.e., posterolateral). Anteroseptal ischemia or infarction with lateral extension is represented by involvement in leads V_1 through V_6, with or without leads I and aVL (Fig. 33-8). This is extensive ischemia or infarction and encompasses a large percentage of the LV. Reciprocal changes can be seen with lateral wall infarctions but only if the high lateral wall (leads I and aVL) is involved. In this setting, the reciprocal changes appear in leads II, III, and aVF (see Figs. 33-7 and 33-8).

Inferior Wall. Acute coronary events involving the inferior wall of the LV are represented by changes in leads II, III, and aVF. These limb leads represent the electrical activity of the heart in the frontal plane and are oriented downward and inferiorly. Reciprocal changes of an inferior wall MI are represented by ST segment depression in leads I and aVL. Myocardial ischemia in this region is typically caused by

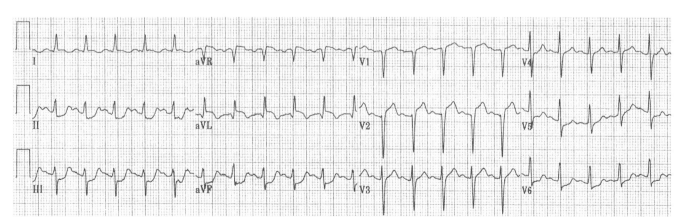

FIGURE 33-5 · Acute myocardial infarction secondary to left main coronary artery disease. This ECG from a 75-year-old man with acute chest pain demonstrates ST segment elevation (STE) in leads V_1 and V_2 as well as leads I and aVL. The precordial leads represent the septal region of the left ventricle and leads I and aVL represent the high lateral wall. Also note the ST segment depression in leads II, III, and aVF. These changes are compatible with reciprocal changes from the infarction of the high lateral wall of the left ventricle. Figures 33-1 through 33-4 do not show reciprocal changes because there are no leads of the standard 12-lead ECG that are anatomically 180 degrees opposite the anterior or septal regions of the left ventricle. This tracing also demonstrates STE in lead aVR that is greater in amplitude than the elevation in lead V_1, a relatively sensitive and specific indicator of left main coronary artery disease.

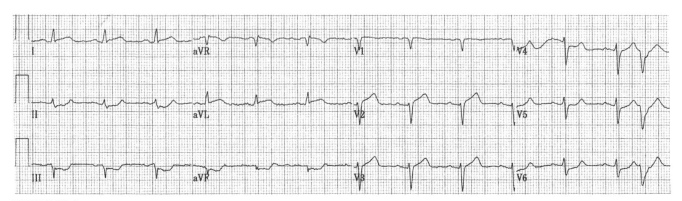

FIGURE 33-6 • **High lateral wall myocardial infarction (MI).** As in other regions of the left ventricle (LV), an isolated lateral wall MI is unusual. This ECG demonstrates ST segment elevation in leads I and aVL. The ST segment depression in leads II, III, and aVF most likely represents reciprocal changes from the high lateral wall MI. On the other hand, the ST segment depression in leads V_5 and V_6 corresponds with myocardial ischemia in the remainder of the lateral wall of the LV.

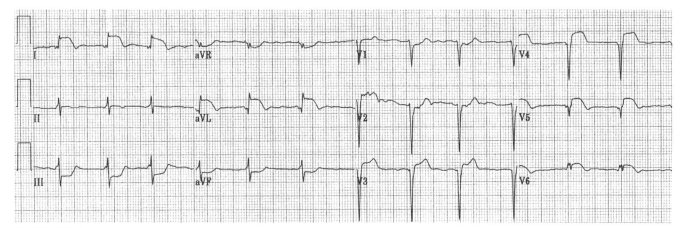

FIGURE 33-7 • **Acute anterolateral myocardial infarction (MI).** This ECG is from a 99-year-old man who presented with chest pain and dyspnea. The tracing shows ST segment elevation in leads V_3 to V_6 as well as in leads I and aVL, and corresponds to an acute anterolateral MI. The ST segment depressions in II, III, and aVF are most likely reciprocal changes from the infarction involving the high lateral wall of the left ventricle.

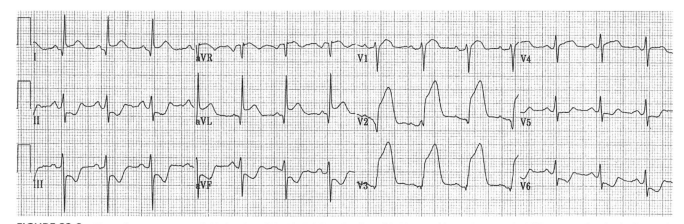

FIGURE 33-8 • **Extensive acute myocardial infarction (MI).** The ECG tracing from this 55-year-old man shows marked ST segment elevation in the septal, anterior, and lateral walls of the left ventricle (LV). The ST segment depression in the inferior leads represents reciprocal changes. The large anatomic region of the LV involved with this MI predicts extensive coronary artery disease.

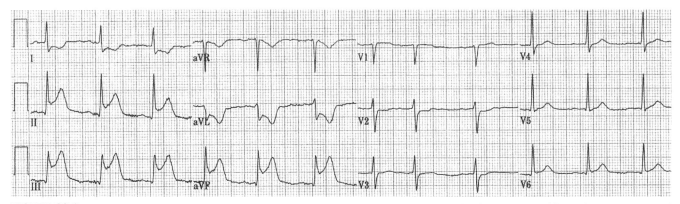

FIGURE 33-9 · **Acute inferior myocardial infarction, right coronary artery (RCA).** This ECG tracing from a 70-year-old man demonstrates marked ST segment elevation (STE) in leads II, III, and aVF. The ST segment depression in leads I and aVL associated with this isolated inferior myocardial infarction represents reciprocal changes in these leads. The STE in lead III that is of greater amplitude than that of lead II suggests an occlusion of the proximal or mid-portion of the RCA.

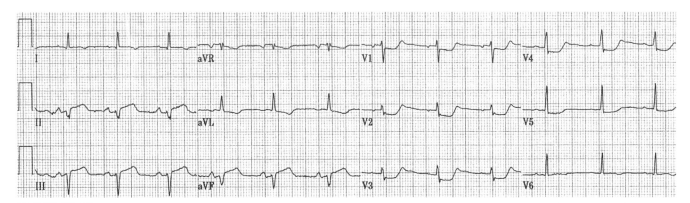

FIGURE 33-10 · **Acute inferior myocardial infarction (MI), left circumflex coronary artery (LCX).** The inferior MI of this 80-year-old woman is associated with ST segment elevation of relatively the same magnitude in leads II and III. This is often a predictor of an occlusion in the LCX. The ST segment depression in leads V_1 to V_5 may represent ischemia of the posterior region of the left ventricle or, more likely, ischemia of the anteroseptal region.

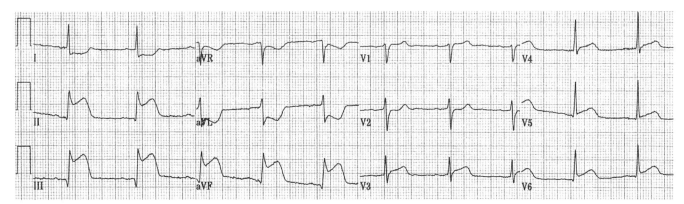

FIGURE 33-11 · **Acute inferior myocardial infarction with extreme coronary artery disease.** This ECG is from a 70-year-old man with chest pain of 3 to 4 hours' duration. The tracing reveals ST segment elevation in leads II, III, and aVF, as well as leads V_3 to V_6, indicating extensive coronary artery disease.

disease of the RCA and, less commonly, the LCX. The presence of STE in lead III exceeding the elevation in lead II can predict an occlusion in the proximal or mid-portion of the RCA (Fig. 33-9). The presence of STE in lead III, equal to that of lead II, is a strong predictor of LCX occlusion[7,8] (Fig. 33-10). This finding is attributable to the anatomic distribution of the respective coronary arteries; the RCA is

more right-sided, leading to greater changes in the right-sided lead III.

Isolated inferior wall involvement can occur but more commonly extends to the lateral wall, posterior wall, or the RV. The involvement of more than just the inferior wall of the LV is an indication of extensive disease. The presence of STE of 2 mm or more in leads V_5 and V_6 (Fig. 33-11), in association

33-1 • ELECTROCARDIOGRAPHIC CRITERIA FOR RIGHT VENTRICULAR INFARCTION

Presence of an inferior wall myocardial infarction
ST segment elevation in lead III > lead II
ST segment elevation in lead V_1
ST segment depression in lead V_2
ST segment elevation >2 mm in lead V_{4R} (leads V_{3R} to V_{6R})

ELECTROCARDIOGRAPHIC PEARLS

- Reciprocal changes are located anatomically 180 degrees away from the involved region of the left ventricle.
- Septal or anteroseptal myocardial infarctions (MIs) with ST segment elevation in lead aVR that is greater than or equal to the ST segment elevation in lead V_1 are often associated with occlusion of the left main coronary artery.
- Anteroseptal MIs associated with lateral wall involvement are associated with extensive coronary artery disease.
- The ST segment elevation of an acute inferior MI that is of greater amplitude in lead III than in lead II is a strong predictor of occlusion of the proximal right coronary artery.
- Acute inferior MI associated with ST segment elevation in lead V_1 is suggestive of right ventricular infarction.
- Posterior MI can be differentiated from septal myocardial ischemia by the presence of an R:S wave amplitude ratio of at least 1.

with an inferior wall MI, is a sensitive and specific indicator of extensive coronary artery disease and a large area of involvement.[9]

Right Ventricle. Approximately one fourth to one third of inferior wall AMIs are associated with RV infarction. The criteria for RV infarction are included in Table 33-1. Approximately 87% of RV infarctions occur in association with inferior wall infarctions and are associated with occlusion of the proximal RCA.[10] Infarction of the RV allows the vector from the interventricular septum to pass unopposed. This vector is usually directed anterior, inferior, and to the right. Lead III lies directly in this vector's path, which causes the STE of an inferior wall MI to be of greater amplitude in lead III than in lead II. Because the unopposed vector from the interventricular septum is directed anterior and to the right, the ST segment in lead V_1 can be elevated (Fig. 33-12).

The STE is usually restricted to lead V_1 but occasionally can extend across the precordial leads.[11–13] At times, the STE in lead V_1 is accompanied by ST segment depression in lead V_2.[14] This depression occurs because the vector originating from the interventricular septum is directed toward the right (lead V_1) and away from the left (lead V_2). Using the right

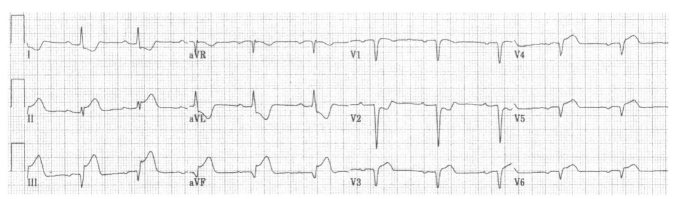

A

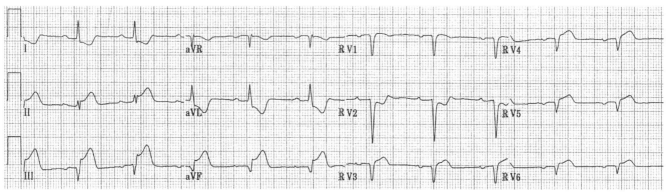

B

FIGURE 33-12 • Inferior wall and right ventricular (RV) infarction. *A,* The inferior myocardial injury pattern of a 60-year-old woman also demonstrates ST segment elevation (STE) in lead V_1. This finding often predicts an associated RV infarction. *B,* Right-sided precordial leads from this patient demonstrate STE in leads V_{3R} to V_{6R}, which strongly suggests an RV infarction. Involvement of the RV is usually associated with occlusion of the proximal right coronary artery. This is also suggested by the STE in lead III that is of greater amplitude than that of lead II.

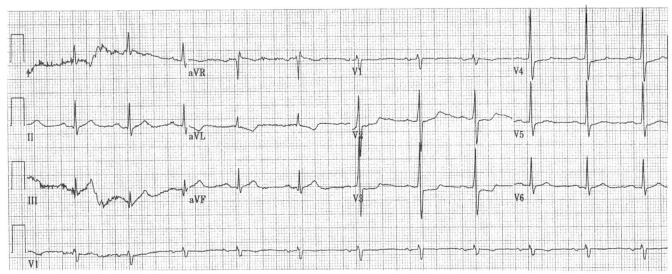

FIGURE 33-13 • **Acute posterior wall myocardial infarction (MI).** This tracing was obtained from a 66-year-old patient who presented with substernal chest pain. It has ST segment depression in primarily leads V_2 and V_3. Because the R wave in lead V_2 is of equal or greater amplitude compared with the S wave in the same lead and the duration of the R wave is greater than 0.03 sec, this tracing represents a true or isolated posterior MI and not ischemia of the anterior or septal regions of the left ventricle.

precordial leads can often make the ECG diagnosis of RV infarction. The right precordial leads are placed as mirror images of the left precordial leads. Although STE can be seen in leads V_{3R} through V_{6R}, STE in lead V_{4R} is most sensitive and specific for RV infarction[11,15] (Fig. 33-12). STE in the right precordial leads is not specific for RV infarction. Infarction of the LV (anteroseptal) as well as pericarditis, blunt chest trauma, and pulmonary embolism may also be associated with similar findings in these leads.[16–19]

Posterior Wall. The posterior wall of the LV is perfused by the posterior descending coronary artery, which usually originates from the RCA and occasionally from the LCX. Isolated, or pure, posterior wall ischemia or infarction is uncommon (Fig. 33-13). Infarction of the posterior wall is more commonly associated with AMI of either the inferior (Fig. 33-14) or lateral walls (Fig. 33-15). The standard 12-lead

ECG does not directly image the posterior wall. Therefore, identifying reciprocal changes in leads that are 180 degrees away from the posterior region, namely, leads V_1 and V_2, establishes the ECG diagnosis of posterior wall MI; in other words, ST segment depression in leads V_1, V_2, or V_3 is strongly suggestive of posterior wall MI. The classic ECG changes in leads V_1 and V_2 associated with a posterior wall MI are tall R waves relative to S waves, ST segment depression, and upright T waves. The R wave in the right precordial leads associated with posterior wall infarction has an R:S amplitude ratio of at least 1. The R waves are wider than normal and usually have a duration of at least 0.03 sec. ST segment depression in the right precordial leads can represent posterior wall infarction or septal ischemia. The ST segment depression of septal ischemia is associated with an R:S amplitude ratio of less than 1 and an R wave width less than 0.03 sec.

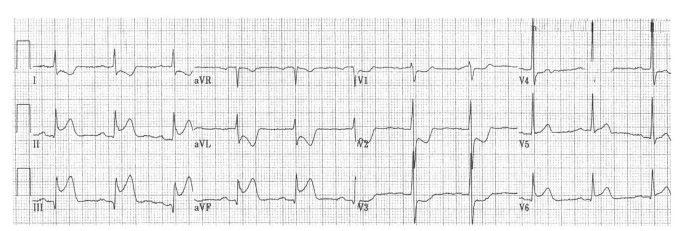

FIGURE 33-14 • **Acute infero-posterolateral myocardial infarction.** This tracing from a 75-year-old man with chest pain, dyspnea, and diaphoresis demonstrates ST segment elevation in the inferior (leads II, III, and aVF) and lateral (leads V_5 and V_6) regions of the left ventricle. The ST segment depression in leads I and aVL are reciprocal changes from the involvement of the inferior wall. The ST segment depression in leads V_1 to V_3 represents infarction of the posterior wall.

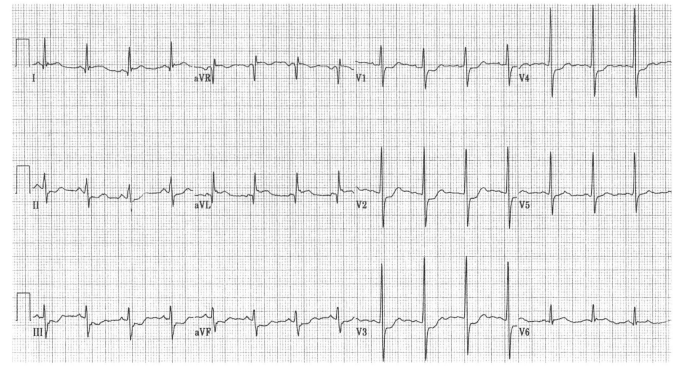

FIGURE 33-15 · **Acute high lateral myocardial infarction with posterior involvement.** This ECG demonstrates ST segment elevations in the high lateral leads (I and aVL) with reciprocal changes in the inferior leads. The ST segment depression in leads V_1 to V_4 is representative of a posterior wall infarction as well. This is confirmed by the large R wave relative to S wave in the same leads.

Using additional ECG leads, namely leads V_7 through V_9, can make the differentiation between posterior infarction and septal ischemia. Leads V_7 through V_9 are located on the same horizontal plane as leads V_4 through V_6. Lead V_7 lies along the posterior axillary line, lead V_8 lies along the inferior angle of the scapula, and lead V_9 is located at the left paraspinal border. Because these leads lie directly over the posterior wall of the LV, they demonstrate the classic STE, abnormal Q wave, and inverted T wave of an AMI. The tall R wave relative to S wave in the right precordial leads is a more reliable indicator of posterior wall infarction than the ST segment or T wave changes in these same leads.[20,21] A tall R wave relative to S wave in lead V_1 is not specific for posterior wall MI and can be seen in other conditions.

References

1. Goldberger AL: Myocardial Infarction: Electrocardiographic Differential Diagnosis, 4th ed. St. Louis, Mosby-Year Book, 1991.
2. Blanke H, Cohen M, Schlueter GU, et al: Electrocardiographic and coronary arteriographic correlations during acute myocardial infarction. Am J Cardiol 1984;54:249.
3. Roberts WC, Gardin JM: Location of myocardial infarcts: A confusion of terms and definitions. Am J Cardiol 1978;42:868.
4. Hindman NB, Schocken DD, Widmann M, et al: Evaluation of a QRS scoring system for estimating myocardial infarct size: V. Specificity and method of application of the complete system. Am J Cardiol 1985;55:1485.
5. Engelsen DJ, Gorgels AP, Cheriex EC, et al: Value of the electrocardiogram in localizing the occlusion site in the left anterior descending coronary artery in acute anterior myocardial infarction. J Am Coll Cardiol 1999;34:389.
6. Yamaji H, Iwasaki K, Kusachi S, et al: Prediction of acute left main coronary artery obstruction by 12-lead electrocardiography: ST segment elevation in lead aVR with less ST segment elevation in lead V_1. J Am Coll Cardiol 2001;38:1348.
7. Zimetbaum PJ, Krishnan S, Gold A, et al: Usefulness of ST-segment elevation in lead III exceeding that of lead II for identifying the location of the totally occluded coronary artery in inferior wall myocardial infarction. Am J Cardiol 1998;81:918.
8. Chia BL, Yip JW, Tan HC, Lim YT: Usefulness of ST segment II/III ratio and ST deviation in lead I for identifying the culprit artery in inferior wall acute myocardial infarction. Am J Cardiol 2000; 86:341.
9. Assali AR, Sclarovsky S, Herz I, et al: Comparison of patients with inferior wall acute myocardial infarction with versus without ST-segment elevation in leads V_5 and V_6. Am J Cardiol 1998;81:81.
10. Kinch JW, Ryan TJ: Right ventricular infarction. N Engl J Med 1994;330:1211.
11. Lopez-Sendon J, Coma-Canella I, Alcasena S, et al: Electrocardiographic findings in acute right ventricular infarction: Sensitivity and specificity of electrocardiographic alterations in right precordial leads V_{4R}, V_{3R}, V_1, V_2 and V_3. J Am Coll Cardiol 1985;6:1273.
12. Andersen HR, Nielsen D, Falk E: Right ventricular infarction: Diagnostic value of ST elevation in lead III exceeding that of lead II during inferior/posterior infarction and comparison with right-chest leads. Am Heart J 1989;117:82.
13. Saw J, Davies C, Fung A, et al: Value of ST elevation in lead III greater than lead II in inferior wall acute myocardial infarction for predicting in-hospital mortality and diagnosing right ventricular infarction. Am J Cardiol 2001;87:448.
14. Lew AS, Laramee P, Shah PK, et al: Ratio of ST-segment depression in lead V_2 to ST-segment elevation in lead aVF in evolving inferior acute myocardial infarction: An aid to the early recognition of right ventricular ischemia. Am J Cardiol 1986;57:1047.

15. Robalino BD, Whitlow PL, Underwood DA, Salcedo EE: Electrocardiographic manifestations of right ventricular infarction. Am Heart J 1989;118:138.
16. Medrano GA, de Micheli A, Osornio Vargas A, Renteria V: Electric signs of experimental pericarditis. Arch Inst Cardiol Mex 1985;55:7.
17. Chia BL, Tan HC, Lim YT: Right sided chest lead electrocardiographic abnormalities in acute pulmonary embolism. Int J Cardiol 1997;61:43.
18. Abundes Velasco A, Navarro Robles J, Autrey Caballero A, et al: Electrocardiographic data suggesting anteroseptal myocardial infarction, in presence of infarction of the left ventricle. Arch Inst Cardiol Mex 1997;67:223.
19. Walsh P, Marks G, Aranguri C, et al: Use of V_{4R} in patients who sustain blunt chest trauma. J Trauma 2001;51:60.
20. Casa RE, Marriott HJ, Glancy DL: Value of leads V_7–V_9 in diagnosing posterior wall acute myocardial infarction and other causes of tall R waves in V_1–V_2. Am J Cardiol 1997;80:508.
21. Zalenski RJ, Cooke D, Rydman R, et al: Assessing the diagnostic value of the ECG containing leads V_{4R}, V_8, and V_9: The 15-lead ECG. Ann Emerg Med 1993;22:786.

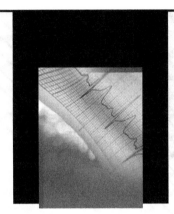

Chapter 34

Acute Myocardial Infarction: Confounding Patterns

William J. Brady and Marc L. Pollack

Significant ST segment changes, including elevation and depression, are frequently seen in the patient with chest pain, resulting from a range of clinical syndromes.[1,2] Acute coronary syndromes (ACS), particularly acute myocardial infarction (AMI), represent a less common cause of these electrocardiographic changes among all other entities.[1,2] In fact, the electrocardiogram (ECG) frequently demonstrates significant abnormality which is unrelated to ACS. These ST segment/T wave changes are due in large part to left bundle branch block (LBBB), left ventricular hypertrophy (LVH), and ventricular paced rhythms (VPR). The physician must be familiar with the ST segment/T wave changes resulting from these confounding patterns. If the clinician is unfamiliar with these changes, these patterns can introduce the potential for diagnostic error. Furthermore, these same patterns reduce the ECG's ability to detect evidence of ACS—these patterns confound the clinician's ability to use the ECG in the evaluation of ACS. LBBB and VPR significantly impair the ECG's capability of demonstrating ECG change; LVH also weakens the ECG's ability to detect ischemic ECG change.

Electrocardiographic Manifestations

Left Bundle Branch Block. In LBBB, the ventricular depolarization pattern is abnormal. The left ventricle (LV) is not depolarized from the left bundle branch; rather, the electrical discharge moves along the right bundle and into the ventricular myocardium, ultimately reaching the LV and producing depolarization. This altered intraventricular conduction produces a number of ECG changes that must be recognized as primary abnormalities of the new pattern and not necessarily the *direct* manifestation of ACS. This statement is true not only for the LBBB presentation but the LVH and VPR scenarios as well.

In the patient with LBBB (Figs. 34-1 and 34-2), the QRS complex is widened to at least 0.12 sec in the adult.[3,4] The ECG demonstrates a broad, mainly negative QS or rS complex in lead V_1. QS complexes are noted in the right to mid-precordial leads, rarely extending beyond lead V_4. QS complexes may also be seen in the inferior leads III and aVF. In the lateral leads (leads I, aVL, V_5, and V_6), a monophasic R wave (positive QRS complex) is seen. The expected ST segment/T wave configurations of the new, abnormal intraventricular conduction are discordant. This statement describes the relationship of the ST segment/T wave and the major, terminal portion of the QRS complex with respect to the isoelectric baseline.

This relationship is called *QRS complex/T wave axis discordance* and the related changes are described by the *rule of appropriate discordance* (Fig. 34-3). According to this rule, leads with either QS or rS complexes (i.e., QRS complexes that are entirely or partially negative) may have markedly elevated ST segments, mimicking AMI; the distribution of

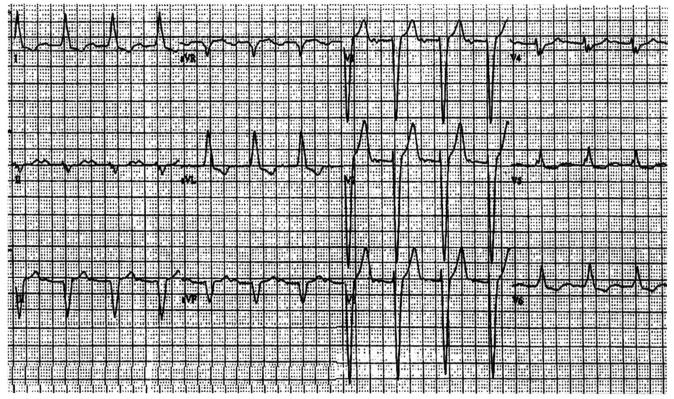

FIGURE 34-1 · **Left bundle branch block (LBBB).** This 12-lead ECG in a 57-year-old patient with LBBB shows "normal" or expected ST segment/T wave changes without ECG evidence of acute myocardial infarction.

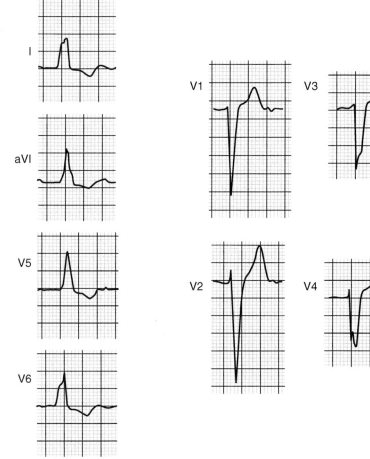

A

B

FIGURE 34-2 · **Left bundle branch block: normal findings.** *A*, A large monophasic R wave is seen in the lateral leads—note the entirely positive QRS complex with ST segment depression and T wave inversion. *B*, The anterior leads show a predominantly negative QRS complex—note the ST segment elevation and upright T wave.

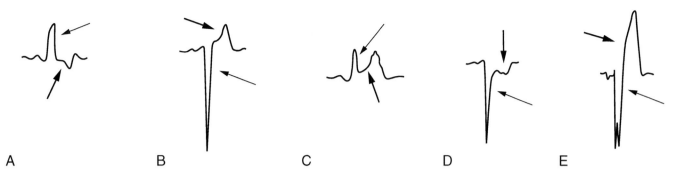

A   B   C   D   E

FIGURE 34-3 · **Rule of appropriate discordance in left bundle branch block setting.** This principle states that the major terminal portion of the QRS complex and the initial, upsloping portion of the ST segment/T wave complex are situated on opposite sides of the isoelectric baseline. *A,* Discordant ST segment depression (normal finding)—the major terminal portion of the QRS complex (*small arrow*) is located on the opposite side of the baseline from the ST segment/T wave (*large arrow*). *B,* Discordant ST segment elevation (STE; normal finding)—the major terminal portion of the QRS complex (*small arrow*) is located on the opposite side of the baseline from the ST segment/T wave (*large arrow*). *C,* Concordant STE (abnormal finding)—the major terminal portion of the QRS complex (*small arrow*) is located on the same side of the baseline as the ST segment/T wave (*large arrow*). *D,* Concordant ST segment depression (abnormal finding)—the major terminal portion of the QRS complex (*small arrow*) is located on the same side of the baseline as the ST segment/T wave (*large arrow*). *E,* Excessive discordant STE (abnormal finding)—the major terminal portion of the QRS complex (*small arrow*) is located on the opposite side of the baseline as the ST segment/T wave (*large arrow*), as is expected, yet the degree of elevation is excessive, greater than 5 mm.

this ECG phenomenon is seen in leads V_1 to V_3 or V_4, as well as leads III and aVF. Conversely, leads with positive QRS complexes (i.e., large monophasic R waves) demonstrate ST segment depression—as seen in leads I, aVL, V_5, and V_6. The T wave, especially in the right to mid-precordial leads, is quite prominent with a vaulting appearance, similar to the hyperacute T wave of early AMI. The T waves in leads with the monophasic R wave are frequently inverted. Loss of this normal QRS complex/T wave axes discordance in patients with LBBB may indicate an ACS[5] (Fig. 34-4).

Sgarbossa et al. have developed a clinical prediction rule to assist in the ECG diagnosis of AMI in the setting of LBBB

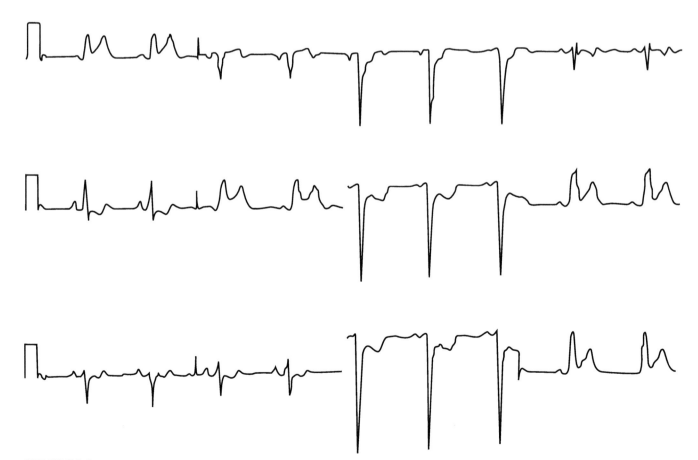

FIGURE 34-4 · **Left bundle branch block (LBBB) with ECG acute myocardial infarction (AMI).** This ECG from a 49-year-old man with LBBB anterolateral AMI shows concordant ST segment elevation in leads I, aVL, V_5, and V_6 as well as concordant ST segment depression in leads V_1 to V_3, violating the rule of appropriate discordance.

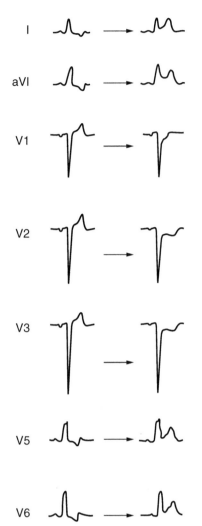

FIGURE 34-5 · **Left bundle branch block with serial development of ECG acute myocardial infarction (AMI).** Normal complexes are shown progressing to complexes encountered in ECG AMI, with the left column of complexes demonstrating the normal, "expected" ST segment/T wave configurations and the right column demonstrating the findings seen in ECG AMI, with violations of the rule of appropriate discordance.

using three specific ECG findings.[6] Criteria suggestive of AMI, ranked with a scoring system based on the probability of such a diagnosis, are as follows: (1) ST segment elevation (STE) greater than or equal to 1 mm concordant with QRS complex (score of 5; see Fig. 34-3C); (2) ST segment depression greater than or equal to 1 mm in leads V_1, V_2, or V_3 (score of 3; see Fig. 34-3D); and (3) STE greater than or equal to 5 mm discordant with the QRS complex (score of 2; see Fig. 34-3E). A total score of 3 or more suggests that the patient is likely experiencing an AMI based on the ECG criteria. With a score less than 3, the ECG diagnosis is less certain, requiring additional evaluation. A comparison with prior ECGs may demonstrate significant change (Fig. 34-5).

Subsequent publications[7–9] have suggested that this clinical prediction rule is less useful than reported, with studies demonstrating decreased sensitivity and inter-rater reliability.[7–9] Even if the Sgarbossa et al. clinical prediction rule is found to be less useful in the objective evaluation of the ECG in the patient with LBBB, the report has merit; it has forced the clinician to review the ECG in detail and casts some degree of doubt on the widely taught belief that the ECG is entirely invalidated in the search for AMI in the patient with LBBB.[6]

Left Ventricular Hypertrophy. An ECG pattern consistent with LVH is seen in approximately 30% of patients with chest pain in the emergency department (ED).[1,2] Similarly, Larsen et al. have shown that the LVH pattern is encountered in approximately 10% of patients with chest pain in the ED initially diagnosed with ACS; after more extensive evaluation in the hospital, only 25% of these admitted patients were found to have ACS—the remainder were diagnosed with non-ACS diagnoses.[10] Of note, the physicians caring for these patients incorrectly interpreted the ECG more than 70% of the time; they frequently did not identify the LVH pattern and therefore attributed the ST segment/T wave changes to ACS, when in fact the observed changes resulted from repolarization abnormalities due to LVH.[10]

In patients with LVH, ST segment/T wave changes are encountered in approximately 70% of cases; these changes result from the altered repolarization of the ventricular myocardium due to LVH and represent the new normal ECG findings in these patients (Figs. 34-6 and 34-7). LVH is

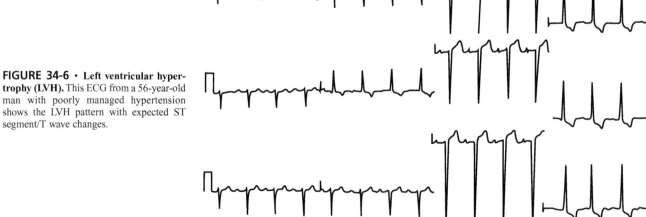

FIGURE 34-6 · **Left ventricular hypertrophy (LVH).** This ECG from a 56-year-old man with poorly managed hypertension shows the LVH pattern with expected ST segment/T wave changes.

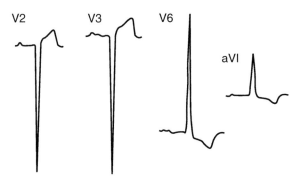

FIGURE 34-7 · Left ventricular hypertrophy (LVH). Prominent ST segment elevation in the right to mid-precordial leads and ST segment depression with T wave inversion in the lateral leads are often seen in LVH.

associated with poor R wave progression in the right to mid-precordial leads, most commonly producing a QS pattern in this distribution. In general, these QS complexes are located in leads V_1 and V_2 and variably so in lead V_3. Marked ST segment elevation with prominent T waves is seen in these leads. The ST segment elevation seen in this distribution is usually 2 to 4 mm in height, although it may reach 5 mm or more. The initial, upsloping portion of the ST segment/T wave complex is frequently concave in LVH, compared with the either flattened or convex pattern observed in the patient with AMI.[11] This morphologic feature is imperfect; AMI may reveal such a concave feature.

The "strain" pattern, characterized by downsloping ST segment depression with asymmetrical, biphasic, or inverted T waves in leads with prominent R waves—the lateral leads I, aVL, V_5, and V_6—is frequently misinterpreted as ACS[4,12] (see Figs. 34-6 and 34-7). The ST segment/T wave complex has been described in the following manner: initially bowed upward (convex upward) followed by a gradual downward sloping into an inverted, asymmetrical T wave with an abrupt return to the baseline. Significant variability may be encountered in the "strain" pattern. The T wave may be minimally inverted or the inversion may be greater than 5 mm in depth. These T wave abnormalities may also be encountered in patients lacking prominent voltage (i.e., large S and R waves).[4,12] Other features of this portion of the ST segment/T wave complex suggestive of LVH-related repolarization change include the following (all favoring a nonischemic diagnosis): (1) depression of the J point; (2) asymmetry of the T wave inversion with a gradual downslope and a rapid return to the baseline; (3) terminal positivity of the T wave, described as "overshoot"; (4) T wave inversion in lead V_6 greater than 3 mm; and (5) T wave inversion greater in lead V_6 than in lead V_4.[4,12,13]

Ventricular Paced Rhythm. In the patient with right VPR, the ECG shares many similarities with the LBBB presentation. The ECG reveals a broad, mainly negative QS or rS complex in leads V_1 to V_6 with either QS complexes or poor R wave progression (Figs. 34-8 and 34-9). A large monophasic R wave is encountered in leads I and aVL and, rarely, in leads V_5 and V_6. QS complexes are frequently encountered in the inferior leads (II, III, and aVF). As with the LBBB pattern, the appropriate ST segment/T wave configurations are discordant with the QRS complex—that is, directed opposite from the terminal portion of the QRS complex (see Fig. 34-9).

Multiple investigators have attempted to characterize diagnostic criteria for ACS in patients with VPR using numerous approaches, including the somewhat similar ECG appearance of VPR and LBBB, the use of past ECGs for comparison, or a complicated analysis of the QRS complex vectors. These investigations did not provide the physician with the necessary tools to evaluate the ECG in the setting of ACS. Sgarbossa et al. have investigated the ECG changes encountered in patients with VPR experiencing AMI.[14] Three ECG criteria were found to be useful in the early diagnosis of AMI, including (1) discordant STE greater than or equal to 5 mm; (2) concordant STE greater than or equal to 1 mm; and (3) ST segment depression greater than or equal to 1 mm in leads V_1, V_2, or V_3 (Fig. 34-10). Unlike the LBBB criteria, the most statistically powerful criterion found in Sgarbossa and colleagues' work is discordant STE of 5 mm or more; this finding violates the rule of appropriate discordance, not with concordant ST segment changes but with an inappropriate degree of discordant STE.[15] Repolarization changes of VPRs should produce STE of less magnitude in the "normal" state. ECG criteria (2) and (3), namely, concordant STE and ST segment depression (limited to leads V_1, V_2, or V_3), are examples of infractions of the rule of appropriate discordance. Sgarbossa and colleagues' article, in contrast to much of the existing cardiology literature, attempts to distinguish between past and acute myocardial infarction; it furthers provides the physician with the interpretive tools to make the early ECG diagnosis of AMI.[15-20]

Summary. Several strategies are available to assist in the correct interpretation of these complicated ECG patterns. A single clinical strategy, however, is probably not applicable in all instances; rather, a combination of a detailed knowledge of the ECG and the use of serial and previous ECGs will enable the clinician to evaluate the patient appropriately. These guidelines provide the physician with the interpretive tools to make the early ECG diagnosis of AMI in patients with confounding patterns. The physician must realize, however, that these ST segment changes only suggest AMI in patients with complicated ECGs; by themselves, these findings are not diagnostic of AMI. Furthermore, their absence does not rule

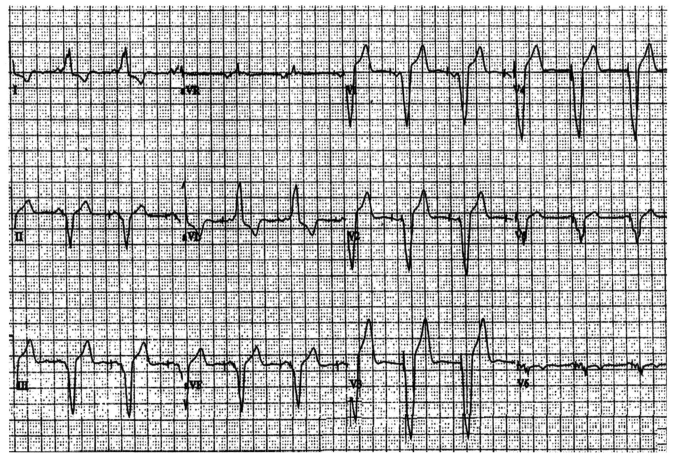

FIGURE 34-8 • **Ventricular paced rhythm.** In this ECG from a 71-year-old woman with a ventricular paced rhythm, the "normal" ST segment/T wave configurations for this form of altered intraventricular conduction are seen.

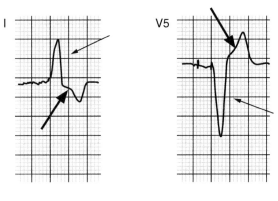

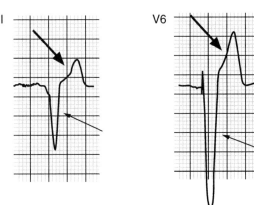

FIGURE 34-9 • **Ventricular paced rhythm: normal findings.** These tracings once again depict the rule of appropriate discordance, with the major terminal portion of the QRS complex (*small arrow*) located on the opposite side of the baseline to the ST segment/T wave (*large arrow*).

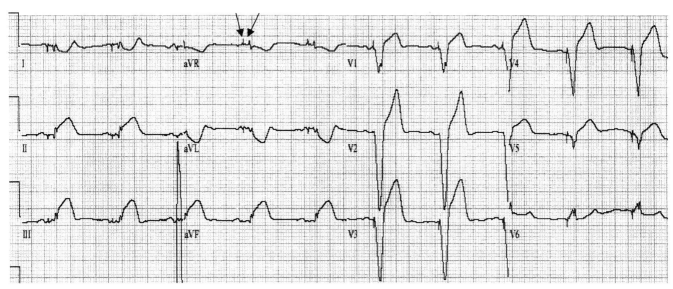

FIGURE 34-10 · Acute myocardial infarction (AMI) in patient with ventricular paced rhythm. There is evidence of a functioning dual chamber artificial pacemaker (*arrows*). Moreover, there is concordant ST segment elevation in leads II, III, and aVF, as well as reciprocal ST segment depression in leads I and aVL. Cardiac enzymes were positive for AMI. Cardiac catheterization revealed a marked stenosis of the proximal right coronary artery.

out the possibility of AMI. Therapeutic decisions must be made with these caveats in mind.

References

1. Brady WJ, Perron AD, Martin ML, et al: Electrocardiographic ST segment elevation in emergency department chest pain center patients: Etiology responsible for the ST segment abnormality. Am J Emerg Med 2001;19:25.
2. Otto LA, Aufderheide TP: Evaluation of ST segment elevation criteria for the prehospital electrocardiographic diagnosis of acute myocardial infarction. Ann Emerg Med 1994;23:17.
3. Marriott HJL: Myocardial infarction. In Marriott HJL (ed): Practical Electrocardiography, 8th ed. Baltimore, Williams & Wilkins, 1988, pp 419–450.
4. Aufderheide TP, Brady WJ: Electrocardiography in the patient with myocardial ischemia or infarction. In Gibler WB, Aufderheide TP (eds): Emergency Cardiac Care. St. Louis, Mosby, 1994, p 169.
5. Brady WJ, Aufderheide TP: Left bundle block pattern complicating the evaluation of acute myocardial infarction. Acad Emerg Med 1997;4:56.
6. Sgarbossa EB, Pinski SL, Barbagelata A, et al: Electrocardiographic diagnosis of evolving acute myocardial infarction in the presence of left bundle branch block. N Engl J Med 1996;334:481.
7. Shapiro NI, Fisher J, Zimmer GD, et al: Validation of electrocardiographic criteria for diagnosing acute myocardial infarction in the presence of left bundle branch block [abstract]. Acad Emerg Med 1998;5:508.
8. Shlipak MG, Lyons WL, Go AS, et al: Should the electrocardiogram be used to guide therapy for patients with left bundle branch block and suspected acute myocardial infarction? JAMA 1999;281:714.
9. Edhouse JA, Sakr M, Angus J, Morris FP: Suspected myocardial infarction and left bundle branch block: Electrocardiographic indicators of acute ischaemia. J Accid Emerg Med 1999;16:331.
10. Larsen GC, Griffith JL, Beshansky JR, et al: Electrocardiographic left ventricular hypertrophy in patients with suspected acute cardiac ischemia: Its influence on diagnosis, treatment, and short-term prognosis. J Gen Intern Med 1994;9:666.
11. Brady WJ, Syverud SA, Beagle C, et al: Electrocardiographic ST segment elevation: The diagnosis of AMI by morphologic analysis of the ST segment. Acad Emerg Med 2001;8:961.
12. Sharkey SW, Berger CR, Brunette DD, Henry TD: Impact of the electrocardiogram on the delivery of thrombolytic therapy for acute myocardial infarction. Am J Cardiol 1994;73:550.
13. Beach C, Kenmure ACF, Short D: Electrocardiogram of pure left ventricular hypertrophy and its differentiation from lateral ischemia. Br Heart J 1981;46:285.
14. Sgarbossa EB, Piniski SL, Gates KB, et al: Early electrocardiographic diagnosis of acute myocardial infarction in the presence of ventricular paced rhythm. Am J Cardiol 1996;77:423.
15. Carp C, Campeanu A, Gutiu I: Electrocardiographic diagnosis of myocardial infarction in patients with pacemakers. Rev Roum Med Med Int 1976;14:257.
16. Thurman M: Vector and electrocardiographic findings of hearts with electrical pacemakers. Am J Med Sci 1967;94:578.
17. Niremberg V, Amikam S, Roguin N, et al: Primary ST changes: Diagnostic aid in patients with acute myocardial infarction. Br Heart J 1977;39:502.
18. Cardenas ML, Sanz G, Linares JC, et al: Diagnostica electrographica de infarto del miocardio en pacientes con estimulacion encocardia del ventriculo derecho par marcapasos. Arch Inst Cardiol Mex 1972;42:345.
19. Castellanos A, Zoble R, Procacci PM, et al: ST-qR pattern: New sign for diagnosis of anterior myocardial infarction during right ventricular pacing. Br Heart J 1973;35:1161.
20. Kozlowski FH, Brady WJ, Aufderheide TP, Buckley RS: The electrocardiographic diagnosis of acute myocardial infarction in patients with entricular paced rhythms. Acad Emerg Med 1998;5:52.

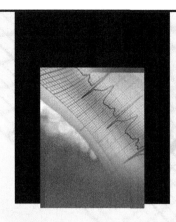

Chapter 35

Ventricular Hypertrophy

Paolo M. Gazoni and Timothy C. Evans

Clinical Features

Cardiac hypertrophy is a compensatory response of the myocardium to increased demand and hemodynamic burden. The overall mass of the heart increases because of an increase in the size, but not the number, of myocytes.[1,2] The overall prevalence of left ventricular hypertrophy (LVH) identified in the Framingham Study is 16% in women and 19% in men.[1]

The pathologic pattern of hypertrophy depends on the stimulus and etiology. Pressure ("systolic") overload, seen in systemic arterial hypertension, aortic stenosis and, occasionally, ischemic heart disease, results in concentric ventricular hypertrophy in which the left ventricular (LV) wall is thickened in a uniform manner at the expense of cavity size. Volume ("diastolic") overload, commonly associated with significant aortic and mitral insufficiency, causes eccentric hypertrophy in which the LV both hypertrophies and dilates.[2,3]

Right ventricular hypertrophy (RVH) often results from chronic right-sided pressure overload. Etiologies of RVH include congenital heart diseases involving right ventricular tract outflow obstruction (e.g., pulmonary atresia, pulmonic stenosis, and tetralogy of Fallot); pulmonary disease (recurrent or massive acute pulmonary embolism [PE], pulmonary hypertension, chronic obstructive pulmonary disease [COPD], and the Pickwickian syndrome); and cardiac etiologies (mitral stenosis and myocardial diseases causing elevated LV end-diastolic pressures).[3–5]

ELECTROCARDIOGRAPHIC HIGHLIGHTS

- The most common ECG feature of ventricular hypertrophy is an increased amplitude of the QRS complex:
  - For left ventricular hypertrophy (LVH), consider the amplitude in leads I, aVL, V_5, V_6.
  - For right ventricular hypertrophy, consider the amplitude in leads V_1 and V_2.
- Repolarization "strain" abnormalities of the ST segment/ T wave complex may also be seen in the same leads.
- Biventricular hypertrophy produces a complex interplay of electrical forces that makes defining characteristic ECG changes difficult.

The identification of LVH on the electrocardiogram (ECG) identifies a population at increased risk for symptomatic coronary heart disease, heart failure, and premature death.[1,6–9] In the Framingham Study, patients with ECG evidence of LVH had 6.6 to 9.3 times the risk of death from cardiovascular causes and 1.6 to 6.2 times the risk of sudden death compared with those without LVH.[8]

Electrocardiographic Manifestations

Left ventricular hypertrophy

QRS Complex. The most characteristic ECG finding in LVH is an increase in the amplitude of the QRS complex. This increase in the QRS voltage reflects the increase in LV mass and a shift in the position of the heart as it enlarges so that the lateral free wall lies closer to the anterior chest wall. In addition, the increased mass of the ventricle and its new position directs electrical activity more toward the left and posteriorly than previously.[3,5]

As a result of these changes, the R wave in leads facing the LV (leads I, aVL, V_5, and V_6) is taller than normal. The S wave in leads overlying the RV (V_1 and V_2) is deeper than normal[3] (Fig. 35-1). Poor progression of the R wave in the right and mid-precordial leads is frequently noted. Occasionally, the R wave is absent in V_1 and V_2, resulting in a QS pattern in these leads.[5] R waves greater than 11 mm in aVL and the combination of a large R wave in lead I and a deep S wave in lead III may also be seen[3,5] (see Fig. 35-1).

Widening and notching of the QRS complex may also be noted. The widening of the QRS complex to beyond 0.11 sec either reflects the increase in time necessary to activate the thickened ventricular wall or a conduction abnormality. A delay in the onset of the intrinsicoid deflection to 0.05 sec or greater in leads V_5 or V_6 and "notching" of the QRS complex have been described in association with LVH.[3–5]

ST Segment/T Wave. Abnormalities in repolarization may result in a variety of ST segment/T wave patterns. The amplitude of the ST segment and the T wave may be normal or increased in the leads with tall R waves. These tall T waves may resemble the "hyperacute" T waves of myocardial ischemia.

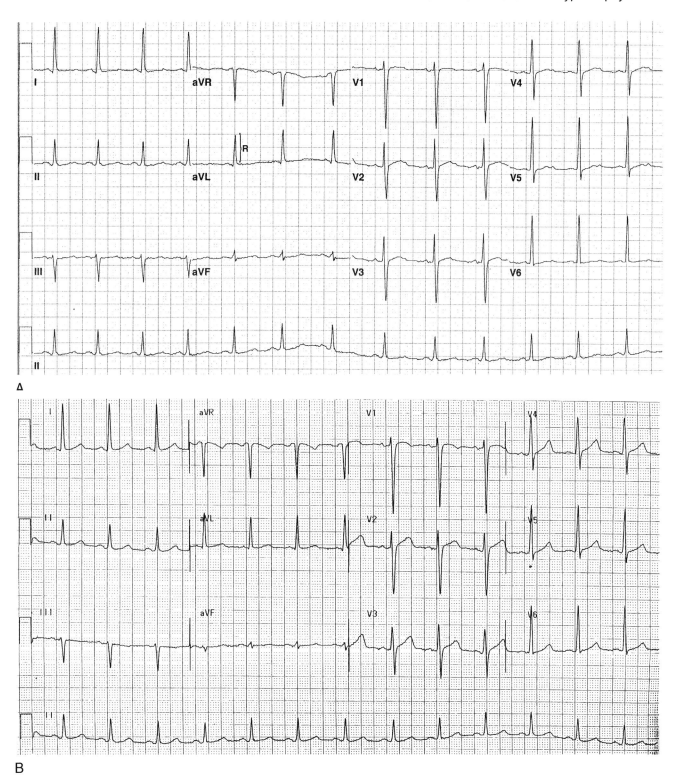

FIGURE 35-1 · **Various examples of left ventricular hypertrophy (LVH) on 12-lead ECG.** *A,* LVH suggested by R wave greater than 11 mm in lead aVL. *B,* LVH criteria met by deep S wave in V₁ and large R waves in leads V₅ and V₆. See Table 35-1 for more specific diagnostic criteria.

With increased myocardial mass, there is often a reversal in direction of the usual electrical vector, resulting in ST segment/T wave changes. These changes can result in ST segment depression with asymmetrical, biphasic, or inverted T waves in leads with prominent R waves, particularly the lateral leads (I, aVL, V₅, and V₆).

The most characteristic changes include depression of the J point, ST segment depression with a bowed morphology (Fig. 35-2), and T wave inversion with the descending portion inscribed slower than the ascending portion. This T wave is usually asymmetrical as opposed to the symmetrical T wave seen in patients with myocardial ischemia. This constellation

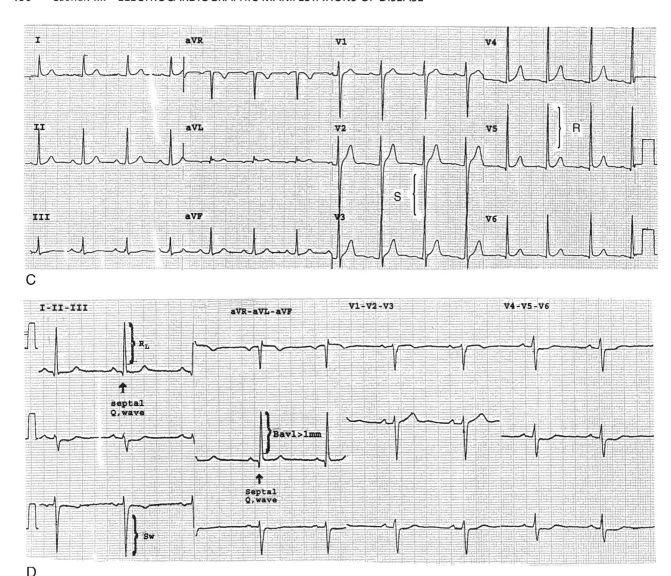

FIGURE 35-1 • **Various examples of left ventricular hypertrophy (LVH) on 12-lead ECG.** *C,* LVH characterized again by tall R wave in lead V_5 and deep S wave in lead V_2. *D,* LVH suggested by the R wave greater than 11 mm in aVL and deep S wave in lead III. See Table 35-1 for more specific diagnostic criteria.

of findings has been called *LVH with strain* (Fig. 35-2). A more appropriate term is *LVH with repolarization abnormality.*

Certain morphologic characteristics of the ST segment/ T wave complex may suggest LVH with repolarization abnormality as opposed to acute coronary syndrome. The initial upsloping of the elevated ST segment is frequently concave in LVH and more likely flat or convex in ST segment elevation myocardial infarction. Additional features of the ST segment/ T wave changes favoring the "strain" pattern of LVH include J point depression, asymmetrical T wave inversion with gradual downsloping and a rapid return to baseline, "overshoot" of the terminal portion of the inverted T wave so that it becomes a positive deflection, and T wave inversions in lead V_6 greater than 3 mm or greater than those in lead V_4[10,11] (see Fig. 35-2). However, there can be significant variation in this pattern, with minimal T wave inversion or inversions greater than 5 mm in patients lacking prominent voltage criteria for LVH.

U Wave. Some investigators report a high incidence of inverted U waves in leads I, V_5, and V_6 in patients with LVH. This finding is not supported in other studies.[5,12]

Diagnostic Criteria. Several sets of diagnostic criteria have been developed in an attempt to improve the ability of ECG to detect LVH. Some of the most commonly used criteria are provided in Table 35-1.[3,5,13] As indicated, these derived criteria tend toward higher specificity at the expense of sensitivity for the diagnosis.

Right ventricular hypertrophy

Normally, because of its larger size, the electrical forces produced by the LV predominate over those generated by the right ventricle (RV).[3] Thus, for the ECG manifestations of RVH to be appreciated, the RV must hypertrophy significantly

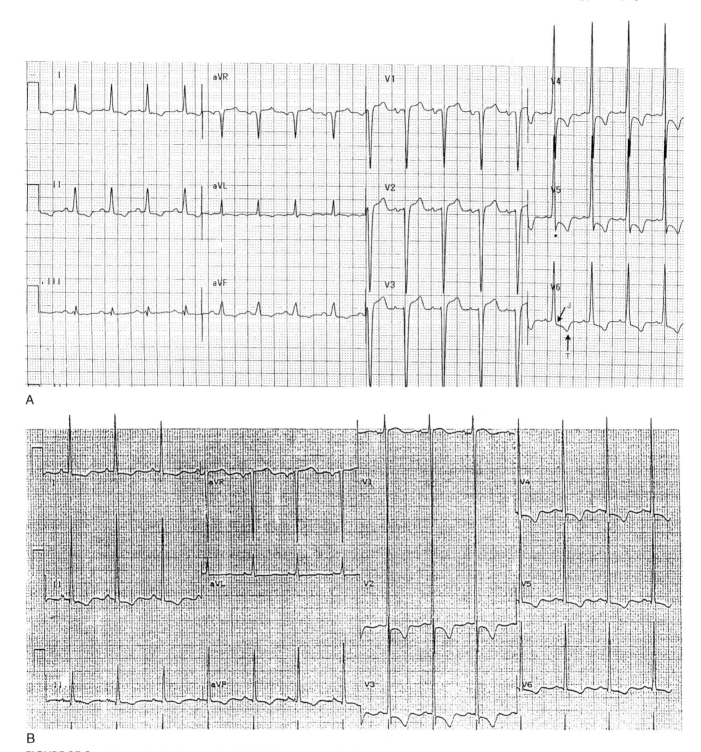

A

B

FIGURE 35-2 · Left ventricular hypertrophy (LVH) with strain. *A*, ECG demonstrating LVH with repolarization abnormalities or "strain." Note the J point depression (J), ST segment depression with downward concavity, and asymmetrical T wave inversions (T). *B*, Another example of LVH with strain. Note the ST segment depression and T wave inversions in leads V₂ to V₆.

35-1 • DIAGNOSTIC CRITERIA FOR LEFT VENTRICULAR HYPERTROPHY WITH APPROXIMATE SENSITIVITIES AND SPECIFICITIES

Criterion	Points	Sensitivity (%)	Specificity (%)
I. Sokolow-Lyon Index			
$S_{V1} + (R_{V5}$ or $R_{V6}) > 35$ mm		22	100
II. Cornell Voltage Criteria			
$S_{V3} + R_{aVL} > 28$ mm (men)		42	96
20 mm (women)			
III. Romhilt and Estes Point Score System		33	94
LVH is present if ≥5 points			
Probable LVH if >4 points			
A. Amplitude (any of the following):	3		
1. Any limb lead R wave or S wave ≥20 mm			
2. S wave in leads V_1 or V_2 ≥30 mm			
3. R wave in leads V_5 or V_6 ≥30 mm			
B. ST segment/T wave changes			
1. LVH with repolarization abnormality without digitalis	3		
2. LVH with repolarization abnormality with digitalis	1		
C. Left atrial abnormality	3		
Present if terminal negativity of P wave in leads V_1 is ≥1mm with a duration of ≥0.04 sec			
D. Left axis deviation ≥ −30 degrees	2		
E. QRS complex duration ≥0.09 sec	1		
F. Intrinsicoid deflection in V_5 or V_6 ≥0.05 sec	1		
IV. $R_I + S_{III} > 25$ mm		11	100
V. R in aVL >11 mm		11	100

LVH, left ventricular hypertrophy.

(to two or three times its normal size and weight) to overcome LV electrical forces.[3–5]

QRS Complex and Frontal Plane Axis. Right axis deviation (RAD) seen in the limb leads is a criterion in diagnosing RVH. In severe RVH, the normal leftward and posterior forces generated by the dominant LV are replaced by anterior and rightward forces generated by the now dominant RV.[5] ECG manifestations include abnormally tall R waves and small S waves in V_1 and V_2, or an R/S ratio in V_1 greater than 1, along with deep S waves and small R waves in V_5 and V_6 (Fig. 35-3). These changes can result in the reversal of the R wave progression across the precordial leads.[3–5,14]

ELECTROCARDIOGRAPHIC PEARLS

- The ECG is not sensitive in diagnosing ventricular hypertrophy, but ECG changes can be specific for it.
- The following features favor left ventricular hypertrophy "strain":
  - J point depression
  - Concave STE; bowed downsloping ST segment depression
  - "Overshoot" of the terminal aspect of T wave
  - Temporal stability

In less severe hypertrophy, the observed ECG manifestations may be limited to rSr′ or qR patterns in V_1. The $S_1S_2S_3$ pattern is also an ECG manifestation of RVH, although it also may be seen in normal patients and patients with COPD. In the $S_1S_2S_3$ pattern, the S wave in lead II has greater amplitude than the S wave in lead III. Other authors have defined this pattern as the R/S ratio being less than or equal to 1 in leads I through III.[3,5]

As with LVH, the QRS complex may widen, indicating the increased time necessary to activate the thickened ventricular wall or damage to the ventricular conduction system. This may be manifest as a complete or incomplete right bundle branch block.[3–5]

ST Segment/T Wave. The repolarization abnormalities encountered in RVH are similar to those in LVH but are most often seen in the right precordial and inferior limb leads. These changes include J point depression with ST segment depression with bowed morphology, and asymmetrical T wave inversion (see Fig. 35-3).

Diagnostic Criteria. There have been several criteria proposed for RVH[3–5,14] (Table 35-2). As in the case of LVH, the ECG criteria have low sensitivities and high specificities. Certain clinical scenarios require specific comment. In COPD, the combination of the more vertical position of the heart in the chest and the insulating effect of the overinflated lungs may produce a reduction in QRS amplitude, RAD, and delay in the usual precordial R wave progression.[5] Significant PE

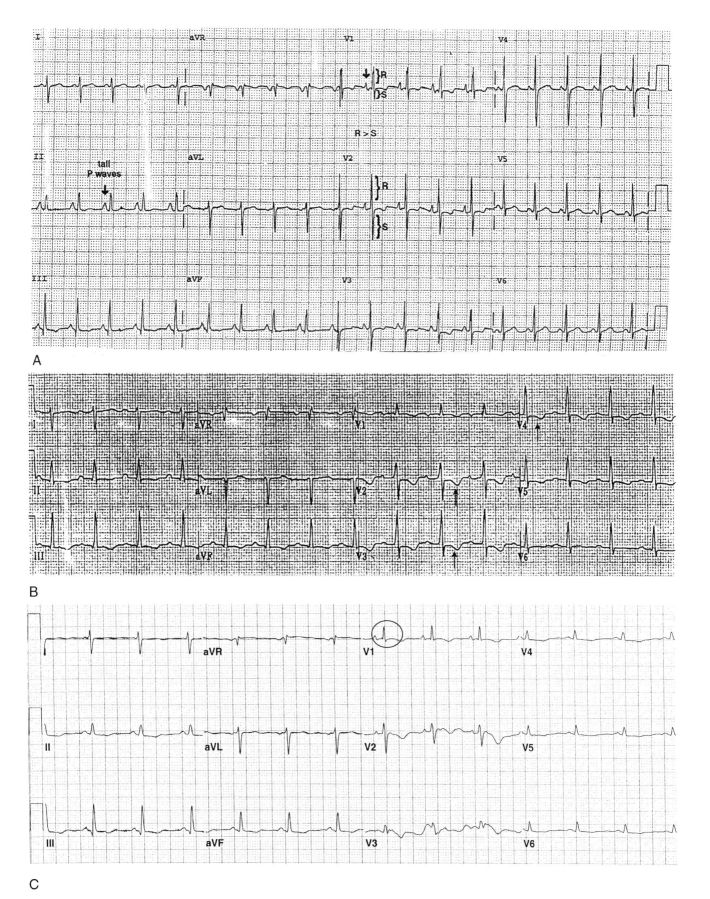

FIGURE 35-3 • Various examples of right ventricular hypertrophy (RVH) on 12-lead ECG. *A*, RVH demonstrated by rightward axis and R waves larger than their corresponding S waves in leads V_1 and V_2. Also note the finding of right atrial abnormality in leads II and V_1 (*arrows*). *B*, RVH with repolarization abnormalities indicated by the right axis deviation (RAD), and prominent R waves with ST segment/T wave changes in the right precordial leads (*arrows*). *C*, RVH suggested by RAD and prominent R wave in lead V_1 (*circle*). Also note repolarization abnormality, best seen in lead V_2. See Table 35-2 for more specific diagnostic criteria.

35-2 • DIAGNOSTIC CRITERIA FOR RIGHT VENTRICULAR HYPERTROPHY

Criterion

1. R/S ratio in leads V_5 or V_6 <1
2. R/S ratio in lead V_1 >1
   (with R >0.7 mm)
3. S in leads V_5 or V_6 >0.7 mm
4. R in lead V_5 or V_6 <0.4 mm
   with S in lead V_1 <0.2 mm
5. Right axis deviation > +110 degrees
6. P pulmonale
7. $S_1S_2S_3$ pattern

producing acute RV pressure overload can result in more specific ECG changes associated with PE (see Chapter 59, Pulmonary Embolism).

Biventricular hypertrophy

The enlargement of both the right and left ventricles produces electrical forces that may serve to counterbalance one another either partially or completely. Therefore, biventricular hypertrophy produces a complex interplay of electrical forces that makes defining characteristic ECG changes difficult. As a general rule, the ECG is an insensitive indicator of biventricular hypertrophy. It may show a modification of the changes associated with LVH. These modifications include tall R waves in both the right and left precordial leads, RAD in the presence of LVH, deep S waves in the left precordial leads in the setting of LVH, and, in the precordial leads a shift in the precordial transition zone to the left in the presence of LVH.[3-5,14]

References

1. Lorell BH, Carabello BA: Left ventricular hypertrophy: Pathogenesis, detection, and prognosis. Circulation 2000;102:470.
2. Siegel RJ: Myocardial hypertrophy. In Bloom S (ed): Diagnostic Criteria for Cardiovascular Pathology. Philadelphia, Lippincott-Raven, 1997, pp 55–59.
3. Mirvis DM, Goldberger AL: Electrocardiography. In Braunwald E (ed): Heart Disease: A Textbook of Cardiovascular Medicine. Philadelphia, WB Saunders, 2001, pp 95–100.
4. Surawicz B: Electrocardiographic diagnosis of chamber enlargement. J Am Coll Cardiol 1986;8:711.
5. Surawicz B, Knilans TK: Chou's Electrocardiography in Clinical Practice: Adult and Pediatric, 5th ed. Philadelphia, WB Saunders, 2001.
6. Kannel WB, Gordon T, Castelli WP, et al: Electrocardiographic left ventricular hypertrophy and risk of coronary heart disease: The Framingham Study. Ann Intern Med 1970;72:813.
7. Kannell WB, Abbott RD: A prognostic comparison of asymptomatic left ventricular hypertrophy and unrecognized myocardial infarction: The Framingham Study. Am Heart J 1986;111:391.
8. Rabkin SW, Mathewson FAL: The electrocardiogram in apparently healthy men and the risk of sudden death. Br Heart J 1982;47:546.
9. Mirvis DM, Graney MJ: The cumulative effects of historical and physical examination findings on the prognostic value of the electrocardiogram. J Electrophysiol 2001;34:215.
10. Beach C, Kenmure ACF, Short D: Electrocardiogram of pure left ventricular hypertrophy and its differentiation from lateral ischemia. Br Heart J 1981;46:285.
11. Brady WJ, Chan TC, Pollack M: Electrocardiographic manifestations: Patterns that confound the ECG diagnosis of acute myocardial infarction-left bundle branch block, ventricular paced rhythm, and left ventricular hypertrophy. J Emerg Med 2000;18:71.
12. Lepeschkin E: The U wave of the electrocardiogram. Mod Concepts Cardiovasc Dis 1969;38:39.
13. Romhilt DW, Estes EH: A point-score system for the ECG diagnosis of left ventricular hypertrophy. Am Heart J 1968;75:752.
14. Murphy ML, Thenabadu PN, de Soyza N, et al: Reevaluation of electrocardiographic criteria for left, right and combined cardiac ventricular hypertrophy. Am J Cardiol 1984;53:1140.

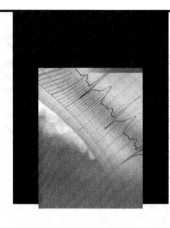

Chapter 36

Cardiomyopathy

Michael J. Bono

Clinical Features

Cardiomyopathy is a disease of the myocardium that causes cardiac dysfunction and ranks as the third most common form of heart disease in the United States, behind coronary heart disease and hypertensive heart disease. Cardiomyopathies are classified based on the dominant physiology: dilated, hypertrophic, restrictive, and the rare dysrhythmogenic right ventricular cardiomyopathy.[1] There are cardiomyopathies that do not fit the specific criteria of these broad classifications, as well as those classified based on specific cardiac or systemic disorders (e.g., amyloidosis, systemic hypertension).

Dilated Cardiomyopathy. Dilated cardiomyopathy is usually idiopathic and represents global myocardial dysfunction. Left and right ventricular function is depressed, and although onset may be insidious, systolic pump failure is the usual presenting feature, with associated signs and symptoms of congestive heart failure.

Hypertrophic Cardiomyopathy. Hypertrophic cardiomyopathy is also known as idiopathic hypertrophic subaortic stenosis, obstructive cardiomyopathy, asymmetrical septal hypertrophy, hypertrophic obstructive cardiomyopathy, and muscular subaortic stenosis. Hypertrophy of the left ventricle without dilatation results in either a small chamber cavity or decreased wall compliance, leading to restricted left ventricular filling. Cardiac output and ejection fractions are normal. Clinical symptoms are the result of restricted left ventricular filling, and include dyspnea on exertion, chest pain, palpitations, and syncope. Hypertrophic cardiomyopathy is a cause of sudden death in young athletes, most of whom have normal coronary arteries at autopsy and a noncontributory family history.[2] Physical examination may reveal a loud S_4 gallop and a midsystolic murmur, which is crescendo–decrescendo. Valsalva maneuver or squatting decreases venous return, which increases the obstructive physiology of hypertrophic cardiomyopathy, and increases the intensity of the murmur.

Restrictive Cardiomyopathy. Restrictive cardiomyopathy is the least common form of cardiomyopathy in developed countries. Most cases are idiopathic, but other diseases that can cause restrictive cardiomyopathy are amyloidosis, sarcoidosis, hemochromatosis, scleroderma, and neoplastic infiltration. Fibrosis or other lesions invade the myocardium,

leading to rigid ventricular walls and limited ventricular filling. Systolic function is normal and ventricular thickness may be normal or increased. Patients present with exercise intolerance, congestive heart failure (left or right sided), and syncope.

Dysrhythmogenic Right Ventricular Cardiomyopathy. An exceedingly rare form of cardiomyopathy, dysrhythmogenic right ventricular cardiomyopathy is a disease process in which myocardial cells in the right ventricle are replaced by fibrofatty tissue. This cardiomyopathy has a familial predilection and patients present at a young age with ventricular dysrhythmias or sudden death.

ELECTROCARDIOGRAPHIC HIGHLIGHTS

Dilated cardiomyopathy

- Left atrial abnormality
- Left ventricular hypertrophy (LVH)
- Left axis deviation (LAD)
- Intraventricular conduction abnormalities, especially left bundle branch block
- Poor precordial R wave progression
- Atrial fibrillation
- Ventricular dysrhythmias

Hypertrophic cardiomyopathy

- LVH
- LAD
- Septal Q waves
- Diminished or absent R waves in lateral leads

Restrictive cardiomyopathy

- LAD
- Low voltage
- Atrial fibrillation
- Ventricular dysrhythmias
- Atrioventricular block
- Complete heart block (sarcoidosis)
- Acute coronary syndrome patterns (sarcoidosis)

Dysrhythmogenic right ventricular cardiomyopathy

- Right bundle branch block

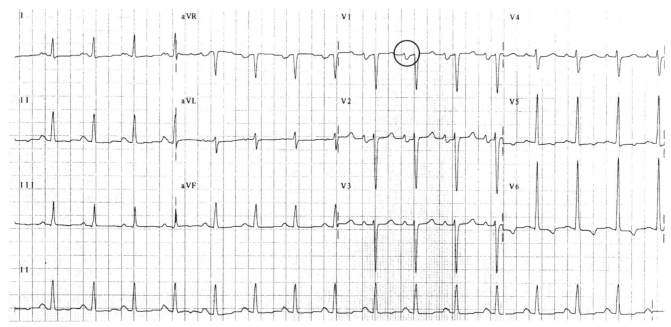

FIGURE 36-1 • **Dilated cardiomyopathy.** Left atrial abnormality (LAA; *circle*), left ventricular hypertrophy (LVH), and nonspecific ST segment/T wave changes in a 19-year-old woman with dilated cardiomyopathy. The degree of LAA, LVH, and ST segment/T wave changes corresponds to the severity of the dilatation.

Electrocardiographic Manifestations

Electrocardiographic (ECG) manifestations of cardiomyopathy include various degrees of ventricular hypertrophy, atrial enlargement, and bundle branch block.

Dilated Cardiomyopathy. ECG changes in dilated cardiomyopathy are nonspecific, but the ECG is always abnormal. Atrial abnormality, particularly, left atrial abnormality (LAA), is very common (Fig. 36-1). Prolongation of the

PR interval can occur. Left ventricular hypertrophy (LVH) and left bundle branch block (LBBB) are common. LVH is evident usually on the basis of QRS complex voltage criteria. In patients with dilated cardiomyopathy, the degree of LVH and left axis deviation (LAD) corresponds roughly to the degree of dilatation and disease. Similarly, nonspecific ST segment/T wave changes are the rule and depend on the amount of dilatation. The anterior precordium may demonstrate poor R wave progression associated with Q or

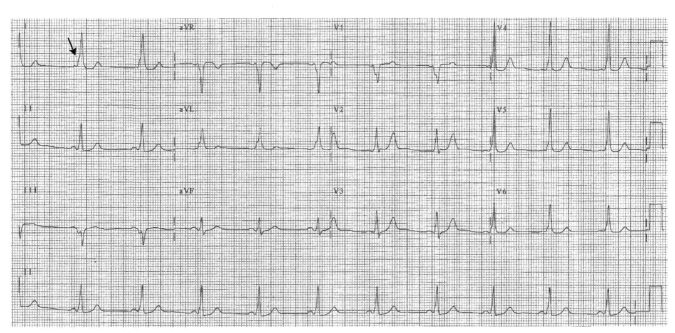

FIGURE 36-2 • **Dilated cardiomyopathy.** Evolving left bundle branch block (LBBB) in a 38-year-old man with dilated cardiomyopathy. Note the similarity to Wolff-Parkinson-White syndrome with respect to the early phase of the QRS complex (*arrow*).

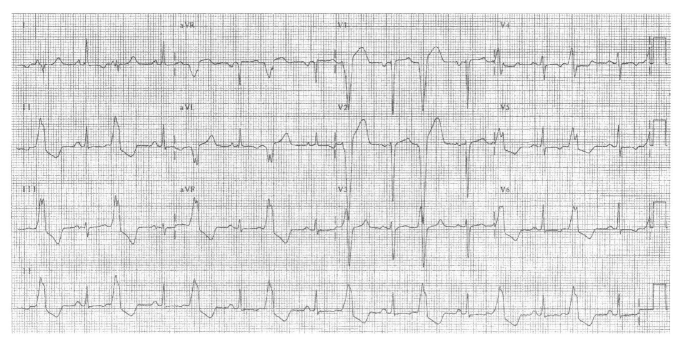

FIGURE 36-3 • **Dilated cardiomyopathy.** Bigeminy in a 44-year-old man with dilated cardiomyopathy due to chronic cocaine abuse. Ventricular ectopy is commonly seen in patients with severely dilated cardiomyopathy.

QS waves, appearing as a pseudoinfarction pattern (see Chapter 35, Ventricular Hypertrophy). Intraventricular conduction delay, particularly LBBB, is common (Fig. 36-2), although right bundle branch block (RBBB) can occur, usually with concomitant LAD.

Because of atrial enlargement, atrial fibrillation is often seen. In addition, ventricular ectopy may be present in cases of severe dilated cardiomyopathy (Fig. 36-3).

Hypertrophic Cardiomyopathy. The ECG is abnormal in 90% of patients with hypertrophic cardiomyopathy. Similar to dilated cardiomyopathy, the dominant ECG findings are LAA and LVH (Fig. 36-4). Enlargement of the septum may produce a large Q wave, called a *septal Q wave*, in the anterior, inferior, or lateral leads, producing a pseudoinfarction pattern (Fig. 36-5). Nonspecific ST segment/T wave changes, T wave inversions, large T waves, and absent R waves in the lateral

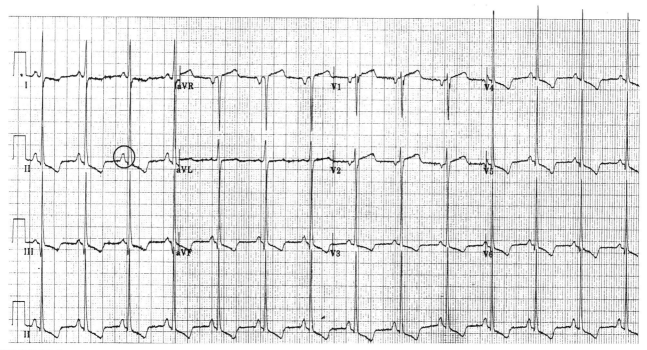

FIGURE 36-4 • **Hypertrophic cardiomyopathy.** Left atrial abnormality and left ventricular hypertrophy with repolarization abnormality in a 17-year-old girl with hypertrophic cardiomyopathy; right atrial abnormality is noted as well (P wave amplitude greater than 2.5 mm in lead II) (*circle*).

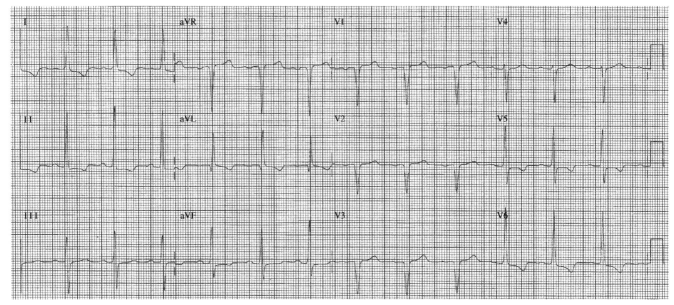

FIGURE 36-5 • **Hypertrophic cardiomyopathy.** Septal QS waves in the anterior precordial leads with upright T waves demonstrating pseudoinfarction in a 72-year-old woman with hypertrophic cardiomyopathy. Also note the inverted T waves laterally (leads I, aVL, V₅, and V₆).

leads are all commonly seen. In patients with hypertrophic cardiomyopathy with septal Q waves, the T wave may help distinguish between infarction and pseudoinfarction. In the leads that have the Q waves, an upright T wave suggests hypertrophic cardiomyopathy, whereas an inverted T wave suggests ischemia. Apical hypertrophic cardiomyopathy is a variant of this disease that produces giant negative T waves in the left precordial leads.[3] Atrial and ventricular dysrhythmias are common, including atrial fibrillation that is poorly tolerated because left ventricular filling is restricted. Other dysrhythmias

include premature atrial contractions, premature ventricular contractions, and multifocal ventricular ectopy.

Restrictive Cardiomyopathy. ECG findings in restrictive cardiomyopathy include nonspecific ST segment/T wave changes and low voltage (Fig. 36-6). LAD may be present. Patients with restrictive cardiomyopathy due to amyloidosis or sarcoidosis may present with atrial fibrillation due to atrial enlargement. Sarcoidosis may feature granulomas, which have a predilection for the interventricular septum, causing conduction abnormalities. These patients may present with

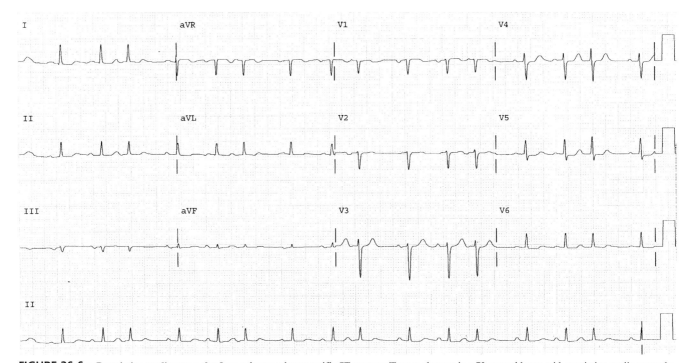

FIGURE 36-6 • **Restrictive cardiomyopathy.** Low voltage and nonspecific ST segment/T wave changes in a 73-year-old man with restrictive cardiomyopathy.

ventricular dysrhythmias or complete heart block, with a high risk of sudden death. Steroid-treated granulomas produce scars that appear as Q waves resembling an old infarct pattern.

Dysrhythmogenic Right Ventricular Cardiomyopathy. The pathologic process in this entity is primarily in the right ventricle; therefore, ECG findings may show a RBBB pattern and precordial T wave inversion.

References

1. Richardson P, McKenna W, Bristow M, et al: Report of the 1995 World Health Organization/International Society and Federation of Cardiology Task Force on the Definition and Classification of Cardiomyopathies. Circulation 1996;93:841.
2. Elliott PM, Poloniecki J, Dickie S, et al: Sudden death in hypertrophic cardiomyopathy: Identification of high risk patients. J Am Coll Cardiol 2000;36:2212.
3. Sakamoto T: Apical hypertrophic cardiomyopathy (apical hypertrophy): An overview. J Cardiol 2001;37(Suppl 1):161.

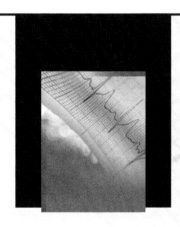

Chapter 37

Myopericarditis

Theodore C. Chan

Clinical Features

Acute and chronic pericarditis or myopericarditis, a diffuse inflammation of the pericardial sac and superficial myocardium, has a number of underlying causes, including infection (primarily viral), immunologic disorders, uremia, trauma, malignancy, and cardiac ischemia and infarction. Patients complain of sharp, pleuritic, precordial, or retrosternal chest pain, which can radiate to the left upper back, shoulder, or arm. The pain is worsened by recumbency, cough, swallowing, and inspiration, and relieved by an upright position and leaning forward. Patients with subacute or chronic pericarditis may develop significant pericardial effusions or progress to constrictive pericarditis.

Electrocardiographic Manifestations

Acute Myopericarditis. Up to 90% of patients have electrocardiographic (ECG) abnormalities with changes in PR segment, ST segment, and T wave morphologies.[1] These changes are a result of repolarization abnormalities in the atrium and ventricle from epicardial inflammation, injury, and ischemia. Depolarization is usually normal and the P wave and QRS complex are usually unaffected.

Classic Four-Stage Progression. The classic four-stage evolution seen in acute myopericarditis was first described by Spodick and others as a progression involving ST segment elevation (STE)/PR segment depression, resolution, T wave inversion, and normalization.[1,2] Less than half of patients, however, evolve through all stages, and atypical progression is common.[3] *Stage I* occurs during the first few days, lasts up to 2 weeks, and is notable for diffuse STE and PR segment depression. Stage I abnormalities are seen more often than those of later stages and are considered "quasidiagnostic," particularly PR segment depression.[4] *Stage II*, characterized by ST segment normalization, is variable in duration, lasting from a few days to several weeks after resolution of stage I.

ELECTROCARDIOGRAPHIC HIGHLIGHTS

Four-staged progression in acute myopericarditis

Stage I (Days to 2 weeks)

- Diffuse PR segment depression (leads I, II, III, aVL, aVF, V_2 to V_6, with reciprocal elevation in leads aVR, V_1)
- Diffuse ST segment elevation (leads I, II, III, aVL, aVF, V_2 to V_6, with reciprocal ST segment depression in leads aVR, V_1)

Stage II (1 to 3 weeks)

- ST segment normalization
- T wave flattening with decreased amplitude

Stage III (3 to several weeks)

- T wave inversion

Stage IV (Several weeks)

- Normalization
- Return to baseline ECG

In addition, T wave amplitude decreases or flattens. *Stage III* occurs in the second or third week of the illness and may be transient or prolonged, lasting from days to several weeks. During this time, full T wave inversion occurs. *Stage IV* is marked by resolution of T wave abnormalities and return to the premyopericarditis ECG.

ST Segment Elevation.   STE is usually less than 5 mm and occurs simultaneously throughout all limb and precordial leads (I, II, III, aVF, aVL, and V_2 to V_6), with the exception of leads aVR and V_1 (which often have reciprocal ST segment depression). Other than postinfarct myopericarditis, where inflammation may be localized, there is no clear territorial distribution. The STE is concave or obliquely flat on its initial upslope, with an indistinct J point. The T wave remains concordant, without flattening or inversion (Figs. 37-1 though 37-5).

Differentiating STE due to acute myopericarditis from other causes of elevation such as benign early repolarization (BER) and acute myocardial infarction (AMI) or ischemia can be difficult. Similar in morphology, with an initial concave and indistinct J point, STE in BER is limited primarily to the precordial leads. BER STE may transiently return to baseline with exercise and does not resolve over days to weeks. In BER, the J point is minimally elevated with a prominent T wave.

In myopericarditis, the J point and STE are more pronounced and the T wave less prominent. One can assess this difference using the ST segment/T wave ratio. Using the end of the PR segment as the baseline to measure STE (at the onset, or J point) and T wave amplitude, an ST segment/T wave ratio of 0.25 or greater suggests myopericarditis,

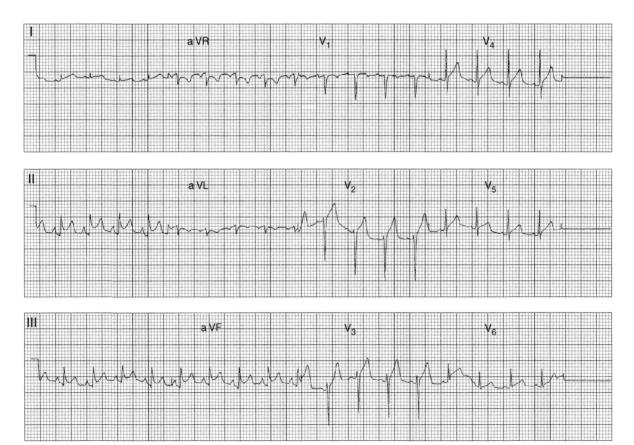

FIGURE 37-1 · Acute viral myopericarditis. This ECG shows sinus tachycardia in a patient with idiopathic myopericarditis after a viral upper respiratory infection, with concave ST segment elevation in leads II, III, aVF, and V_2 to V_5, and reciprocal ST segment depression in lead aVR. PR segment depression is seen in leads II, III, and aVF, and reciprocal elevation in lead aVR.

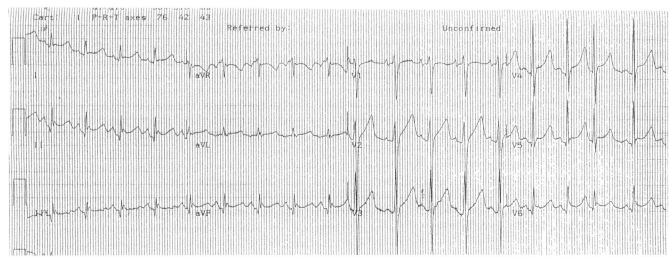

FIGURE 37-2 · **Uremic myopericarditis.** This ECG shows sinus tachycardia in a patient with uremic myopericarditis with numerous ECG changes consistent with pericarditis: (1) ST segment elevation in leads I, II, aVF, and V_2 to V_6; (2) PR segment depression in leads II, III, aVF, and V_3 to V_6; and (3) reciprocal PR segment elevation in lead aVR.

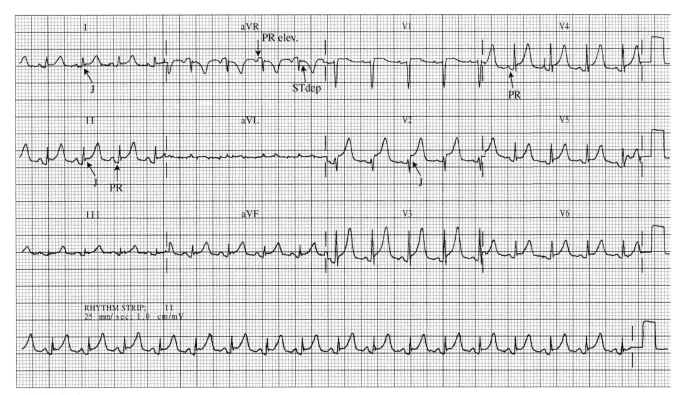

FIGURE 37-3 · **Drug-induced acute myopericarditis.** Note the ST segment elevation and J point elevation (J) in leads I, II, III, aVF, and V_2 to V_6; the PR segment depression in leads I, II, aVF, and V_2 to V_6 (PR); the reciprocal ST segment depression in lead aVR (ST dep); and the reciprocal PR segment elevation in lead aVR (PR elev).

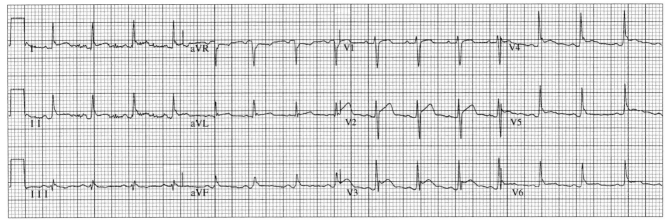

FIGURE 37-4 · Acute myopericarditis in a patient with chest pain. Note the diffuse ST segment elevation that could be confused with ischemia. PR segment depression is most notable in lead II, with reciprocal PR segment elevation in lead aVR.

whereas a ratio less than 0.25 suggests BER.[5] This finding is most reliably seen in lead V_6, but can be seen in leads V_4, V_5, and I, although with less sensitivity and specificity (Fig. 37-6) (see Chapter 40, Benign Early Repolarization).

Initial ST segment morphology is often convex or obliquely flat in AMI. Moreover, STE distribution is usually territorial. T wave inversion often occurs with STE in AMI, but occurs only after resolution in myopericarditis (Fig. 37-7).

The presence of Q waves suggests AMI, whereas PR segment depression suggests myopericarditis. In addition, the ECG abnormalities evolve over a much shorter time with AMI (hours to a few days) than with myopericarditis. There are few conditions that produce acute onset ST segment depression other than ischemia or myopericarditis. Although localized ST segment depression in lead V_1 occurs with posterior MI, it is usually not associated with ST segment depression in lead aVR, diffuse PR segment depression, or STE, as seen with myopericarditis (see Chapter 32, Acute Coronary Syndromes: Acute Myocardial Infarction and Ischemia).

PR Segment Depression.   PR segment depression is usually transient and may be the earliest and most specific sign of acute myopericarditis.[6] Like STE, PR segment depression occurs diffusely in the limb and precordial leads (most prominently in leads II, V_5, and V_6), except leads aVR and V_1, which may have reciprocal elevation. In assessing the PR segment, it is important to use the TP segment as baseline; otherwise, the depression may be misinterpreted as STE (see Figs. 37-3 and 37-5).

T Wave Inversion.   T wave inversions are encountered diffusely in later stages, only after STE has resolved. Abnormal T wave persistence or gradual reversal of T wave deflection suggests postinfarct pericardial inflammation.

Electrocardiographic Rhythm.   The most common rhythm associated with acute myopericarditis is normal sinus or sinus tachycardia. Because of the proximity of the sinus node to the pericardium, it was previously thought the inflammation could precipitate atrial fibrillation or flutter. Recent studies suggest the sinus node is virtually immune to surrounding

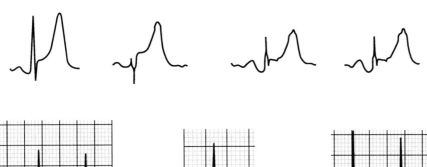

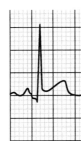

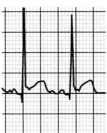

FIGURE 37-5 · Morphologic changes in acute myopericarditis. These tracings are single-beat examples of PR segment depression, J point elevation, and concave ST segment elevation seen in acute myopericarditis.

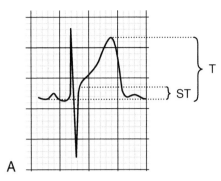
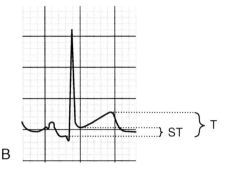

FIGURE 37-6 · The ST segment/T wave amplitude ratio. The end of the PR segment is used as the reference for the calculation. Ratios of ST segment elevation (measured at the J point) to T wave height greater than or equal to 0.25 strongly suggest acute myopericarditis (*B*), whereas ratios less than 0.25 are associated with benign early repolarization (*A*). This calculation is best performed in lead V_6, as well as leads I, V_4, and V_5.

inflammation. Moreover, although myopericarditis can occur in conjunction with dysrhythmias (most commonly supraventricular dysrhythmias), these disturbances are attributable to underlying cardiac disease.[7]

Chronic Pericarditis. ECG abnormalities seen with chronic pericarditis are usually related to the presence of a pericardial effusion or progression to constrictive pericarditis. Pericardial effusions result in diminished voltage amplitude in all leads and affect all deflections, including the P-QRS-T complex. In subacute pericarditis, the T waves may remain inverted or flattened, as described in stage III. Electrical alternans, a beat-to-beat variation in the QRS complex (and potentially the P and T waves) caused by shifting fluid and heart position, may occur with larger effusions and cardiac tamponade. Similar ECG manifestations are seen in constrictive pericarditis from either the chronic effusion or thick fibrin layer deposition in the pericardial sac. Electrical alternans, however, does not occur. With significant diastolic dysfunction, left atrial abnormality may occur, resulting in typical P wave abnormalities (see Chapter 10, P Wave).

Chronic pericarditis and myxedema can both present with diminished-amplitude QRS complex deflections and low-voltage or inverted T waves. Myxedema usually results in

---

ELECTROCARDIOGRAPHIC PEARLS

- Classic four-stage progression is seen in less than half of patients and atypical progression is common.
- PR segment depression is most characteristic of acute myopericarditis.
- ST segment elevation is usually less than 5 mm, concave, and diffuse, and resolves before discordant T wave inversions.
- Serial ECGs may be helpful in differentiating from acute myocardial infarction; ST segment/T wave ratio may be helpful in differentiating from benign early repolarization.
- Normal sinus rhythm or sinus tachycardia is the most common rhythm. Supraventricular and other dysrhythmias are related to underlying cardiac disease.
- Diffuse low-voltage QRS complexes and other deflections are seen in subacute/chronic pericarditis.

---

bradycardia, whereas pericarditis usually manifests with tachycardia. Other causes of pericardial effusion must also be considered along with chronic pericarditis (see Chapter 43, Pericardial Effusion).

References

1. Shabetai R: Acute myopericarditis. Cardiol Clin 1990;8:639.
2. Spodick DH: Acute Myopericarditis. New York, Grune and Stratton, 1959.
3. Marinella MA: Electrocardiographic manifestations and differential diagnosis of acute myopericarditis. Am Fam Physician 1990;57:699.
4. Spodick DH: Diagnostic electrocardiographic sequences in acute myopericarditis: Significance of PR segment and PR vector changes. Circulation 1973;48:575.
5. Ginzton LE, Laks MM: The differential diagnosis of acute myopericarditis from the normal variant: New electrocardiographic criteria. Circulation 1982;65:1004.
6. Baljepally R, Spodick DH: PR-segment deviation as the initial electrocardiographic responses in acute myopericarditis. Am J Cardiol 1998;812:1505.
7. Spodick DH: Significant arrhythmias during myopericarditis are due to concomitant heart disease. J Am Coll Cardiol 1998;32:551.

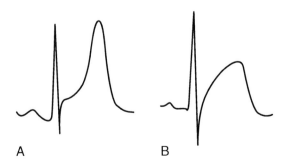

FIGURE 37-7 · Differentiating acute myopericarditis from acute myocardial infarction (AMI). *A,* This tracing was obtained from a patient with acute myopericarditis; note the PR segment depression with concave ST segment elevation (STE). *B,* This tracing represents AMI; note the convex morphology to the STE.

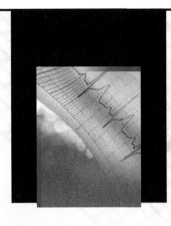

Chapter 38

Myocarditis

Douglas S. Ander and Katherine L. Heilpern

Clinical Features

Myocarditis is defined as an inflammation of the heart muscle. A number of infectious agents (bacterial, viral, protozoan), systemic diseases (e.g., lupus, acquired immunodeficiency syndrome),[1,2] medications, and toxins have been associated with the development of myocarditis. The most common infectious agents in North America and Europe are viruses, whereas worldwide, Chagas' disease is the most common cause of myocarditis. It is generally believed that myocarditis results from an immunologic and cytotoxic cascade of events precipitated by the infectious agents, rather than from the actual primary infection.

The clinical presentation of myocarditis is extremely variable, ranging from asymptomatic to severe cardiogenic shock. Patients may also present with sudden cardiac death. Because of disturbances of the conduction system, patients with atrioventricular (AV) blocks or dysrhythmias may present with syncope or palpitations. Most patients complain of an antecedent flulike illness.[3] Another possible presentation is chest pain that may be atypical, pleuritic, or ischemic in nature. Myocarditis may even mimic acute myocardial infarction (AMI) with ischemic-like chest pain, electrocardiographic (ECG) changes, and increased cardiac enzymes.

The diagnosis of myocarditis is difficult. The sensitivity of laboratory findings is low. Endomyocardial biopsy, considered the gold standard for diagnosis, is required to confirm myocarditis. Current treatment of myocarditis incorporates all the current therapies for patients with heart failure, and immunosuppressive therapy for autoimmune myocarditis.

Electrocardiographic Manifestations

The potential ECG changes seen with myocarditis are broad and not pathognomonic for myocarditis. Myocarditis should be considered in any patient with chest pain, antecedent viral-type complaints, and ECG changes. The ECG changes in myocarditis include various dysrhythmias, abnormalities of the conduction system, and ischemic ST segment/T wave changes. More severe forms of these changes may cause palpitations, syncope, or sudden cardiac death.

Dysrhythmias. The most common ECG finding in myocarditis is sinus tachycardia[4] (Fig. 38-1). Myocarditis is also associated with supraventricular and ventricular dysrhythmias.[5,6]

Conduction Abnormalities. Various forms of conduction delays and blocks have been noted in myocarditis, including left bundle branch block (LBBB) and various degrees of AV block.[5–10] In patients with Chagas' disease, the most characteristic finding is right bundle branch block[11] (Fig. 38-2).

Changes Consistent with Acute Coronary Syndrome. A pseudoinfarction pattern has been noted in patients with the diagnosis of myocarditis. Studies have identified patients presenting with chest pain and ST segment elevation consistent with AMI, later identified as biopsy-proven myocarditis[12–15] (Fig. 38-3). Other potential ECG changes that might be interpreted as ischemic in nature are T wave inversions, pathologic Q waves, poor R wave progression, LBBB, and ST segment depression.[6–8,10,13–15] Nonspecific ST segment/T wave changes may occur as well.[7]

Evolution of Electrocardiographic Abnormalities. An association may exist between the onset of symptoms and the ECG abnormalities.[6] Patients with less than 1 month of symptoms have AV block and repolarization abnormalities as the predominant findings on admission. In comparison, left atrial abnormality, atrial fibrillation, left ventricular hypertrophy, and LBBB were noted more commonly in patients with symptoms of longer duration.[6] A pseudoinfarction pattern heralds a rapidly fatal clinical course.

Differentiating Myocarditis from Acute Coronary Syndrome and Pericarditis. Differentiation between

---

ELECTROCARDIOGRAPHIC HIGHLIGHTS

- Sinus tachycardia the most common ECG abnormality
- Supraventricular and ventricular dysrhythmias
- Atrioventricular block (first, second, third degree)
- Intraventricular and bundle branch blocks
- ST segment/T wave abnormalities

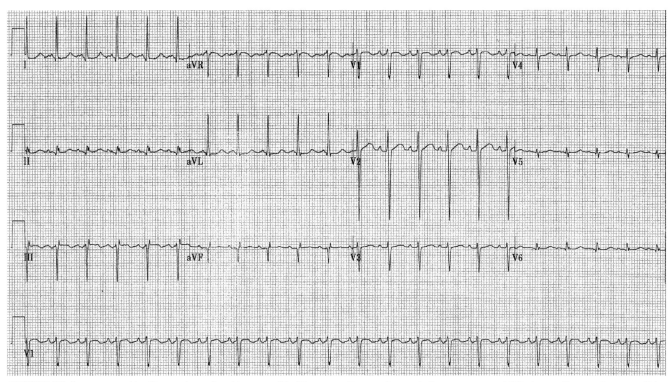

FIGURE 38-1 • **Myocarditis.** Sinus tachycardia with nonspecific ST segment/T wave changes is the most common ECG abnormality seen in myocarditis.

myocarditis from other causes of ST segment and T wave changes, such as acute coronary syndrome and pericarditis, is difficult. With myocarditis and AMI, patients can present with chest pain and ST segment elevations on the ECG. In one case series, eight patients had localized ECG findings and only one had segmental wall motion abnormalities by echocardiogram.[14]

The diagnosis of myocarditis is suggested by diffuse wall motion abnormalities on echocardiography and regional ECG changes. Myocarditis should also be considered if there are ischemic ECG changes that involve more than a single vascular distribution. Similarly, myocarditis should be suspected in patients presenting with chest pain and an ECG revealing

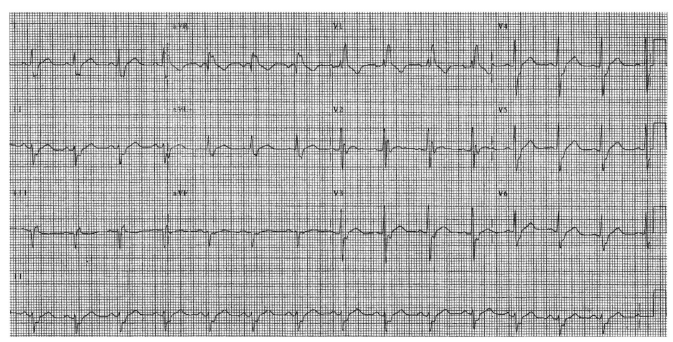

FIGURE 38-2 • **Chagas' disease.** A right bundle branch block pattern with rsR′ pattern in lead V_1 and slurred S waves in leads I and V_6 can present in many forms of myocarditis, but particularly in Chagas' disease.

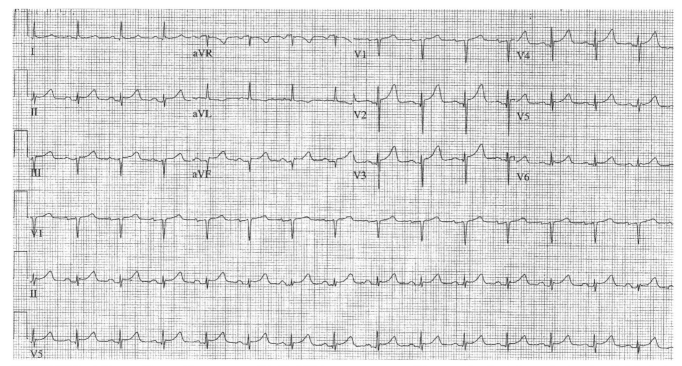

FIGURE 38-3 • **A 51-year-old man with acute myocarditis.** The ECG demonstrates concave ST segment elevation in the anterior, lateral, and inferior leads.

ELECTROCARDIOGRAPHIC PEARLS

- The ECG changes seen with myocarditis are broad and are not pathognomonic for the disease.
- ST segment and T wave changes may create a "pseudo-infarction" pattern on ECG.
- Myocarditis ECG changes do not evolve as rapidly as those of acute coronary syndrome.

---

ischemic damage beyond one vascular distribution.[13,14] Also, failure of ECG changes to evolve in a typical AMI pattern may assist the clinician in pursuing the diagnosis of myocarditis.[10] Myocarditis is more likely in patients with prolonged chest pain and antecedent flulike symptoms. Pericarditis can present with many of the same ECG manifestations as myocarditis.

References

1. Reilly JM, Cunnion RE, Anderson DW, et al: Frequency of myocarditis, left ventricular dysfunction and ventricular tachycardia in the acquired immune deficiency syndrome. Am J Cardiol 1988;62:789.
2. Anderson DW, Virmani R, Reilly JM, et al: Prevalent myocarditis at necropsy in the acquired immunodeficiency syndrome. J Am Coll Cardiol 1988;11:792.
3. Myocarditis Treatment Trial Investigators: Incidence and clinical characteristics of myocarditis [abstract]. Circulation 1991;84:2.
4. Fuster V, Alexander RW, O'Rourke RA, et al (eds): Hurst's the Heart, 10th ed. New York, McGraw-Hill, 2001.
5. Karjalaninen J, Viitasalo M, Kala R, Heikkila J: 24-hour electrocardiographic recordings in mild acute infectious myocarditis. Ann Clin Res 1984;16:34.
6. Morgera T, DiLenarda A, Dreas L, et al: Electrocardiography of myocarditis revisited: Clinical and prognostic significance of electrocardiographic changes. Am Heart J 1992;124:455.
7. Hayakawa M, Inoh T, Yokota Y, et al: A long-term follow-up study of acute myocarditis: An electrocardiographic and echocardiographic study. Jpn Circ J 1984;48:1362.
8. Take M, Sekiguchi M, Hiroe M, Hirosawa K: Long-term follow-up of electrocardiographic findings in patients with acute myocarditis proven by endomyocardial biopsy. Jpn Circ J 1982;46:1227.
9. Toshima H, Ohkita Y, Shingu M: Clinical features of acute coxsackie B viral myocarditis. Jpn Circ J 1979;43:441.
10. Nakashima H, Honda Y, Katayama T: Serial electrocardiographic findings in acute myocarditis. Intern Med 1994;33:659.
11. Chou T, Knilans TK (eds): Electrocardiography in Clinical Practice: Adult and Pediatric, 4th ed. Philadelphia, WB Saunders, 1996.
12. Angelini A, Calzolari V, Calabrese F, et al: Myocarditis mimicking acute myocardial infarction: Role of endomyocardial biopsy in the differential diagnosis. Heart 2000;84:245.
13. Narula J, Khaw BA, Dec W, et al: Brief report: Recognition of acute myocarditis masquerading as acute myocardial infarction. N Engl J Med 1993;328:100.
14. Dec GW, Waldman H, Southern J, et al: Viral myocarditis mimicking acute myocardial infarction. J Am Coll Cardiol 1992;20:85.
15. Miklozek CL, Crumpacker CS, Royal HD, et al: Myocarditis presenting as acute myocardial infarction. Am Heart J 1988;115:768.

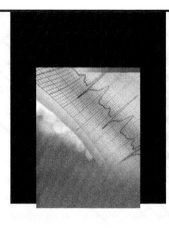

Chapter 39

Endocarditis

Varnada A. Karriem-Norwood and Katherine L. Heilpern

Clinical Features

In 1846, Virchow first described infective endocarditis as bacterial vegetations of the cardiac valves. Endocarditis is usually a bacterial infection, but can occasionally be caused by fungi, viruses, or other pathogens. In some cases, the infecting organism is never determined, as is the case in culture-negative endocarditis. The incidence of endocarditis varies from 1.6 per 100,000 to 11.6 per 100,000 per year, and occurs primarily in patients with known valvular disease, prosthetic heart valves, certain congenital anomalies, or intravenous drug use.[1]

The initial trigger to the development of endocarditis is a period of bacteremia, fungemia, or viremia. Vegetations are formed when microorganisms attach to susceptible valvular surfaces and multiply. Virulence factors give certain organisms vigorous adherence qualities and a propensity to attach to native valves in association with certain disease states, prosthetic valves, or, in the extreme, normal valves.

Endocarditis may be categorized into acute and subacute endocarditis. Acute endocarditis is associated with acute onset of symptoms and rapid destruction of tissue. It primarily involves native valves; *Staphylococcus aureus* is the most common pathogen. Subacute endocarditis is associated with a more insidious onset of symptoms and usually occurs on prosthetic valves or in patients with underlying valvular disease. Subacute endocarditis is typically caused by *Streptococcus viridans*. In cases involving prosthetic valves, *Staphylococcus epidermidis* is the most common organism. In patients with a history of intravenous drug use, *S. aureus* is the most common pathogen.

Patients usually present with nonspecific symptoms of systemic infection, including fever, chills, night sweats, anorexia, myalgias, arthralgias, and general malaise. Physical examination findings are variable and characterized by findings associated with valvular disease and infectious illness. Low-grade fever is common in all types of endocarditis, and a new or different murmur is present in most patients with endocarditis. Extracardiac manifestations are usually the result of embolic phenomena and occur more commonly in subacute bacterial endocarditis. These classic manifestations may be absent in acute bacterial endocarditis and are actually rare in patients with subacute endocarditis. Abscess formation is a major complication of bacterial endocarditis. Vegetations may extend to involve the paravalvular tissue or conducting system. Extension of disease, abscess formation, edema, and embolization are all implicated in the development of conduction abnormalities, congestive heart failure, and cardiac ischemia.[2–4]

Electrocardiographic Manifestations

Electrocardiographic (ECG) changes in endocarditis are variable and nonspecific. Findings include tachycardia, ectopy, conduction abnormalities, including atrioventricular (AV) block and bundle branch blocks (BBB), lower QRS complex voltage, and nonspecific ST segment/T wave changes; ECG changes may be consistent with acute coronary syndrome (ACS) due to actual ischemic injury caused by septic embolization. Although abnormalities are common, none can be considered pathognomonic of endocarditis.

Conduction Abnormalities. Conduction abnormalities occur in 4% to 26% of patients with endocarditis, with the highest incidence in patients with prosthetic valves and those with aortic valve involvement.[3–7] The incidence of conduction abnormalities is not influenced by age, sex, pathogen type, intravenous drug use, extensive disease, or abscess formation.[2,3,6]

ELECTROCARDIOGRAPHIC HIGHLIGHTS

- Bundle branch block (most common ECG finding)
- Conduction abnormalities
- First, second, and third degree atrioventricular blocks.
- Intraventricular conduction delay and bundle branch block
- Rhythm changes, including sinus tachycardia, supraventricular tachycardia, and ectopy (premature atrial contractions, premature ventricular contractions).
- Nonspecific and ischemic ST segment and T wave changes
- Low QRS complex voltage

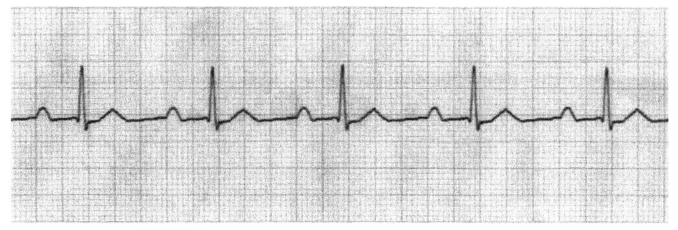

FIGURE 39-1 · **Endocarditis.** First degree atrioventricular block in a patient with endocarditis.

Surrounding edema, fistulae, and embolization have been implicated as causative factors in the development of conduction abnormalities or ischemia. Morbidity and mortality are higher in patients in whom conduction abnormalities develop.

Specific conduction abnormalities in endocarditis include AV blocks (first, second, and third degree blocks), as well as BBB. First degree AV block occurs in 31% of cases (Fig. 39-1), most commonly associated with disturbance in the AV node.[7] The abnormality involves the atrial tissue or His-Purkinje system less commonly (such cases are usually distinguished by prolongation of the QRS complex). Second-degree heart block represents 8% of ECG abnormalities seen in patients with endocarditis. The anatomic abnormality is usually in the AV node. Third degree AV block occurs in approximately 11% of endocarditis cases.[7] It is always associated with paravalvular extension of disease or abscess formation. The development of type II second degree block or third degree block is an ominous finding. These

ECG abnormalities usually are seen in patients who require permanent pacemaker placement or emergent valve replacement.[8]

Intraventricular conduction abnormalities noted in endocarditis include left BBB (Fig. 39-2), right BBB, and left anterior fascicular block. Intraventricular conduction abnormalities occur in up to 50% of endocarditis cases, with or without associated AV conduction disturbances, and are associated with congestive heart failure and higher morbidity and mortality.[7,9]

Ischemic Changes. There are a few reported cases of cardiac ischemia or infarction associated with endocarditis. These may occur when there is septic embolization of a vegetation to one of the coronary arteries, or from underlying coronary artery disease. ECG characteristics include all typical changes associated with ACS, including hyperacute T waves, T wave inversion, ST segment depression, ST segment elevation, or Q waves in various leads, depending on the artery involved.[8,10,11]

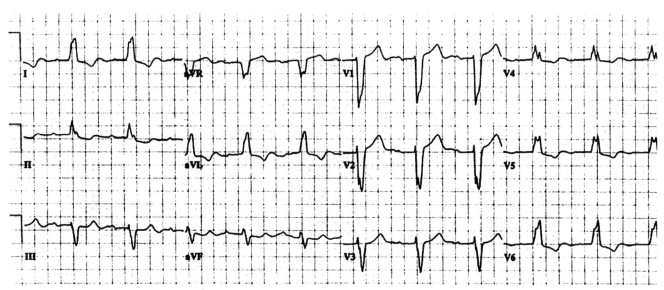

FIGURE 39-2 · **Endocarditis.** New left bundle branch block in a patient with endocarditis.

ELECTROCARDIOGRAPHIC PEARLS

- The presence of conduction abnormalities is associated with higher morbidity and mortality in endocarditis.
- Third degree atrioventricular (AV) block in endocarditis is always associated with paravalvular extension or abscess formation.
- Development of type II second degree AV block or third degree AV block may indicate the need for temporary pacemaker placement and possibly emergent surgery.
- Endocarditis can lead to acute coronary syndrome.

Other Findings.   Numerous additional ECG findings have been described in patients with endocarditis, including low-voltage QRS complex, nonspecific ST segment/T wave changes, supraventricular tachycardia, and other dysrhythmias.

References

1. Fuster V, Alexander RW, O'Rourke RA, et al: Hurst's the Heart, 10th ed. New York, McGraw-Hill, 2001.

2. Blumberg EA, Karalis DA, Chandrasekaran K, et al: Endocarditis-associated paravalvular abscess: Do clinical parameters predict the presence of abscess? Chest 1995;107:898.

3. Wu Y-J, Hong TC, Hou CJ, et al: *Bacillus popilliae* endocarditis with prolonged complete heart block. Am J Med Sci 1999;317:263.

4. Weiss AB, Khan M: The relationship between new cardiac conduction defects and extension of valve infection in native valve endocarditis. Clin Cardiol 1990;13:337.

5. DiNubile MJ: Heart block during bacterial endocarditis: A review of the literature and guidelines for surgical intervention. Am J Med Sci 1984;287:30.

6. Myamoto MI, Hutter AM Jr, Blum JH, et al: Cardiac conduction abnormalities preceding transesophageal echocardiographic evidence of perivalvular extension of infection in a case of *Salmonella* prosthetic valve endocarditis. Heart 1997;78:416.

7. Trip M, Meine TJ, Nettles RE, et al: Cardiac conduction abnormalities in endocarditis defined by the Duke criteria. Am Heart J 2001;142:281.

8. Jeremias A, Casserly I, Estess JM, et al: Acute myocardial infarction after aortic valve endocarditis. Am J Med 2001;110:417.

9. DiNubile MJ, Calderwood SB, Steinhaus DM, et al: Cardiac conduction abnormalities complicating native valve active infective endocarditis. Am J Cardiol 1986;58:1213.

10. Perera R, Noack S, Dong W: Acute myocardial infarction due to septic coronary embolism. N Engl J Med 2000;342:997.

11. Berk WA: Electrocardiographic findings in infective endocarditis. J Emerg Med 1988;6:129.

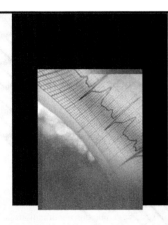

Chapter 40

Benign Early Repolarization

William J. Brady and Marcus L. Martin

Clinical Features

The syndrome of benign early repolarization (BER) is thought to be a normal variant, not indicative of underlying cardiac disease.[1]

BER has been reported in men and women of all age groups in people of varying ethnic background. The general population has early repolarization on the electrocardiogram (ECG) in approximately 1% of cases[2]; it is also a common finding in athletes.[3] For unknown reasons, BER is seen at an increased frequency and is encountered in 13% of patients with chest pain in the emergency department.[4] In a large population-based study of BER, the mean age of patients with BER was 39 years, with a range of 16 to 80 years; it was seen predominantly in those patients younger than 50 years of age and rarely encountered in individuals older than 70 years of age (3.5%).[2] For unknown reasons, BER is more often encountered in black men from the ages of 20 to 40 years,[5] although other authors dispute such a tendency in African Americans.[2]

The physiologic basis for this ECG normal variant is poorly understood and a subject of ongoing controversy.[6] Suggested mechanisms of BER include early repolarization of the subepicardium, relatively earlier repolarization of the anterior wall of the left ventricle compared with the posterior wall, regional differences in sympathetic tone, and sympathetic–parasympathetic tone imbalances.[6]

Electrocardiographic Manifestations

The ECG definition of BER (Figs. 40-1 and 40-2) includes the following characteristics: (1) ST segment elevation (STE);

ELECTROCARDIOGRAPHIC HIGHLIGHTS

- ST segment elevation
- Upward concavity of the initial portion of the ST segment
- Notching or slurring of the terminal QRS complex
- Symmetrical, concordant T waves of large amplitude
- Widespread or diffuse distribution of ST segment elevation
- Relative temporal stability

(2) concavity of the initial portion of the ST segment; (3) notching or slurring of the terminal QRS complex (Fig. 40-3); (4) symmetrical, concordant T waves of large amplitude; (5) widespread or diffuse distribution of STE on the ECG; and (6) relative temporal stability.[1]

ST Segment Elevation. The STE begins at the "J" (or junction) point—the portion of the ECG cycle where the QRS complex ends and the ST segment begins. The degree of J point elevation is usually less than 3.5 mm.[2] This STE morphologically appears as if the ST segment has been evenly lifted upward from the isoelectric baseline at the J point[1] (see Figs. 40-1 and 40-2). This elevation results in a preservation of the normal concavity of the initial, upsloping portion of the ST segment/T wave complex—a very important ECG feature used to distinguish BER-related STE from STE associated with acute myocardial infarction (AMI). The J point itself is frequently notched or irregular in contour and is considered highly suggestive—but not diagnostic—of BER[1,2,7] (Fig. 40-3).

The STE encountered in BER is usually less than 2 mm but may approach 5 mm in certain individuals (see Fig. 40-2). Eighty to 90% of individuals demonstrate STE of less than 2 mm in the precordial leads and less than 0.5 mm in the limb leads; only 2% of cases of BER manifest STE greater than 5 mm.[2,8] The degree of STE related to BER is usually greatest

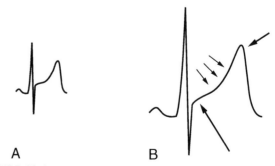

A   B

FIGURE 40-1 · Benign early repolarization (BER). *A,* This single ECG complex illustrates BER. Note the elevated J point with concave, elevated ST segment, and prominent T wave. *B,* An enhanced version of the ECG complex from *A* emphasizes the J point elevation (*large arrow*), concave morphology to the elevated ST segment (*small, grouped arrows*), and prominent T waves (*intermediate arrow*).

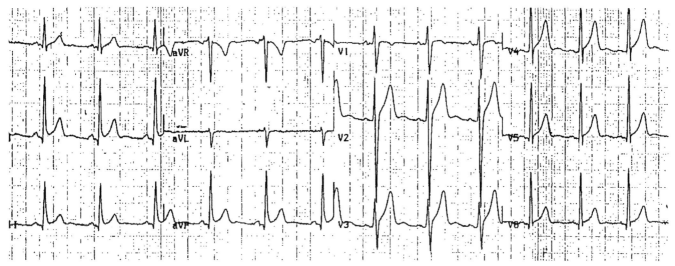

FIGURE 40-2 · Benign early repolarization. This 12-lead ECG is from a 42-year-old man with chest pain. Note the ST segment elevation with concave morphology (leads V_1 to V_6, II, III, and aVF) and prominent T waves (leads V_2 to V_4). The J point is slightly irregular in lead II.

in the mid- to left precordial leads (leads V_2 to V_5). The ST segments of the remaining ECG leads are less often elevated to the extent observed in leads V_2 through V_5. The limb leads are less often observed to demonstrate STE; one large series reported that the limb leads revealed STE in only 45% of cases of BER. Lead aVR does not demonstrate STE due to BER.[8] "Isolated" BER in the limb leads (i.e., no precordial STE) is a very rare finding.[2,8] Such isolated STE in the inferior or lateral leads should prompt consideration of another explanation for the observed ST segment abnormality.

Acute pericarditis and BER are often difficult to distinguish on ECG. Both demonstrate an initial concavity of the upsloping ST segment/T wave complex. In acute pericarditis, however, the PR segment is often depressed and the T wave more likely to be normal in amplitude and morphology (Fig. 40-4). One can assess this difference using the ST/T ratio (ratio of ST segment to T wave amplitude in lead V_6). Using the end of the PR segment to measure STE (at the onset, or J point) and T wave amplitude, an ST/T ratio of 0.25 or greater suggests myopericarditis, whereas a ratio of less than 0.25 suggests BER[9] (Fig. 40-5).

STE from AMI can be confused with that of BER. However, in BER the normal concavity of the initial, upsloping portion of the ST segment/T wave complex is preserved, unlike in STE from AMI, where the elevation is usually either flattened or convex in morphology (Fig. 40-4).

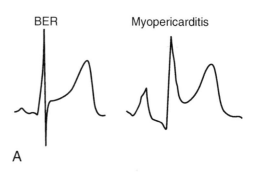

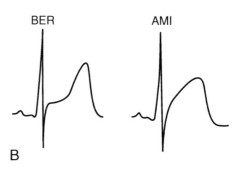

FIGURE 40-4 · A comparison of ECG structures of benign early repolarization (BER), acute myopericarditis, and acute myocardial infarction (AMI). *A,* BER and myopericarditis. Both structures have ST segment elevation with a concave morphology. Myopericarditis often has PR segment depression, a useful feature to help distinguish between the two entities. *B,* BER and AMI. Once again, both entities have ST segment elevation. The important difference centers on the morphology of the elevated ST segment. In BER, the elevated ST segment is concave in morphology, as opposed to the ST segment in AMI, which is often convex in shape. This morphologic difference is reasonably useful in distinguishing between AMI and non-AMI causes of ST segment elevation.

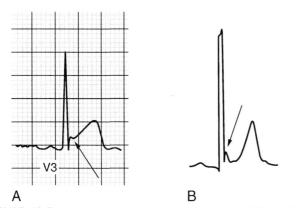

FIGURE 40-3 · J point in benign early repolarization (BER). *A,* This tracing demonstrates the irregularity of the J point in BER. *B,* In this complex, notching of the J point in BER can be seen.

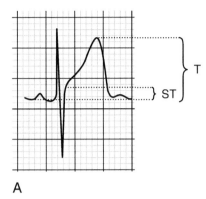

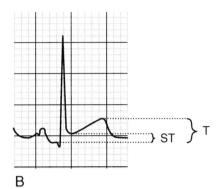

A   B

FIGURE 40-5 • The ST segment/T wave amplitude ratio. The end of the PR segment is used as the reference point for the calculation. Ratios of ST segment to T wave height of 0.25 or greater strongly suggest acute myoperi-carditis (*B*), whereas ratios of less than 0.25 are associated with benign early repolarization (*A*). This calculation is best performed in lead V_6; leads I, V_4, and V_5 perform almost as well if lead V_6 is unavailable or uninterpretable (e.g., secondary to artifact).

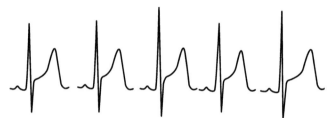

FIGURE 40-6 • Temporal stability. This serial ECG is from the 42-year-old man with chest pain whose 12-lead ECG is depicted in Figure 40-2. Lead II is depicted here, demonstrating P-QRS-T complexes over a number of hours. Note the lack of change in both the magnitude of the ST segment elevation and the morphology of the ST segment itself. This lack of change in the ECG strongly suggests a non–acute myocardial infarction etiology of the elevated ST segment.

ELECTROCARDIOGRAPHIC PEARLS

- Realize that benign early repolarization (BER) is the patient's baseline ECG pattern.
- The most difficult ECG distinction is acute pericarditis.
- Beware of diagnosing BER in patients with ST segment elevation isolated to the inferior leads.
- Exercise caution when attributing ST segment elevation to BER in patients older than age 50 years.

Temporal Stability. The chronic nature of the STE is helpful in the diagnosis of BER (Fig. 40-6). Patients tend to demonstrate the BER pattern consistently over time in most cases. Exceptions to this statement, however, must be made. Certain individuals, when electrocardiographically observed over prolonged periods, demonstrate a changing magnitude of STE with transient fluctuations in the pattern. The magnitude of BER may also lessen over time as the patient ages. In 25% to 30% of patients with BER previously noted on the ECG, additional ECG analysis many years later reveals a complete disappearance of the pattern.[2,8]

T Wave. Prominent T waves (Fig. 40-2) of large amplitude and slightly asymmetrical morphology are also encountered; the T waves may appear "peaked," suggestive of the hyperacute T wave encountered in patients with AMI. The T waves are concordant with the QRS complex and are usually found in the precordial leads. The height of the T waves in BER ranges from approximately 6.5 mm in the precordial distribution to 5 mm in the limb leads.[1,2,10]

References

1. Wasserburger RM, Alt WJ, Lloyd C: The normal RS-T segment elevation variant. Am J Cardiol 1961;8:184.
2. Mehta MC, Jain AC: Early repolarization on scalar electrocardiogram. Am J Med Sci 1995;309:305.
3. Hanne-Paparo N, Drory Y, Schoenfeld Y: Common ECG changes in athletes. Cardiology 1976;61:267.
4. Brady WJ, Perron AD, Martin ML, et al: Electrocardiographic ST segment elevation in emergency department chest pain center patients: Etiology responsible for the ST segment abnormality. Am J Emerg Med 2001;19:25.
5. Thomas J, Harris E, Lassiter G: Observations on the T wave and S-T segment changes in the precordial electrocardiogram of 320 young negro adults. Am J Cardiol 1960;5:468.
6. Mirvis DM: Evaluation of normal variations in S-T segment patterns by body surface isopotential mapping: S-T segment elevation in absence of heart disease. Am J Cardiol 1982;50:122.
7. Goldberger AL: Myocardial Infarction: Electrocardiographic Differential Diagnosis, 4th ed. St. Louis, Mosby, 1991.
8. Kabara H, Phillips J: Long-term evaluation of early repolarization syndrome (normal variant RS-T segment elevation). Am J Cardiol 1976;38:157.
9. Ginzton LE, Laks MM: The differential diagnosis of acute pericarditis from the normal variant: New electrocardiographic criteria. Circulation 1982;65:1004.
10. Aufderheide TP, Brady WJ: Electrocardiography in the patient with myocardial ischemia or infarction. In Gibler WB, Aufderheide TP (eds): Emergency Cardiac Care. St. Louis, Mosby, 1994, p 169.

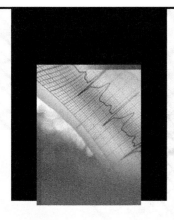

Chapter 41

Ventricular Aneurysm

Richard J. Harper

Clinical Features

Understanding the natural history of ventricular aneurysms and the incidence of electrocardiographic (ECG) manifestations is limited by the lack of a consensus on the definition.[1] Narrowly defined, an aneurysm is a confined area of ventricle displaying local dyskinesis with paradoxical systolic expansion. Defined more broadly, it may simply consist of an area of scar, either dyskinetic or akinetic.[2] Such wider perspective results in a higher rate of reported postinfarction aneurysm, but a lower reported incidence of physiologic consequences.[3]

Aneurysms may be congenital or due to causes such as cardiomyopathy, infection, and infarction.[4] Most, however, result from transmural myocardial infarction. The most common location is the anterior wall, resulting from proximal left anterior descending artery (LAD) stenosis or total LAD occlusion.[5] In particular, the apex is susceptible to aneurysm formation because it is composed of only three muscle layers, compared with four at the base.[1] Right ventricular aneurysms are rare owing to better ischemic tolerance by the thin wall and the lower intracavitary pressures.[6]

The presence of a ventricular aneurysm predisposes a patient to increased risk of death from ventricular dysrhythmias and congestive heart failure. Thromboembolic risk also increases because thrombus often forms within the aneurysm, but the value of anticoagulation remains uncertain.[7]

Changes in the treatment of acute myocardial infarction (AMI) have influenced the rate of aneurysm formation. Fibrinolytic therapy and acute percutaneous intervention have been documented to decrease the rate of aneurysm formation.[8]

Other therapies aimed at control of remodeling have also decreased the rate of aneurysm formation.

On occasion, rather than scarring, the ventricular wall ruptures but is contained by adherent pericardium and scar tissue, forming a pseudoaneurysm.[9] Technically difficult to differentiate from aneurysm, pseudoaneurysms have a graver prognosis. Untreated, the risk of rupture is approximately 30% to 45%.[9] Pseudoaneurysms most frequently result from inferior–posterior myocardial infarction.

Electrocardiographic Manifestations

The ECG of ventricular aneurysm is often described as one of persistent ST segment elevation (STE). Because of variable definitions of aneurysm and a lack of specific criteria for diagnostic STE, the reported incidence of persistent STE in patients with postinfarction ventricular aneurysm varies dramatically.

Raskoff et al. define STE as a convex segment 2 mm above the baseline, 0.04 sec after the J point. Using these criteria, they find STE to be insensitive for detecting ventricular aneurysm.[10] When combining pathologic Q waves with STE, the sensitivity for ventricular aneurysm is 38%, with a specificity of 84%. Persistent STE is, in this definition, limited to the anterior precordial leads despite the presence of significant dyssynergy in the inferior wall (Figs. 41-1 and 41-2).

Although the ECG does not appear accurately to reflect the presence of ventricular aneurysm, the presence of persistent STE in the anterior precordial leads does appear to be predictive of advanced anterior wall damage and resultant dyssynergy.[10–12] As a result, any reference to ventricular aneurysm, based on persistent anterior ST segment abnormality, should be interpreted as advanced contraction abnormality rather than true ventricular aneurysm.

The early time course of STE determines the long-term ECG pattern. STE after AMI resolves within 2 weeks in 95% of patients with inferior infarction, but in only 40% of patients with anterior infarction[11] (Fig. 41-3). If STE persists at 2 weeks, it will become permanent. Surgery to repair the aneurysm reduces STE in approximately one fourth of patients.[13]

Patients with persistent STE frequently have other conduction system abnormalities. Left anterior fascicular block is

---

<table>
<tr><td colspan="1">ELECTROCARDIOGRAPHIC HIGHLIGHTS</td></tr>
<tr><td>

• Persistent ST segment elevation
  - Usually found in anterior leads
  - Usually associated with pathologic Q waves
  - May exhibit convex or concave morphology
  - Usually not associated with reciprocal changes
  - Static, not evolving
  - T wave has small amplitude relative to the QRS complex

</td></tr>
</table>

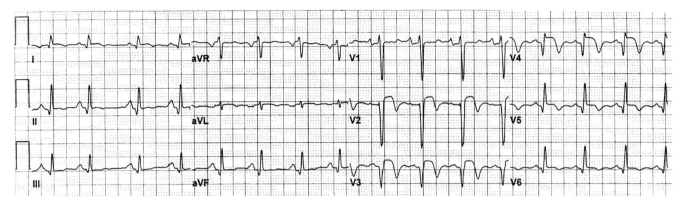

FIGURE 41-1 • **Anterior-apical aneurysm.** This is an ECG from a patient with a long-standing anterior-apical aneurysm. ST segment elevation is present from leads V_2 to V_6. ST segment morphology is convex. Mild ST segment elevation is noted in lateral leads I and aVL. Pathologic Q waves are seen in leads I and V_3 to V_6. T waves are abnormal across the precordium. The computer reading of this ECG was acute myocardial infarction.

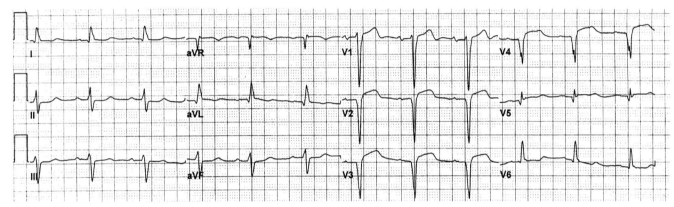

FIGURE 41-2 • **Anterior aneurysm.** This ECG was obtained during a surgical hospitalization from a patient with an anterior aneurysm. ST segment elevation is present from leads V_1 to V_5. Pathologic Q waves are noted in leads V_2 to V_5. ST segment morphology is flat with upright T waves. QT interval prolongation unrelated to the aneurysm is noted. The computer reading of this ECG was acute myocardial infarction.

often found in association with ventricular aneurysm.[14] The presence of left bundle branch block (LBBB) complicates the interpretation of ST segment changes[15] (Fig. 41-3). Criteria for diagnosis of ventricular aneurysm in the setting of LBBB have been proposed.[16] Ventricular aneurysm produces STE primarily in lead V_5, although changes in leads V_4 and V_6 may be noted. In the diagnosis of aneurysm in patients without a LBBB, the criteria noted are specific but not sensitive.

Left ventricular pseudoaneurysm may also produce persistent STE, but at a lower rate. Most patients have only nonspecific ST segment abnormalities. Only 20% of patients have persistent STE.[9]

Persistent STE may be the greatest challenge for physicians concerned about the possibility of AMI. When presented with tracings demonstrating STE, the ECG most commonly misinterpreted by emergency physicians as AMI (72%) is that of left ventricular aneurysm.[17] This is hardly surprising because the ST segment profile cannot differentiate between AMI and ventricular aneurysm, especially in the absence of the clinical scenario.

Persistent STE due to ventricular aneurysm is usually limited to the anterior leads. It may be concave or convex in morphology and may be associated with normal or abnormal T waves. Reciprocal ST segment depression is rarely present.

Most important, the changes with ventricular aneurysm are static over time (although the morphology may vary owing to heart rate, electrolytes, and other circumstances). If the clinician can obtain timely historical information regarding previous myocardial infarction and obtain copies of previous ECGs, the static changes of aneurysm may be differentiated from acute and evolving changes resulting from myocardial infarction.

Recently, the ratio of T wave to QRS amplitude has been advanced as a means to discriminate anterior AMI from left ventricular aneurysm. If any single lead has a T wave/QRS

ELECTROCARDIOGRAPHIC PEARLS

• The ST segment changes are indistinguishable from anterior acute myocardial infarction, but changes (unlike acute infarction) are stable over time. An old ECG is the best tool to assist in differentiating the cause of the changes.

• A history of previous myocardial infarction is an early clue to possible aneurysm.

• Most patients with aneurysm have significant left ventricular dyssynergy and as a result have a history of heart failure.

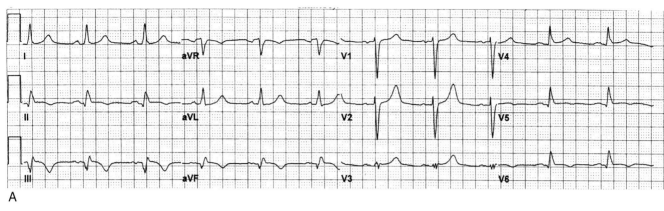

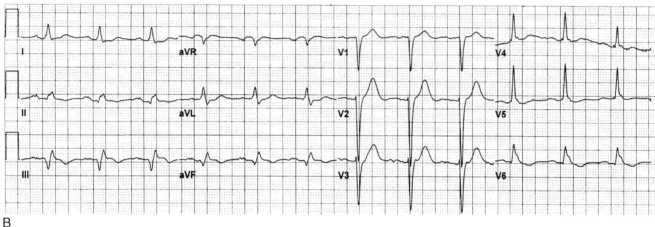

FIGURE 41-3 • **Inferior aneurysm.** *A,* This unusual ECG shows persistent ST segment elevation (STE) in the inferior leads 2 weeks after acute myocardial infarction. Pathologic Q waves are present in the same leads. The patient has a very large true aneurysm of the inferior surface of the heart. Inferior aneurysms are less common than anterior aneurysms and usually do not produce persistent STE. STE of leads V_3 to V_6 is likely a result of aneurysmal extension to the lateral wall. *B,* The patient later developed a complete left bundle branch block with persistent STE in leads III and aVF.

complex amplitude ratio of greater than 0.36, it is likely to be AMI, whereas if all leads feature a T wave/QRS complex ratio of less than 0.36, the findings likely reflect ventricular aneurysm.[18]

References

1. Baalbaki HA, Clements SDJ: Left ventricular aneurysm: A review. Clin Cardiol 1989;12:5.

2. Lee DCS, Johnson RA, et al: Angiographic predictors of survival following left ventricular aneurysmectomy. Circulation 1977;56(Suppl II):12.

3. Davidson HH, Lindsay J: Redefining true ventricular aneurysm. Am J Cardiol 1989;64:1192.

4. Toda G, Iliev I, et al: Left ventricular aneurysm without coronary artery disease, incidence and clinical features: Clinical analysis of 11 cases. Intern Med 2000;39:531.

5. Tikiz H, Balbay Y, et al: The effect of thrombolytic therapy on left ventricular aneurysm formation in acute myocardial infarction: Relationship to successful reperfusion and vessel patency. Clin Cardiol 2001;24:656.

6. Nahas C, Jones JW, et al: Right ventricular aneurysm associated with postinfarction ventricular septal defect. Ann Thorac Surg 1996;61:737.

7. Diet F, Erdmann E: Thromboembolism in heart failure: Who should be treated? Eur J Heart Fail 2000;2:355.

8. Stawicki S: Long term echocardiographic evaluation of thrombolytic therapy effect on regional function of and aneurysm formation in the left ventricle in myocardial infarction. Pol Arch Med Wewn 1993;90:192.

9. Frances C, Romero A, et al: Left ventricular pseudoaneurysm. J Am Coll Cardiol 1998;32:557.

10. Raskoff W, Smith GLJ, et al: Sensitivity and specificity of electrocardiographic diagnosis of ventricular motion disorders: Studies in patients recovered from myocardial infarction. Chest 1976;69:148.

11. Mills RMJ, Young E, et al: Natural history of S-T segment elevation after acute myocardial infarction. Am J Cardiol 1975;35:609.

12. Lindsay JJ, Dewey RC, et al: Relation of ST-segment elevation after healing of acute myocardial infarction to the presence of left ventricular aneurysm. Am J Cardiol 1984;54:84.

13. Hashway TJ, Lewis RC: The electrocardiogram after ventricular aneurysmectomy. Cleve Clin Q 1979;46:125.

14. Levy S, Gerard R, et al: Pure left anterior hemiblock: hemodynamic and arteriographic aspects in patients with coronary artery disease. Eur J Cardiol 1978;8:553.

15. Sgarbossa EB, Pinski SL, et al: Electrocardiographic diagnosis of evolving acute myocardial infarction in the presence of left bundle branch block. N Engl J Med 1996;334:481.

16. Madias JE, Ashtiani R, et al: Diagnosis of myocardial infarction-induced ventricular aneurysm in the presence of complete left bundle branch block. J Electrocardiol 2001;34:147.

17. Brady WJ, Perron AD, et al: Electrocardiographic ST-segment elevation: Correct identification of acute myocardial infarction (AMI) and non-AMI syndromes by emergency physicians. Acad Emerg Med 2001;8:349.

18. Smith SW, Nolan M: Ratio of T amplitude to QRS amplitude best distinguishes acute anterior MI from anterior left ventricular aneurysm [abstract]. Acad Emerg Med 2003;10:516.

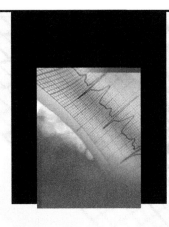

Chapter 42

Valvular Disorders

Christopher F. Richards and Richard J. Harper

Anatomically, valvular disorders of the heart can involve any of the four valves; functionally, these disorders may result in either stenosis, regurgitation, or a combination of dysfunction. The clinical and electrocardiographic (ECG) manifestations reflect the underlying pathophysiologic process and the physiologic response to the hemodynamic stressors. Most disorders result in hypertrophy of one or more chambers, with atrial enlargement often leading to atrial dysrhythmias.

TRICUSPID VALVE DISEASE

Clinical Features

Tricuspid valve disease can be due to intrinsic disease of the valve or secondary to right ventricular (RV) dysfunction.

Tricuspid Stenosis. Tricuspid stenosis (TS) is most often caused by rheumatic heart disease (usually associated with mitral stenosis [MS]) followed by carcinoid tumors, which usually originate in the gastrointestinal tract. Other causes include eosinophilic myocarditis, infective endocarditis, trauma from indwelling catheters or pacemaker leads, and tumors, both intrinsic or extracardiac.

Tricuspid Regurgitation. Tricuspid regurgitation (TR) is associated with intrinsic conditions such as rheumatic heart disease, carcinoid heart disease, trauma, infective endocarditis, right atrial myxoma, connective tissue disorders, eosinophilic myocarditis, and congenital heart disease

(e.g., Ebstein's anomaly, cleft tricuspid leaflet). Secondary RV dysfunction resulting in TR is usually due to processes that cause increased pulmonary pressures such as primary or secondary pulmonary hypertension, pulmonary embolism, collagen vascular disease, sleep apnea, agents causing anorexia (e.g., fenfluramine or phentermine), and left-sided ventricular failure, or right ventricular failure due to RV infarct, cardiomyopathy, radiation therapy, or RV endomyocardial fibrosis.

Electrocardiographic Manifestations

Isolated TS, producing right atrial abnormality (RAA), can cause a large peaked P wave in lead II, a frontal plane P wave axis of greater than +75 degrees, or a positive initial deflection of the P wave in leads V_1 or V_2 of greater than 0.15 mV (Fig. 42-1). TS associated with MS may result in a wide notched P wave in lead II or a peaked biphasic P in V_1—both suggestive of additional left atrial abnormality (LAA). Associated RV hypertrophy (RVH) is present in many cases.[1] With TR, an rSR′ in lead V_1 consistent with incomplete right bundle branch block and delayed activation can be present, RVH is present, and atrial fibrillation is common.

PULMONIC VALVE DISEASE

Clinical Features

Pulmonic Stenosis. Pulmonic stenosis (PS) is usually congenital. Carcinoid heart disease, rare cases of rheumatic disease isolated to the pulmonic valve, and extrinsic compression from mediastinal masses are less common causes of PS.[2,3] Long-standing or congenital PS invariably leads to RVH (Fig. 42-2), but carcinoid heart disease or stenosis due to extrinsic compression frequently is present without RVH.[4]

Pulmonic Regurgitation. Pulmonic regurgitation is usually associated with RV volume overload and hypertrophy. Pulmonary valve dysfunction secondary to primary pulmonary hypertension or primarily pulmonary vascular bed problems (e.g., pulmonary emboli) present differently from

---

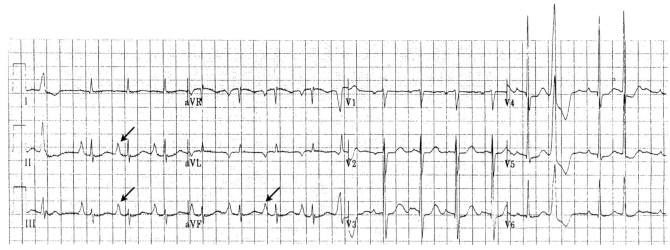

FIGURE 42-1 · Tricuspid stenosis. Narrow peaked P waves in the inferior leads (*arrows*) suggest right atrial abnormality, without evidence of right ventricular hypertrophy, typical of tricuspid stenosis.

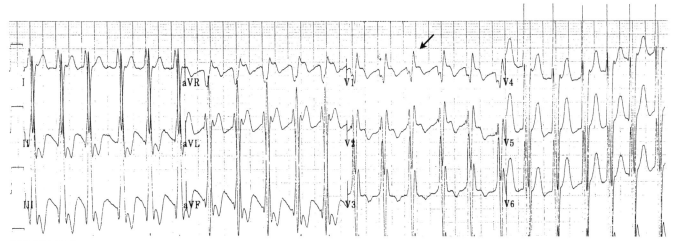

FIGURE 42-2 · Right ventricular hypertrophy (RVH). Evidence of RVH is typical of either tricuspid regurgitation, pulmonic stenosis, or pulmonic regurgitation, if chronic. This tracing shows RVH as evidenced by R > S in lead V_1 (*arrow*) and deep S waves in lead V_6. Rightward QRS frontal plane axis and right atrial abnormality also suggest RVH.

those due to mitral valve disease or other causes of left heart failure.

Electrocardiographic Manifestations

Pulmonic valve disease may result in manifestations of RVH on the ECG. Frontal plane QRS right axis deviation is frequently seen, usually greater than 100 degrees (see Chapter 35, Ventricular Hypertrophy). With PS, the degree of RVH reflects the severity and chronicity of the lesion. Acute PS may have a normal ECG, whereas moderate PS with moderate RVH causes a qR in lead V_1, and severe PS leads to an rSR' in lead V_1. Severe PS also results in RAA and possibly atrial fibrillation. Regurgitant lesions of the pulmonary valve also cause RVH, with rSR' in lead V_1 in severe cases.

MITRAL VALVE DISEASE

Clinical Features

Mitral Stenosis.   MS is almost invariably a result of chronic rheumatic heart disease. The typical patient with MS contracts rheumatic fever at the age of 12 years, acquires a murmur 20 years later, and acquires symptoms, typically dyspnea on exertion or atrial fibrillation, in the fourth and fifth decades. Valvular stenosis results in left atrial enlargement, elevated left-sided pressures and pulmonary edema, atrial fibrillation, and pulmonary hypertension.

Mitral Regurgitation.   Mitral regurgitation (MR) is more complicated and may be chronic or acute in nature. Chronic MR can result from such diseases as rheumatic heart disease, systemic lupus erythematosus, Marfan's syndrome, Ehlers-Danlos syndrome, amyloidosis, ankylosing spondylitis, endocarditis, hypertrophic or dilated cardiomyopathy, or congenital valvular disease. It causes progressive left atrial and ventricular volume overload and eventual left ventricular failure. Acute MR caused by trauma or a ruptured chordae tendineae (e.g., due to ischemia or infection) causes acute increases in preload and decreases in afterload and rapidly progressive pulmonary edema.

Electrocardiographic Manifestations

Early MS may manifest as LAA. The P wave is greater than 0.12 sec in duration and either biphasic (especially in lead V_1, with a large negative deflection) or bifid (P mitrale) in the limb leads. Most patients with MS have atrial fibrillation. Left ventricular hypertrophy (LVH) is absent, but RVH may be present. The combination of LAA with signs of RVH or right axis deviation on the ECG suggests MS.[1]

MR results in LAA and also often results in atrial fibrillation. In contrast to MS, MR is almost always associated with LVH (Fig. 42-3). Patients with acute-onset MR either have a nonspecific ECG, or manifestations of the underlying

pathologic process (e.g., myocardial infarction with papillary muscle dysfunction).

AORTIC VALVE DISEASE

Clinical Features

Aortic Stenosis. Idiopathic degeneration of a bicuspid or tricuspid aortic valve is the most common cause of aortic stenosis (AS).[5] One percent of people are born with a bicuspid valve, but one third of these experience gradual degeneration.[6] Patients with congenital AS usually experience symptoms in the third decade of life; those with rheumatic heart disease in the fifth decade; those with congenital bicuspid aortic valves in the sixth decade; and those with degenerative bicuspid valves usually experience symptoms in the sixth and seventh decades of life.[7]

Aortic Regurgitation. Aortic regurgitation (AR) may result from leaflet failure or aortic root disease. The primary causes of AR are rheumatic heart disease, bicuspid valve, and infective endocarditis. Diseases of the aortic root include atherosclerosis, Marfan's syndrome, osteogenesis imperfecta,

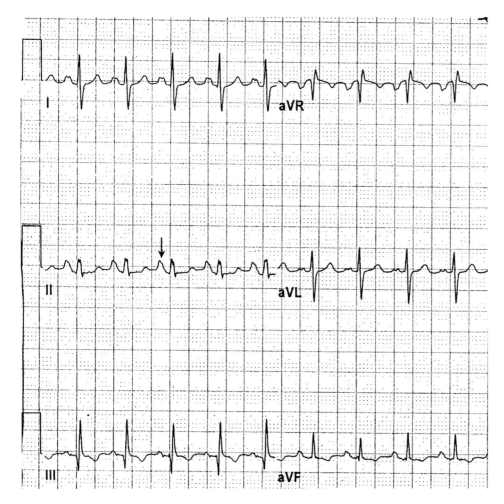

FIGURE 42-3 · **Left atrial abnormality in mitral stenosis (LAA).** LAA (P mitrale; *arrow*) without left ventricular hypertrophy in mitral stenosis. Limb leads only are shown in this figure.

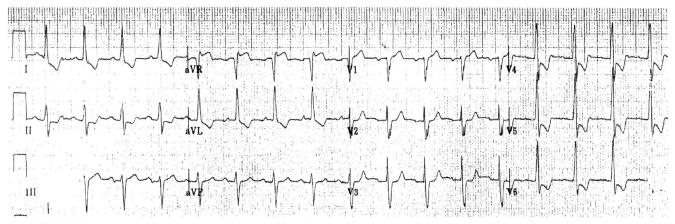

FIGURE 42-4 · **Left ventricular hypertrophy (LVH).** LVH with repolarization abnormality, consistent with both aortic stenosis or regurgitation.

> ### ELECTROCARDIOGRAPHIC PEARLS
>
> • Atrial fibrillation is commonly seen in valvular disease, particularly that involving the mitral valve.
> • ECG manifestations of valvular disease are usually nonspecific.
> • Aortic stenosis may present with significant ST segment/T wave changes that may not be related to acute coronary syndrome.

systemic lupus erythematosus, aortic dissection, hypertension, and syphilitic aortitis.

Electrocardiographic Manifestations

Although the pathophysiologic processes of AS (pressure overload) and AR (volume overload) are different, both forms of aortic valve dysfunction present with LVH as well as LAA on the ECG (Fig. 42-4). In general, these include prominent left-sided forces (i.e., large R waves in left-sided limb and precordial leads), prominent S waves in right-sided precordial leads, and evidence of leftward frontal plane QRS axis deviation and LAA. ST segment/T wave changes consistent with repolarization abnormality or "strain" may be evident (Fig. 42-4; see Chapter 35, Ventricular Hypertrophy).

References

1. Surawicz B, Knilans TK: Chou's Electrocardiography in Clinical Practice: Adult and Pediatric, 5th ed. Philadelphia, WB Saunders, 2001.
2. Altrichter PM, Olson LJ, Edwards WD, et al: Surgical pathology of the pulmonary valve: A study of 116 cases spanning 15 years. Mayo Clin Proc 1989;64:1352.
3. Viseur P, Unger P: Doppler echocardiographic diagnosis and follow-up of acquired pulmonary stenosis due to external cardiac compression. Cardiology 1995;86:80.
4. Putterman C, Gilon D, Uretzki G, et al: Right ventricular outflow obstruction due to extrinsic compression by non-Hodgkin's lymphoma: Importance of echocardiographic diagnosis and follow-up. Leuk Lymphoma 1992;7:211.
5. Pasik CS, Ackerman DM, Pluth JR, Edward WD: Temporal changes in the causes of aortic stenosis: A surgical pathologic study of 646 cases. Mayo Clin Proc 1987;62:119.
6. Fenoflio JJ Jr, McAllister HA Jr, DeCastro CM, et al: Congenital bicuspid aortic valve after age 20. Am J Cardiol 1977;39:164.
7. Campbell M: Calcific aortic stenosis and congenital bicuspid aortic valves. Br Heart J 1968;30:606.

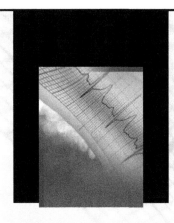

Chapter 43

Pericardial Effusion

Francis L. Counselman

Clinical Features

The pericardium is a fibroserous sac consisting of an inner serous layer (visceral pericardium) tightly adherent to the heart's surface, and a flask-shaped fibrous outer layer (parietal pericardium). The pericardial space normally contains up to 50 mL of clear serous fluid.[1]

A pericardial effusion occurs when there is an excessive amount of fluid because of abnormal production or drainage of pericardial fluid[1] from numerous conditions (uremia, collagen vascular diseases, human immunodeficiency virus infection/acquired immunodeficiency syndrome, neoplasms, and iatrogenic causes).[1–5]

Effusions can be classified as symptomatic or asymptomatic (incidental), or in terms of volume (small, moderate, and large). Symptoms do not always correlate with the size of the effusion.[6] As little as 100 mL of fluid entering the pericardial space rapidly may result in hemodynamic compromise (as in a penetrating injury), whereas effusions of 1 L or more that accumulate over a prolonged period (as in myxedema) may be associated with minimal or no symptoms. Cardiac tamponade occurs when fluid accumulation results in increased intrapericardial pressure, progressive limitation of ventricular diastolic filling, and reduction of stroke volume and cardiac output.[6]

Patients without tamponade may be asymptomatic or present with symptoms related to pericardial inflammation (e.g., chest pain, fever) or the underlying process responsible for the effusion. Large pericardial effusions can compress adjacent anatomic structures (e.g., trachea, esophagus) and cause cough, hoarseness, hiccups, dysphagia, orthopnea, and shortness of breath. If tamponade is present, complaints will usually be more severe, and include generalized weakness, dyspnea, chest discomfort, dizziness, and even syncope.

On physical examination, tachycardia, tachypnea, and hypotension occur if the effusion results in cardiac compression. A pericardial friction rub can often be heard. Beck's triad, defined as hypotension, increased jugular venous pressure, and muffled heart sounds, is considered the classic presentation of tamponade, but occurs only in one third of cases.[7,8] Pulsus paradoxus is observed commonly in cardiac tamponade.

Electrocardiographic Manifestations

In general, the electrocardiogram (ECG) is poorly diagnostic of pericardial effusion and cardiac tamponade because findings are often too few, subtle, insensitive, and nonspecific.[9,10] However, the following ECG manifestations of pericardial effusion and cardiac tamponade may be present and suggest the diagnosis.

Electrocardiographic findings of myopericarditis

Because pericardial effusion is frequently present in the setting of myopericarditis, associated ECG findings, such as diffuse ST segment elevation, PR segment depression, or T wave inversion, may be present (see Chapter 37, Myopericarditis).

ELECTROCARDIOGRAPHIC HIGHLIGHTS

- Sinus tachycardia
- ECG findings of myopericarditis at times
- Reduced QRS complex and T wave voltage
- Electrical alternans
  - QRS complex only
  - QRS-T complex alternation (2:1)
  - P-QRS-T complex alternation (extremely rare)
- Pulseless electrical activity

DIFFERENTIAL DIAGNOSIS OF REDUCED VOLTAGE

- Pneumothorax
- Pleural effusion
- Chronic obstructive pulmonary disease
- Body habitus with increased anteroposterior diameter (e.g., extreme kyphosis)
- Congestive heart failure
- Infiltrative cardiomyopathy
- Nephrotic syndrome
- Hypothyroidism and myxedema
- Anasarca
- Obesity

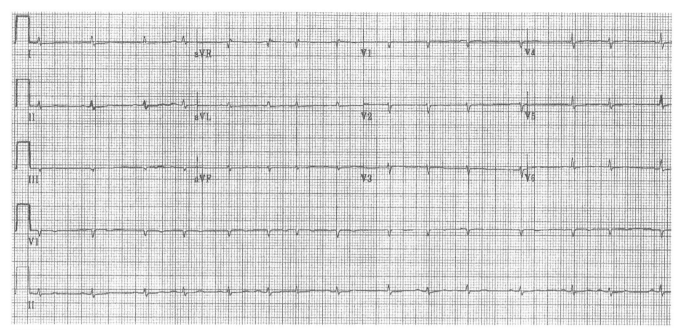

FIGURE 43-1 · **Reduced QRS-T voltage.** Note the low QRS complex and T wave voltage in all leads and nonspecific ST segment/T wave changes in this patient with a large pericardial effusion.

Sinus Tachycardia. Sinus tachycardia is a common but non-specific finding, and is observed more frequently in large pericardial effusions and cardiac tamponade until just before cardiac arrest, when there is bradycardia.

Low Voltage. In the presence of large effusions and tamponade, some reduction in the amplitude of the QRS complex and T wave has been described; the P wave is normally spared. Low QRS voltage has a moderate association with cardiac tamponade, but only a mild association with large and moderate pericardial effusions.[9] Low voltage is a nonspecific finding, and can be observed in fluid retention states (e.g., anasarca, congestive heart failure, nephrotic syndrome, myxedema), obesity, left pleural effusions, and infiltrative cardiomyopathies[10-12] (Table 43-1). Several mechanisms have been proposed to explain the association of pericardial effusion and low QRS complex voltage, including internal short-circuiting of the electrical current by pericardial fluid; change in position of the heart; increased distance from the current generator to the recording electrodes; decreased cardiac chamber size and volume; and changes in the generation and propagation of myocardial electrical currents[13] (Fig. 43-1).

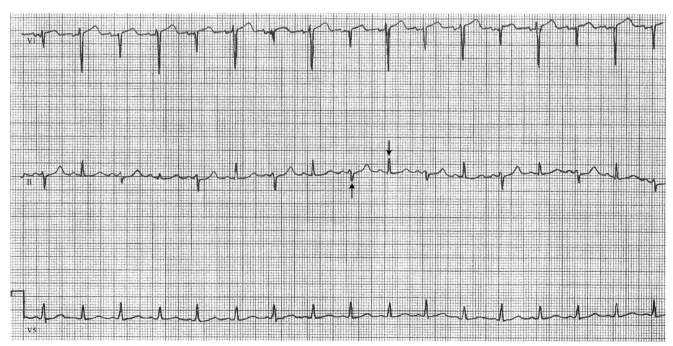

FIGURE 43-2 · **Electrical alternans.** Note the alternation in QRS amplitude in lead V₁ and polarity in lead II (*arrows*) in this patient with cardiac tamponade.

DIFFERENTIAL DIAGNOSIS OF ELECTRICAL ALTERNANS

- Hypothermia
- Electrolyte imbalance
- Prolonged QT syndromes
- Paroxysmal tachycardia
- Bradycardia
- Wolff-Parkinson-White syndrome
- Coronary artery spasm/occlusion
- Hypertension
- Cor pulmonale
- Rheumatic heart disease

ELECTROCARDIOGRAPHIC PEARLS

- The ECG is frequently normal in pericardial effusion and can be normal in cardiac tamponade. No ECG finding is sensitive or specific enough to be considered diagnostic.
- A reduction in ECG voltage, compared with a previous ECG, in the proper clinical setting, suggests pericardial effusion.
- Total electrical alternans (P-QRS-T complex) is a very rare ECG finding, but highly suggestive of cardiac tamponade.

Electrical Alternans. Electrical alternans, although commonly associated with pericardial effusion and tamponade, has been found to be neither a sensitive nor specific ECG finding for these entities[9,10,14] (Table 43-2). If present, it may be observed in some or all leads as an alternate change (usually 2:1) in pattern or magnitude of the ECG complex. Best seen in the mid-precordial leads, ventricular electrical alternans due to pericardial effusion is attributed to phasic alteration in the spatial axis of the QRS complex due to the swinging of the heart while the ECG electrodes remain in place.[15] On occasion, both the QRS complex and T wave alternate. The alternation of the P-QRS-T complex (simultaneous electrical alternation or total electrical alternans) is extremely rare and seen almost exclusively in cardiac tamponade[9,16] (Fig. 43-2).

Pulseless Electrical Activity/Electromechanical Dissociation. This is observed in severe cardiac tamponade and is usually a terminal event without immediate drainage of the pericardial sac.

References

1. Karam N, Patel P, deFilippi C: Diagnosis and management of chronic pericardial effusions. Am J Med Sci 2001;322:79.
2. Colombo A, Olson HG, Egan J, et al: Etiology and prognostic implications of a large pericardial effusion in men. Clin Cardiol 1988;11:389.
3. Corey GR, Campbell PT, Van Trigt P, et al: Etiology of large pericardial effusions. Am J Med 1993;95:209.
4. Sagristá-Sauleda J, Mercé J, Permanyer-Miralda G, et al: Clinical clues to the causes of large pericardial effusions. Am J Med 2000;109:95.
5. Heidenreich PA, Eisenberg MJ, Kee LL, et al: Pericardial effusion in AIDS. Incidence and survival. Circulation 1995;92:3229.
6. Tsang TSM, Oh JK, Seward JB: Diagnosis and management of cardiac tamponade in the era of echocardiography. Clin Cardiol 1999;22:446.
7. Guberman BA, Fowler NO, Engel PJ, et al: Cardiac tamponade in medical patients. Circulation 1981;64:633.
8. Beck CS: Two cardiac compression triads. JAMA 1935;104:714.
9. Eisenberg MJ, Munoz de Romeral L, Hiedenreich PA, et al: The diagnosis of pericardial effusion and cardiac tamponade by 12-lead ECG: A technology assessment. Chest 1996;110:318.
10. Meyers DG, Bagin RG, Levene JF: Electrocardiographic changes in pericardial effusion. Chest 1993;104:1422.
11. Unverferth DV, Williams TE, Fulkerson PK: Electrocardiographic voltage in pericardial effusion. Chest 1979;75:157.
12. Spodick DH: "Low voltage ECG" and pericardial effusion [letter]. Chest 1979;75:113.
13. Bruch C, Schmermund A, Dagres N, et al: Changes in QRS voltage in cardiac tamponade and pericardial effusion. Reversibility after pericardiocentesis and after anti-inflammatory drug treatment. J Am Coll Cardiol 2001;38:219.
14. Smith JM, Clancy EA, Valeri CR, et al: Electrical alternans and cardiac electrical instability. Circulation 1988;77:110.
15. Spodick DH: Electrocardiographic abnormalities in pericardial disease. In Spodick DH (ed): The Pericardium: A Comprehensive Textbook. New York, Marcel Dekker, 1997, p 58.
16. Sotolongo RP, Horton JD: Total electrical alternans in pericardial tamponade. Am Heart J 1981;101:853.

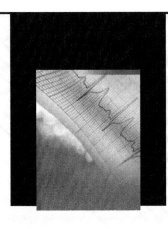

Chapter 44

Cardiac Transplant

Robert A. VerNooy and James D. Bergin

Clinical Features

In cardiac allograft hearts, new electrophysiologic conditions result from several unique factors, including the procurement procedure, the surgical transplantation techniques, the denervated state of the transplanted heart, and ongoing potential for immunologic rejection. For example, in the standard orthotopic heart transplant (OHT), residual atrial tissue of the patient (recipient atrium) remains and is surgically attached to the donor heart and donor atrium. Therefore, specific electrocardiographic (ECG) changes may be seen, most notably those representing rhythm and conduction abnormalities.

Electrocardiographic Manifestations

Heart Rate. In the cardiac allograft patient, sympathetic and parasympathetic denervation results in long-term higher resting heart rates of 90 to 110 beats/minute, with limited heart rate variability. In hemodynamic states of stress such as exercise, transplant heart rate responses and heart rate variability are blunted by reliance on circulating catecholamines for chronotropic and inotropic effects.

Increased heart rate variability over time is considered a sign of reinnervation, and can be further evidenced clinically by lower resting and nocturnal heart rates and increased circadian variability.[1] In general, the reinnervation is primarily sympathetic and not parasympathetic, and thus patients rarely respond to medications that affect the parasympathetic system, such as atropine and digoxin.

ELECTROCARDIOGRAPHIC HIGHLIGHTS

- Higher resting heart rates and decreased heart rate variability
- Right bundle branch block seen frequently
- Two P waves seen; the recipient is often slower and dissociated from the QRS complexes
- Sinus bradycardia early after transplantation, junctional bradycardia more common later
- Premature atrial contractions, atrial fibrillation, and atrial flutter common
- Ventricular dysrhythmias less common

Two P Waves. Another cardinal ECG finding after the standard biatrial procedure of OHT may be the presence of dual P waves. If dual P waves are noted, one P wave should be dissociated from the QRS complexes, representing the activity of the remaining part of the recipient atrium, and the other P wave should have a 1:1 P-to-QRS relationship, representing the activity of the donor atrium (Fig. 44-1). The rate of the remnant sinoatrial (SA) nodal tissue is often slower than that of the donor atrial pacemaker cells because of intact vagal tone regulation. In a study following long-term ECG findings in heart transplant recipients, the recipient P wave can be seen in 68% at 1 month, and in 23% at 5 years.

Studies suggest the recipient atrial electrical activity may become mechanically entrained (i.e., recipient and donor atrial contraction synchronization) over time, may be of lower-amplitude voltage, may become more disorganized toward fibrillation, or may cease altogether.[2] In some patients, a donor P wave or atrioventricular (AV) conduction fails to develop, making rhythm interpretation difficult, and is seen as donor complete heart block (Fig. 44-2).

Right Bundle Branch Block. The most common ECG abnormality in OHT recipients, occurring in up to 70% of individuals, is some variety of right bundle branch block[2] (RBBB; Fig. 44-3). This finding likely results from higher right atrial pressures secondary to a combination of increased pulmonary resistance and procurement-related ischemia.[3] The clinical implications of new conduction abnormalities, such as RBBB, after cardiac transplantation are controversial.[2] In general, the presence of RBBB in a given patient has not been shown to be associated with acute rejection, transplant coronary artery disease, or mortality.[2] However, one study looking at the 1-year follow-up of 97 heart transplant recipients identifies the finding of "a progressive RBBB" (i.e., the QRS complex width increased by 0.5 mm over time) as an independent predictor of long-term mortality.[4] Another study of 87 patients followed for a mean of 2 years showed that stable or progressive QRS complex widening (fascicular blocks or complete bundle branch blocks) was associated with left ventricular dysfunction and increased long-term mortality, probably secondary to sudden death.[5]

Bradydysrhythmias. Bradydysrhythmias are the most common type of rhythm disturbance, seen in up to 20% to

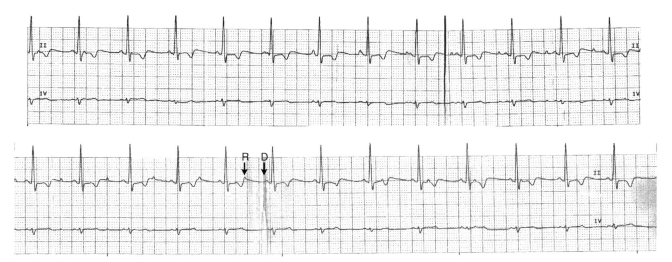

FIGURE 44-1 • **Dual P waves in orthotopic heart transplant (OHT).** This telemetry tracing shows the characteristic dual P waves often seen after OHT representing recipient and donor atrial tissue, with donor P waves (D) conducting and followed by QRS complexes, whereas the recipient P wave (R) is dissociated from the QRS complexes.

40% of patients.[6] Most of the time, bradydysrhythmias are seen early in the postoperative setting, involve the SA rather than AV node, and follow a transient course of days to weeks. Possible causes include increased donor ischemic time, physical trauma to the conduction system during procurement and implantation, abnormalities of the SA nodal artery, and preoperative treatment with amiodarone.[6] Early sinus node dysfunction does not seem to be associated with allograft rejection.[7]

Temporary pacing is often necessary after surgery; however, if symptomatic bradycardia persists 3 weeks after surgery, permanent pacing is often instituted.[7] The incidence of late symptomatic bradycardia greater than 1 year after transplantation is 5% and appears more often to be due to disease of the AV node and not associated with transplant rejection.[6] Overall, symptomatic bradycardia requiring permanent pacemaker implantation varies in reported incidence from 4% to 29%.[7]

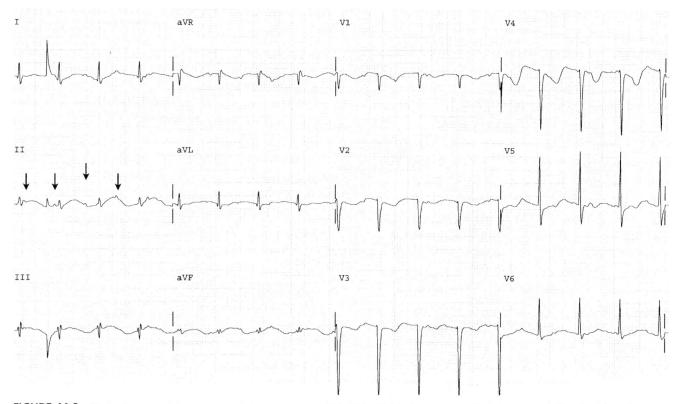

FIGURE 44-2 • **Native P wave activity in orthotopic heart transplant.** This 12-lead ECG shows a P wave (recipient; *arrows*) dissociated from the narrow complex QRS. The P wave represents underlying recipient asynchronous atrial P wave activity at a rate of 125 beats per minute. Furthermore, no donor P waves are seen, resulting in accelerated junctional escape rhythm.

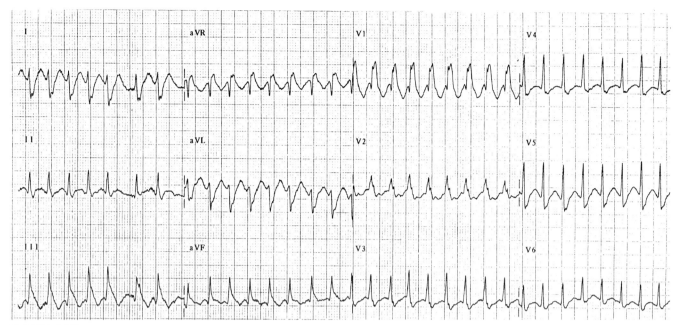

FIGURE 44-3 • **Wide-complex tachycardia in orthotopic heart transplant (OHT).** This 12-lead ECG on a patient 10 days after OHT shows a wide-complex tachycardia with a right bundle branch block morphology and an irregular, rapid rate secondary to atrial fibrillation, a common dysrhythmia early after transplantation.

In the first 3 weeks post-transplantation, supersensitivity of the transplanted heart to adenosine can result in severe bradycardia or even asystole that has been successfully reversed in some cases with theophylline.[8]

Supraventricular Tachydysrhythmias. On the other hand, tachydysrhythmias after cardiac transplantation are less common. Importantly, atrial tachydysrhythmias such as atrial fibrillation or flutter may herald a risk of acute rejection of between 30% to 70%[9,10] (Fig. 44-4). An increase in atrial

conduction times or in the terminal force of the P wave in lead V_1 has been shown to have a high predictive value for rejection in the atrium, and also in predicting the occurrence of atrial fibrillation and flutter.[10,11] Atrial fibrillation may occur more frequently in the immediate postoperative period secondary to pericardial irritation and increased adrenergic state. In contrast, atrial flutter may occur more commonly in later stages and is often associated with allograft rejection or transplant vasculopathy with ischemia or infarction.[11]

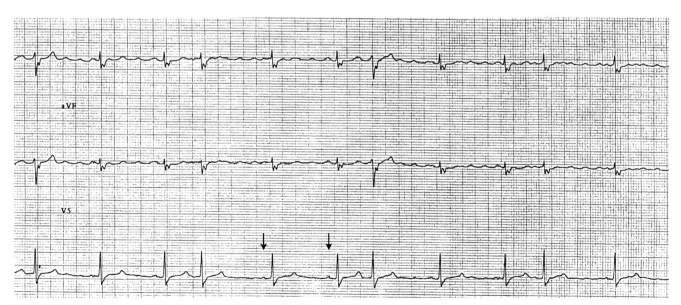

FIGURE 44-4 • **Supraventricular dysrhythmia.** This three-lead rhythm ECG shows seemingly coarse atrial activity and regularly irregular ventricular rhythm. Further analysis of the ECG shows likely donor sinus P waves (*arrows*) with supraventricular trigeminy and probable coarse atrial fibrillation of the remnant recipient atrium.

ELECTROCARDIOGRAPHIC PEARLS

- Higher resting heart rates are indicative of autonomic denervation, with transplant hearts more sensitive to circulating catecholamines.
- Early after transplantation, bradydysrhythmias are very common and not associated with allograft rejection.
- Adenosine administration can result in significant bradydysrhythmia and asystole in recently transplanted hearts.
- RBBB is quite common, but not clearly associated with a worse long-term prognosis.
- Atrial tachyarrhythmias are common and can be associated with acute allograft rejection.
- New QTc interval prolongation can be a sign of acute allograft rejection.

The type of surgical anastomosis with OHT seems to have an impact on the occurrence of atrial flutter, but not atrial fibrillation. The standard OHT procedure with a recipient-atrial–to–donor-atrial anastomosis may have a higher late incidence of atrial flutter compared with a total OHT with a bicaval anastomotic technique.[11,12] Longer donor ischemic times immediately before transplantation also have been shown to correlate with the increased incidence of atrial flutter and atrial fibrillation.[11] Rarely, recipient-to-donor atrioatrial conduction has been reported as a cause of symptomatic atrial tachydysrhythmias (including atrial premature beats and atrial tachycardia, flutter, and fibrillation) after heart transplantation.[13] Normally, the remnant native atrium beats independently of the donor atrium and is electrically isolated from the donor right atrial tissue by the atrioatrial anastomosis.

Ventricular Dysrhythmias. Because of the autonomically denervated state, the predilection of the transplanted heart to ventricular dysrhythmias is reduced. In fact, in long-term survivors of cardiac transplantation, the denervated heart shows little ventricular ectopic activity compared with normal hearts.[14]

QT Interval. Finally, a progressive increase in the corrected QT interval (QT_C) in a given patient may be an early marker of transplant vasculopathy and acute allograft rejection.[15,16] Successful treatment of rejection is followed by a shortening of the QT_C, and a normal or unchanged QT_C in any given patient indicates mild or no rejection requiring no treatment.[16]

References

1. Halpert I, Goldberg AD, Levine AB, et al: Reinnervation of the transplanted human heart as evidenced from heart rate variability studies. Am J Cardiol 1996;77:180.
2. Golshayan D, Seydoux C, Berguer DG, et al: Incidence and prognostic value of electrocardiographic abnormalities after heart transplantation. Clin Cardiol 1998;21:680.
3. Villa A, de Marchena EJ, Myerburg RJ, et al: Comparison of paired orthotopic cardiac transplant donor and recipient electrocardiograms. Am Heart J 1994;127:70.
4. Osa A, Almenar L, Arnau MA, et al: Is the prognosis poorer in heart transplanted patients who develop a right bundle branch block? J Heart Lung Transplant 2000;19:207.
5. Leonelli FM, Dunn JK, Young JB, et al: Natural history, determinants, and clinical relevance of conduction abnormalities following orthotopic heart transplantation. Am J Cardiol 1996;77:47.
6. Weinfeld M, Kartashov A, Piana R, et al: Bradycardia: A late complication following cardiac transplantation. Am J Cardiol 1996;78:969.
7. Scott CD, Dark JH, McComb J: Sinus node function after cardiac transplantation. J Am Coll Cardiol 1994;24:1334.
8. Redmond JM, Zehr KJ, Gillinov MA, et al: Use of theophylline for treatment of prolonged sinus node dysfunction in human orthotopic heart transplantation. J Heart Lung Transplant 1993;12:133.
9. Pavri BB, O'Nunain SS, Newell JB, et al: Prevalence and prognostic significance of atrial arrhythmias after orthotopic cardiac transplantation. J Am Coll Cardiol 1995;25:1673.
10. Cui G, Kobashigawa J, Chung T, et al: Atrial conduction disturbance as an indicator of rejection after cardiac transplantation. Transplantation 2000;70:223.
11. Guanggen C, Tung T, Kobashigawa J, et al: Increased incidence of atrial flutter associated with the rejection of heart transplantation. Am J Cardiol 2001;88:280.
12. Brandt M, Harringer W, Hirt S, et al: Influence of bicaval anastomoses on late occurrence of atrial arrhythmia after heart transplantation. Ann Thorac Surg 1997;64:70.
13. Lefroy D, Fang J, Stevenson L, et al: Recipient-to-donor atrioatrial conduction after orthotopic heart transplantation: Surface electrocardiographic features and estimated prevalence. Am J Cardiol 1998;82:444.
14. Alexopoulus D, Yusuf S, Bostock J, et al: Ventricular arrhythmias in long term survivors of orthotopic and heterotopic cardiac transplantation. Br Heart J 1988;59:648.
15. Ali A, Mehra M, Malik F, et al: Insights into ventricular repolarization abnormalities in cardiac allograft vasculopathy. Am J Cardiol 2001;87:367.
16. Richartz BM, Radovancevic B, Bologna MT, et al: Usefulness of the QTc in predicting acute allograft rejection. Thorac Cardiovasc Surg 1998;46:217.

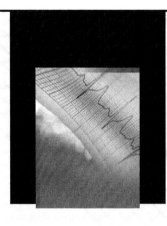

Chapter 45

Dextrocardia

Moss Mendelson

Clinical Features

Dextrocardia is defined as a cardiac position that is a mirror image of normal anatomy. A description of the visceroatrial orientation (anatomic positioning of the heart and viscera) is often appended to the description of heart position. Congenital disorders of the heart can be associated with dextrocardia. In dextrocardia with situs solitus or situs ambiguus, the rate of congenital heart disease is very high—approximately 90% or more.[1] If the great vessels or atria are discordant with the ventricles, severe physiologic dysfunction is present.

This chapter generally considers dextrocardia found in patients with situs inversus. These patients have great vessel/atrial/ventricular physiologic concordance, and usually have no heart disease. Many are asymptomatic and undiagnosed until an electrocardiogram (ECG) or chest radiograph is done for other reasons.

Dextrocardia with situs inversus is seen infrequently, with a reported incidence of 1:5000 to 1:10,000 and a slight male predominance. Congenital heart disease can occur in approximately 3% to 5% of these patients.[1] It is unclear if there is any difference in the incidence of acquired cardiac disease in these patients compared with patients with normal cardiac anatomy. Dextrocardia has been described in association with heart block,[2–5] familial prolonged QT syndrome,[6] and coronary artery disease.[7–10] Kartagener's syndrome, in which ciliary function is impaired, refers to the triad of dextrocardia with situs inversus, sinusitis, and bronchiectasis. Kartagener's syndrome is present in approximately 20% of patients with dextrocardia and situs inversus.

Electrocardiographic Manifestations

Traditional lead placement in patients with dextrocardia and situs inversus leads to a number of easily recognized abnormalities on the ECG (Fig. 45-1).

P Wave Vector. With a mirror image location of the atrial pacemaker, the atrial impulse starts on the left and proceeds rightward (reversed from normal), giving the frontal plane P wave vector a rightward axis (around +135 degrees). Thus, the P wave is inverted in leads I and aVL[11] (Fig. 45-1).

QRS Morphology. The initial QRS vector results from septal depolarization and proceeds right to left (reversed from normal) in patients with dextrocardia and situs inversus. Thus, normal, small septal q waves are not seen in leads V_5 or V_6, but are present in leads V_{5R} and V_{6R} (see Fig. 45-1).

The second phase of the ventricular depolarization also proceeds in a reversed fashion in patients with dextrocardia. This vector proceeds left to right, producing profound right axis deviation. In addition, a prominent R wave in lead V_1 is seen and poor R wave progression through the precordial leads is present. Leads aVR and aVL show reversal of their normal QRS complex configuration, with a predominantly upright QRS complex in lead aVR and a downward QRS complex in lead aVL. Leads II and III are likewise reversed. Lead aVF remains unaffected. Low voltage in traditional left precordial leads is seen because the majority of ventricular mass is right sided[11–13] (Fig. 45-1).

Lead Reorientation. For a patient with known dextrocardia, reversal of the arm leads results in a "normal" P wave pattern and QRS axis in the frontal plane limb leads. In addition,

---

<table>
<tr><td>

ELECTROCARDIOGRAPHIC HIGHLIGHTS

- Total inversion of lead I (inverted P-QRS-T)
- Right axis deviation of P wave and QRS complex
- Prominent R wave in lead V_1, with poor R wave progression/low voltage in left precordial leads
- Leads aVR and aVR appear reversed
- Leads II and III appear reversed

</td><td>

ELECTROCARDIOGRAPHIC PEARLS

- Repositioning of ECG leads (Fig. 45-3) allows "normal" ECG interpretation. Arm leads are reversed and right-sided precordial leads are used.
- ECG manifestations of heart disease in patients presenting with undiagnosed dextrocardia may be confusing owing to their mirror image appearance.

</td></tr>
</table>

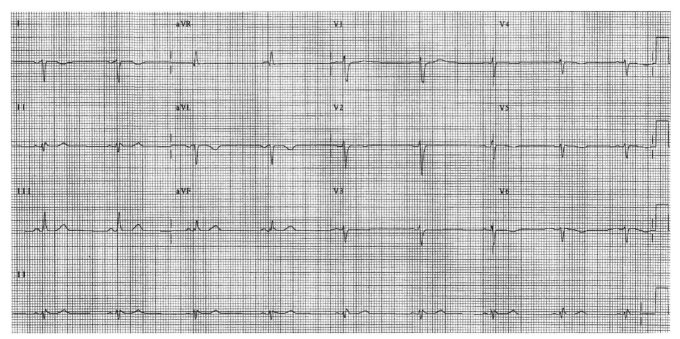

FIGURE 45-1 · **Twelve-lead ECG in a patient with dextrocardia and situs inversus totalis.** Note inverted P wave and QRS complex in lead I, upright QRS complex in lead aVR and downward QRS complex in lead aVL, and poor R wave progression through the precordial leads.

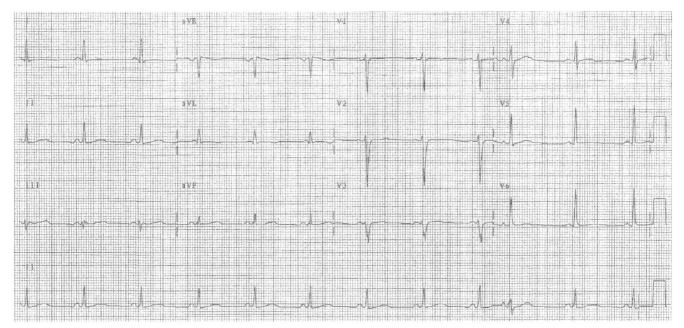

FIGURE 45-2 · **ECG in patient from Figure 45-1 with adjusted lead placement.** Note normalization of the frontal plane and precordial findings—in essence, the "typical" ECG appearance of an adult patient.

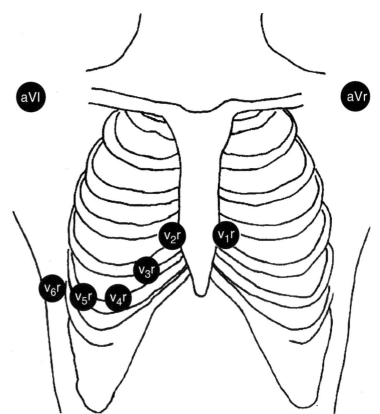

FIGURE 45-3 · **Suggested lead placement in patients with dextrocardia.** Arm leads are reversed and right-sided precordial leads are used.

reorientation of precordial leads to a right-sided approach, to create leads V_{1R} through V_{6R} (Fig. 45-2), results in the appearance of a typical pattern of septal depolarization and R wave progression on the 12-lead ECG. This right-sided positioning of the precordial leads allows a conventional approach to interpretation[13] (Fig. 45-3).

References

1. Schlant RC, Alexander R, O'Rourke RA, et al: The Heart Arteries and Veins. New York, McGraw-Hill, 1994.
2. Badui E, Lepe L, Solorio S, et al: Heart block in dextrocardia with situs inversus: A case report. Angiology 1995;46:537.
3. Brito MR, Miranda CE, Barros VC, et al: Heart block in dextrocardia and situs inversus: A case report. Ann Noninvas Electrocardiol 2001;6:369.
4. Garcia OL, Metha AV, Pickoff AS, et al. Left isomerism and complete atrioventricular block: A report of six cases. Am J Cardiol 1981;48:1103.
5. Yang J, Russell DA, Bourdeau JE: Case report: Ranitidine-induced bradycardia in a patient with dextrocardia. Am J Med Sci 1996;312:133.
6. Corcos AP, Tzivoni D, Medina A: Long QT syndrome and complete situs inversus: Preliminary report of a family. Cardiology 1989;76:228.
7. Bhat PS, Ojha JP, Sinha VK, et al: Myocardial infarction with dextrocardia and situs inversus: A rare case report. Indian Heart J 1980;32:190.
8. Liem KL, ten Veen JH: Inferior myocardial infarction in a patient with mirror-image dextrocardia and situs inversus totalis. Chest 1976; 69:239.
9. Robinson N, Golledge P, Timmis A: Coronary stent deployment in situs inversus. Heart 2001;86:E15.
10. Yamazaki T, Tomaru A, Wagatsuma K, et al: Percutaneous transluminal coronary angioplasty for morphologic left anterior descending artery lesion in a patient with dextrocardia: A case report and literature review. Angiology 1997;48:451.
11. Rao PS: Dextrocardia: Systematic approach to differential diagnosis. Am Heart J 1981;102:389.
12. Mattu A, Brady WJ, Perron AD, Robinson DA: Prominent R wave in lead V1: Electrocardiographic differential diagnosis. Am J Emerg Med 2001;19:504.
13. Wagner GS: Marriott's Practical Electrocardiography, 9th ed. Philadelphia, Lippincott Williams & Wilkins, 2001.

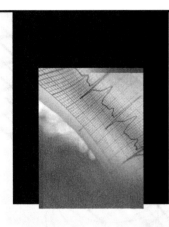

Chapter 46

Cardiac Trauma

Brian F. Erling and Jeffrey S. Young

Clinical Features

Direct myocardial injury involves those mechanisms that directly affect the anatomic and physiologic function of the heart. Myocardial contusion is the most common direct cardiac injury, followed by less common processes secondary to coronary artery trauma. These can include spasm, thrombosis, and dissection of the coronary arteries. Penetrating myocardial trauma is universally serious, where the conduction abnormalities and subsequent electrocardiographic (ECG) changes are the least of the victim's medical problems. Electrical injury can result in a spectrum of clinical and ECG morbidity with variable outcomes. Commotio cordis, another form of myocardial trauma, is the induction of ventricular fibrillation after relatively minor blunt trauma delivered precisely during the susceptible phase of ventricular repolarization.[1] Unlike myocardial contusion (i.e., actual myocardial injury), it is the timing of the blow in the electric cycle of depolarization/repolarization in commotio cordis that produces the fibrillation rather than direct injury to the cardiac musculature.

Indirect myocardial injury is the subsequent ischemia and possible infarction experienced by a nontraumatized heart as a result of the physiologic stresses of trauma and hemorrhage. This injury can be difficult to differentiate from other types of direct injury because myocardial contusion can mimic acute coronary syndrome (ACS) and coronary artery trauma can have similar clinical features to an acute myocardial infarction (AMI). Indirect cardiac injury is much more common in susceptible, diseased hearts.

Electrocardiographic Manifestations

Blunt Trauma. The ECG response to the insult can be equally diverse, ranging from a normal ECG and subtle, inconsequential changes, to sudden death. The most frequently encountered abnormalities include sinus tachycardia with nonspecific ST segment/T wave changes. Although less frequent, conduction system malfunction is another ECG indicator of myocardial injury; such injury is manifested by either right bundle branch block (Fig. 46-1) or nonspecific intraventricular conduction delay. Significant ST segment changes, including both elevation (Fig. 46-2) and depression (Fig. 46-3), and T wave abnormalities (Fig. 46-4) are also seen in such trauma patients. The entire range of dysrhythmias, including sinus tachycardia as noted previously, is seen. After sinus tachycardia, frequent premature ventricular depolarizations represent another commonly seen rhythm disturbance. One prospective study of echocardiographic abnormalities after trauma reported a 54% incidence of

---

ELECTROCARDIOGRAPHIC HIGHLIGHTS

Blunt trauma

Myocardial contusion

- Dysrhythmias
- Axis changes
- Nonspecific ST segment/T wave changes
- ST segment elevation/T wave changes consistent with acute coronary syndrome (ACS)
- Heart block
- Unexplained sinus tachycardia

Coronary artery spasm/Thrombosis/Dissection

- ST segment elevation/T wave changes consistent with ACS

Penetrating trauma

- ST segment/T wave changes consistent with ACS
- Low voltage
- Sinus tachycardia
- Electrical alternans

Electrical injury

- Sinus tachycardia
- Nonspecific ST segment/T wave changes
- Ventricular fibrillation (severe alternating current injury)
- Asystole (severe direct current injury, e.g., lightning)
- Heart block
- Bundle branch block
- Premature ventricular contractions and ventricular dysrhythmias
- Premature atrial contractions and atrial fibrillation
- Prolonged QT interval

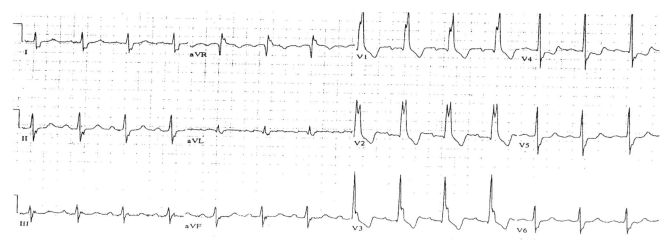

FIGURE 46-1 · **Right bundle branch block (RBBB) from myocardial contusion.** Twelve-lead ECG from a 29-year-old patient status post-motor vehicle crash. The patient noted significant chest pain with onset after the impact. This ECG demonstrates a new RBBB.

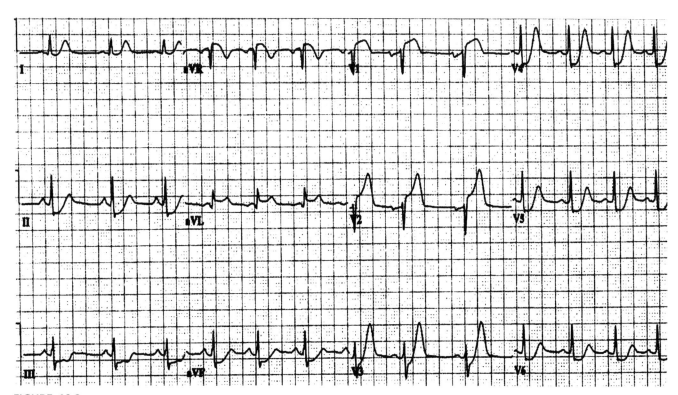

FIGURE 46-2 · **Myocardial contusion mimicking acute myocardial infarction.** Twelve-lead ECG from a 34-year-old motor vehicle crash victim with hypotension and multiple anterior rib fractures. This ECG demonstrates significant ST segment/T wave abnormalities. ST segment depression is seen in leads II, III, aVF, V_3, V_4, V_5, and V_6; ST segment elevation is noted in leads I, aVL, V_2, and V_3; and prominent T waves are seen in leads V_2 and V_3. Serum troponin values were elevated and an echocardiogram demonstrated inferior and anterior wall motion abnormalities. Subsequent cardiac catheterization, performed 1 week later, revealed normal wall motion and no evidence of significant coronary artery disease.

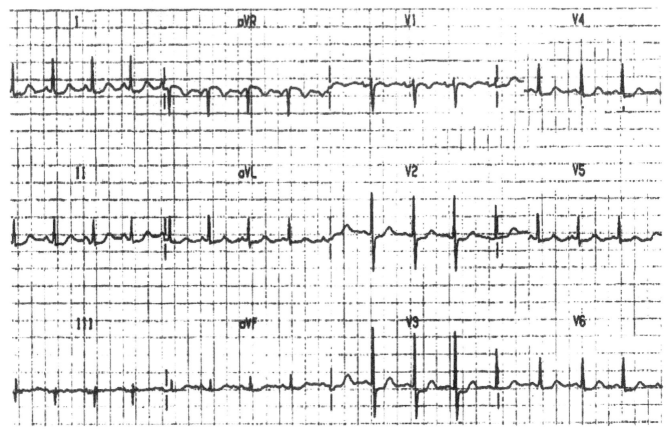

FIGURE 46-3 · **ST segment depression from traumatic injury.** Twelve-lead ECG from an adult patient who sustained a 20-foot-fall with impact on the anterior chest. The ECG demonstrates minimal ST segment depression in the inferior and anterior leads.

ECG changes. Forty-nine percent of the abnormalities were nonspecific ST segment depression and T wave changes, whereas the remainder constituted conduction abnormalities, axis deviation, and dysrhythmias[2] (Fig. 46-5).

Although an ECG lacks sensitivity and specificity for myocardial injury, most of the literature supports the use of an initial ECG as an effective screening tool to identify those patients at risk for significant cardiac disease either resulting from the trauma directly or secondary to traumatic triggering of underlying myocardial disease.[3–7]

Penetrating Trauma. Penetrating cardiac trauma is frequently a surgical emergency that mandates treatment to

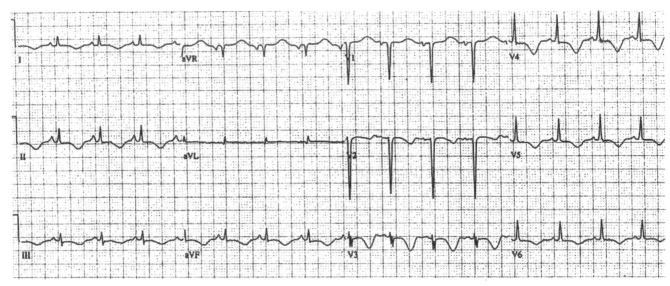

FIGURE 46-4 · **Diffuse T wave changes after blunt trauma.** Twelve-lead ECG from an adult motor vehicle crash victim demonstrating widespread T wave inversions.

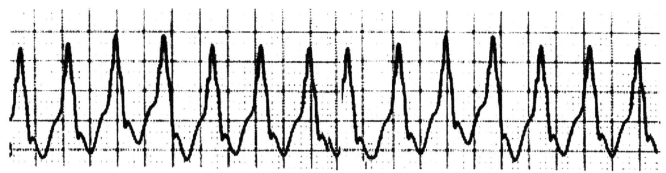

FIGURE 46-5 · **Wide QRS complex tachycardia.** ECG rhythm strip demonstrating a wide-complex tachycardia likely due to ventricular tachycardia in a patient who sustained blunt injury to the chest.

alleviate the hemorrhage and possible tamponade. In the case of major penetrating trauma, rarely is there time for an ECG, nor would its results change management. In the case of minor, nonfatal penetrating trauma, the ECG may reveal ST segment changes suggestive of ACS. A retrospective review of penetrating cardiac trauma revealed multiple patterns in the presenting ECGs; approximately 10% of patients had changes consistent with AMI (Fig. 46-6). In addition, pericarditis was evident in 27% of patients and repolarization changes were seen in 35%.[8] Injury to the pericardium may also present with ECG changes consistent with pericardial effusion or tamponade. Tachycardia, low voltage, or electrical alternans may precede any clinical deterioration secondary to tamponade.

Electrical Injury. The most common result of electrical insult to the heart is acute dysrhythmia, which can be due to direct electrical effects to the myocardium or damage to the conduction system itself. Direct heat injury to the myocardium,

as well as coronary artery thrombosis, have been reported, yet are rare.[9,10] It has been reported that alternating current is more likely to produce ventricular fibrillation, whereas direct current or very high alternating current is more likely to produce asystole.[11] Although these dramatic rhythms are the most feared, the most common post-electrical shock ECG findings are sinus tachycardia and nonspecific ST segment/T wave changes.[12,13] Heart block, bundle branch block, premature ventricular contractions, premature atrial contractions, prolonged QT interval, and atrial fibrillation have also been seen.[14,15]

Lightning strikes can result in a transient ventricular asystole that spontaneously reverts to a normal sinus rhythm if the coexisting respiratory arrest is treated. If the apnea is not addressed, the temporarily recovered rhythm may deteriorate to ventricular fibrillation.[16] Transient nonspecific changes may be seen over the 48 hours after the lightning strike.

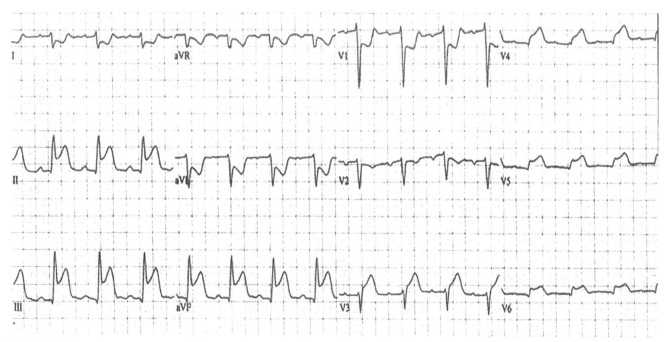

FIGURE 46-6 · **Extensive acute myocardial infarction (AMI) from penetrating coronary artery injury.** Twelve-lead ECG from a 17-year-old patient who received a stab wound to the left lateral chest. Urgent surgery revealed a laceration to the left ventricle with injury to the proximal left circumflex artery. The patient experienced an extensive AMI because of this coronary artery injury. Significant ST segment changes are seen, with depression in leads I, aVL, and V_1 and elevation in leads II, III, aVF, and V_3 through V_6.

ELECTROCARDIOGRAPHIC PEARLS

- The most common ECG findings after blunt myocardial traumatic injury are sinus tachycardia and nonspecific ST segment/T wave changes.
- The ECG is of initial value in the evaluation of traumatic cardiac injury.
- ST segment elevation may be due to myocardial contusion or acute myocardial infarction in the trauma patient.

Many of the more benign rhythms associated with lightning strikes, however, can be refractory to treatment because of areas of patchy myocardial necrosis. These focal anatomic changes result in resistant dysrhythmogenic foci. Damage to the atrioventricular or sinus node is common, and may be permanent. Acute inferior myocardial infarction is the most common infarction pattern, possibly owing to the close proximity of the right coronary artery to the anterior chest wall.[17]

The myocardial dysfunction after prolonged electrical injury can be secondary to direct blast-wave myocardial contusion, infarction, thermal necrosis, or conduction disturbance. The degree of recovery is variable, and permanent sequelae are common. The diagnosis of myocardial injury must be suspected when significant body surface burns are present, and when the course of the electrical injury from entrance to exit is vertical. In a study of 24 patients with electrical injury, 13 of the 24 had elevated cardiac enzymes, with 10 of the 13 showing ECG changes. Of the 11 patients without serologic evidence of myocardial injury, 4 of the 11 demonstrated worrisome ECG changes, including dysrhythmia and ST segment/T wave changes. In several cases where the electricity was determined to course through the thorax, delayed ventricular dysrhythmias were seen as late as 8 to 12 hours postinjury. As for the more common cases of household electric shock, it has been well demonstrated that a healthy patient with a normal ECG can be safely discharged without further monitoring.[18]

References

1. Perron AD, Brady WJ, Erling BF: Commotio cordis: An underappreciated cause of sudden cardiac death in young patients. Assessment and management in ED. Am J Emerg Med 2001;19:406.
2. Helling TS, Duke P, Beggs CW, et al: A prospective evaluation of 68 patients suffering blunt chest trauma for evidence of cardiac injury. J Trauma 1989;29:961.
3. Maenza RL, Seaberg D, DiAmico F: A meta-analysis of blunt cardiac trauma: Ending myocardial confusion. Am J Emerg Med 1996;14:237.
4. Dowd MD, Krug S: Pediatric blunt cardiac injury: Epidemiology, clinical features, and diagnosis. Pediatric Emergency Medicine Collaborative Research Committee: Working Group on Blunt Cardiac Injury. J Trauma 1996;40:61.
5. Miller FB, Shumate CR, Richardson JD: Myocardial contusion: When can the diagnosis be eliminated? Arch Surg 1989;124:805.
6. Wisner DH, Reed WH, Riddick RS: Suspected myocardial contusion: Triage and indications for monitoring. Ann Surg 1990;212:82.
7. Illig KA, Swierzewski MJ, Feliciano DV, et al: A rational screening and treatment strategy based on electrocardiogram alone for suspected cardiac contusion. Am J Surg 1991;162:537.
8. Duque HA, Florez LE, Moreno A, et al: Penetrating cardiac trauma: follow-up study including electrocardiography, echocardiography, and functional test. World J Surg 1999;23:1254.
9. Jain S, Bandi V: Electrical and lightning injuries. Crit Care Clin 1999;15;319.
10. Kinney TJ: Myocardial infarction following electrical injury. Ann Emerg Med 1982;11:622.
11. Lown B, Neuman J, Amarasingham R, et al: Comparison of alternating current with direct current electroshock across the closed chest. Am J Cardiol 1962;10:223.
12. Solem L, Fischer RP, Strate RG: The natural history of electrical injury. J Trauma 1977;17:487.
13. Kobernick M: Electrical injuries: Pathophysiology and emergency management. Ann Emerg Med 1982;11:633.
14. DiVincenti FC, Moncrief JA, Pruitt BA: Electrical injuries. A review of 65 cases. J Trauma 1969;9:497.
15. Das KM: Electrocardiographic changes following electric shock. Indian J Pediatr 1974;41:192.
16. Ravitch MM, Lane R, Safar P, et al: Lightning stroke: Report of a case with recovery after cardiac massage and prolonged artificial respiration. N Engl J Med 1961;264:36.
17. Carleton SC: Cardiac problems associated with electrical injury. Cardiol Clin 1995;13:263.
18. Cunningham PA: The need for cardiac monitoring after electrical injury. Med J Aust 1991;154:765.

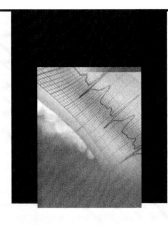

Chapter 47

Long QT Syndromes

Jesse M. Pines and William J. Brady

Clinical Features

The long QT syndrome represents a collection of diseases involving cardiac ion channel dysfunction that results in prolonged repolarization of the myocyte. This lengthened repolarization time leaves the ventricle more susceptible to an early afterdepolarization, which can precipitate a variety of dysrhythmias. This electrophysiologic event is commonly known as the "R-on-T" phenomenon and predisposes the patient to ventricular dysrhythmia, the most common of which is torsades de pointes[1] (Fig. 47-1). Clinically, patients with long QT syndrome are usually asymptomatic (other than findings associated with the various congenital forms of long QT syndrome). These syndromes present clinically when sudden cardiac dysrhythmias occur, causing syncope, seizures, and death.

Regarding etiology, the long QT syndrome can be divided into the congenital and acquired forms. The congenital, or inherited, forms of the disease are estimated to be present in approximately 1 in 5000 to 7000 people and are thought to result from a defect in cardiac potassium and sodium channels. Congenital syndromes include the Romano-Ward syndrome and the Jervell/Lange-Nielsen syndrome (Figs. 47-2 and 47-3). Clinical symptoms are often precipitated by exercise, emotion, or other adrenergic stimuli, although up to one third of individuals with these syndromes may never experience symptoms.

Acquired long QT syndromes are usually caused by myocyte potassium channel dysfunction as a result of a variety of agents and conditions. Although once rare, acquired long QT syndromes are now more common than the congenital form, primarily as a result of the increasing numbers of medications that prolong the QT interval (see Chapters 49 through 57 for discussion of the toxicologic effects of medications). Many medications and combinations of medications affecting the QT interval can interact through common metabolism in the cytochrome P-450 pathway and result in a prolonged QT interval. In addition, a prolonged QT interval is associated with some bradycardias, cocaine abuse, organophosphate poisoning, and electrolyte disturbances such as hypokalemia[2] (see Chapter 58, Electrolyte Abnormalities).

Electrocardiographic Manifestations

The QT Interval. The QT interval represents the period from the depolarization to the repolarization of the ventricles. It begins with the first phase of the QRS complex and ends with the completion of the T wave. The QRS interval reflects the activation of the ventricles, whereas the ST segment reflects the repolarization of the ventricles.

The QT interval varies with heart rate; as heart rate increases, the length of the QT interval tends to decrease. A number of formulas have been developed to account for this variability. Originally developed by Bazett in 1920, a corrected QT interval (QT_C) can be calculated as follows:

$$QT_C \text{ (seconds)} = QT \text{ (seconds)}/\sqrt{RR} \text{ (seconds)}$$

The Bazett formula predicts an increasing velocity of repolarization with increasing heart rate and a slower velocity with decreasing heart rate. Many other formulas that include hyperbolic, exponential, and logarithmic functions for the correction of the QT interval have been suggested, all of which have their inherent limitations.[3] These formulas do not account for the effect of autonomic tone on the QT interval that can occur independent of rate.[4]

The risk of life-threatening dysrhythmias is exponentially related to the length of the Bazett QT_C interval.[5] Typically, the upper range of normal for the QT_C interval is no greater than 0.44 sec in adults. Some studies have suggested 0.46 sec as the upper limit in women. The clinician can approximate the maximum normal QT interval without the need for advanced calculation of the QT_C. In general, the normal QT interval should be less than one-half the R-R interval for normal sinus rhythm between 60 and 100 bpm. With slow rates, the normal

ELECTROCARDIOGRAPHIC HIGHLIGHTS

- Prolonged QT interval
- T wave alternans
- Bifid or notched T waves
- Sinus bradycardia
- Polymorphic ventricular tachycardia

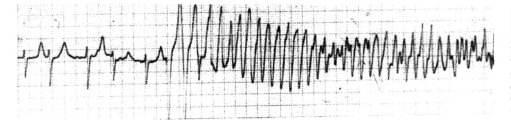

FIGURE 47-1 · Torsades de pointes in patient with long QT syndrome. An ECG rhythm strip from a 15-year-old boy with congenital long QT syndrome. This ECG shows the development of torsades de pointes during an exercise examination. (From Vincent GM: Long QT syndrome. Cardiol Clin 2000;18:319, with permission.)

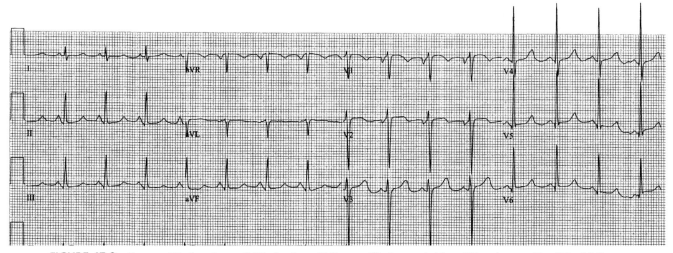

FIGURE 47-2 · Romano-Ward syndrome. ECG of patient with Romano-Ward congenital long QT syndrome, with a QT_C of 0.53 sec.

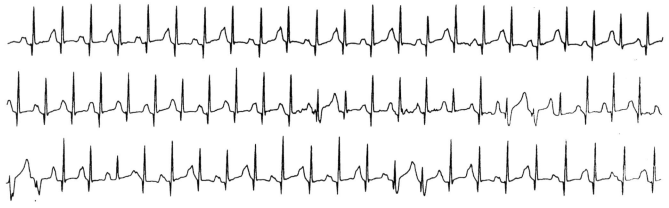

FIGURE 47-3 · Jervell/Lange-Nielsen syndrome. The rhythm strip demonstrates prolonged QT interval and T wave alternans.

QT is progressively less than half the R-R interval. With fast rates, the normal QT is progressively longer than half the R-R interval. If the QT interval is of greater duration than one-half the R-R interval, than the QT interval is abnormally prolonged for the given heart rate.

The QT interval duration can also be lead dependent, a phenomenon known as *QT interval dispersion*, and is typically longest in leads V_3 and V_4. This variability may be due to electrical instability and also may be a risk factor for

---

ELECTROCARDIOGRAPHIC PEARLS

- The normal QT interval varies with heart rate.
- With normal sinus rhythm at normal rates, the normal QT interval should not exceed one-half the R-R interval.
- Some patients with long QT syndrome may have borderline or nearly normal QT intervals on ECG.

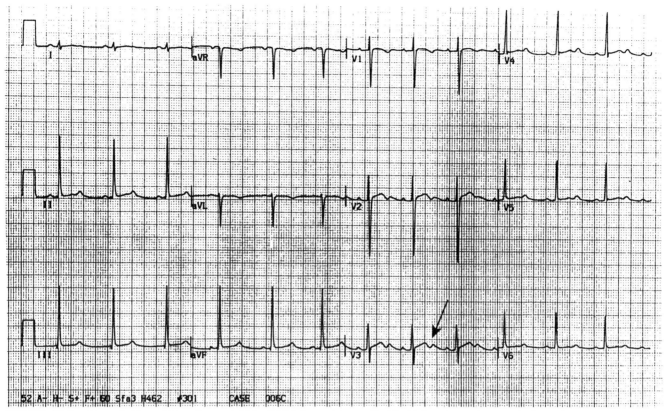

FIGURE 47-4 · Congenital long QT syndrome. A 12-lead ECG from a 16-year-old girl with long QT syndrome. This disease is characterized by bifid T waves (*arrow*), particularly present in inferior and lateral precordial leads. The QT interval is barely prolonged at 0.43 sec, and the QT_C is 0.47 sec, demonstrating the intermittent nature of prolongation. (From Vincent GM: Long QT syndrome. Cardiol Clin 2000;18:319, with permission.)

47-1 · DIAGNOSTIC CRITERIA FOR LONG QT SYNDROME

Criterion	Point Score
ECG	
QT_C prolonged	
>0.48 sec	3
0.46–0.48 sec	2
<0.46 sec (men only)	1
Torsades de pointes	2
T wave alternans	1
Notched T wave (in three leads)	1
Low heart rate for age	0.5
Clinical	
Syncope	
With stress	2
Without stress	1
Congenital deafness	0.5
Family History	
Family member with syndrome	1
Unexplained sudden death (immediate family member younger than age 30 years)	0.5

The scoring system is as follows: ≥4, high probability for the diagnosis; 2–3, intermediate probability; ≤1, low probability. A high-probability score is interpreted as indicating the definite presence of the syndrome. A low-probability score is interpreted as indicating the syndrome is highly unlikely to be present. Intermediate scores require additional consideration and investigation.[9]

dysrhythmias by causing regional differences in refractoriness (see Chapter 73, QT Dispersion).[6-8]

Besides the actual QT duration, there are other electrocardiographic (ECG) criteria for the syndrome, as noted in the 1993 Long QT Syndrome Criteria for congenital forms of the syndrome. These criteria include (1) T wave alternans—a regular alternation in amplitude or in polarity of two different T wave configurations while the R-R interval is constant (Fig. 47-3); and (2) bifid or notched T waves (Fig. 47-4). The diagnosis of congenital long QT syndrome can be made using diagnostic criteria in the form of a point score using ECG criteria, clinical history, and family history[9] (Table 47-1).

With congenital forms, however, there is variable penetrance, and not all patients who have the gene will necessarily meet strict ECG diagnostic criteria for the disorder. In fact, only approximately 70% of patients actually meet ECG criteria; the remaining 30% have borderline long or entirely normal QT_C intervals[10] (Fig. 47-4).

References

1. Vincent GM: Long QT syndrome. Cardiol Clin 2000;18:309.
2. Khan IA: Long QT syndrome: Diagnosis and management Am Heart J 2002;143:7.
3. Molnar J, Weiss J, Zhang F, et al: Evaluation of five QT correction formulas using a software-assisted method for continuous QT measurements from 24-hour Holter recordings. Am J Cardiol 1996;78:920.

4. Mirvis BM, Goldberger AL: Electrocardiography. In Braunwald E, Zipes DP, Libby P (eds): Heart Disease: A Textbook of Cardiovascular Medicine, 6th ed. Philadelphia, WB Saunders, 2001, p 89.
5. Moss AJ: Measurement of the QT interval and the risk associated with QTc interval prolongation: A review. Am J Cardiol 1993;72:23B.
6. Day CP, McComb JM, Campbell RWF: QT dispersion: An indicator of arrhythmia risk in patients with long QT intervals. Br Heart J 1990;63:342.
7. Franz MR, Zabel M: Electrophysiological basis of QT dispersion measurements. Prog Cardiovasc Dis 2000;47:311.
8. Perkiomaki JS, Koistinen J, Yli-Mayry S, et al: Dispersion of QT interval in patients with and without susceptibility to ventricular tachyarrhythmias after previous myocardial infarction. J Am Coll Cardiol 1995;26:174.
9. Schwartz PJ, Moss AJ, Vincent GM, Crampton RS: Diagnostic criteria for the long QT syndrome: An update. Circulation 1993;88:782.
10. The Sudden Death Arrhythmia Foundation web page: Available at http://www.sads.org.

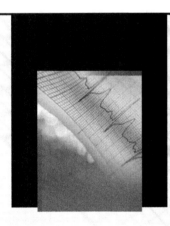

Chapter 48

Congenital Heart Disease

Renee Yvette Friday, Pamela A. Ross, and Nancy L. McDaniel

Clinical Features

Congenital heart disease (CHD) is defined as a structural or functional anomaly of the heart or great vessels; such an anomaly is present in nearly 1 in every 100 infants born (1% of all births).[1-3] Early identification of the infant with serious or life-threatening heart disease is essential for optimal outcome. The evaluation of neonates should focus on the three cardinal signs of neonatal cardiovascular distress: cyanosis, decreased systemic perfusion, and tachypnea.

The electrocardiogram (ECG) provides an evaluation of the electrical characteristics of the heart and is but one of the cardiovascular tests obtained in the evaluation and diagnosis of CHD; unfortunately, it is not a very specific diagnostic procedure for the presence of CHD.[1,3] Unless a dysrhythmia is present, an ECG is usually of limited value in making a specific diagnosis of a congenital heart lesion at birth.

Electrocardiographic Manifestations

The most important point to be made about the ECG in patients with CHD is that it will not make the diagnosis.[1-3] The ECG lacks sensitivity and specificity necessary for the identification of the complex anatomic and hemodynamic characteristics of various CHD lesions. The role of the ECG is one of providing a parameter to follow changes in the degree and progression of cardiac flow obstruction and atrial or ventricular hypertrophy, and the development of dysrhythmias associated with the congenital lesion. It is important to

have a systematic, step-by-step means of interpreting ECGs and a familiarity with changes that are age dependent. The Electrocardiographic Highlights Box lists common CHD lesions and their associated ECG findings.

Normal electrocardiograms in the presence of congenital heart disease

CHD can exist in the presence of a normal ECG[1-3] (Table 48-1).

Patent ductus arteriosus (PDA) occurs in 5% to 10% of cases of CHD and has a female-to-male predominance of 3:1. The physiologic consequence is left-to-right shunting from the aorta to the pulmonary artery, except when pulmonary hypertension exists. Patients are typically asymptomatic, and the most common finding in physical examination is a continuous murmur. Small infants may have signs of pulmonary congestion. Although PDA can result in a normal ECG, the typical finding is one of left ventricular hypertrophy (LVH) with tall R wave in lead V_6[1-3] (Fig. 48-1).

Abnormal electrocardiograms in the presence of congenital heart disease

Right Ventricular Hypertrophy. Right ventricular hypertrophy (RVH) is the most common abnormality in young patients with CHD. It is present in pulmonary stenosis, Tetralogy of Fallot, transposition of the great arteries, and in ventricular septal defects (VSDs) with pulmonary stenosis or pulmonary hypertension. It is often difficult to distinguish from normal

ELECTROCARDIOGRAPHIC HIGHLIGHTS

Congenital Heart Defect	Axis	LAA	RAA	RAD	LAD	RVH	LVH	RsR' (in Lead V1)	T wave
Atrial septal defect	+95 to +170		+	+		+		+	
Ventricular septal defect						+	+		
Patent ductus arteriosus						+			
Atrioventricular canal defect	−30 to −150	+/−	+/−		+	+	+		
Aortic stenosis							+		+ Inversion
Pulmonary stenosis				+		+			
Coarctation of the aorta						+ Newborn	+ Adults		
Hypertrophic cardiomyopathy							++		+ Inversion
Tetralogy of Fallot				+		+			
Transposition of the great arteries				+		+			
Tricuspid atresia	0 to −180		+		+		+		
Pulmonary valve atresia	+30 to +90						+		
Hypoplastic left heart syndrome	+90 to +120					+			

LAA, left atrial abnormality; LAD, left axis deviation; LVH, left ventricular hypertrophy; RAA, right atrial abnormality; RAD, right axis deviation; RVH, right ventricular

48-1 • CONGENITAL HEART DEFECTS WITH NORMAL ELECTROCARDIOGRAMS

Patent ductus arteriosus
Mild valvular pulmonary stenosis
Moderate valvular pulmonary stenosis (10%)
Coarctation of the aorta (20%)
d-Transposition of the great arteries
Atrial septal defect
Ventricular septal defect

48-2 • CONGENITAL HEART DEFECTS WITH POSSIBLE RIGHT VENTRICULAR HYPERTROPHY

Large ventricular septal defect (increased pulmonary vascular resistance)
Tetralogy of Fallot
Pulmonary stenosis
Coarctation of the aorta (newborn)
d-Transposition of the great arteries
Pulmonary valve atresia
Atrioventricular canal defect
Hypoplastic left heart syndrome
Atrial septal defect

in the neonate but becomes more apparent in the older infant and child. The most useful diagnostic feature is the lack of normal regression of the right ventricular forces in lead V_1[3] (Table 48-2).

Pulmonary stenosis is a form of right ventricular outflow tract obstruction that can be valvular, subvalvular, supravalvular, or peripheral. Mild to moderate stenosis produces few or no symptoms. However, severe stenosis may produce cyanosis as a result of right-to-left shunting at the atrial level through a patent foramen ovale or atrial septal defect (ASD). On physical examination, a systolic ejection murmur may be heard. The ECG may be normal or may show right axis deviation and RVH in cases of mild pulmonary stenosis. In moderate pulmonary stenosis, a normal ECG is rare. The axis is normal with tall R waves of RVH in the right precordial leads (V_1). In cases of severe pulmonary stenosis, there are tall R waves in lead V_1 with negative or upright T waves. There may be right atrial abnormality (RAA) from hypertrophy resulting in peaked P waves in lead II[2,3] (Figs. 48-2 and 48-3).

Tetralogy of Fallot consists of VSD, pulmonary stenosis, aortic override of the interventricular septum, and RVH; it represents 10% of congenital heart lesions. The degree of right-to-left shunting depends on the degree of pulmonary outflow obstruction resulting in a variable clinical condition.

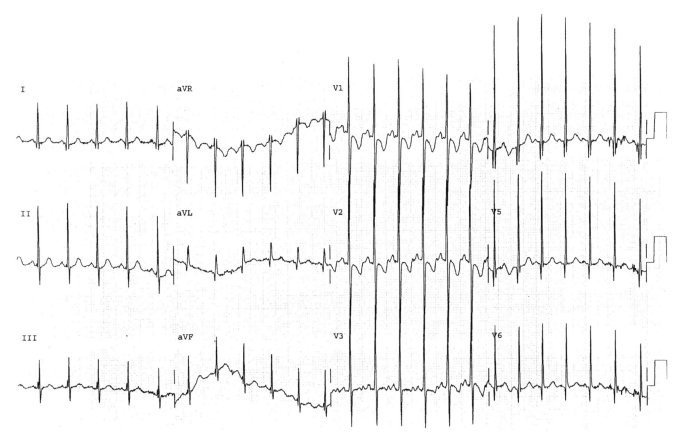

FIGURE 48-1 • Patent ductus arteriosus (PDA). This ECG from a 23-month-old demonstrates findings of mild right atrial abnormality, right ventricular hypertrophy (tall R wave in lead V_1), and left ventricular hypertrophy with a deep S wave in leads V_1 and V_2 and tall R waves in leads V_5 and V_6. This ECG is suggestive of left-to-right shunt lesion in an infant. PDA or ventricular septal defect would be the likely diagnosis.

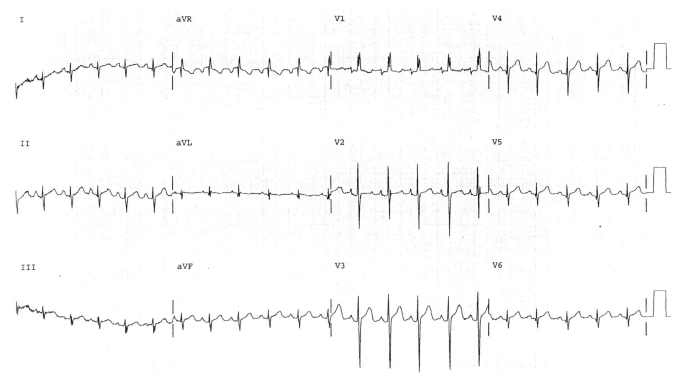

FIGURE 48-2 • **Pulmonary stenosis.** This ECG from a 19-month-old demonstrates a QRS axis that is more rightward than expected. Lead V$_1$ demonstrates the rSR′ pattern.

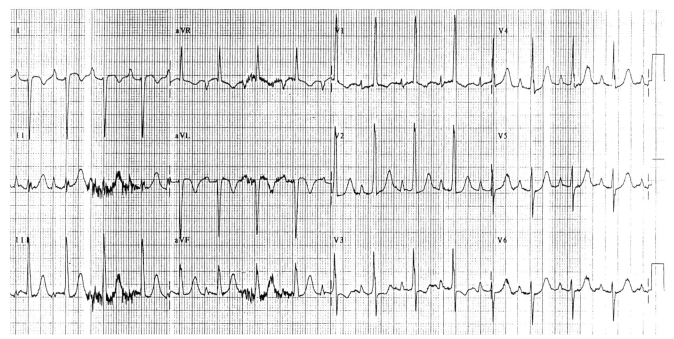

FIGURE 48-3 • **Pulmonary stenosis.** This ECG from an 11-year-old demonstrates right axis deviation, right atrial abnormality, and marked right ventricular hypertrophy. Note the very tall R wave in leads V$_1$ and V$_2$ and deep S waves in leads V$_5$ and V$_6$. There is first degree atrioventricular block (PR prolongation) and left atrial abnormality as well.

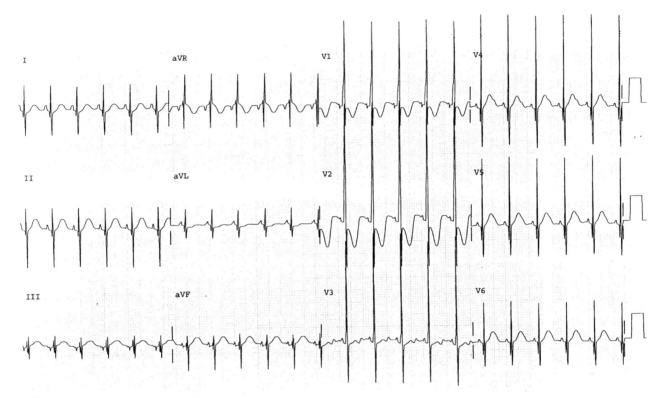

FIGURE 48-4 · Tetralogy of Fallot. This ECG from a 4-month-old demonstrates extreme axis deviation and significant right ventricular hypertrophy (tall R wave in leads V_1 and V_2, deep S waves in leads V_5 and V_6). In addition, there is a tall R wave in lead V_5, suggesting left ventricular hypertrophy as well.

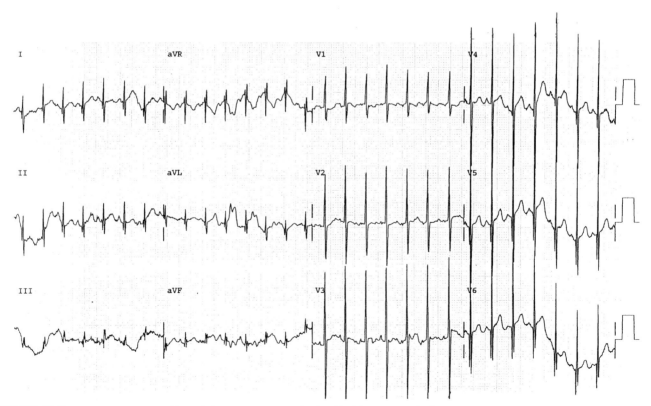

FIGURE 48-5 · Tetralogy of Fallot. This ECG demonstrates a normal axis with right (RVH) and left ventricular hypertrophy. The RVH is not as striking because the child was only 8 weeks old, and right ventricular forces are prominent in infants.

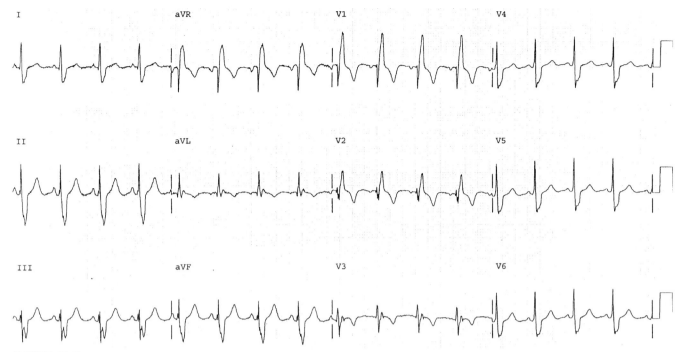

FIGURE 48-6 • **Tetralogy of Fallot (TOF).** This ECG from an adult with repaired TOF shows normal sinus rhythm with a short PR interval, left axis deviation, and bifascicular block (right bundle branch block and left anterior fascicular block).

The ECG looks similar to any normal ECG seen in a newborn. There is RVH and right axis deviation. The RVH is rarely extreme and thus may be considered normal for age. If the pulmonary stenosis is mild to moderate, there may be significant right-to-left shunt and LVH on the ECG. Right bundle branch block (RBBB) is common after surgical repair[1,2] (Figs. 48-4 through 48-6).

Transposition of the great arteries consists of the aorta arising from the right ventricle and the pulmonary artery arising off of the left ventricle, occasionally with associated VSD, ASD, and PDA. As a result, the right ventricle supplies the systemic circulation and the left ventricle supplies the pulmonary circulation, with unoxygenated blood supplying the body and oxygenated blood being supplied to the pulmonary circulation. It represents 5% of congenital heart lesions and has a male-to-female predominance of 3:1. The atrial and ventricular masses are normal and the position of the heart in the thorax is normal. The ECG is usually normal for age in the first days of life, with right axis deviation. There can be RVH or combined ventricular hypertrophy, although these findings vary considerably depending on age and anatomic and physiologic factors[1] (Fig. 48-7).

Ventricular septal defects are congenital lesions or holes in the ventricular septum. VSD represents 20% of CHD lesions. The physiologic results of these lesions are based on defect size, degree of left-to-right shunting of blood, and pulmonary vascular resistance, which increase the volume of blood circulating through the lungs. Small VSDs usually present with no symptoms, although moderate and large VSDs may have symptoms of pulmonary congestion. On physical examination, a loud holosystolic murmur and diastolic rumble of the apex may be heard.[1-3]

The ECG is usually normal in small VSDs, although an RSR′ can appear in lead V_1. The RSR′ pattern is sometimes called *incomplete bundle branch block* and is found in 5% to 10% of normal 5-year-olds. In the case of moderate-sized VSDs, there may be mild or moderate elevation of right ventricular pressure, resulting in RVH, and seen on ECG in lead V_1 as an rsR′ pattern with increasing R′ amplitude. LVH is a prominent feature of moderate to large VSDs with significant right-to-left shunt and pulmonary hypertension (Figs. 48-8 and 48-9).

Hypoplastic left heart syndrome is a complex congenital heart lesion that consists of underdevelopment of the left heart structures, including the mitral valve, left ventricle, aortic valve, and ascending aorta. It occurs in 7% of congenital heart lesions and has a male-to-female predominance of 2:1. Systemic circulation and cardiac output depend on right-to-left flow provided by the ductus arteriosus. If the ductus arteriosus closes, circulatory collapse results in poor perfusion, cyanosis, and death. The ECG in this case is nondiagnostic, showing RVH. The QRS axis is +90 to +210 degrees. There may also be peaked P waves, indicating RAA. The left precordial leads usually display a paucity of left ventricular forces. There may be diffuse ST segment abnormalities, which may reflect coronary insufficiency secondary to inadequate retrograde aortic blood flow[1,3] (Fig. 48-10).

Left Ventricular Hypertrophy. LVH is seen in patients with CHD with small right ventricles (tricuspid atresia, pulmonary atresia with intact ventricular septum) and those with left ventricular outflow tract obstruction (aortic stenosis, coarctation of the aorta, hypertrophic cardiomyopathy). It is also common in adolescent boys, even in the absence of systemic hypertension. The ECG features are a tall R wave in the left precordial leads (V_5 and V_6), deep S waves in lead V_1, and tall R waves in the inferior leads (II, III and aVF)[1-3] (Table 48-3, Figs. 48-11 and 48-12).

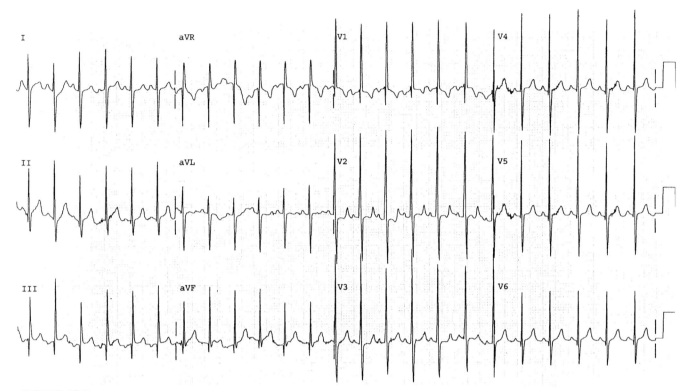

FIGURE 48-7 · **Transposition of the great arteries.** This ECG from a 5-month-old demonstrates features of both left and right ventricular hypertrophy.

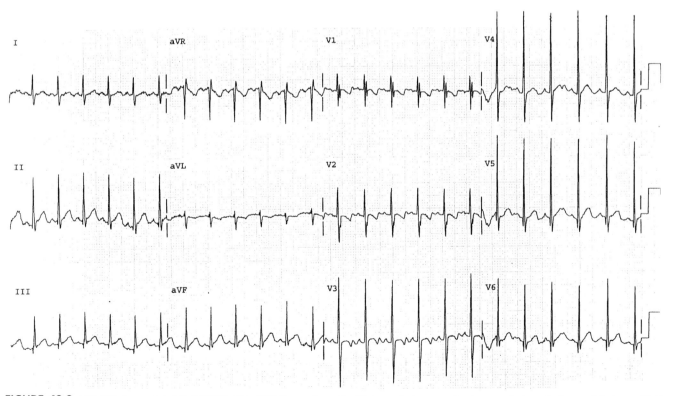

FIGURE 48-8 · **Ventricular septal defect (VSD).** This ECG from a 9-month-old demonstrates normal axis, normal sinus rhythm, and features of left ventricular hypertrophy (tall R waves in leads V_5 and V_6). Note the RSr′ in lead V_1, with the first deflection (R) being taller than the second (r). This can be seen in normal children and in small VSDs. The pattern is also called incomplete right bundle branch block or terminal conduction delay.

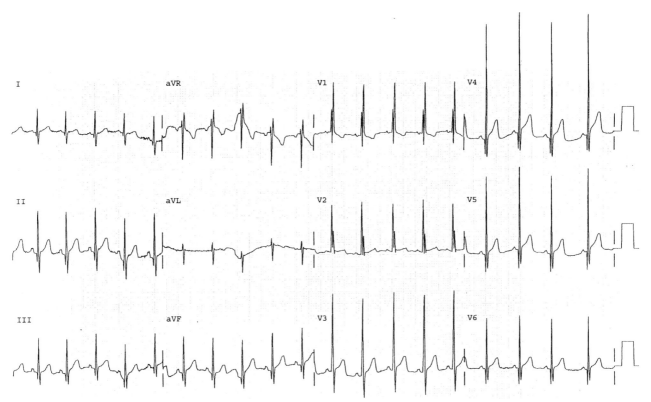

FIGURE 48-9 · Ventricular septal defect. This ECG from an 8-month-old demonstrates normal axis and biventricular hypertrophy. Note the rSR′ pattern, with the first deflection (r) being smaller than the second positive deflection (R).

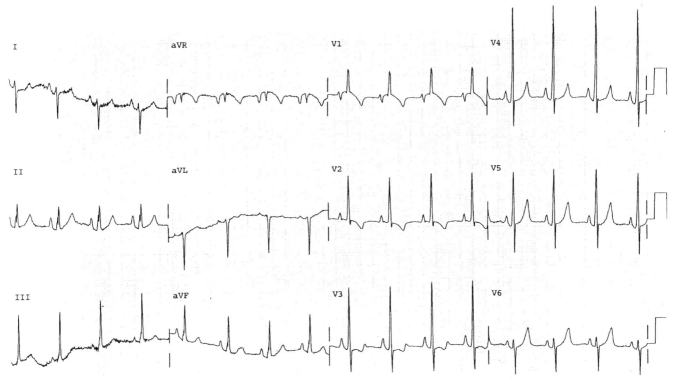

FIGURE 48-10 · Hypoplastic left heart syndrome. This ECG from a 3-year-old demonstrates right axis deviation, right atrial abnormality (tall p waves in lead II), and right ventricular hypertrophy. There is abnormal R wave progression with decreased left ventricular forces in lead V_6.

48-3 • CONGENITAL HEART LESIONS WITH LEFT VENTRICULAR HYPERTROPHY

Tricuspid atresia
Moderate to large ventricular septal defect and atrioventricular
canal defects
Patent ductus arteriosus (older child)
Coarctation of the aorta
Pulmonary atresia with intact ventricular septum
Aortic stenosis
Hypertrophic obstructive cardiomyopathy

Tricuspid atresia is agenesis of the tricuspid valve and represents 2% of cases of CHD. Associated defects may include ASDs, small right ventricle, malposition of the great arteries, VSDs, and pulmonary stenosis. Cyanosis may be mild to severe, depending on the relation of great arteries and degree of pulmonary stenosis. There is always a right-to-left shunt at the atrial level. On physical examination, there may be a holosystolic murmur of a VSD or a systolic ejection murmur of pulmonary stenosis. Occasionally there may be excessive pulmonary blood flow and congestive heart failure. The ECG shows a left or extreme QRS axis deviation, with RAA and LVH. In tricuspid atresia, left axis deviation is caused by early right ventricular activation with a relative delay, primarily on the base of the left ventricle.[3]

Pulmonary atresia with intact ventricular septum consists of an underdeveloped right ventricle and an imperforate pulmonary valve, and comprises 1% of congenital heart defects. The most common physiologic result is severe cyanosis in the newborn period. All have right-to-left shunts at the atrial level. Pulmonary blood flow is supplied by the PDA and circulatory collapse occurs once the ductus closes.

The ECG shows normal sinus rhythm and may show a lack of right ventricular forces and LVH. There may also be RAAs and ST segment abnormalities (Fig. 48-13).

Aortic stenosis is a congenital heart defect in which left ventricular output is obstructed by a narrowed aortic valve. The level of the obstruction may be valvular, subvalvular, or supravalvular. Valvular stenosis is the most common and is most commonly secondary to a bicuspid valve. It represents 5% of cases of CHD, with a male-to-female predominance of 4:1. Symptoms occur in those with moderate to severe stenosis, and include exercise intolerance, chest pain, syncope, and congestive heart failure. The classic ECG findings are similar in all cases of left-sided outflow tract obstructive lesions. There is LVH with small Q waves, tall R waves, and negative T waves in lateral precordial leads (V_5 and V_6) when the stenosis worsens[1-3] (Fig. 48-14).

Coarctation of the aorta consists of a narrowed area of the aortic arch at the level of the ductus arteriosus (or ligamentum), represents 8% of congenital heart lesions, and has a male-to-female predominance of 2:1. Physiologically there is an obstruction to left ventricular systemic cardiac output with upper body hypertension. LVH, a compensatory mechanism that develops when there is obstruction of cardiac output, may develop over time. Patients are usually asymptomatic but can present with cardiovascular collapse and shock. Interestingly, the ECG is usually normal. Infants may have RVH. The ECG in older children reflects the effects of long-standing left ventricular pressure overload represented by LVH (tall R waves in lead V_6 and deep S waves in the right precordial leads). ST segment and T wave depression may indicate the presence of aortic valve or subvalve stenosis, which is commonly associated. Associated intracardiac lesions also affect the ECG findings, adding to the difficulty of making a specific diagnosis[1-3] (Fig. 48-15).

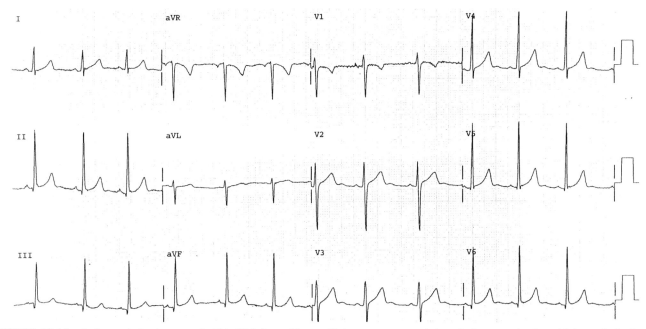

FIGURE 48-11 · Left ventricular hypertrophy. This ECG from a 13-year-old demonstrates normal sinus rhythm, normal axis, and left ventricular forces at the upper limits of normal. In addition, note the ST segment elevation in all of the leads where the T wave is positive. This is a condition called *J point elevation* or *early repolarization phenomenon.* This is a normal variant in childhood.

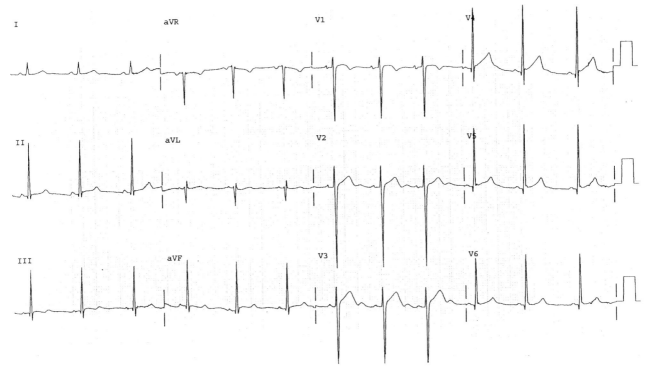

FIGURE 48-12 · Left ventricular hypertrophy (LVH). This ECG from a 13-year-old demonstrates LVH. Note the deep S waves in lead V_2 and prominent R waves in leads V_4 through V_6.

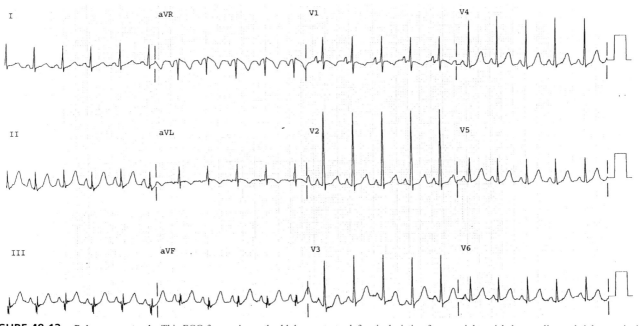

FIGURE 48-13 · Pulmonary atresia. This ECG from a 4-month-old demonstrates left axis deviation for age, right atrial abnormality, and right ventricular hypertrophy (note the R wave in lead V_2).

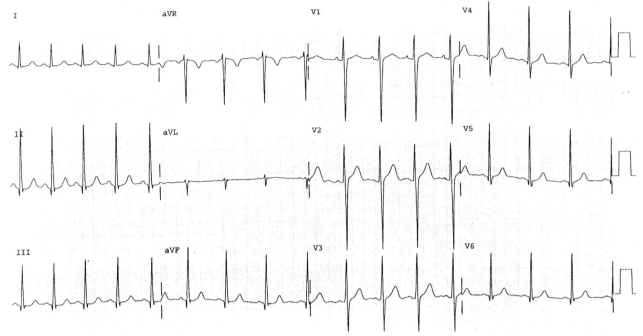

FIGURE 48-14 · **Aortic stenosis.** This ECG from an 11-year-old demonstrates left ventricular hypertrophy (deep S wave in lead V_2).

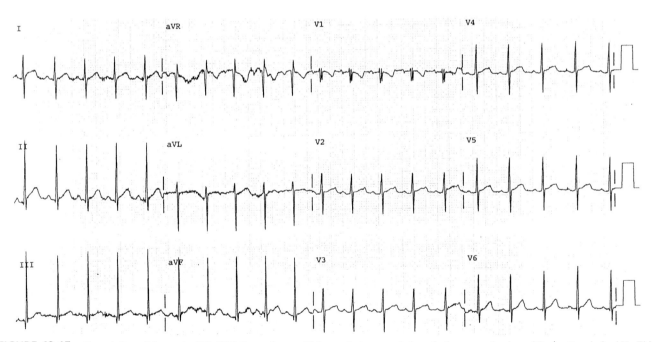

FIGURE 48-15 · **Coarctation of the aorta.** This ECG from a 2-year-old demonstrates normal sinus rhythm, normal axis, and Rsr′ pattern in lead V_1. This child has bicuspid aortic valve and had coarctation of aorta repair in infancy.

Hypertrophic cardiomyopathy is a complex left ventricular outflow tract obstructive lesion that is progressive and clinically asymptomatic for a long period. Unfortunately, the first appearance of clinical symptoms may be the last, with sudden death being the initial indicator of disease. Only in cases of significant outflow tract obstruction is a systolic murmur present. The ECG findings are nonspecific, with LVH, ST segment alterations with ventricular strain patterns, abnormal Q waves, and diminished R waves in the right precordial leads. Unfortunately, the ECG pattern does not reliably discriminate between patients with or without obstruction to left ventricular outflow or those at risk for sudden death; however, those patients with an LVH pattern on ECG more commonly show greater wall thickening on echocardiography[3] (Fig. 48-16).

Right Axis Deviation. Right axis deviation is present when the QRS axis is more positive (rightward) than normal for age[1-3] (Table 48-4).

Atrial septal defect is a congenital heart defect that consists of a hole in the atrial septum between the left and right atria; it represents 5% to 10% of congenital lesions and has a female-to-male predominance of 2:1. The primary physiologic consequence is left-to-right shunting with volume overload of the right atrium, right ventricle, and pulmonary artery. The patient is usually asymptomatic, and a nonspecific systolic ejection murmur of increased pulmonary blood flow and a fixed split second heart sound may be the only findings on physical examination. The ECG may show normal sinus rhythm, although a junctional or supraventricular tachycardia, such as atrial flutter, can be seen. There may be right axis deviation of the QRS axis, + 95 to +170 degrees. P wave changes may suggest RAA or right atrial hypertrophy. An rsR′ or incomplete RBBB pattern in lead V_1 is usually seen and

48-4 • CONGENITAL HEART DEFECTS WITH RIGHT AXIS DEVIATION
Atrial septal defect
Tetralogy of Fallot
Coarctation of the aorta (newborn)
d-Transposition of the great arteries
Pulmonary stenosis

indicates right ventricular volume overload. The QRS duration is normal[1-3] (Figs. 48-17 and 48-18).

Left Axis Deviation. Left axis deviation is present when the QRS axis is more leftward than the normal range (Table 48-5). As previously mentioned, isolated left axis deviation has no clinical significance in asymptomatic patients (Fig. 48-19).

Extreme Axis Deviation. Superior axis deviation is present when the QRS axis is between +180 and +240 degrees, with a negative R wave in both leads I and aVF commonly seen in partial or complete atrioventricular canal defects (AVC). AVC is a congenital heart defect derived from failure of endocardial cushion development. These defects represent 2% of cases of CHD, with 30% of AVCs occurring in children with trisomy 21. The common physiologic result is left-to-right shunting at the atrial or ventricular septal levels with right-sided volume overload and pulmonary congestion. Clinical symptoms are variable; patients may present with failure to thrive and congestive heart failure symptoms resulting from pulmonary overcirculation. The murmur is often soft and nonspecific. The classic ECG demonstrates an extreme QRS axis. Right ventricular volume overload results in RVH and some variation of rsR′, as previously described, in the right precordial chest leads. Patients with mitral valve insufficiency or

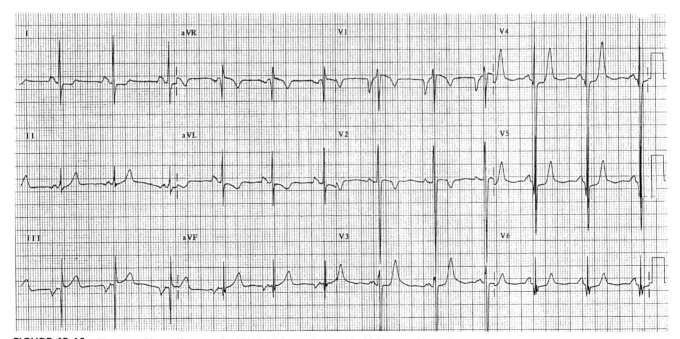

FIGURE 48-16 • **Hypertrophic cardiomyopathy.** This ECG from a 6-year-old with hypertrophic cardiomyopathy demonstrates left ventricular hypertrophy and left atrial abnormality. Note the very deep narrow Q wave in lead III that is associated with cardiac hypertrophy. The P axis is also abnormal, suggesting a low atrial pacemaker.

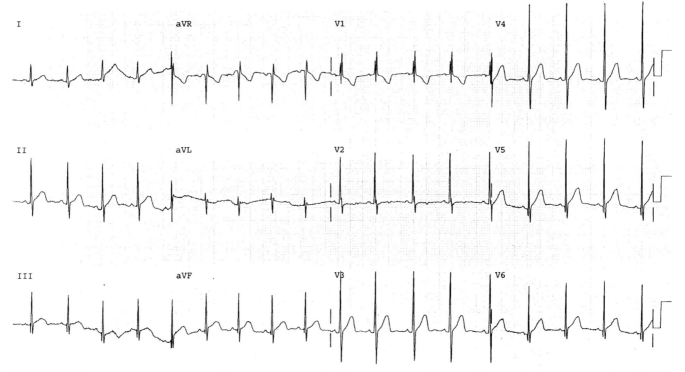

FIGURE 48-17 · **Atrial septal defect (ASD).** This ECG from a 21-month-old demonstrates the rSR′ pattern of right ventricular hypertrophy. This child could have an ASD or could have normal cardiac anatomy.

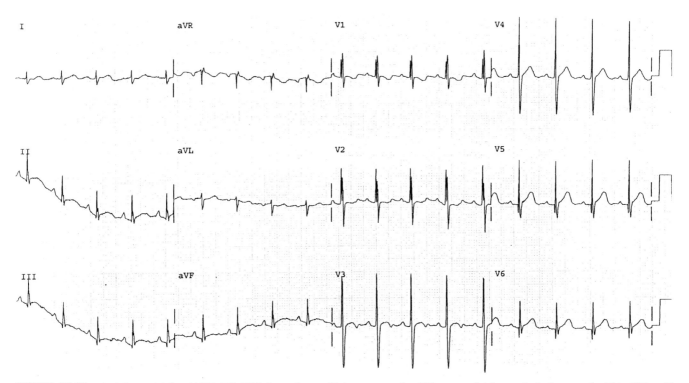

FIGURE 48-18 · **Atrial septal defect (ASD).** This ECG from a 3-year-old demonstrates the rSR′ pattern of right ventricular hypertrophy. This child could have an ASD or could have normal cardiac anatomy.

	48-5 • CONGENITAL HEART DEFECTS WITH POSSIBLE LEFT AXIS DEVIATION

Complete atrioventricular canal defect
Ventricular septal defect (large)
Tricuspid atresia
d-Transposition of the great arteries

large left-to-right shunts often have additional evidence of LVH (Fig. 48-20).

Right Atrial Abnormality.   Lesions that result in large left-to-right shunts and volume overload of the right atrium can result in RAA (Table 48-6). Determination of RAA is usually based on increased P wave voltage of greater than 2.5 mV or a P wave duration greater than 100 msec. Effects of atrial

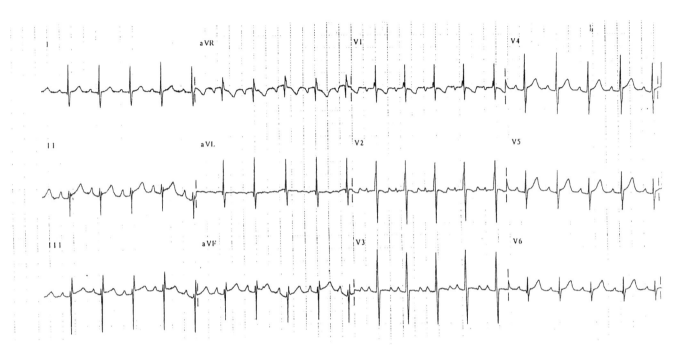

FIGURE 48-19 · **Left axis deviation (LAD).** This ECG from a normal 13-month-old demonstrates LAD. There is borderline right atrial abnormality. The P wave in lead V_1 has a slow terminal portion, suggesting left atrial abnormality as well. There is no ventricular hypertrophy.

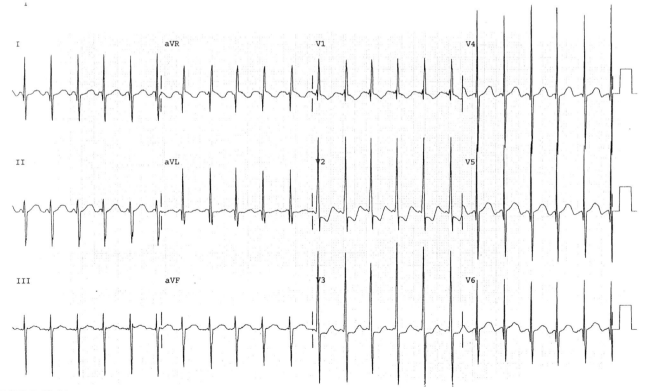

FIGURE 48-20 · **Possible atrioventricular canal defect.** This ECG from a 6-week-old demonstrates an abnormal axis and biventricular hypertrophy. This pattern is suspect for an atrioventricular canal defect.

48-6 • CONGENITAL HEART DEFECTS WITH RIGHT ATRIAL ABNORMALITY

Atrial septal defect
Complete atrioventricular canal defect
Tricuspid atresia
Ebstein's anomaly
Severe pulmonary stenosis

48-7 • CONGENITAL HEART DEFECTS WITH LEFT ATRIAL ABNORMALITY

Complete atrioventricular canal defect
Mitral valve disease (stenosis or insufficiency)
Left heart obstruction

enlargement may manifest in the early (right) or the late (left) portion of the P wave. Increased voltage in leads II, V_1, and V_2 indicates RAA (Fig. 48-21).

Left Atrial Abnormality. Left atrial abnormality occurs with significant right-to-left and left-to-right shunts, mitral valve insufficiency or stenosis, and left ventricular outflow tract obstruction with left ventricular failure (Table 48-7, Fig. 48-21).

Right Bundle Branch Block. One difficulty in determining the CHD cause of RBBB is distinguishing between variants of the normal involution of right ventricular forces (especially in lead V_1) and mild degrees of RVH produced by right ventricular

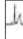

48-8 • CONGENITAL HEART DEFECTS WITH INCOMPLETE RIGHT BUNDLE BRANCH BLOCK (rsR' OR RSR')

Atrial septal defects
Complete atrioventricular canal defect
Small ventricular septal defect
Tetralogy of Fallot (after repair)

volume overload conditions such as ASDs. The RSR' pattern associated with RBBB is present in 5% to 10% of normal 5-year-olds, and is also similar to the pattern seen in patients with ASDs. This finding is often referred to as an incomplete RBBB pattern, but of shorter duration. If the second positive deflection, the R', is taller than the R (rsR'), it is more likely to represent actual RVH[1-3] (Table 48-8).

References

1. Gutgesell H, Atkins D, Barst R, et al: Cardiovascular monitoring of children and adolescents receiving psychotropic drugs. Circulation 1999;99:979–982.
2. Davignnon A: ECG standards for children. Pediatr Cardiol 1979/80; 1:133–152.
3. Van Hare GF, Dubin A: The normal electrocardiogram. In Allen H, Gutgesell H, Clarke E, Driscoll D (eds): Moss and Adam's Heart Disease in Infants, Children, and Adolescents: Including the Fetus and Young Adult, 6th ed. Philadelphia, Lippincott Williams & Wilkins, 2001.

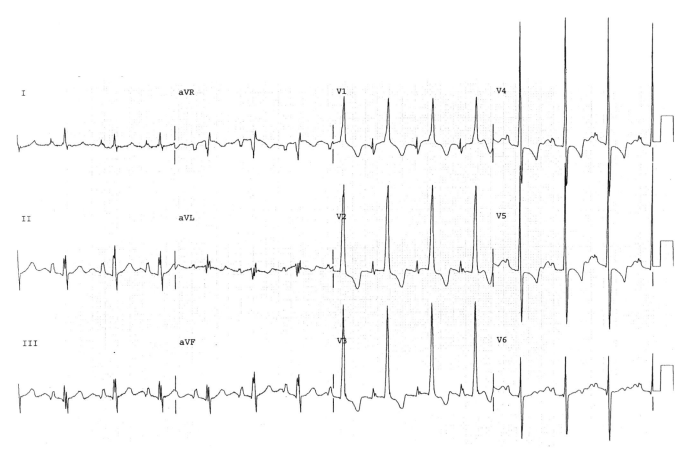

FIGURE 48-21 • **Biatrial abnormality.** This ECG from a 10-year-old demonstrates many abnormal features, including sinus rhythm with prolonged PR interval, intraventricular conduction delay, biventricular hypertrophy and marked right and left atrial enlargement. The QT is mildly prolonged, likely associated with the conduction delay.

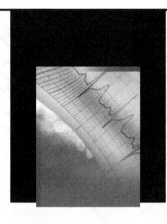

TOXICOLOGY AND SYSTEMIC DISEASE

Chapter 49
Toxicology Section: Introduction

Theodore C. Chan

Toxicologic, medication- and drug-induced changes and abnormalities on the 12-lead electrocardiogram (ECG) are common. Discussion of all medications and drugs that can cause cardiac and ECG abnormalities is beyond the scope of this text. Alternatively, this section focuses on the most important cardioactive agents that cause significant ECG abnormalities, regardless of whether those changes occur at therapeutic or toxic levels of the agent.

Accordingly, this section is organized into a number of chapters based on cardiac effect. Chapters 50, 51, 52, and 53 discuss those agents with significant direct cardioactive effects, and include digitalis compounds, beta-blocking adrenergic agents, calcium channel antagonists, and other cardioactive agents such as clonidine and other medications. Chapters 54, 55, and 56 discuss other agents that affect the cardiac cycle,

and in particular, the myocyte ion channels, that can result in electrocardiographic changes. These drugs include tricyclic antidepressants, antipsychotic agents, and other sodium channel blockers. Chapter 57 covers the electrocardiographic findings associated with sympathomimetic agents, including cocaine.

Many of these agents act on the myocyte ion channels that control depolarization and repolarization across the cardiac cell membrane (Figure 49-1). In its resting state, the myocyte membrane is impermeable to sodium (Na^+), and Na^+ ions are actively pumped out of the cell to maintain a negative transmembrane electric potential (phase 4 of the cardiac action potential). Depolarization occurs with the rapid opening of Na^+ channels and the subsequent massive Na^+ influx (phase 0). The peak of the action potential is marked by the closure of the Na^+ channels and activation of potassium (K^+) and calcium (Ca^+)

49-1 • TOXICOLOGIC DIFFERENTIAL DIAGNOSIS OF A PROLONGED QT INTERVAL

Antidysrhythmics:	Type Ia	Type Ic	Type III	
	Disopyramide	Encainide	Amiodarone	
	Procainamide	Flecainide	Bretylium	
	Quinidine	Propafenone	Sotalol	
		Moricizine	Dofetilide	
			Ibutilide	
Calcium channel antagonists:	Bepridil, isradipine, nicardipine			
Sympathomimetics:	Cocaine			
Neurologic agents:	Carbamazepine, fosphenytoin, sumatriptan, zolmitriptan, naratriptan			
Anti-infective agents:	Some fluoroquinolones (gatifloxacin, sparfloxacin, moxifloxacin), erythromycin, clarithromycin, pentamidine, amantadine, tetracyclines, foscarnet, quinine, chloroquine			
Psychopharmacologic agents:	Phenothiazines	Butyrophenones	Others	Antidepressants
	Chlorpromazine	Droperidol	Risperidone	Tricyclic antidepressants
	Mesoridazine	Haloperidol	Quetiapine	Fluoxetine
	Thioridazine		Ziprasidone	Sertraline
				Venlafaxine
Antihistamines:	Diphenhydramine			
Organophosphates				
Opioids:	Levo-α-acetyl methadyl (LAAM), methadone			
Gastrointestinal medications:	Cisapride, ipecac, octreotide, dolasetron			
Miscellaneous:	Arsenic, tacrolimus, tamoxifen, probucol, tizanidine, salmeterol			

Electrolyte flux

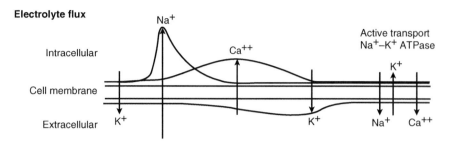

Action potential

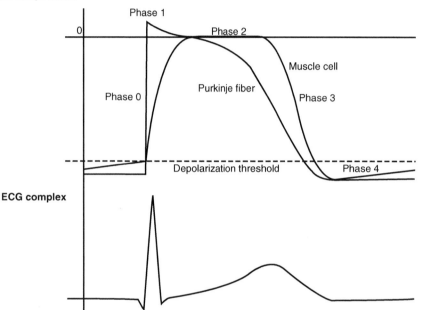

FIGURE 49-1 • Relationship of electrolyte movement across the cell membrane to the action potential and the surface ECG recording. (Adapted from Clancy C: Electrocardiographic evaluation of the poisoned patient. In Goldfrank LR, Flomenbaum NE, Levin NE. et al: Goldfrank's Toxicological Emergencies, 6th ed. Stamford, Appleton and Lange, 1998, p. 106.)

channels (phase 1). Calcium influx results in a plateau in the action potential (phase 2), followed by K⁺ efflux and a return to the negative potential (phase 3) (see Figure 49-1).

Agents that act on the various different types of ion channels alter the action potential of the cardiac cycle and the depolarization and repolarization of cardiac tissue. For example, agents that block Na⁺ channels cause a delay and slowing in phase 0 of depolarization, resulting in a wide QRS complex.

Many of these agents have multiple cardiac effects not easily categorized into single mechanisms. For example, tricyclic antidepressants can cause sodium channel blockade, adrenergic blockade, and anticholinergic effects. As a result, many agents cause similar, typical changes in the ECG. Two of the most common findings associated with these agents include QT prolongation and wide-complex tachycardia. Accordingly, this introduction provides a toxicologic differential diagnosis for both of these ECG findings (Tables 49-1 and 49-2).

49-2 • TOXICOLOGIC DIFFERENTIAL DIAGNOSIS OF A WIDE-COMPLEX TACHYCARDIA

Antidysrhythmics:	**Type IA**	**Type IC**
	Disopyramide	Encainide
	Procainamide	Flecainide
	Quinidine	Propafenone
		Moricizine
Tricyclic antidepressants		
Antipsychotics:	Piperidine phenothiazines	
	Mesoridazine	
	Thioridazine	
Sympathomimetics:	Cocaine	
Beta-adrenergic blocking agents:	Acebutolol, propranolol	
Opioids:	Propoxyphene	
Antimalarials:	Quinine, chloroquine	
Anticonvulsants:	Carbamazepine	
Antihistamines:	Diphenhydramine	
Muscle relaxants:	Cyclobenzaprine	

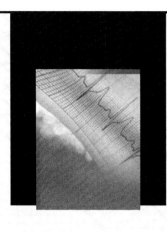

Chapter 50

Digitalis

Christopher P. Holstege and Mark A. Kirk

Clinical Features

Digitalis and other cardiac glycosides occur naturally in plants such as foxglove, lily of the valley, oleander, red squill, and hellebore. Therapeutically, digitalis derivatives are used to slow conduction through the atrioventricular (AV) node (such as in patients with supraventricular tachydysrhythmias) or increase myocardial contractility and inotropy (such as in patients with congestive heart failure). Digoxin is the major cardiac glycoside used for medicinal purposes, although its use has been decreasing as newer agents have been developed.

The incidence of digoxin toxicity in patients on the medication has been reported to range from 2% to 23% in hospitalized patients.[1–3] In 2001, the American Association of Poison Centers reported 2977 cardiac glycoside exposures. Of these, 652 (22%) were considered to have moderate to major effects, with 13 deaths (<1%) reported.[4]

Identification of digitalis toxicity is a challenge because the clinical presentation is often subtle and varies depending on whether the toxicity is due to a single acute ingestion or chronic toxicity. Moreover, electrolyte disturbances such as hypokalemia or hypomagnesemia (such as from concomitant diuretic use) can exacerbate the cardiotoxicity associated with digitalis.

In acute poisonings, nausea, vomiting, and cardiotoxicity are most prominent. Diagnosing chronic digitalis toxicity is more difficult because the presentation may mimic common illnesses, such as influenza or gastroenteritis, or have been precipitated by another clinical illness. Common symptoms include fatigue, weakness, nausea, anorexia, headache, vertigo, syncope, seizures, memory loss, confusion, disorientation, delirium, depression, and hallucinations. The most frequently reported visual disturbances are cloudy or blurred vision and loss of vision; yellow-green halos (xanthopsia) are classic, but rare.[5,6]

Cardiac glycosides act by binding specific receptor sites and inactivating the sodium–potassium adenosine triphosphatase pump (Na^+-K^+-ATPase).[7] This pump maintains the electrochemical membrane potential, vital to conduction tissues, by concentrating sodium extracellularly and potassium intracellularly. When the Na^+-K^+-ATPase is inhibited, the sodium–calcium exchanger removes accumulated intracellular sodium in exchange for calcium. This exchange increases sarcoplasmic calcium and is the mechanism responsible for the positive inotropic effect of digitalis. These intracellular changes also impair conduction through the AV node and simultaneously increase cardiac automaticity.[8]

Electrocardiographic Manifestations

Cardiac glycoside toxicity results from an exaggeration of its therapeutic action.

In digoxin-intoxicated patients, increased vagal tone and direct AV depression produce conduction disturbances. The decreased refractory period of the myocardium increases automaticity.[7,9] Intracellular calcium overload in digitalis-intoxicated patients causes delayed afterdepolarizations and gives rise to triggered dysrhythmias.[7] The end result is an increased propensity toward automaticity accompanied by slowed conduction through the AV node. As a result, electrocardiographic manifestations of digitalis toxicity are common, with an extremely wide variety of dysrhythmias reported.

Differentiating electrocardiographic abnormalities due to digitalis toxicity from those due to another etiology is often difficult. Patients on digitalis therapy often have numerous chronic disease processes, placing them at risk for electrolyte abnormalities and primary cardiac events. For example, it is frequent to manage a patient with acute renal failure, an elevated digoxin level, hyperkalemia, and cardiac dysrhythmia. The cardinal electrocardiographic features of digitalis toxicity are increased automaticity and ectopy combined with AV conduction block. A patient with atrial fibrillation and a seemingly "well-controlled" rate—even bradycardic—may be digitalis intoxicated.

Digitalis Effect. Digitalis at therapeutic doses has been associated with a number of electrocardiographic changes that are consistent with the presence of digitalis at therapeutic levels, but do not indicate or correlate with toxicity.

The earliest finding of "digitalis effect" is changes to the T wave, including flattening, inversion, and other abnormal waveforms. These T wave changes, in combination with ST segment depression, are frequently described as a "sagging"

ELECTROCARDIOGRAPHIC HIGHLIGHTS

"Digitalis effect" associated with therapeutic levels

- T wave changes (flattening, inversion, biphasic)
- ST segment depression (scooped appearance)
- QT interval shortening
- PR interval prolongation
- U wave

Digitalis toxicity

ECTOPIC RHYTHMS

- Atrial tachycardia with block
- Nonparoxysmal junctional tachycardia
- Premature ventricular contractions
- Ventricular tachycardia, flutter, and fibrillation
- *Bidirectional* ventricular tachycardia

DEPRESSION OF PACEMAKERS

- Sinoatrial arrest

DEPRESSION OF CONDUCTION

- Atrioventricular block
- Ectopic rhythms with depressed conduction

TRIGGERED AUTOMATICITY

- Accelerated junctional rhythms after premature ectopic impulses
- Ventricular dysrhythmias triggered by supraventricular dysrhythmias
- Junctional tachycardia triggered by ventricular tachycardia

---

or "scooped" ST segment/T wave (Fig. 50-1). This finding is most pronounced in leads with tall R waves and is a common indication of digitalis effect.

In addition, QT interval shortening can occur as a result of decreased ventricular repolarization time. Other findings associated with digitalis effect include lengthening of the PR interval as a result of increased vagal activity, and the development of, or increase in, U wave amplitude.

Premature Ventricular Contractions. As a result of increased automaticity, ectopy is a common manifestation of digitalis toxicity. Premature ventricular contractions, both unifocal and multifocal, are the most common electrocardiographic findings in adult digitalis intoxication, with bigeminy and trigeminy also reported (Fig. 50-2). Similarly, premature atrial contractions also may be seen with toxicity.

Bradydysrhythmias and Conduction Block. Because digitalis can have a suppressant effect on both impulse formation and conduction, a number of bradycardic rhythms have been reported. Sinus bradycardia from increased vagal tone, and even sinoatrial (SA) node arrest, have been reported. Variable AV conduction block, ranging from first degree to complete heart block, is common with digitalis toxicity. In fact, marked slowing of the ventricular response in a patient with atrial fibrillation on digoxin should suggest the possibility of toxicity (Fig. 50-3). Because digitalis has little effect on the bundle branches, bundle branch blocks are rare.

Tachydysrhythmias. Because of increased automaticity, digitalis can lead to a number of tachydysrhythmias. These include supraventricular tachycardias, such as paroxysmal

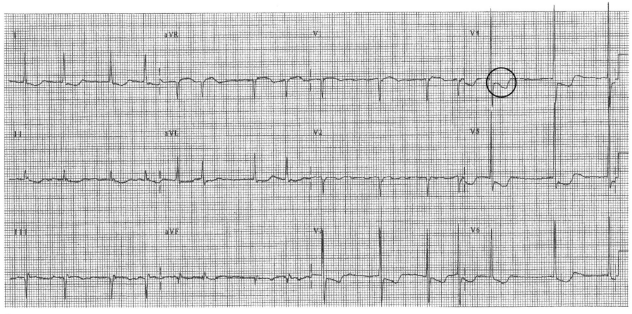

A

FIGURE 50-1 • *A,* **Digitalis effect.** Note the sagging or scooped ST segments with inverted T waves (*circle*). This finding is especially pronounced in those leads with a tall R wave.

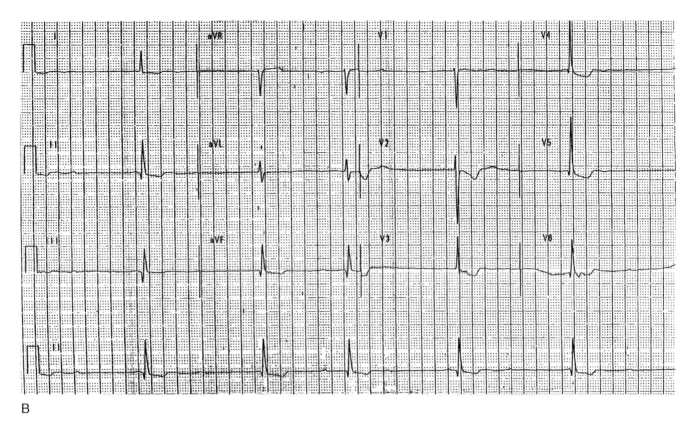

FIGURE 50-1 · *B*, **Coexistent digitalis effect and toxicity.** Digitalis effect on ST segment/T waves is noted in leads I, II, and V₃ through V₆. Also note the third degree atrioventricular block resulting in a junctional bradycardia with atrial activity.

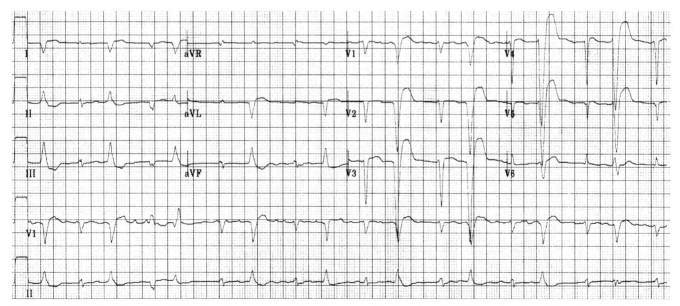

FIGURE 50-2 · **Digitalis toxicity.** Marked ventricular ectopy results in bigeminy with alternating wide QRS complexes in a digitalis-intoxicated patient.

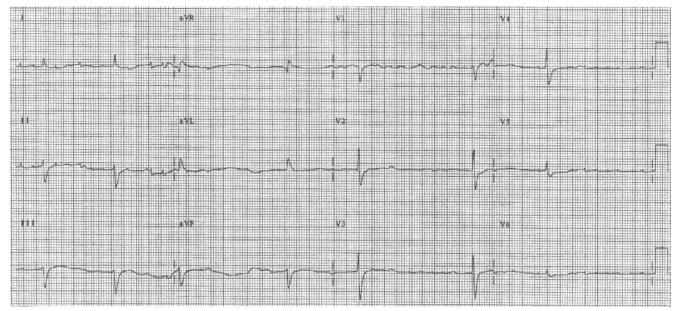

FIGURE 50-3 • **High grade atrioventricular (AV) block from digitalis toxicity.** Atrial fibrillation/flutter with AV block results in bradycardia in a digitalis-intoxicated patient.

atrial tachycardia, junctional tachycardias, and ventricular tachycardia and fibrillation. These tachydysrhythmias are often associated with variable AV block that also is a result of digitalis toxicity. Thus, classic electrocardiographic rhythms associated with toxicity include paroxysmal tachycardia with block, junctional tachycardia, ventricular tachycardia, and bidirectional ventricular tachycardia.

Paroxysmal Atrial Tachycardia with Block. Atrial tachycardia (enhanced automaticity) with variable AV block (impaired conduction) is highly suggestive, and even considered

pathognomonic for digitalis toxicity. The atrial rate usually ranges between 150 and 250 bpm. The degree of AV block varies, with second degree being the most common form (Fig. 50-4).

Junctional Tachycardia. AV junctional escape rhythms occur as a result of SA node suppression. Accelerated junctional rhythms at rates higher than 60 bpm are common with digitalis toxicity and, as with paroxysmal tachycardia with block, variable degrees of block can occur (Fig. 50-5).

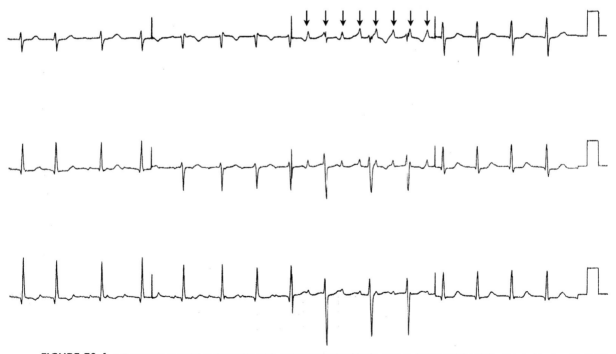

FIGURE 50-4 • **Paroxysmal atrial tachycardia with atrioventricular block.** *Arrows* denote atrial activity at a rapid rate with AV block.

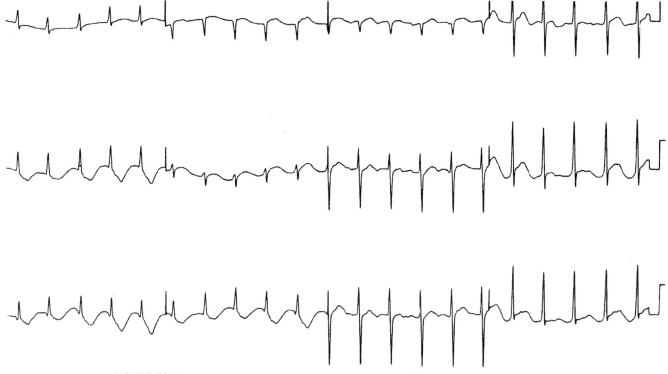

FIGURE 50-5 · **Junctional tachycardia from digitalis poisoning.** Note the accelerated junctional rate.

Ventricular Tachycardia. With increasing ectopy, ventricular rhythms, such as ventricular tachycardia, ventricular bigeminy, torsades de pointes, and even ventricular fibrillation (usually late manifestations of digitalis toxicity), can occur.

Bidirectional Ventricular Tachycardia. Bidirectional ventricular tachycardia is specific for digitalis toxicity but extremely

rare. Impulses arising from the AV junction or high ventricle are conducted through the anterior and posterior fascicles of the left bundle with beat-to-beat variation, resulting in an alternating QRS axis and morphology. These alternating QRS complexes are often narrow with a right bundle branch block morphology at rates of 90 to 160 bpm (Fig. 50-6).

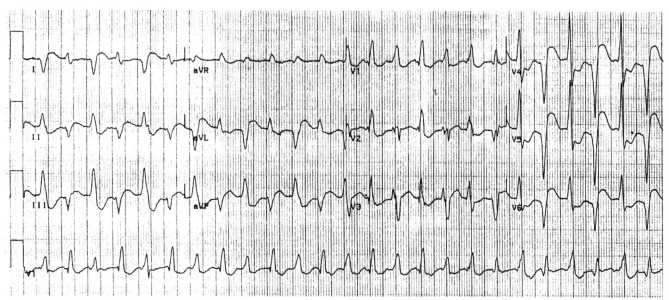

FIGURE 50-6 · **Bidirectional ventricular tachycardia in a case of severe digoxin toxicity.** Note the alternating QRS axis and right bundle branch block morphology.

ELECTROCARDIOGRAPHIC PEARLS

- The electrocardiogram can neither rule in nor rule out digitalis toxicity.
- Electrocardiographic manifestations of digitalis toxicity are common, with an extremely wide variety of dysrhythmias reported.
- Paroxysmal atrial tachycardia with variable atrioventricular (AV) block and accelerated junctional rhythm are highly suggestive of digitalis toxicity.
- Bidirectional ventricular tachycardia is specific for digitalis toxicity but extremely rare.
- Electrolyte disturbances such as hypokalemia or hypomagnesemia (such as from concomitant diuretic use) can exacerbate the cardiotoxicity associated with digitalis.
- The cardinal electrocardiographic feature of digitalis toxicity is increased automaticity combined with AV conduction block. A patient with atrial fibrillation and a seemingly "well-controlled" rate—even bradycardic—may be digitalis intoxicated.

References

1. Mahdyoon H, Battilana G, Rosman H, et al: The evolving pattern of digoxin intoxication: Observations at a large urban hospital from 1980 to 1988. Am Heart J 1990;120:1189.
2. Gheorghiade M, Rosman H, Mahdyoon H, et al: Incidence of digitalis intoxication. Primary Cardiol 1988;1:5.
3. Kernan WN, Castellsague J, Perlman GD, et al: Incidence of hospitalization for digitalis toxicity among elderly Americans. Am J Med 1994;96:426.
4. Litovitz TL, Klein-Schwartz W, Rodgers GC, et al: 2001 annual report of the American Association of Poison Control Centers Toxic Exposure Surveillance System. Am J Emerg Med 2002;20:391.
5. Closson RG: Visual hallucinations as the earliest symptom of digoxin intoxication. Arch Neurol 1983;40:386.
6. Dubnow MH, Burchell HB: A comparison of digitalis intoxication in two separate periods. Ann Intern Med 1965;62:956.
7. Smith TW: Digitalis: Mechanisms of action and clinical use. N Engl J Med 1988;18:358.
8. Ma G, Brady WJ, Pollack M, Chan TC: Electrocardiographic manifestations: Digitalis toxicity. J Emerg Med 2001;20:145.
9. Fisch C, Knoebel SB: Digitalis cardiotoxicity. J Am Coll Cardiol 1985;5:91A.

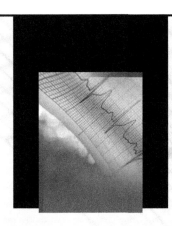

Chapter 51

Beta-Adrenergic Blocking Agents

James Dave Barry and Saralyn R. Williams

Clinical Features

Beta-adrenergic blocking agents are categorized as class II antidysrhythmics in the Vaughan Williams classification, and act by antagonizing beta-adrenergic receptor sites. These medications have become an important component of the treatment of cardiac conditions, including hypertension, angina pectoris, tachydysrhythmias, and acute myocardial infarction (AMI). Noncardiac uses include management of glaucoma, anxiety, essential tremor, migraine headaches, and pheochromocytoma.[1]

There are three types of beta-adrenergic receptors that have been identified. Beta$_1$ receptors are located primarily in the myocardium. Beta$_2$ receptors are found mainly in the smooth muscle of bronchioles, arterioles, and the uterus.

Beta$_2$ receptors also modulate insulin secretion, glycogenolysis, and lipolysis in the pancreas, liver, and adipose tissue, respectively. The role of the beta$_3$ receptor has not been fully elucidated.[2] Beta receptors generate their physiologic responses through a G protein that activates adenylate cyclase, which in turn increases the production of cyclic adenosine monophosphate and increases intracellular and sarcoplasmic reticular calcium concentrations.

Conversely, beta blockade causes decreased intracellular calcium concentrations. Blockade of beta$_1$ receptors decreases automaticity, contractility, and conduction velocity in heart muscle cells—this encompassing the therapeutic benefit of most beta-adrenergic blocking agents. Beta$_2$ blockade produces many of the notable side effects caused by these agents, including bronchospasm in susceptible individuals,

---

ELECTROCARDIOGRAPHIC HIGHLIGHTS

- Sinus bradycardia
- Atrioventricular blockade (first degree, third degree)
- Second degree atrioventricular block, right bundle branch block, intraventricular conduction delay (rare)
- QRS complex widening (propranolol)
- QT interval prolongation (sotalol)
- Ventricular dysrhythmias, including torsades de pointes (propranolol, sotalol)

51-1 • DIFFERENTIAL DIAGNOSIS FOR ELECTROCARDIOGRAPHIC EFFECTS OF BETA-ADRENERGIC BLOCKING AGENTS

Hyperkalemia
Myocardial infarction
Sick sinus syndrome
Vasovagal episode
Hypothermia
Other toxidromes
    Calcium channel blocker toxicity
    Digitalis glycoside toxicity
    Alpha$_2$ agonist (clonidine) toxicity
    Cholinergic agent (organophosphate) toxicity
    Sodium channel blocker toxicity
    Sedative-hypnotic (barbiturates) or opioid toxicity

---

peripheral vasoconstriction, impaired ability to recover from hypoglycemia, and moderate increases in serum potassium.

Although beta subunit selectivity is important, other pharmacologic properties that can significantly affect the therapeutic and toxic cardiac actions of beta-adrenergic blocking agents include alpha-adrenergic blocking activity, sodium channel blocking properties, and potassium channel blocking properties. A few beta-adrenergic blocking agents, such as labetalol and carvedilol, possess alpha$_1$ blocking activity in addition to their beta blocking activity. Propranolol and other beta-adrenergic blocking agents can cause fast sodium channel blockade, whereas sotalol can result in potassium channel blockade, both of which can affect cardiac conduction. As such, beta-adrenergic blocking agents—in both therapeutic and toxic scenarios—can cause a variety of electrocardiographic (ECG) changes.

Electrocardiographic Manifestations

Table 51-1 lists some of the conditions that can produce the same ECG manifestations as beta-adrenergic blocking agents.

Bradycardia. The cardiac effects of beta-adrenergic blocking agents are mainly a manifestation of their beta$_1$ antagonism. Blockade of beta$_1$ receptors decreases automaticity, contractility, and conduction velocity in heart muscle cells. At therapeutic dosing, this leads to a decrease in heart rate, usually sinus bradycardia, and a drop in systolic blood pressure,

decreasing myocardial oxygen demand[3] (Fig. 51-1). Toxicity may lead to profound sinus bradycardia with hemodynamic compromise, as well as sinus pause or sinus arrest. However, recent reports suggest that bradycardia may be absent more often than expected with beta-adrenergic blocking agent toxicity.[4]

Atrioventricular Block. Therapeutic doses of beta-adrenergic blocking agents may prolong atrioventricular (AV) conduction time enough to cause first degree AV block. In fact, a PR interval greater than 0.20 sec has been reported to be the most common finding on ECG for symptomatic overdoses.[4] Severe toxicity can lead to second and third degree block. Junctional rhythms, right bundle branch block, and intraventricular conduction delays have also been reported[1] (Fig. 51-2).

QRS Complex Widening. Certain beta-adrenergic blocking agents also possess membrane-stabilizing activity (MSA), which has been attributed to the blockade of fast sodium channels in myocardial cells by these agents. Sodium channel blockade prolongs the action potential and is manifested on the ECG by a widened QRS complex greater than 0.12 sec.

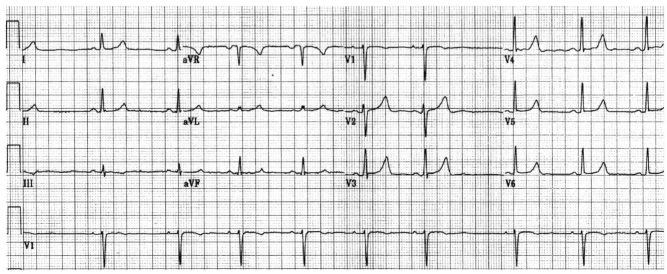

FIGURE 51-1 • Propranolol toxicity. Sinus bradycardia with sinus arrhythmia caused by propranolol toxicity.

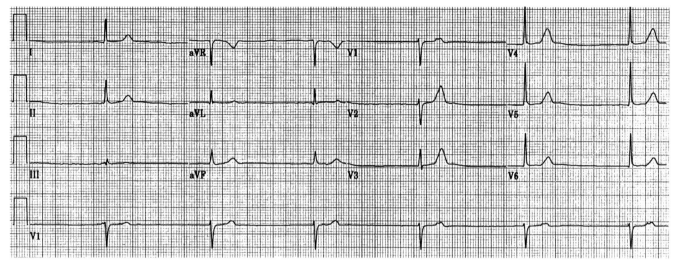

FIGURE 51-2 · Atenolol toxicity. Junctional rhythm at a rate of 36 bpm caused by atenolol toxicity. Note the absence of P wave activity.

In addition, sodium channel blockade further depresses myocardial function and places the patient at risk for tachydysrhythmias, including torsades de pointes. Exposure to a beta-adrenergic blocking agent with MSA is associated with an increased risk of cardiovascular morbidity.[5] Beta-adrenergic blocking agents with MSA include propranolol, labetalol, acebutolol, metoprolol, and pindolol. Of these agents, propranolol possesses the highest MSA and is responsible for a disproportionately high percentage of fatalities.[6] Acebutolol has also been reported to cause QRS complex widening at a disproportionately high rate.[4]

QT Interval Prolongation. Sotalol, a class III antidysrhythmic agent with beta-adrenergic blocking effects, is unique because of its additional actions on the potassium channel. Sotalol prolongs the action potential and lengthens repolarization, manifested on the ECG by a prolonged QT interval. Sotalol usually prolongs the QT interval with minimal effect on the QRS complex width. Like other drugs that prolong the QT interval, sotalol toxicity places the patient at risk for torsades de pointes and ventricular dysrhythmias. Another important characteristic of sotalol is its relatively long half-life, which makes delayed or prolonged toxicity a significant risk.[7,8] Acebutolol has also been reported to prolong the QT interval and, unlike sotalol, also prolongs the QRS complex width.[4]

Ventricular Dysrhythmias. As a result of the QRS complex widening or QT interval prolongation noted previously with certain beta-adrenergic blocking agents, patients may be at risk for ventricular dysrhythmias, including ventricular tachycardia and torsades de pointes. In particular, sotalol and acebutolol may predispose patients to ventricular tachydysrhythmias characteristic of other medications that prolong ventricular repolarization.

References

1. Kerns W, Kline J, Ford MD: β-Blocker and calcium channel blocker toxicity. Emerg Med Clin North Am 1994;12:365.
2. Hoffman BB: Catecholamines, sympathomimetic drugs and adrenergic receptor antagonists. In Hardman JG, Limbird LE (eds): Goodman and Gilman's The Pharmacological Basis of Therapeutics, 10th ed. New York, McGraw-Hill, 2001, pp 249–260.
3. Frishman WH: β-Adrenergic blockers. Med Clin North Am 1988;72:37.
4. Love JN, Enlow B, Howell JM, et al: Electrocardiographic changes associated with beta-blocker toxicity. Ann Emerg Med 2002;40:603.
5. Love JN, Howell JM, Litovitz TL, et al: Acute beta blocker overdose: Factors associated with the development of cardiovascular morbidity. Clin Toxicol 2000;38:275.
6. Love JN, Litovitz, Howell JM, et al: Characterization of fatal beta blocker ingestion: A review of the American Association of Poison Control Centers data from 1985 to 1995. Clin Toxicol 1997;35:353.
7. Snook CP, Otten EJ: Effect of toxins on the heart. In Gibler WB, Aufderheide TP (eds): Emergency Cardiac Care. St. Louis, Mosby-Year Book, 1994, pp 552–554.
8. Hohnloser SH, Woosley RL: Sotalol. N Engl J Med 1994;331:31.

ELECTROCARDIOGRAPHIC PEARLS

- Hypotension and bradycardia are classic symptoms of beta-adrenergic blocking agent toxicity.
- Widening of the QRS complex is indicative of membrane-stabilizing activity (MSA) with sodium channel blockade. Propranolol is the beta-adrenergic blocking agent with the highest MSA.
- Prolonged QT interval is indicative of potassium channel blockade (class III antidysrhythmics). Sotalol is the beta-adrenergic blocking agent with class III actions.
- Sotalol may present with delayed and prolonged toxicity because of its long half-life.

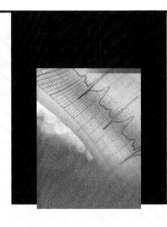

Chapter 52
Calcium Channel Antagonists

Steven R. Offerman and Binh T. Ly

Clinical Features

Calcium channel antagonists (CCAs) are commonly prescribed for the treatment of hypertension and tachydysrhythmias. Undesirable and life-threatening cardiovascular effects may occur with therapeutic dosing, medication interactions, or overdose.

The therapeutic and toxic effects of CCAs are caused by the blockade of slow, voltage-sensitive "L-type" calcium channels in vascular smooth muscle and cardiac tissues. These channels allow calcium to enter the vascular smooth muscle cells and bind calmodulin, resulting in muscle contraction and vasoconstriction. In cardiac myocytes, calcium entering through these channels triggers further entry through other membrane channels as well as release of previously stored calcium from the sarcoplasmic reticulum, resulting in greater cardiac contractility. L-type calcium channels are also critical for impulse propagation in cardiac conduction tissues, including the sinoatrial (SA) and atrioventricular (AV) nodes, where they are responsible for phase 4 depolarization and spontaneous impulse generation.[1] Overall, blockade results in vascular smooth muscle relaxation, decreased cardiac contractility, slowing of cardiac impulse propagation, and inhibition of spontaneous depolarization in the SA and AV nodes. Clinically, these effects may manifest as decreased blood pressure, bradycardia, or cardiac conduction blocks.

At therapeutic doses, CCAs may show selectivity for various tissues. Cardioselective agents, like verapamil or diltiazem, have more pronounced effects on cardiac conduction and contractility. On the other hand, agents with less cardiac selectivity, like nifedipine, preferentially block vascular calcium channels and cause vasodilatation. At supratherapeutic doses this selectivity is lost and both cardiac and vascular effects can be expected.

Although the toxic effects of CCAs usually manifest within 6 hours of overdose, ingestion of sustained-release CCAs, which are responsible for as many as half of all overdoses, may result in delayed onset of toxicity greater than 12 hours after ingestion.[1–3]

Because most CCAs exert vascular effects at low doses, hypotension is the earliest and most commonly encountered toxic effect.[2,4,5] Alteration in mental status is another common finding and may occur despite normal blood pressure; seizures may also occur. Because insulin release is mediated by L-type calcium channels on pancreatic beta cells, hyperglycemia is commonly encountered. Overdose of cardioselective agents, like verapamil, results in cardiac conduction abnormalities more commonly than with the vascular-selective agents.[6]

Electrocardiographic Manifestations

Electrocardiographic patterns indicative of CCA toxicity include bradycardia with hypotension, cardiac conduction blocks, and sinus bradycardia.

Reflex Sinus Tachycardia. Peripheral vasodilatation due to blockade of vascular calcium channels may precipitate hypotension and reflex tachycardia. Although common, this is a very nonspecific finding.

ELECTROCARDIOGRAPHIC HIGHLIGHTS

- Reflex sinus tachycardia
- Sinus bradycardia
- Partial atrioventricular (AV) block (first or second degree)
- Complete heart block (third degree AV block)
- Sinus node arrest/junctional rhythm

ELECTROCARDIOGRAPHIC PEARLS

- Electrocardiographic (ECG) findings associated with calcium channel antagonist (CCA) toxicity usually are not specific. Bradycardia in the setting of hypotension is, however, indicative.
- ECG abnormalities may be delayed after CCA overdose (up to 12 hours after overdose of sustained-release preparations). Initial lack of ECG findings does not exclude toxicity.[1]
- Toxicity from cardioselective agents, like verapamil, is more likely to result in cardiac conduction disturbances.
- In overdose, tissue selectivity may be lost. Therefore, overdose of any CCA agent may lead to cardiac toxicity.

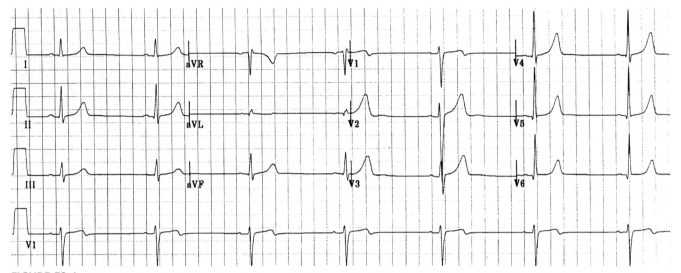

FIGURE 52-1 · **Sinus bradycardia.** Calcium channel antagonist toxicity resulting in sinus bradycardia at a rate of 41 bpm, despite ongoing hypotension in this patient.

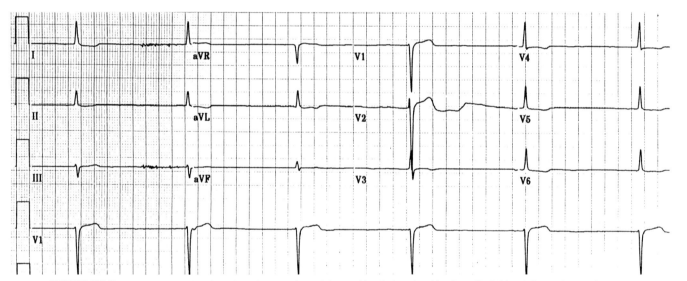

FIGURE 52-2 · **Bradycardia.** Calcium channel antagonist toxicity resulting in junctional bradycardia (34 bpm) due to sinus node arrest.

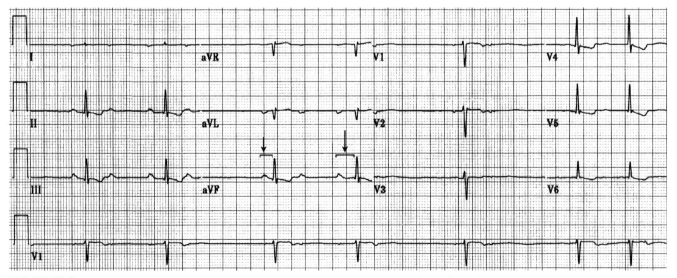

FIGURE 52-3 · **Atrioventricular (AV) block.** Second degree AV block, Mobitz type I. Note the increasing PR interval (*arrows*), as well as the group beating of QRS complexes. In addition, there appear to be sinus pauses.

Sinus Bradycardia.   L-type calcium channels in pacemaker cells of the SA node are responsible for spontaneous depolarization. Blockade of these channels in the SA node may result in sinus bradycardia even in the presence of hypotension (Fig. 52-1).

Sinus Arrest/Junctional Bradycardia.   In cases of severe poisoning, calcium channel blockade at the sinus node may cause complete SA node arrest. Cardiac impulses due to intrinsic automaticity may then originate at or below the AV node (Fig. 52-2).

Atrioventricular Block.   Calcium channels located in AV nodal tissues are responsible for impulse propagation. Blockade of these channels may result in partial or complete inhibition of impulses through the AV node. First degree, second degree, or third degree AV blocks may occur (Fig. 52-3).

References

1. Proano L, Chiang WK, Wang RY: Calcium channel blocker overdose. Am J Emerg Med 1995;13:444.
2. Ramoska EA, Spiller HA, Winter M, et al: A one year evaluation of calcium channel blocker overdoses: Toxicity and treatment. Ann Emerg Med 1993;22:196.
3. Spiller HA, Myers A, Ziemba T, et al: Delayed onset of cardiac arrhythmias from sustained-release verapamil. Ann Emerg Med 1991;20:201.
4. Hofer CA, Smith JK, Tenholder MF: Verapamil intoxication: A literature review of overdose and discussion of therapeutic options. Am J Med 1993;95:431.
5. Pearigen PD, Benowitz NL: Poisoning due to calcium antagonists: Experience with verapamil, diltiazem, and nifedipine. Drug Saf 1991;6:408.
6. Ramoska EA, Spiller HA, Myers A: Calcium channel blocker toxicity. Ann Emerg Med 1990;19:649.

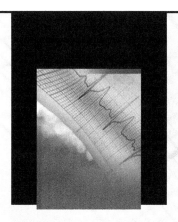

Chapter 53

Other Cardioactive Agents

Aaron B. Schneir and Richard F. Clark

Centrally Acting Antihypertensives.   Clonidine, methyldopa, guanabenz

Vasodilators.   Angiotensin-converting enzyme (ACE) inhibitors, alpha$_1$ antagonists, arteriolar vasodilators

Class III Antidysrhythmics.   Amiodarone, ibutilide, dofetilide, sotalol, bretylium

Clinical Features

Toxicity with diverse agents occurs both in the setting of therapeutic intent, particularly when agents are combined, and less commonly with inadvertent or intentional overdose. Most of these agents are used as antihypertensive agents. Clinical manifestations of toxicity are usually extensions of intended therapeutic effects and are primarily cardiovascular. Paradoxically, hypertension may precede hypotension with both the centrally acting agents and bretylium.[1] If other clinical manifestations occur, such as depressed level of consciousness, they are more likely the result of systemic hypoperfusion rather than direct drug effects. Exceptions include the "centrally acting

antihypertensives"[2] and two of the class III antidysrhythmics, bretylium[3] and sotalol,[4] which may have direct central nervous system (CNS) effects. Clonidine poisoning may resemble that from opioids, and manifest depressed level of consciousness, hypoventilation, and miosis.[5]

This group of medications can be categorized by the location at which their effects are mediated, and include the CNS, the peripheral vasculature, and the heart. Those that exert their effects through the CNS are considered "centrally acting" antihypertensives, and include clonidine, methyldopa, and guanabenz. All are agonists at the presynaptic alpha$_2$ receptor and act to decrease sympathetic outflow from the CNS.

Agents acting on the peripheral vasculature cause vasodilatation, and include the popular angiotensin-converting enzyme (ACE) inhibitors, angiotensin II receptor antagonists, alpha$_1$ receptor antagonists (prazosin, doxazosin, terazosin), arteriolar vasodilators (hydralazine, minoxidil), and combined venous and arteriolar vasodilators (diazoxide, nitroprusside). Angiotensin II is a potent vasoconstrictor and stimulator of aldosterone secretion. By inhibiting the production

---

ELECTROCARDIOGRAPHIC HIGHLIGHTS

Reflex tachycardia

- Angiotensin-converting enzyme inhibitors
- Angiotensin II receptor antagonists
- Hydralazine
- Minoxidil
- Diazoxide
- Alpha$_1$ antagonists (not common)

Bradycardia

- Centrally acting agents
  - Clonidine
  - Methyldopa
  - Guanabenz
- Class III antidysrhythmics
  - Sotalol
  - Amiodarone

AV block

- Clonidine
- Methyldopa
- Amiodarone
- Sotalol

QT interval prolongation and torsades de pointes

- Amiodarone
- Ibutilide
- Dofetilide
- Sotalol

---

of angiotensin II, ACE inhibitors cause vasodilatation and act to decrease circulating volume.

The class III (Vaughan-Williams classification) antidysrhythmics exert their effect directly on the heart and include amiodarone, bretylium, ibutilide, dofetilide, and sotalol. Each drug in this class has unique activity, but all share the property of prolonging the cardiac action potential by extending the duration of repolarization without decreasing the rate or amplitude of phase zero depolarization.[6] The common mechanism is inhibition of the delayed potassium rectifier channel.

Amiodarone has properties of all antidysrhythmic classes.[7] Bretylium is unusual in that it initially induces norepinephrine release (leading to hypertension) followed by sympathetic ganglionic blockade (leading to hypotension).[1] Ibutilide uniquely promotes the influx of sodium through slow inward channels during the plateau phase of the action potential and is increasingly used for the acute termination of atrial fibrillation and flutter.[8] Sotalol is notable for its nonselective beta-antagonist property that helps to explain the severity of toxicity with this agent.[4]

Electrocardiographic Manifestations

The predominant electrocardiographic (ECG) findings of patients manifesting toxicity from the aforementioned centrally acting and peripheral vasodilating agents are primarily either sinus tachycardia or sinus bradycardia. Although some characteristic ECG findings have been reported and are highlighted in the following, most are uncommon and rarely require specific treatment.

Tachycardia.   The agents that dilate peripheral vasculature manifest reflex tachycardia when hypotension occurs. The alpha$_1$ antagonists are unusual in that despite peripheral vasodilatation, reflex tachycardia is not typical.[9]

Bradycardia.   The centrally acting antihypertensive agents characteristically cause bradycardia in toxicity.[2,10] The bradycardia may initially be a reflex to the paradoxical hypertension induced by nonspecific alpha-adrenergic agonism and resulting peripheral vasoconstriction. More commonly, it coincides with hypotension and is a reflection of decreased sympathetic tone. Frequently, bradycardia is observed in toxicity with both amiodarone and particularly sotalol.[4] Amiodarone possesses properties of all classes of antidysrhythmics, including calcium channel and beta receptor blocking activity, both of which may contribute to bradycardia. Sotalol is a nonselective beta adrenergic blocking agent and predictably manifests mild to severe bradycardia in toxicity (Fig. 53-1).

QT Interval Prolongation.   Amiodarone, ibutilide, dofetilide, and sotalol are all associated with dose-related QT interval prolongation that predisposes to the development of torsades de pointes (Fig. 53-2). With ibutilide, the QT interval returns to baseline 2 to 4 hours after the infusion is complete.[11] Bretylium is unusual in that despite being a class III antidysrhythmic, it does not prolong the QT interval and torsades de pointes has not been associated with its use. The major ECG manifestation with bretylium is increased ventricular ectopy associated with initial norepinephrine release after large inadvertent infusions.[4]

Torsades de Pointes.   This is the major life-threatening complication associated with amiodarone, ibutilide, dofetilide, and sotalol. Although torsades de pointes has been reported with amiodarone, it is much less common than with the other agents.[12] The incidence of torsades de pointes with ibutilide administration is 4.3%, and almost all cases occur within 40 minutes of infusion initiation.[11]

Atrioventricular Block.   All types of atrioventricular (AV) blocks (first degree, both types of second degree, and third degree) and sinus arrest have been reported with clonidine.[13–15] First and second degree blocks have also been reported with methyldopa.[16–18] The sympatholytic effect of these agents likely explains these actions. First degree AV block has also been associated with amiodarone.[4]

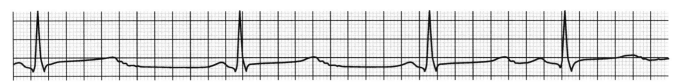

FIGURE 53-1 · Sotalol toxicity. This rhythm strip demonstrates the presence of bradycardia and QT interval prolongation, both classic for sotalol toxicity.

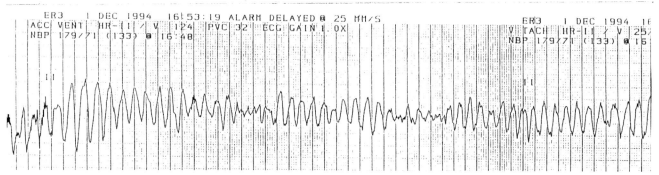

FIGURE 53-2 • **Torsades de pointes.** This is the major dysrhythmia associated with amiodarone, ibutilide, dofetilide, and sotalol toxicity.

ELECTROCARDIOGRAPHIC PEARLS

• The most common ECG abnormality seen with this diverse group of agents is either sinus tachycardia or bradycardia.

• Vasodilators cause a reflex tachycardia, with a few notable exceptions.

• Centrally acting agents and type III antidysrhythmics may manifest significant bradycardia.

• Amiodarone, sotalol, dofetilide, and ibutilide can cause QT interval prolongation and predispose to torsades de pointes. Bretylium does not usually result in QT prolongation or torsades de pointes.

• Risk for torsades de pointes with ibutilide infusion occurs within the first 2 hours after medication administration.

ST Segment Changes. Toxicity from the vasodilators minoxidil, hydralazine, and diazoxide has been associated with ST segment depression with corresponding hypotension and reflex tachycardia.[19–21] Overdose of the alpha₁ antagonist doxazosin has been reported with transient bradycardia and ST segment elevation.[22]

T Wave Changes. In a prospective study using therapeutic minoxidil, 90% of patients were noted to have flattening or inversion of T waves that was slight to very marked.[23]

T wave inversions have also been observed in the setting of minoxidil overdose and are associated with ST segment depression.[19]

References

1. Bodnar T, Nowak R, Tomlanovich MC, et al: Massive intravenous bolus bretylium tosylate. Ann Emerg Med 1980;9:630.
2. Zarifis J, Lip GYH, Ferner RE: Poisoning with anti-hypertensive drugs: Methyldopa and clonidine. J Hum Hypertens 1995;9:787.
3. Gibson JS, Munter DW: Intravenous bretylium overdose. Am J Emerg Med 1995;13:177.
4. Leatham EW, Holt DW, McKenna WJ: Class III antiarrhythmics in overdose. Drug Saf 1993;9:450.
5. Wiley JF, Wiley CC, Torrey SB, et al: Clonidine poisoning in young children. J Pediatr 1990;116:654.
6. Bauman JL: Class III antiarrhythmic agents: The next wave. Pharmacotherapy 1997;17:76S.
7. Nattel S: Comparative mechanisms of action of antiarrhythmic drugs. Am J Cardiol 1993;72:13F.
8. Rogers KC, Wolfe DA: Ibutilide: A class III rapidly acting antidysrhythmic for atrial fibrillation or atrial flutter. J Emerg Med 2001;20:67.
9. Lip GYH, Ferner RE: Poisoning with anti-hypertensive drugs: Alpha-adrenoceptor antagonists. J Hum Hypertens 1995;9:523.
10. Hall AH, Smolinske BS, Kulig KW, et al: Guanabenz overdose. Ann Intern Med 1985;102:787.
11. Naccarelli GV, Lee KS, Gibson JK, et al: Electrophysiology and pharmacology of ibutilide. Am J Cardiol 1996;78(Suppl 8a):12.
12. Lazzara R: Amiodarone and torsade de pointes. Ann Intern Med 1989;111:549.
13. Kibler LE, Gazes PC: Effect of clonidine on atrioventricular conduction. JAMA 1977;238:1930.
14. Williams PL, Krafcik JM, Potter BB, et al: Cardiac toxicity of clonidine. Chest 1977;72:784.
15. Schwartz E, Friedman E, Mouallem M, et al: Sinus arrest associated with clonidine therapy. Clin Cardiol 1987;11:53.
16. Sadjadi SA, Leghari RU, Berger AR: Prolongation of the PR interval induced by methyldopa. Am J Cardiol 1984;54:675.
17. Gould L, Reddy R, Singh BK, et al: Electrophysiologic properties of methyldopa in man. Chest 1979;3:310.
18. Cregler LL, Mark H: Second-degree atrioventricular block and alpha-methyldopa: A probable connection. Mt Sinai J Med 1987;54:168.
19. Poff SW, Rose SR: Minoxidil overdose with ECG changes: Case report and review. J Emerg Med 1992;10:53.
20. Smith BA, Ferguson DB: Acute hydralazine overdose: Marked ECG abnormalities in a young adult. Ann Emerg Med 1992;21:126.
21. Abe I, Kawasaki T, Kawazoe N, et al: Acute electrocardiographic effects of captopril in the initial treatment of malignant or severe hypertension. Am Heart J 1983;106:558.
22. Gokel Y, Dokur M, Paydas S: Doxazosin overdosage. Am J Emerg Med 2000;18:638.
23. Hall D, Charocopos F, Froer KL, et al: ECG changes during long-term minoxidil therapy for severe hypertension. Arch Intern Med 1979;139:790.

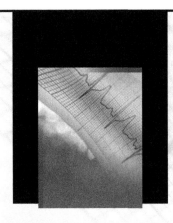

Chapter 54

Antipsychotic Agents and Lithium

Leslie S. Carroll

ANTIPSYCHOTIC AGENTS

Clinical Features

Antipsychotic agents can cause severe neurologic and cardiovascular toxicity. These agents include the phenothiazines (e.g., chlorpromazine, trifluoperazine, perphenazine, thioridazine), butyrophenones (e.g., haloperidol, droperidol), and other structural classes such as the thioxanthene and benzisoxazole derivatives. Newer agents include risperidone, olanzapine, quetiapine, and ziprasidone. Neurologically, the antipsychotic agents may produce sedation, coma, seizures, and extrapyramidal side effects. The antipsychotic agents may lead to serious cardiovascular toxicity, including hypotension and dysrhythmias. The electrocardiogram (ECG) is an essential diagnostic tool in assessment and management of antipsychotic poisoning.

Antipsychotic agents possess diverse neurotransmitter receptor antagonism and ion channel blocking properties. They antagonize dopamine, histamine, alpha-adrenergic, serotonin, and muscarinic acetylcholine receptors. Dopamine antagonism may produce the undesirable extrapyramidal syndromes (EPS) including dystonias, parkinsonism, akathisia, and tardive dyskinesia. Serotonin antagonism decreases EPS by disinhibition of central dopaminergic neurons.[1,2] Histamine antagonism leads to central nervous system depression. Anticholinergic poisoning manifestations include a change in mental status, mydriasis, tachycardia, decreased gastrointestinal motility, and urinary retention. Alpha-adrenergic receptor antagonism produces miosis, priapism, orthostasis, hypotension, and reflex tachycardia.

The cardiovascular toxicity of antipsychotic agents is attributed to blockade of both neurotransmitter receptors and cardiac ion channels, including (1) muscarinic acetylcholine receptor blockade, (2) alpha-adrenergic receptor blockade, (3) cardiac potassium channel blockade, (4) cardiac fast sodium channel blockade, and (5) cardiac L-type calcium channel blockade. Potassium channel blockade produces a prolonged QT interval.[3] Fast sodium channel blockade exerts a "quinidine-like" effect on the myocardium, which widens the QRS complex.[4,5] L-type calcium channel blockade properties have been demonstrated in vitro and may produce in vivo effects of bradycardia, heart block, and negative inotropy.[5,6]

Electrocardiographic Manifestations

Sinus Tachycardia. Reflex sinus tachycardia results from peripheral alpha-adrenergic receptor blockade, as well as muscarinic acetylcholine receptor antagonism. Normally, acetylcholine released from the vagus nerve binds to postsynaptic muscarinic receptors linked to potassium channels, resulting in potassium efflux. This hyperpolarization makes depolarization more difficult and results in bradycardia. Antipsychotic agents antagonize these vagally mediated effects, producing tachycardia.[7]

QT Interval Prolongation. Antipsychotic agents can cause an acquired form of the long QT syndrome (Fig. 54-1) secondary to blockade of the delayed rectifier potassium current. Blocking the delayed rectifier current prolongs repolarization

---

ELECTROCARDIOGRAPHIC HIGHLIGHTS

Antipsychotics

- Sinus tachycardia common
- QRS complex interval widening
- QT interval prolongation occurs with some antipsychotics in therapeutic use as well as toxicity
- QT interval prolongation predisposes to torsades de pointes

Lithium

- T wave flattening and inversions at both therapeutic and toxic levels
- U wave
- Sinus node dysfunction (bradycardia, junctional escape rhythms)

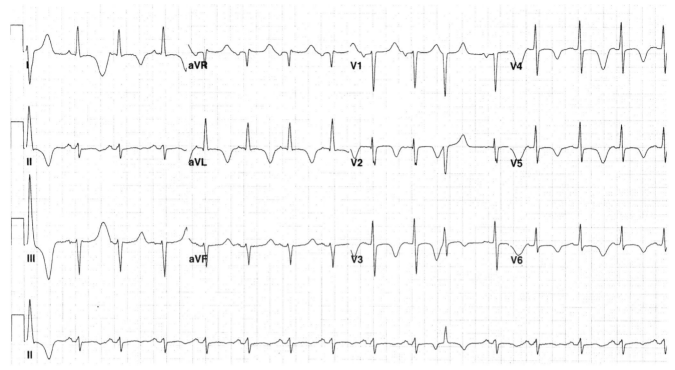

FIGURE 54-1 · **Antipsychotic agent toxicity.** Prolonged corrected QT interval greater than 0.60 sec associated with antipsychotic agent.

and thereby lengthens the QT interval.[8–10] This QT interval prolongation can exceed 0.50 sec and predisposes individuals to ventricular tachycardia, torsades de pointes, and cardiac arrest.

QRS Complex Widening.   Antipsychotic agents block cardiac fast sodium channels, leading to widening of the QRS complex. This effect has been demonstrated in guinea pig myocytes and case reports of overdose, and occurs especially with thioridazine.[4,5] Similar to other agents that act by blocking sodium channels, the QRS complex interval prolongation is usually responsive to bicarbonate therapy.

Torsades de Pointes.   Prolongation of the QT interval predisposes patients to torsades de pointes (Fig. 54-2). Episodes of torsades de pointes may go unrecognized, recur in rapid succession, or degenerate into ventricular fibrillation, leading to syncope and death. The ECG features of torsades de pointes include a long QT interval followed by an early afterdepolarization, which triggers the dysrhythmia. Progressive twisting of the QRS complex occurs around an imaginary baseline, with amplitudes of the QRS complexes changing in a sinusoidal fashion. Heart rate is 150 to 300 bpm.[11]

LITHIUM TOXICITY

Clinical Features

Lithium is an extremely effective agent in the treatment of mania. Lithium can produce severe neurologic but rarely life-threatening cardiac toxicity. Neurologic manifestations of toxicity include tremor, hyperreflexia, clonus, confusion, seizures, coma, extrapyramidal reactions, and cerebellar dysfunction.[12] Severe cardiac manifestations of lithium toxicity are usually secondary to sinus node dysfunction.[13]

Electrocardiographic Manifestations

T Wave Abnormalities and U Waves.   T wave flattening or inversion on the ECG is reported to occur in 20% to 100% of patients therapeutically on lithium and is occasionally accompanied by U waves.[14,15] Intracellular potassium displacement by lithium is thought to induce T wave changes and generate U waves.[15,16] Severe toxicity can produce diffuse T wave inversion[12] (Fig. 54-3).

Sinus Node Dysfunction.   Sinus node dysfunction is the most common conduction defect occurring with lithium.[13] Sinus node dysfunction manifested as sinus bradycardia, sinus arrest, or asystole can occur with therapeutic and toxic

---

ELECTROCARDIOGRAPHIC PEARLS

- The ECG should be scrutinized for rate, QRS complex width, and QT interval prolongation in the face of antipsychotic toxicity or cardiovascular symptoms in patients on these agents.
- QT interval prolongation can be exacerbated by concomitant electrolyte disorders, hereditary prolonged QT syndromes, and additional use of other agents that cause QT interval prolongation.
- Thioridazine is an older antipsychotic agent classically linked to "quinidine-like" effects and sodium channel blockade that can manifest with QRS complex interval prolongation.
- Newer antipsychotics can cause QT interval prolongation as well (risperidone and quetiapine in toxicity; ziprasidone in therapeutic dosing).
- The most significant cardiac effect of lithium is sinus node dysfunction. Ventricular dysrhythmias are rare with lithium.

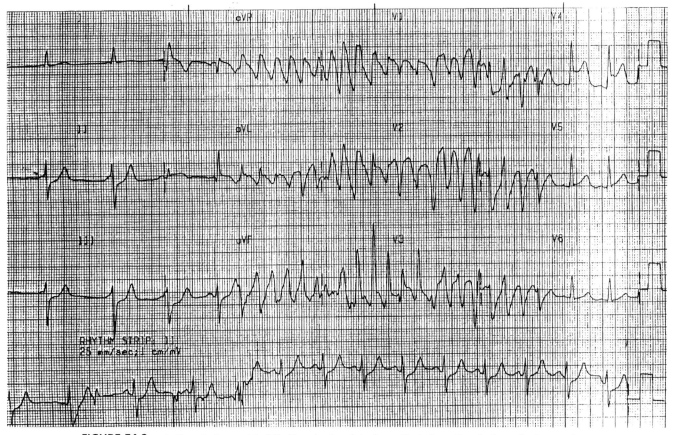

FIGURE 54-2 • **Antipsychotic agent toxicity.** Torsades de pointes in a patient after antipsychotic medication overdose.

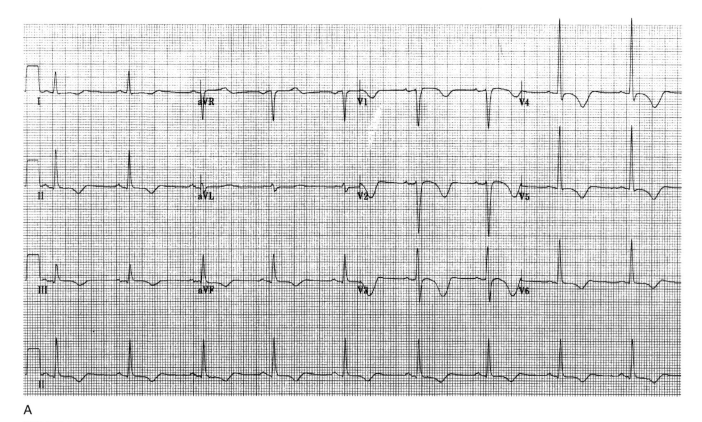

A

FIGURE 54-3 • **Lithium toxicity.** *A,* Sinus bradycardia with diffuse T wave inversion in a patient with a lithium level of 4.5 mmol/L. This ECG demonstrates both sinus node dysfunction and T wave changes.

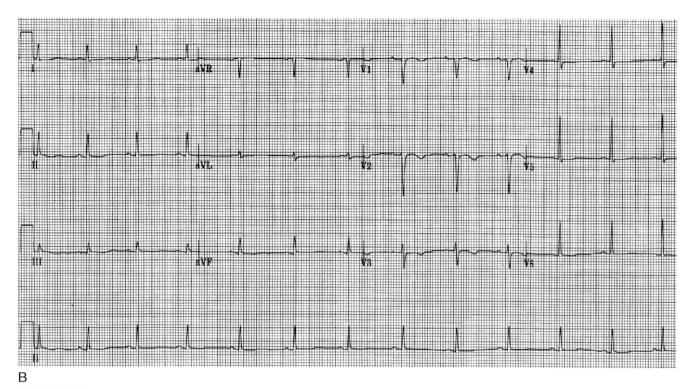

B

FIGURE 54-3 · **Lithium toxicity.** *B,* Same patient after dialysis with a lithium level of 1.0 mmol/L. Patient is now in a normal sinus rhythm. The deep T wave inversions have resolved and now show flattening or minimal inversion, typical of a therapeutic lithium level.

concentrations of lithium.[17] Occasionally a junctional escape rhythm arises.[18,19] Sinus node dysfunction is usually reversible upon lithium withdrawal but may persist despite cessation of the drug.[20] Permanent pacemaker placement has been used in patients with severe lithium-induced sinus node dysfunction.[19,21,22]

Ventricular Dysrhythmias. Lithium-associated ventricular dysrhythmias are rare. Three case reports of lithium-induced ventricular dysrhythmias have appeared in the literature.[23–25] One case demonstrated torsades de pointes in a patient on lithium and thioridazine, a phenothiazine known to induce QT interval prolongation and subsequent torsades de pointes.[23] The other cases report premature ventricular contractions (PVCs) and ventricular fibrillation in patients on lithium.[24,25] Discontinuation of lithium abolished the PVCs, which returned with reintroduction of the drug. Tilkian et al. have noted increased PVCs in patients therapeutically on lithium.[26]

Myocarditis. Four cases of lithium-associated myocarditis have been reported in the literature.[27] Although the etiology of the myocarditis could not definitively be attributed to lithium, the clinical scenario was consistent with a toxin-induced myocarditis. Three of these four cases demonstrated T wave changes, namely, flattening or inversion, which are consistent with either lithium therapy or myocarditis. Although lithium-induced myocarditis may exist, the condition is extremely rare.

References

1. Kapur S, Remington G: Serotonin-dopamine interaction and its relevance to schizophrenia. Am J Psychiatry 1996;153:466.
2. Lieberman JA, Mailman RB, Duncan G, et al: Serotonergic basis of antipsychotic drug effects in schizophrenia. Biol Psychiatry 1998;44:1099.
3. Welch R, Chue P: Antipsychotic agents and QT changes. J Psychiatry Neurosci 2000;25:154.
4. Ogata N, Narahashi T: Block of sodium channels by psychotropic drugs in single guinea-pig cardiac myocytes. Br J Pharmacol 1989;97:905.
5. Schmidt W, Lang K: Life-threatening dysrhythmias in severe thioridazine poisoning treated with physostigmine and transient atrial pacing. Crit Care Med 1997;25:1925.
6. Flaim SF, Brannan MD, Swigart SC, et al: Neuroleptic drugs attenuate calcium influx and tension development in rabbit thoracic aorta: Effects of pimozide, penfluridol, chlorpromazine, and haloperidol. Proc Natl Acad Sci USA 1985;82:1237.
7. Curry SC, Mills KC, Graeme KA: Neurotransmitters. In Goldfrank LR, Flomenbaum NE, Lewin NA, et al (eds): Goldfrank's Toxicologic Emergencies, 6th ed. Stamford, Conn, Appleton and Lange, 1998, p 137.
8. Suessbrich H, Schonherr R, Heinemann SH, et al: The inhibitory effect of the antipsychotic drug haloperidol on HERG potassium channels expressed in *Xenopus* oocytes. Br J Pharmacol 1997;120:968.
9. Rampe D, Murawsky MK, Grau J, Lewis EW: The antipsychotic agent sertindole is a high affinity antagonist of the human cardiac potassium channel HERG. J Pharmacol Exp Ther 1998;286:788.
10. Kang J, Wang L, Cai F, Rampe D: High affinity blockade of the HERG cardiac K+ channel by the neuroleptic pimozide. Eur J Pharmacol 2000;392:137.
11. Tan LH, Hou CJY, Lauer MR, Sung RJ: Electrophysiologic mechanism of the long QT interval syndromes and torsades de pointes. Ann Intern Med 1995;122:701.
12. Timmer RT, Sands JM: Lithium intoxication. J Am Soc Nephrol 1999;10:666.
13. Riccioni N, Roni P, Bartolomei C: Lithium-induced sinus node dysfunction. Acta Cardiol 1983;2:133.
14. Mitchell JE, Mackenzie TB: Cardiac effects of lithium therapy in man: A review. J Clin Psychiatry 1982;43:47.
15. Kochar MS, Wang RIH, D'Cunha GF: Electrocardiographic changes simulating hypokalemia during treatment with lithium carbonate. J Electrocardiol 1971;4:371.
16. Tilkian AG, Schroeder JS, Kao JJ, Hultgren HN: The cardiovascular effects of lithium in man. Am J Med 1976;61:665.

17. Brady HR, Horgan JH: Lithium and the heart, unanswered questions. Chest 1988;93:166.
18. Ong ACM, Handler CE: Sinus arrest and asystole due to severe lithium intoxication. Int J Cardiol 1991;30:364.
19. Roose SP, Nurnberger JI, Dunner DL, et al: Cardiac sinus node dysfunction during lithium treatment. Am J Psychiatry 1979;136:804.
20. Terao T, Abe H, Abe K: Irreversible sinus node dysfunction induced by resumption of lithium therapy. Acta Psychiatr Scand 1996;93:407.
21. Hagman A, Arnman K, Rydén L: Syncope caused by lithium treatment. Acta Med Scand 1979;205:467.
22. Kast R: Reversal of lithium-related cardiac repolarization delay by potassium. J Clin Psychopharmacol 1990;10:304.
23. Rosenquist RJ, Brauer WW, Mork JN: Recurrent major ventricular arrhythmias. Minn Med 1971;54:877.
24. Tangedahl TN, Gau GT: Myocardial irritability associated with lithium carbonate therapy. N Engl J Med 1972;287:867.
25. Worthley LIG: Lithium toxicity and refractory cardiac arrhythmia treated with intravenous magnesium. Anaesth Intensive Care 1974;11:357.
26. Tilkian AG, Schroeder JS, Hultgren H: Effect of lithium on cardiovascular performance: Report on extended ambulatory monitoring and exercise testing before and during lithium therapy. Am J Cardiol 1976;38:701.
27. Arana GW, Dupont RM, Clawson LD: Is there clinical evidence that lithium toxicity can induce myocarditis? J Clin Psychopharmacol 1984; 4:364.

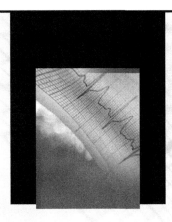

Chapter 55

Tricyclic Antidepressant Agents

Richard A. Harrigan

Clinical Features

Tricyclic antidepressant agents (TCAs) can cause serious neurologic and cardiovascular toxicity. Life-threatening manifestations include seizures, altered mental status, hypotension, and cardiac dysrhythmias. In the absence of a rapidly available laboratory test to predict toxicity, the electrocardiogram (ECG) has emerged as an indirect, easy, noninvasive screening tool for toxicity from these drugs.

TCAs pose a quadruple threat to cardiovascular function: (1) peripheral and central nervous system inhibition of presynaptic neurotransmitter reuptake; (2) alpha-adrenergic receptor blockade; (3) anticholinergic effects at the muscarinic receptor; and (4) blockade of the fast sodium channels, causing a "quinidine-like" effect on the myocardium.[1,2]

ELECTROCARDIOGRAPHIC HIGHLIGHTS

- Sinus tachycardia
- Widening of the QRS complex
- Rightward deviation of the terminal 40-msec frontal plane QRS vector (prominent R wave in lead aVR)
- Prolongation of the corrected QT interval—although this is seen in both therapeutic and toxic scenarios[7]

Collectively, these four effects contribute in varying degrees to the cardiovascular changes seen with TCA toxicity.

Electrocardiographic Manifestations

TCAs produce a number of ECG changes related to the four previously mentioned actions. Neurotransmitter reuptake inhibition, alpha-adrenergic blockade, and antimuscarinic effects can result in cardiac rhythm disturbances. "Quinidine-like" sodium channel blockade can decrease cardiac automaticity and impair conduction, resulting in cardiac rhythm and morphologic changes. Findings on ECG include sinus tachycardia, QRS complex widening, rightward deviation of the QRS axis, and QT interval prolongation.

Sinus Tachycardia.   Initially, the hyperadrenergic state produced from reuptake inhibition of biogenic amines (e.g., serotonin, dopamine, and norepinephrine) produces a tachycardia. Reflex tachycardia, due to the peripheral vasodilatation resulting from alpha-adrenergic antagonism, also contributes to increasing the heart rate. However, the principal cause of the sinus tachycardia frequently seen in TCA toxicity is the anticholinergic effects of these agents. This finding is extremely nonspecific.[1,2]

QRS Complex Widening.   The sodium channel blocking effect of the drug causes progressive widening of the QRS complex. A number of studies suggest that QRS complex

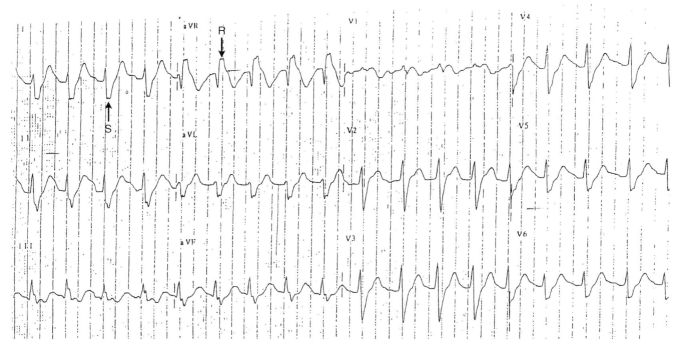

FIGURE 55-1 · Tricyclic antidepressant toxicity. This 12-lead ECG shows sinus tachycardia with widened QRS complex (0.17 sec) and a very prominent R wave in lead aVR (R); note also the deep S wave in lead I (S). (Adapted from Harrigan RA, Brady WJ. ECG abnormalities in tricyclic antidepressant ingestion. Am J Emerg Med. 1999 Jul;17(4):387-393.)

widening greater than 0.1 sec may be useful in predicting significant TCA toxicity, with one group reporting 100% sensitivity of this finding for subsequent seizures and dysrhythmias (although this finding lacks specificity).[3] Others have found that a narrow QRS complex did not preclude the development of seizures or ventricular dysrhythmias from TCA toxicity.[4] More recently, maximal limb lead QRS complex duration of 0.1 sec or more was found to have a sensitivity and specificity for seizures or ventricular dysrhythmias of 82% and 58%, respectively[5] (Fig. 55-1).

Rightward Deviation of the Terminal 40-msec Frontal Plane QRS Axis. Nieman and colleagues[6] found TCA-positive patients had a significantly more rightward terminal 40-msec frontal plane QRS vector (T40) on computer-assisted analysis of ECGs. Recognizing that a rightward deviation in T40 could be inferred from the presence of a negative deflection (S wave) in lead I and a positive terminal deflection (R wave) in lead aVR (Figs. 55-1 and 55-2), Liebelt and associates[5] prospectively found that an R wave height in lead aVR of at least 3 mm to be 81% and 73% sensitive specific for TCA-induced seizures and ventricular dysrhythmias. Increasing the threshold to 5 mm raised the specificity to 97%, but diminished the sensitivity to 50%.[5]

TCAs are known preferentially to delay conduction on the right side of the heart, and toxicity may be manifested by the development of a right bundle branch block (RBBB).[5] Because of the variability seen in the ECGs of normal children (especially with regard to right axis deviation and RBBB), rightward T40 axis deviation has not been found to be useful in predicting pediatric TCA ingestion or toxicity.

Prolongation of the QT Interval. The corrected QT interval may be prolonged in TCA toxicity; however, it may well be prolonged at therapeutic levels of the medication. It tends

to be more prolonged in the face of toxicity, but it has not been found to be a valuable discriminator or predictor of adverse outcome between overdose with TCA agents and other drugs.[7]

Time Course. Early in the course of TCA poisoning, the ECG may simply show sinus tachycardia. Widening of the QRS complex and deviation to the right of the T40 axis may or may not develop; if they do, the presentation invokes the differential diagnosis of wide-complex tachycardia. When presented with a wide-complex tachycardia, the clinical scenario (likelihood of cardiac, metabolic, or toxicologic precipitants) should be considered, and the morphologies of the QRS complex in leads I and aVR should be scrutinized.

For most patients, peak duration of QRS complex width and maximum rightward deviation of T40 are evident at the time of presentation (80% and 86% of cases, respectively). For those TCA-poisoned patients whose ECG worsened after presentation, there was a median delay of 3 hours before worsening was evident (range, 1 to 5 hours for peak rightward deviation of T40 and 1 to 9 hours for peak QRS complex width).[8]

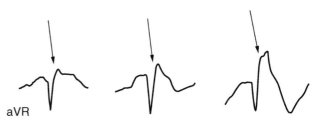

FIGURE 55-2 · Terminal R wave in lead aVR. Progressive growth of the pathologic R wave in lead aVR is seen in tricyclic antidepressant toxicity. (Adapted from Harrigan RA, Brady WJ. ECG abnormalities in tricyclic antidepressant ingestion. Am J Emerg Med. 1999 Jul;17(4):387-393.)

ELECTROCARDIOGRAPHIC PEARLS

- The ECG can neither rule in nor rule out tricyclic antidepressant (TCA) toxicity definitively.
- Peak duration of QRS complex width and maximum rightward deviation of T40 occur most frequently at presentation (80% and 86% of cases, respectively).[8]
- Those TCA-poisoned patients whose ECG worsened after presentation had a median delay of 3 hours before worsening was evident (range, 1 to 5 hours for peak rightward deviation of T40 and 1 to 9 hours for peak QRS complex width).[8]
- Resolution of ECG abnormalities after TCA poisoning occurs at varying time intervals; it usually occurs along with, or sometime after, clinical improvement.[8]
- Rightward T40 axis deviation has not been found to be useful in predicting pediatric TCA ingestion or toxicity.[9]
- Sodium bicarbonate has been shown effectively to treat the cardiac conduction abnormalities and seizures that may result from TCA toxicity.[1]

Serial ECGs may be used to assess patients at risk for toxicity from suspected TCA ingestion. Several studies suggest that asymptomatic individuals in whom serial ECG monitoring shows no tachycardia, QRS complex widening, rightward QRS T40 axis, or QT interval prolongation over 6 hours of observation are at low risk for toxicity.[10]

References

1. Newton EH, Shih RD, Hoffman RS: Cyclic antidepressant overdose: A review of current management strategies. Am J Emerg Med 1994;12:376–379.
2. Harrigan RA, Brady WJ: ECG abnormalities in tricyclic antidepressant ingestion. Am J Emerg Med 1999;17:387–393.
3. Boehnert MT, Lovejoy FH: Value of the QRS duration versus the serum drug level in predicting seizures and ventricular arrhythmias after an acute overdose of tricyclic antidepressants. N Engl J Med 1985;313:474–479.
4. Foulke GE, Albertson TE: QRS interval in tricyclic antidepressant overdosage: Inaccuracy as a toxicity indicator in emergency settings. Ann Emerg Med 1987;16:160–163.
5. Liebelt EL, Francis PD, Woolf AD: ECG lead aVR versus QRS interval in predicting seizures and arrhythmias in acute tricyclic antidepressant toxicity. Ann Emerg Med 1995;26:195–201.
6. Nieman JT, Bessen HA, Rothstein RJ, Laks MM: Electrocardiographic criteria for tricyclic antidepressant cardiotoxicity. Am J Cardiol 1986;57:1154–1159.
7. Caravati EM: The electrocardiogram as a diagnostic discriminator for acute tricyclic antidepressant poisoning [editorial]. J Toxicol Clin Toxicol 1999;37:113–115.
8. Liebelt EL, Ulrich A, Francis PD, Woolf A: Serial electrocardiographic changes in acute antidepressant overdoses. Crit Care Med 1997;25:1721–1726.
9. Berkovitch M, Matsui D, Fogelman R, et al: Assessment of the terminal 40-millisecond QRS vector in children with a history of tricyclic antidepressant ingestion. Pediatr Emerg Care 1995;11:75–77.
10. Banaham BF, Schelkum PH: Tricyclic antidepressant overdose: Conservative management in a community hospital with cost-saving implications. J Emerg Med 1990;8:451–458.

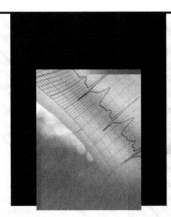

Chapter 56

Other Sodium Channel Blocking Agents

Christopher P. Holstege and Alexander B. Baer

Clinical Features

In the heart, sodium (Na$^+$) channel blockade activity has been described as a *membrane-stabilizing effect*, a *local anesthetic effect*, or a *quinidine-like effect*. Myocardial Na$^+$ channel blocking drugs comprise a diverse group of pharmaceutical agents (Table 56-1). As a result, patients poisoned with these agents have a variety of clinical presentations. For example,

diphenhydramine, propoxyphene, and cocaine may result in anticholinergic, opioid, and sympathomimetic syndromes, respectively.[1–3] In addition, these agents may affect not only the myocardial Na$^+$ channels, but other myocardial ion channels, such as the calcium (Ca^{2+}) influx and potassium (K$^+$) efflux channels.[4,5] This may result in electrocardiographic (ECG) changes and rhythm disturbances not related entirely to Na$^+$ channel blocking activity. However, all the agents

---

ELECTROCARDIOGRAPHIC HIGHLIGHTS

- QRS complex widening
- QT interval prolongation
- Ventricular dysrhythmias
- Bradydysrhythmias (rare, with ominous prognostic implications)

56-1 • DRUGS WITH Na⁺ CHANNEL BLOCKADE PROPERTIES

Amantadine	Loxapine
Amitriptyline	Maprotiline
Amoxapine	Moricizine
Carbamazepine	Nortriptyline
Chloroquine	Orphenadrine
Citalopram	Phenothiazines
Cocaine	Procainamide
Desipramine	Propranolol
Diltiazem	Propafenone
Diphenhydramine	Propoxyphene
Disopyramide	Thioridazine
Doxepin	Quinidine
Encainide	Quinine
Flecainide	Venlafaxine
Hydroxychloroquine	Verapamil
Imipramine	

---

listed in Table 56-1 are similar in that they may induce myocardial Na⁺ channel blockade.

Electrocardiographic Manifestations

As noted previously, in its resting state, the myocyte membrane is impermeable to Na⁺, and sodium ions are actively pumped out of the cell to maintain a negative transmembrane electric potential (phase 4 of the cardiac action potential). Depolarization occurs with the rapid opening of Na⁺ channels and the subsequent massive Na⁺ influx (phase 0). Because of the important role of Na⁺ in myocyte depolarization, a number of ECG findings have been reported after Na⁺ channel blocking agent poisoning.

QRS Complex Widening.   Sodium channel blocking agents bind to the transmembrane Na⁺ channels and decrease the number available for depolarization, delaying phase 0 of depolarization and causing QRS complex prolongation (Fig. 56-1). In some cases, the QRS complexes may take the pattern of recognized bundle branch blocks.[6] In the most severe cases, the QRS complex prolongation becomes so profound that it is difficult to distinguish between ventricular and supraventricular rhythms (Fig. 56-2). Continued prolongation of the QRS complex may result in a sine wave pattern (Fig. 56-3) and eventual asystole.

Differentiating QRS complex prolongation meditated by Na⁺ channel blockade from other nontoxic etiologies is difficult. Rightward axis deviation of the terminal 0.04 sec of the frontal plane QRS axis has been associated with tricyclic antidepressant poisoning.[7] The occurrence of this finding in other Na⁺ channel blocking agents is unknown. Sodium bicarbonate and hypertonic saline have been shown to be beneficial in Na⁺ channel blocker toxicity, often resulting in a narrowing of a widened QRS complex interval in poisoned patients[1,8,9] (Fig. 56-4).

Ventricular Dysrhythmias.   Sodium channel blocking agents may also induce a monomorphic ventricular tachycardia. It has been theorized that Na⁺ channel blocking agents can cause slowed intraventricular conduction, unidirectional conduction block, the development of a reentrant circuit, and

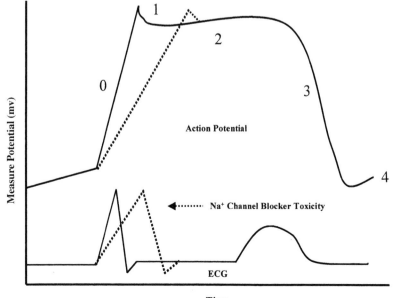

FIGURE 56-1 · **Action potential of a myocardial cell and corresponding ECG.** Agents that block the myocardial Na⁺ channels (*dotted lines*) cause delay of the upslope of depolarization (phase 0) and subsequent QRS complex widening.

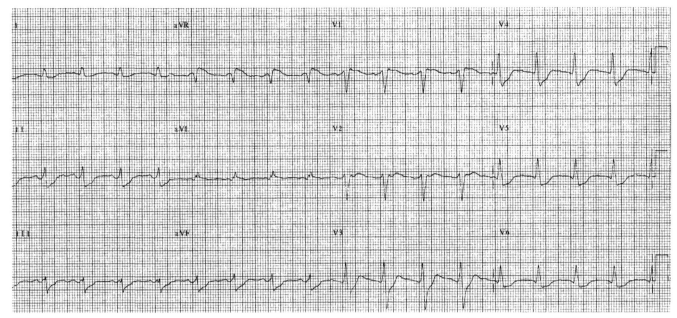

FIGURE 56-2 · **Sodium channel blocking agent overdose.** Sinus tachycardia with widened QRS complex (0.140 sec) and a left bundle branch block pattern in a patient with Na^+ channel blockade.

a resulting ventricular tachycardia, which can then degenerate into ventricular fibrillation.[10] In addition, many Na^+ channel blocking agents also bind to K^+ channels and prevent efflux. Agents with this dual activity include phenothiazines, antihistamines, and type IA antidysrhythmics.[5,11] Prolonged repolarization (phase 3) results in the development of QT interval prolongation and the potential for polymorphic ventricular tachycardia (torsades de pointes).

Bradydysrhythmias. Because many of the Na^+ channel blocking agents are also anticholinergic or sympathomimetic agents, bradydysrhythmias are rare. However, these agents can affect cardiac pacemaker cells. Bradycardia may occur because of slowed depolarization of pacemaker cells that depend on entry of Na^+. In Na^+ channel blocking agent poisoning by anticholinergic and sympathomimetic drugs, the combination of a wide QRS complex and bradycardia is an ominous sign and may indicate a profound Na^+ channel blockade that overwhelms any coexistent muscarinic antagonism or adrenergic agonism.[12]

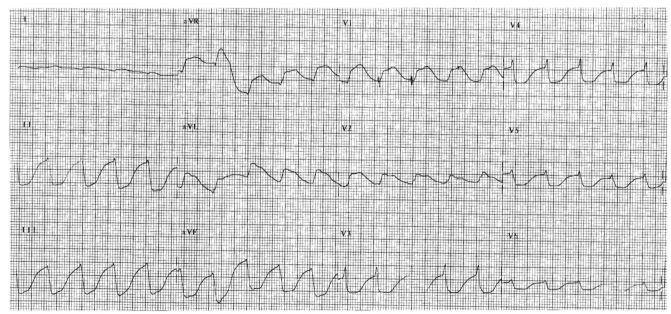

FIGURE 56-3 · **Sine wave pattern from Na^+ channel blockade.** Marked prolongation of the QRS complex resulting in a sine wave pattern.

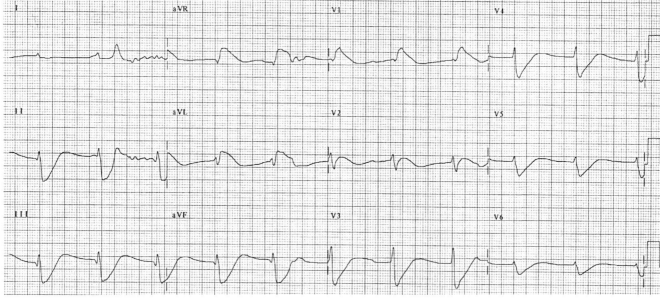

A

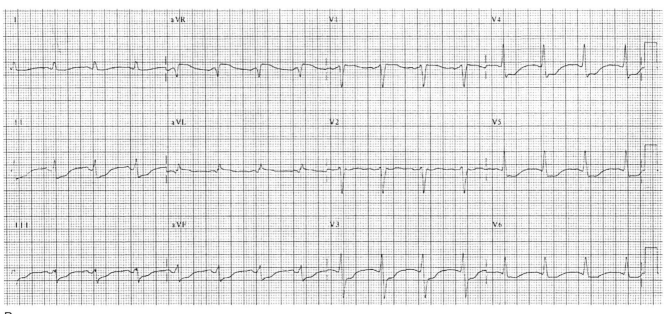

B

FIGURE 56-4 • **Hydroxychloroquine toxicity.** Twelve-lead ECGs in a case of hydroxychloroquine poisoning before (*A*) and after (*B*) sodium bicarbonate therapy.

ELECTROCARDIOGRAPHIC PEARLS

- The ECG can neither rule in nor rule out toxicity from Na⁺ channel blocking agents.
- Tachycardia may occur as a result of concomitant anticholinergic or sympathomimetic actions of various agents with Na⁺ channel blocking activity; as a result, bradydysrhythmias from Na⁺ channel blockade are an ominous sign.
- In some overdoses of Na⁺ channel blocking agents, the QRS complexes may take the pattern of recognized bundle branch blocks.
- Sodium bicarbonate and hypertonic saline have been shown effectively to treat the cardiac conduction abnormalities that can occur from Na⁺ channel blocking agent toxicity.

References

1. Stork CM, Redd JT, Fine K, et al: Propoxyphene-induced wide QRS complex dysrhythmia responsive to sodium bicarbonate: A case report. J Toxicol Clin Toxicol 1995;33:179.
2. Clark RF, Vance MV: Massive diphenhydramine poisoning resulting in a wide-complex tachycardia: Successful treatment with sodium bicarbonate. Ann Emerg Med 1992;21:318.
3. Chakko S, Sepulveda S, Kessler KM, et al: Frequency and type of electrocardiographic abnormalities in cocaine abusers (electrocardiogram in cocaine abuse). Am J Cardiol 1994;74:710.
4. Tanen DA, Ruhah AM, Curry SC, et al: Hypertonic sodium bicarbonate is effective in the acute management of verapamil toxicity in a swine model. Ann Emerg Med 2000;36:547.
5. Kim SY, Benowitz NL: Poisoning due to class IA antiarrhythmic drugs: Quinidine, procainamide and disopyramide. Drug Saf 1990;5:393.

6. Snider RD. Case report: Left bundle branch block—a rare complication of citalopram overdose. J S C Med Assoc 2001;97:380.

7. Wolfe TR, Caravati EM, Rollins DE: Terminal 40-ms frontal plane QRS axis as a marker for tricyclic antidepressant overdose. Ann Emerg Med 1989;18:348.

8. Keyler DE, Pentel PR: Hypertonic sodium bicarbonate partially reverses QRS prolongation due to flecainide in rats. Life Sci 1989;45:1575.

9. Curry SC, Connor DA, Clark RF: The effect of hypertonic sodium bicarbonate on QRS duration and blood pressure in rats poisoned with chloroquine. J Toxicol Clin Toxicol 1996;34:73.

10. Brugada J, Boersma L, Kirchhof C, Allessie M: Proarrhythmic effects of flecainide: Experimental evidence for increased susceptibility to reentrant arrhythmias. Circulation 1991;84:1808.

11. Welch P, Chue R: Antipsychotic agents and QT changes. J Psychiatry Neurosci 2000;25:154.

12. Kolecki PF, Curry SC: Poisoning by sodium channel blocking agents. Crit Care Clin 1997;13:829.

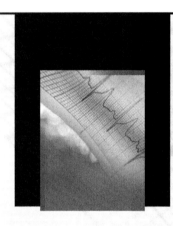

Chapter 57

Cocaine and Other Sympathomimetics

Joshua G. Schier and Robert S. Hoffman

Clinical Features

Sympathomimetic drugs are those agents that cause or mimic increased adrenergic activity. Direct stimulation of alpha- or beta-adrenergic receptors is produced by drugs such as albuterol, dobutamine, norepinephrine, epinephrine, and ergots. Drugs such as cocaine, amphetamines, phencyclidine, and theophylline act indirectly by increasing release of endogenous catecholamines. Mixed-acting agents, such as dopamine and ephedrine, are able to act both directly and indirectly. Certain drugs are able to raise catecholamine concentrations in the synapse through reuptake inhibition and others, such as monoamine oxidase inhibitors, can inhibit enzymatic degradation of released catecholamines. Subsequently, all are able to cause multiple electrocardiographic (ECG) changes through their increased adrenergic stimulatory effects.

Cocaine (benzoylmethylecgonine) is a naturally occurring alkaloid that is extracted from the leaves of the *Erythroxylon coca* shrub. Cocaine is unique in that it has local anesthetic properties like lidocaine (blocking fast sodium channels) but also increases adrenergic stimulation. Cocaine toxicity is known to cause multiple effects, including cerebrovascular, gastrointestinal, and myocardial ischemia and infarction. It also may cause dysrhythmias, rhabdomyolysis, hyperthermia, seizures, and hypertension.

Amphetamines were first synthesized in 1887 and belong to a family of compounds known as phenylethylamines. There are multiple substitutions possible to the base structure, resulting in a large number of amphetamine-like compounds. In addition, many dietary supplements include ephedra alkaloids, which are amphetamine-like compounds.[1] Amphetamines increase the release, block reuptake, and interfere with enzymatic degradation of catecholamines such as dopamine, norepinephrine, and serotonin. Subsequent catecholaminergic stimulation of central and peripheral adrenergic receptors may

---

ELECTROCARDIOGRAPHIC HIGHLIGHTS

- Paroxysmal ventricular contractions
- Tachycardias (sinus, supraventricular or ventricular, atrial fibrillation)
- Prolongation of the QRS complex
- Terminal 40-msec rightward deviation in the frontal plane QRS axis
- Prolongation of the QT interval
- Atrioventricular conduction delays
- ST segment depression or elevation

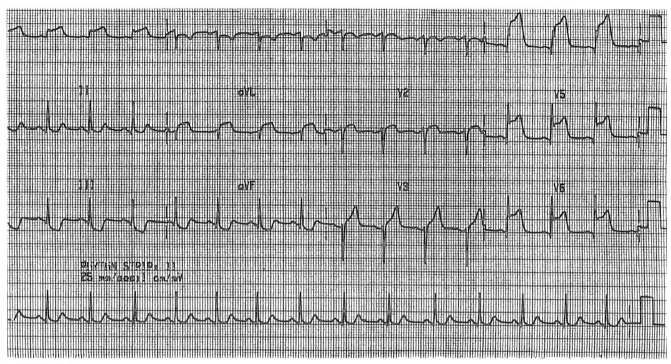

FIGURE 57-1 • **Cocaine-induced myocardial infarction.** ST segment elevation is evident in the anterior-lateral leads (V_2 through V_6 as well as I and aVL) with reciprocal changes in the inferior leads II, III, and aVF.

result in tachycardia, hypertension, mydriasis, hyperthermia, hallucinations, dysrhythmias, psychosis, and seizures.

Electrocardiographic Manifestations

Sympathomimetic toxicity may result in a wide spectrum of ECG manifestations. This spectrum is a reflection of the multiple effects of various sympathomimetics on cardiac tissue primarily through adrenergic stimulation. ECG manifestations vary from paroxysmal ventricular complexes to dysrhythmias, such as sinus and ventricular tachycardia, to ventricular fibrillation.[2]

Cocaine is unique among sympathomimetic drugs in its ability to antagonize fast sodium channels. The ECG manifestations of cocaine result from direct vagal nerve nuclei stimulation, its local anesthetic effects, increased release of norepinephrine and epinephrine with interference of normal catecholamine reuptake by the neuron, and, finally, direct stimulation of certain adrenergic receptors.[3]

Paroxysmal Ventricular Contractions. Increased adrenergic stimulation secondary to elevated levels of circulating catecholamines may result in paroxysmal ventricular contractions.

Initial Sinus Bradycardia. Stimulation of the vagal nucleus may result in a sinus bradycardia, which is the initial effect on the cardiac conduction system from cocaine.[3,4] This early dysrhythmia is extremely short lived and usually not clinically evident.

Sinus Tachycardia. Increased release of catecholamines (especially norepinephrine and epinephrine) in conjunction with impaired normal neuronal reuptake mechanisms and a central sympathetic stimulatory effect can result in a sinus tachycardia. This rhythm is extremely nonspecific and commonly encountered with sympathomimetic use. This dysrhythmia may also result from psychomotor agitation or hyperthermia and may therefore be independent of catecholaminergic effects.

ST Segment Changes. ST segment changes are a common finding in patients with cocaine-associated chest pain. Physician interpretation of the ECG is often problematic because these changes may represent a normal variant or possible ischemia.

Both ST segment elevation and depression may result from myocardial ischemia and infarction after cocaine and amphetamine toxicity[2-6] (Fig. 57-1). This effect is multifactorial and results from increased myocardial oxygen demand, premature atherosclerosis, enhanced platelet aggregation, and, predominantly, coronary vasoconstriction secondary to the alpha-adrenergic effects of increased catecholamine levels. Indeed, the alpha-adrenergic blocking agent phentolamine has been reported to reverse cocaine-induced coronary vasospasm, whereas the beta-adrenergic blocking agent propranolol has been shown to potentiate cocaine-induced coronary vasoconstriction.[7,8] Accordingly, beta-adrenergic blocking agent therapy should be avoided in patients with suspected sympathomimetic toxicity owing to the potential for unopposed alpha-adrenergic vasoconstriction.

Although the patient with cocaine-associated chest pain frequently has an abnormal ECG, it is often a normal variant. Hollander et al. report a very high incidence of abnormal variants, most commonly early repolarization, in patients with cocaine-associated chest pain (typically in young men with thin chest walls).[9] Gitter et al. report on the ECGs of 101 patients with cocaine-associated chest pain. Forty-three percent

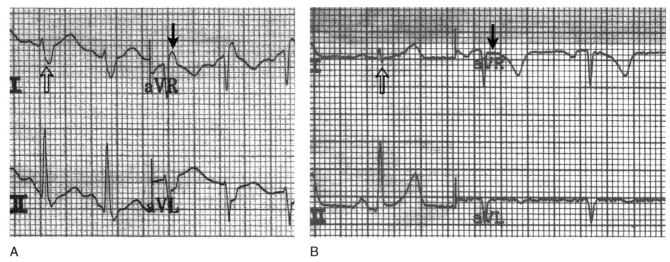

A   B

FIGURE 57-2 • **Sodium channel blocking effects of cocaine.** *A,* Prolongation of the QRS interval accompanied by a prominent R wave in lead aVR (*black arrow*) and a large terminal S wave in lead I (*clear arrow*) due to cocaine toxicity. The latter two effects represent a terminal 40-msec rightward deviation in the frontal plane QRS axis. *B,* The effect of sodium bicarbonate administration on the ECG from *a.* Note the reversal of the prolonged QRS and absence of an R wave in lead aVR (*black arrow*) and S wave in lead I (*clear arrow*).

of the study population had ST segment elevation meeting the criteria for fibrinolysis, but unfortunately did not have the diagnosis of myocardial infarction.[10]

QRS Complex Prolongation. Cocaine and cocaethylene are unique among the sympathomimetic drugs because of their local anesthetic properties. Their ability to antagonize fast sodium channels results in effects similar to those of class I antidysrhythmic drugs.[3,4,11–13] This effect stabilizes neuronal axons and delays phase 0 depolarization of the myocyte action potential. The second effect is manifest as an increased QRS complex interval and a prominent R wave in lead aVR or a larger than normal S wave in lead aVL. The latter two changes are representative of a terminal 40-msec deviation to the right in the frontal plane QRS axis, similar to tricyclic antidepressant toxicity. Similar to other drug-induced ventricular dysrhythmias from sodium channel blockade, the QRS complex width will shorten with sodium bicarbonate therapy (Fig. 57-2).

QT Interval Prolongation. Cocaine's ability to block fast sodium channels can also subsequently increase the QT interval.[11,12] Torsades de pointes has been reported in a patient with idiopathic long QT syndrome after cocaine use.[14]

Wide Complex Dysrhythmias. Ventricular tachycardia and fibrillation are also associated with cocaine toxicity.[3,4,15] These dysrhythmias may result from sodium channel blocking effects or myocardial ischemia from coronary vasoconstriction. Furthermore, acidosis and hyperthermia (both of which commonly occur in toxicity) may potentiate cocaine's anesthetic effects.

Multiple dysrhythmias such as ventricular tachycardia and fibrillation may also result from amphetamine and amphetamine-like compounds.[2] These dysrhythmias, however, are typically due to a hyperadrenergic state induced by the drugs, sometimes with concomitant hyperthermia and acidosis, rather than a local anesthetic effect.

Atrioventricular Conduction Delay. Delayed conduction through the atrioventricular node has been reported experimentally with cocaine use and is represented by an increased PR interval.[11]

Atrial Fibrillation. Atrial fibrillation has been reported after cocaine use and may be due to the adrenergic effects of excessive catecholamines.[16]

Brugada Syndrome. Brugada syndrome is characterized by a right bundle branch block pattern with coved or saddle-back ST segment elevation in the anteroseptal leads. This syndrome has been associated with cocaine use and carries a propensity for ventricular tachycardia, fibrillation, and sudden cardiac death[17,18] (Fig. 57-3).

ELECTROCARDIOGRAPHIC PEARLS

- Sinus tachycardia and paroxysmal ventricular contractions are the most commonly encountered ECG manifestations of sympathomimetic toxicity.
- Dysrhythmias may occur because of direct adrenergic stimulation or as a result of myocardial ischemia from coronary vasoconstriction and platelet aggregation.
- Early repolarization abnormalities commonly occur in patients with cocaine-associated chest pain and may mimic cardiac ischemia.
- Sodium bicarbonate and lidocaine reverse cocaine's sodium channel blocking effects.
- Beta-adrenergic blocking agent therapy should be avoided in patients with suspected sympathomimetic toxicity because of the potential for unopposed alpha-adrenergic vasoconstriction.

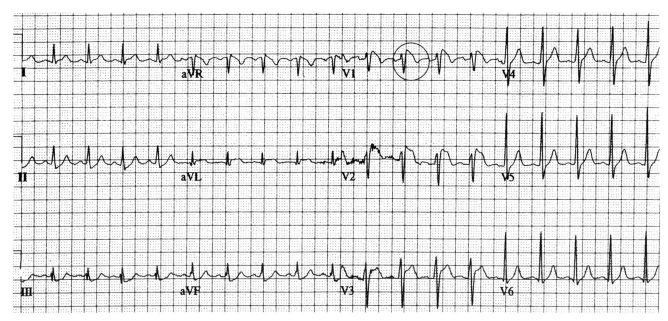

FIGURE 57-3 · Cocaine-induced Brugada pattern. Note the prominent right bundle branch pattern in lead V_1 (*circle*) and the coved-type ST segment elevations in leads V_1 through V_3. (Reproduced with permission from Littmann L, Monroe MH, Svenson RH: Brugada-type electrocardiographic pattern induced by cocaine. Mayo Clin Proc 2000;75:846.)

References

1. Traub SJ, Hoyek W, Hoffman RS: Dietary supplements containing ephedra alkaloids [letter]. N Engl J Med 2001;344:1096.
2. Chiang WK: Amphetamines. In Goldfrank LR, Flomenbaum NE, Lewin NA, et al (eds): Goldfrank's Toxicologic Emergencies, 6th ed. New York, McGraw-Hill, 1998, pp 1091–1103.
3. Hollander JE, Hoffman RS: Cocaine. In Goldfrank LR, Flomenbaum NE, Lewin NA, et al (eds): Goldfrank's Toxicologic Emergencies, 6th ed. New York, McGraw-Hill, 1998, pp 1071–1089.
4. Goldfrank LR, Hoffman RS: The cardiovascular effects of cocaine. Ann Emerg Med 1991;20:165.
5. Minor RL Jr, Scott BD, Brown DD, et al: Cocaine-induced myocardial infarction in patients with normal coronary arteries. Ann Intern Med 1991;115:797.
6. Smith HWB III, Liberman HA, Brody SL, et al: Acute myocardial infarction temporally related to cocaine use. Ann Intern Med 1987;107:13.
7. Lange RA, Cigarroa RG, Yancy CW Jr, et al: Cocaine-induced coronary-artery vasoconstriction. N Engl J Med 1989;321:1557.
8. Lange, RA, Cigarroa RG, Flores ED, et al: Potentiation of cocaine-induced coronary vasoconstriction by beta-adrenergic blockade. Ann Intern Med 1990;112:897.
9. Hollander JE, Lozano M, Fairweather P, et al: "Abnormal" electrocardiograms in patients with cocaine-associated chest pain are due to "normal" variants. J Emerg Med 1994;12:199.
10. Gitter MJ, Goldsmith SR, Dunbar DN, et al: Cocaine and chest pain: Clinical features and outcome of patients hospitalized to rule out myocardial infarction. Ann Intern Med 1991;115:277.
11. Winecoff AP, Hariman RJ, Grawe JJ, et al: Reversal of the electrocardiographic effects of cocaine by lidocaine: Part 1. Comparison with sodium bicarbonate and quinidine. Pharmacotherapy 1994;14:698.
12. Schwartz AB, Janzen D, Jones RT, et al: Electrocardiographic and hemodynamic effects of intravenous cocaine in awake and anesthetized dogs. J Electrocardiol 1989;22:159.
13. Erzouki HK, Baum I, Goldberg SR, et al: Comparison of the effects of cocaine and its metabolites on cardiovascular function in anesthetized rats. J Cardiovasc Pharmacol 1993;22:557.
14. Schrem SS, Belsky P, Schwartzman D, et al: Cocaine-induced torsades de pointes in a patient with the idiopathic long QT syndrome. Am Heart J 1990;120:980.
15. Isner JM, Estes NAM III, Thompson PD, et al: Acute cardiac events temporally related to cocaine abuse. N Engl J Med 1986;315:1438.
16. Monticciolo R, Sirop PA: Atrial fibrillation after the use of intranasal cocaine. Hosp Physician 1988;24:48.
17. Littmann L, Monroe MH, Svenson RH: Brugada-type electrocardiographic pattern induced by cocaine. Mayo Clin Proc 2000;75:845.
18. Ortega-Carnicer J, Bertos-Polo J, Gutierrez-Tirado C: Aborted sudden death, transient Brugada pattern, and wide QRS dysrhythmias after massive cocaine ingestion. J Electrocardiol 2001;34:345.

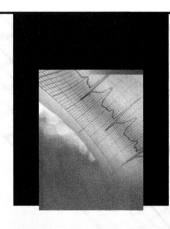

Chapter 58

Electrolyte Abnormalities

George M. Shumaik

Cardiac electrical activity is mediated by ionic shifts across cellular membranes. It is intuitive to expect that aberrations in normal electrolyte homeostasis would be associated with alterations in cardiac conduction. These may be limited to clinically insignificant changes in the surface ECG or result in life-threatening dysrhythmias.

Fluid, acid–base, and electrolyte physiology is complex and can be altered by numerous disease states. Although the laboratory is indispensable in making definitive diagnoses, the bedside electrocardiogram (ECG) can often provide immediate insight and prompt life-saving care.

The clinical syndromes that create high and low concentrations of potassium, calcium, and magnesium are associated with the most common and clinically important disturbances of cardiac rhythm related to electrolyte abnormality. Although the different electrolytes are discussed individually, there is a dynamic physiologic interrelationship to electrolyte homeostasis and that aberration in one "compartment" may affect another.

POTASSIUM

Potassium (K^+) is a predominantly intracellular cation with tightly regulated homeostasis. In the steady state, excretion matches dietary intake, with 90% of ingested K^+ excreted by the kidney. The kidney is better adapted at increasing K^+ excretion than conserving K^+. Hypokalemia and hyperkalemia are the most commonly encountered electrolyte abnormalities in hospitalized patients.[1]

Hypokalemia

Hypokalemia can occur from inadequate intake as well as abnormal losses. The most common etiology of K^+ depletion is the use of diuretics. Other causes include diarrhea, metabolic alkalosis, uncontrolled diabetes, mineralocorticoid excess, renal tubular acidosis, and magnesium depletion. Relative hypokalemia can be created by intracellular shift caused by beta-adrenergic agonists, methylxanthines, insulin, hyperthyroidism, and congenital disorders of K^+ transport. Hypokalemia is usually well tolerated but can be associated

with cardiac rhythm disturbances, particularly in patients with ischemia or cardiac glycoside use. Rhabdomyolysis and ascending paralysis can be seen with severe hypokalemia ($[K^+] < 2.5$ mEq/L).

Electrocardiographic Manifestations— Hypokalemia

The key ECG features of hypokalemia are ST segment depression, T wave flattening, and increased U wave prominence. Although the exact genesis of the U wave is unknown, there is evidence that it is generated by myocardial M cells, which make up approximately 30% of the ventricular wall and normally have a longer action potential and repolarization duration.[2] Hypokalemia further delays action potential

---

ELECTROCARDIOGRAPHIC HIGHLIGHTS

- Hypokalemia
  - Prominent U wave
  - Prolongation of the QT_C (U) interval
  - Torsades de pointes
- Hyperkalemia
  - Tall, "tented" symmetric T waves
  - PR segment lengthening and QRS complex widening
  - Loss of P wave
  - Escape rhythms
  - "Sine wave" pattern
  - Ventricular fibrillation
  - Asystole
- Hypocalcemia
  - Prolongation of the QT_C
  - Torsades de pointes
- Hypercalcemia
  - Shortening of the QT_C
- Hypomagnesemia
  - No uniquely diagnostic features, although a key modulating cation
  - Torsades de pointes
- Hypermagnesemia
  - No uniquely diagnostic features or clinically important dysrhythmias

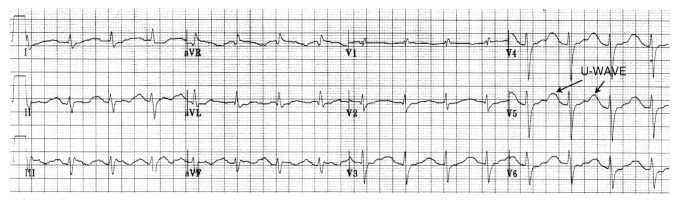

FIGURE 58-1 • **Hypokalemia.** A patient with long-standing renal tubular acidosis. The serum [K+] was 1.8 mEq/L. Note the giant U waves most prominently seen in the lateral precordial leads. Their amplitude is greater than the T waves, for which they could be mistaken. The ST segments are globally depressed and right bundle branch block is present.

duration and recovery, creating the environment for the genesis of early afterdepolarization, increased automaticity, and the potential for triggered dysrhythmias.[3] Prominent U waves can blend or mask the flattening T wave prolonging the corrected QT interval (QT_C). There is no consensus about including the U wave in calculating the QT (U) interval.[4] Patients with severe hypokalemia are at risk for development of polymorphic ventricular tachycardia because of ventricular irritability (Figs. 58-1, 58-2, and 58-3).

Hyperkalemia

Hyperkalemia is less common than hypokalemia but associated with greater morbidity, particularly when severe (e.g., [K+] >6.0 mEq/L). Renal insufficiency is responsible for the vast majority of hyperkalemia cases.[1] There is often an associated precipitant, typically the use of potassium supplements or drug therapy that impairs K+ excretion. Other causes of hyperkalemia include mineralocorticoid deficiency, acute metabolic acidosis, nonsteroidal anti-inflammatory agents, congenital disorders of K+ transport, severe burns, or crush injury. A common clinical problem is factitious hyperkalemia caused by hemolysis during blood sampling. Modest hyperkalemia is usually tolerated well. Severe hyperkalemia is

associated with life-threatening cardiac rhythm disturbances (Table 58-1).

58-1 • ELECTROCARDIOGRAPHIC MANIFESTATIONS RELATED TO HYPERKALEMIA	
Potassium Concentration	**ECG Abnormality**
Mild elevation: [K+] 5.5–6.5 mEq/L	Tall, symmetric, peaked T waves
Moderate elevation: [K+] 6.5–8.0 mEq/L	P wave amplitude decreases
	PR interval lengthens
	QRS complex widens
	Peaked T waves persist
Severe elevation: [K+] >8.0 mEq/L	P wave absent
	Intraventricular, fascicular, bundle branch blocks
	QRS complex widens, progressing to "sine wave"
	Ventricular fibrillation
	Asystole

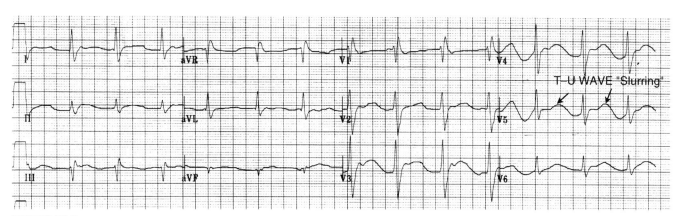

FIGURE 58-2 • **Hypokalemia.** A patient with familial periodic paralysis who presented with global muscle weakness but was otherwise asymptomatic. The serum [K+] was 1.4 mEq/L. Note the prominent U waves masking the P waves. The QT (U) interval is prolonged and the T and U waves appear to merge or have "slurring." Right bundle branch block is present.

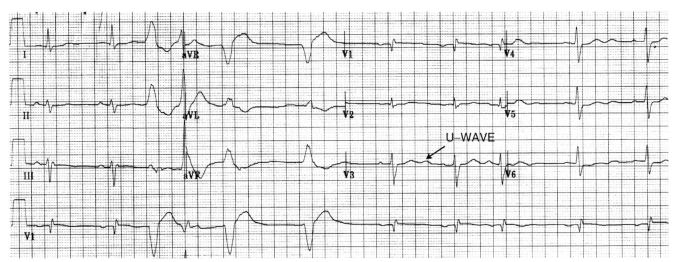

FIGURE 58-3 • **Hypokalemia.** Patient with renal tubular acidosis from Figure 58-1. The serum [K⁺] on this date was 2.0 mEq/L. Although the U waves are clearly apparent in the precordial leads, the more worrisome feature of the tracing is the ventricular "irritability" noted early in the recording.

Electrocardiographic Manifestations— Hyperkalemia

Rising levels of serum K⁺ result in relatively predictable and progressive changes in the ECG (Table 58-1). The earliest and best known manifestation of hyperkalemia is the presence of tall, symmetrically peaked T waves (Figs. 58-4 and 58-5). These are usually best seen in the precordial leads, with "tenting" being the classic descriptor. These changes are caused by changes in the normal transmembrane gradient resulting in acceleration of terminal repolarization. With escalating levels of K⁺, there is further loss of conduction through adjacent myocytes and the Purkinje system. Impairment of sinoatrial nodal automaticity and atrioventricular (AV) nodal conduction can result in loss of the P wave, and the development of a sinoventricular rhythm. Sinus node firing conducts the impulse through intranodal tracks, but the hyperkalemia poisons cell-to-cell atrial transmission and the P wave disappears (Fig. 58-6). With progressive loss of the transmembrane gradient, the QRS complex widens, finally merging with the T wave and creating the classic "sine wave" pattern (Fig. 58-7). This can rapidly deteriorate into ventricular fibrillation

and asystole. When ECG changes suggest hyperkalemia, rapid laboratory confirmation is a must, although treatment should not be withheld while waiting for laboratory verification. The ECG cannot, however, be used to exclude hyperkalemia. Significant hyperkalemia without apparent changes on the ECG has been well described.[5]

CALCIUM

The human body has a nearly inexhaustible reservoir of calcium (Ca²⁺) stored as hydroxyapatite in skeletal bone. Approximately half is protein bound primarily to albumin, a small fraction forms complexes with various anions, and the remainder is ionized (free). Extracellular Ca²⁺ concentrations are tightly controlled through a complex homeostasis mediated primarily by parathyroid hormone and modulated through effector cells in kidney, bone, and intestine. Ca²⁺ is important in a myriad of regulatory mechanisms, skeletal muscle contraction, and control of enzymatic reactions, and is a key ion in myocardial electrical activity and muscle contraction.[6]

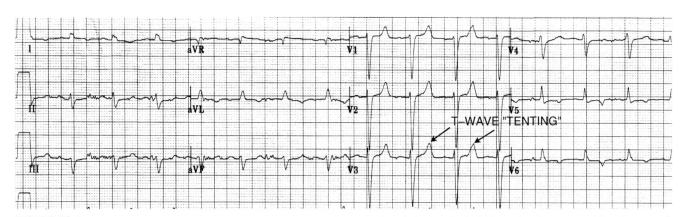

FIGURE 58-4 • **Hyperkalemia.** Asymptomatic patient on renal dialysis with modest hyperkalemia at [K⁺] of 6.3 mEq/L. The T waves, although not prominent, demonstrate the classic symmetric tented appearance in leads V₁ to V₃. The left axis deviation, lateral ST segment changes, and incomplete left bundle branch block were chronic.

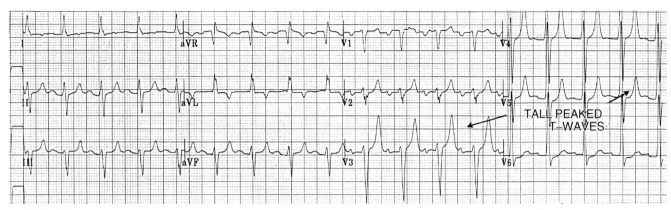

FIGURE 58-5 • **Hyperkalemia.** Another patient on renal dialysis who missed several scheduled treatments. Note the tall, narrow, symmetric T waves, particularly in the precordial leads. The patient's [K⁺] was 9.1 mEq/L.

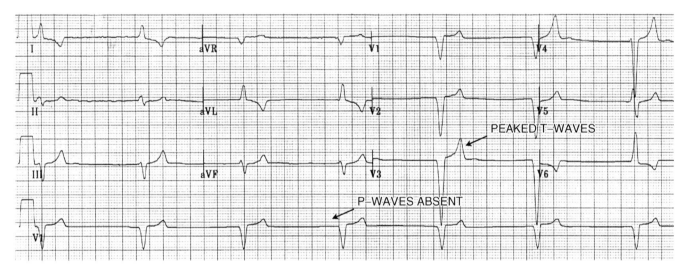

FIGURE 58-6 • **Hyperkalemia.** A 90-year-old patient presenting with dehydration and acute renal failure. Note the absence of P waves and a sinoventricular rhythm. Peaked T waves are noted in leads V_3 and V_4. The patient's [K⁺] was 9.0 mEq/L.

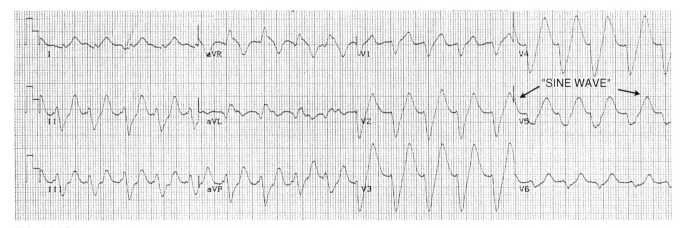

FIGURE 58-7 • **Hyperkalemia.** A patient with diabetic ketoacidosis. Although P waves cannot be identified with certainty, the underlying rhythm is likely sinus tachycardia. Note the marked QRS complex widening with a near "sine wave" appearance. The patient's [K⁺] was 7.8 mEq/L.

Hypocalcemia

Hypocalcemia is classically seen with hypoparathyroidism, either as absolute hormone deficiency (e.g., postparathyroidectomy) or related to one of the "pseudo" syndromes. Other causes include vitamin D deficiency, congenital disorders of Ca^{2+} metabolism, and critical illness (e.g., sepsis). Hypocalcemia is often associated with hypomagnesemia. Neuromuscular irritability is the cardinal feature of hypocalcemia, with carpopedal spasm being the classic physical sign that may progress to frank tetany, laryngospasm, or tonic-clonic seizure activity. ECG conduction abnormalities are common but serious dysrhythmias are not.[6]

Electrocardiographic Manifestations— Hypocalcemia

The primary ECG manifestation of hypocalcemia is lengthening of the QT_C (Fig. 58-8). Hypocalcemia prolongs phase 2 of the ventricular action potential, with the impact modulated by the rate of change of the $[Ca^{2+}]$ and the function of the calcium channels. Prolongation of the QT_C is associated with early after-repolarizations and triggered dysrhythmias. Torsades de pointes potentially can be triggered by hypocalcemia but is much less common than with hypokalemia or hypomagnesemia.[3] Hypocalcemia is commonly seen in critically ill patients, with a reported incidence of as high as 50%.[6] The development of dysrhythmias, however, is relatively uncommon in this population unless associated with other comorbidities such as structural heart disease or ischemia, or with drug therapy (e.g., digitalis, catecholamines).

Hypercalcemia

Hypercalcemia is the principal feature of hyperparathyroidism. It is typically chronic, mild, and well tolerated. Severe hypercalcemia ($[Ca^{2+}] >14$ mg/dL) can be precipitated in these patients by dehydration from gastrointestinal losses or diuretic therapy, or ingestion of large amounts of calcium salts. The most common clinical presentation of hypercalcemia is in patients with metastatic nonparathyroid cancers.[7] Accelerated bone resorption dramatically increases the load of filtered Ca^{2+}. Renal sodium reabsorption becomes impaired, creating a cascade of decreased glomerular filtration, volume depletion, and worsening hypercalcemia. Patients with hypoalbuminemia

may mask significant elevations in the ionized Ca^{2+}. Symptoms of hypercalcemia can be relatively vague, including fatigue, lethargy, motor weakness, anorexia, nausea, constipation, and abdominal pain. Cardiac conduction abnormalities may occur, with bradydysrhythmias being the most common.[7]

Electrocardiographic Manifestations— Hypercalcemia

Hypercalcemia's effect on the ECG is the intuitive obverse of hypocalcemia, with shortening of the QT_C being the hallmark finding. Clinically significant rhythm disturbances associated with hypercalcemia are rare because elevation of extracellular $[Ca^{2+}]$ is not associated with triggered dysrhythmias.[3] Osborn or J waves have also been noted in extreme hypercalcemia[8] (Fig. 58-9).

MAGNESIUM

Magnesium (Mg^{2+}) is primarily an intracellular cation. It participates in hundreds of enzymatic reactions and in essentially all hormonal regulation. It is important in the maintenance of cellular ionic balance, with the modulation of sodium, potassium, and calcium all being Mg^{2+} dependent. It requires ongoing dietary intake to maintain normal levels. There is no known regulatory mechanism to mobilize Mg^{2+} to support extracellular levels.

Hypomagnesemia

Hypomagnesemia is the most common clinically encountered aberration of Mg^{2+} homeostasis and is caused by decreased intake, increased losses, or altered intracellular–extracellular distribution. Unlike other electrolyte disturbances, there is no classic syndrome associated with hypomagnesemia. Moreover, measurement of serum Mg^{2+} either as the total or ionized fraction does not correlate well with clinical manifestations. Hypomagnesemia is associated with far-reaching adversity across the physiologic spectrum, including central nervous system (CNS) effects (seizures, mental status changes), cardiovascular effects (dysrhythmias, vasospasm), endocrine effects (hypokalemia, hypocalcemia), and muscle effects (bronchospasm, muscle weakness).

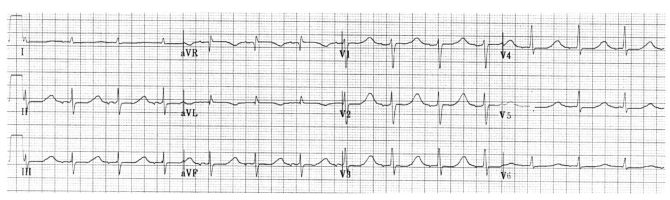

FIGURE 58-8 • **Hypocalcemia.** Patient with a serum calcium of 6.8 mEq/L. The QT_C is prolonged to 0.62 sec.

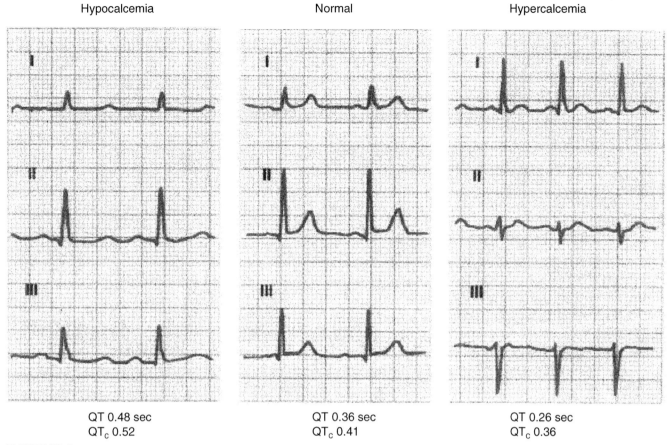

Hypocalcemia	Normal	Hypercalcemia
QT 0.48 sec	QT 0.36 sec	QT 0.26 sec
QT$_C$ 0.52	QT$_C$ 0.41	QT$_C$ 0.36

FIGURE 58-9 • **Changes in QT$_C$ in hypocalcemia and hypercalcemia.** (From Goldberger AL: Clinical Electrocardiography: A Simplified Approach, 6th ed. St. Louis, CV Mosby, 1999.)

Hypermagnesemia

Hypermagnesemia is primarily seen in patients with renal failure who ingest large amounts of magnesium salts, and is usually well tolerated. Symptomatic hypermagnesemia is most often iatrogenic in origin and associated with errors in dosing in intensive care unit settings or in the management of eclampsia. Severe symptoms include CNS depression, areflexia, respiratory failure, and, rarely, cardiac arrest.

Electrocardiographic Manifestations— Magnesium Disturbance

There are no unique ECG effects that can be attributed specifically to either hypomagnesemia or hypermagnesemia. It is

---

ELECTROCARDIOGRAPHIC PEARLS

- Hypokalemia
  - Prominent U wave may be misidentified as T wave.
  - Think "Q-T-U" when evaluating QT interval.
- Hyperkalemia
  - Typically tall, symmetric, peaked T waves
  - If asymmetric, think ischemia
- Hypocalcemia, hypokalemia
  - QT$_C$ prolonged—think comorbid disease or drug effect, and check magnesium level.

---

well known that both supraventricular and ventricular dysrhythmias can be potentiated if not directly caused by hypomagnesemia. If hypomagnesemia is not known to affect the ECG directly (specifically, the QT$_C$), it nonetheless predisposes to both hypocalcemia and hypokalemia, both of which can prolong the QT$_C$.[8]

References

1. Gennari FJ: Disorders of potassium homeostasis: Hypokalemia and hyperkalemia. Crit Care Clin 2002;18:273.
2. Drouin E, Charpentier F, Gauthier C, et al: Electrophysiological characteristics of cells spanning the left ventricular wall of human heart: Evidence for the presence of M cells. J Am Coll Cardiol 1995;26:185.
3. Ramaswamy K, Hamdan M: Ischemia, metabolic disturbances, and arrhythmogenesis: Mechanisms and management. Crit Care Med 2000;28:151.
4. Anderson ME, Al-Khatib SM, Roden DM, et al: Cardiac repolarization: Current knowledge, critical gaps, and new approaches to drug development and patient management. Am Heart J 2002;144:769.
5. Mattu A, Brady WJ, Robinson DA: Electrocardiographic manifestations of hyperkalemia. Am J Emerg Med 2000;18:721.
6. Carlstedt F, Lind L: Hypocalcemic syndromes. Crit Care Clin 2001;17:139.
7. Ziegler R: Hypercalcemic crisis. J Am Soc Nephrol 2001;12(Suppl 17):S3.
8. Surawicz B, Knilans TK: Chou's Electrocardiography in Clinical Practice: Adult and Pediatric, 5th ed. Philadelphia, WB Saunders, 2001.

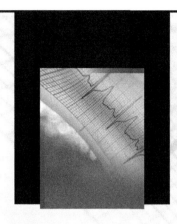

Chapter 59

Pulmonary Embolism

Kurt R. Daniel and Jeffrey A. Kline

Clinical Features

The annual incidence of pulmonary embolism (PE) in the United States ranges from 100,000 to over 600,000 cases, resulting in at least 50,000 deaths each year. The classic clinical description of acute PE includes sudden onset of pleuritic chest pain accompanied by dyspnea in a patient with a risk factor for thrombosis (hypercoagulability, venous stasis, or vascular injury). However, PE rarely presents in such a classic manner and, furthermore, commonly imitates and is imitated by other disorders. In addition, PE produces a highly variable degree of cardiopulmonary stress, ranging from undetectable effects (normal vital signs in a comfortable patient) to proximal pulmonary arterial occlusion and pulseless electrical activity.[1] Patients with PE often complain of nonspecific cardiopulmonary symptoms (shortness of breath with variable severity of chest pain) and manifest nonspecific signs (rapid breathing and pulse rate).

Electrocardiographic Manifestations

There are no pathognomonic electrocardiographic (ECG) changes that enable the diagnosis of PE or its exclusion. However, the ECG plays an essential role in the evaluation of suspected PE primarily because it can diagnose myocardial injury, and therefore provide rapid, noninvasively obtained evidence of an alternative cause of symptoms. Presence of an alternative diagnosis can substantially lower the likelihood of PE.[1] Also, PE that is severe enough acutely to increase the

systolic pulmonary arterial pressure by approximately 50% will begin to produce ECG changes.

In the setting of an acute PE, a completely normal ECG has been reported in 9% to 26% of patients.[2] The most important and common ECG abnormalities are described, and the prevalence of these findings is summarized in Table 59-1.

Tachycardia. Sinus tachycardia (Fig. 59-1) is probably the most common ECG alteration caused by PE. Significant obstruction of the pulmonary tree, often along with acute tricuspid regurgitation, leads to an acute fall in left ventricular end-diastolic volume. Thus, tachycardia occurs as a reflex response to the resulting reduction in cardiac output and low pressure in the baroreceptor system. However, this finding is

---

ELECTROCARDIOGRAPHIC HIGHLIGHTS

- Sinus tachycardia—most common finding in pulmonary embolism (PE)
- ST segment and T wave abnormalities—also very common in PE
- $S_1Q_3T_3$ pattern—occasional finding, but not very helpful
- T wave inversion in leads V_1 to V_4—associated with PE severity
- Incomplete or complete right bundle branch block—associated with mortality
- P pulmonale—uncommon, of little significance
- QRS axis deviation

59-1 • FREQUENCY OF COMMON ELECTROCARDIOGRAPHIC FINDINGS IN PULMONARY EMBOLISM							
Normal	Tachycardia	Anterior T Wave Inversion	Right Bundle Branch Block*	$S_1Q_3T_3$ Pattern	P Pulmonale	Right Axis Deviation	Atrial Fibrillation/ Flutter
18%	44%	34%	18%	20%	9%	16%	8%

*Complete or incomplete.

These data were compiled from 11 published studies, representing 820 total patients with pulmonary embolism.[3,8,9,11–18] Not all criteria were reported in every study. Thus, the data presented represent the available data for each criterion.

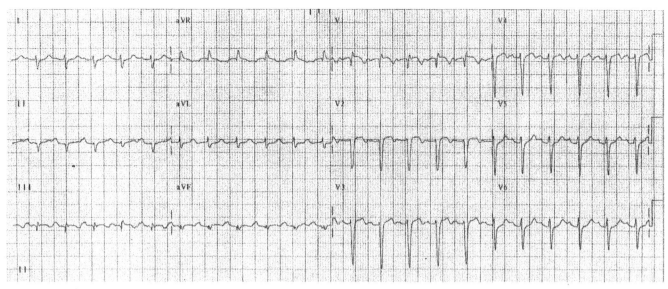

FIGURE 59-1 • $S_1Q_3T_3$ **pattern.** This is a tracing from an 82-year-old patient with rapid progression of chest pain and dyspnea.

too nonspecific to be helpful, especially because tachycardia does not develop in some patients with PE.

Other Rhythm Disturbances. Other rhythm disturbances reported with PE include first degree atrioventricular block, premature atrial contractions, and premature ventricular contractions. Atrial fibrillation and flutter have been reported to occur in anywhere from 0% to 35% of patients with acute PE.[2]

Right Bundle Branch Block. The development of complete and incomplete right bundle branch block (RBBB) has been associated with increased mortality in patients with PE (Fig. 59-2). Patients with PE and progressive RBBB are more likely to have severe pulmonary vascular obstruction that causes acute cor pulmonale with refractory shock. In one study of 18 patients with fatal PE who had more than one ECG before death, 11 (61%) had either a new incomplete RBBB or progressed from incomplete RBBB to complete RBBB.[3] The clinician should view the development of either incomplete RBBB or RBBB with concern in that such

patients not infrequently suffer significant morbidity and mortality.

$S_1Q_3T_3$ Pattern. First reported by McGinn and White in 1935, this is still considered the classic ECG finding[4] (Fig. 59-1). The classic $S_1Q_3T_3$ pattern, mistakenly considered pathognomonic for acute PE by many clinicians, is seen less frequently; 2% to 25% of patients ultimately diagnosed with PE have this pattern. In fact, this pattern can also be seen in many patients who do not have a PE and is neither sensitive nor specific for the diagnosis of PE.[5] The clinician must realize that its presence neither confirms nor negates the diagnosis of PE.

Few experimental data exist to verify the mechanism for this pattern. One frequently proposed mechanism for the S_1 and the Q_3 is clockwise rotation of the heart in response to right ventricular dilation. As a result, when the septum depolarizes during the initial phase of the QRS complex, the electrical impulse travels away from lead III, producing a Q wave.

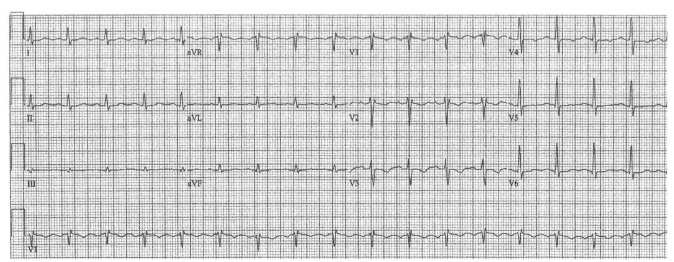

FIGURE 59-2 • **Incomplete right bundle branch block.** A subtle RSR' pattern developed in leads V_1 and V_2 in a patient with a PE whose condition worsened.

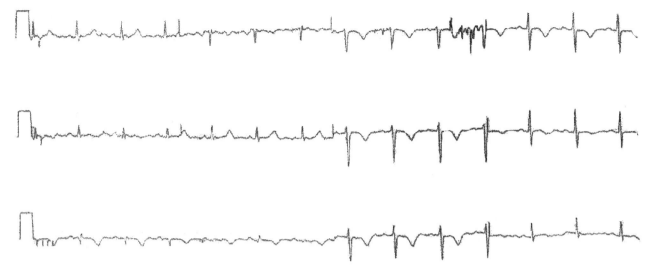

FIGURE 59-3 · Anterior T wave inversions. Note the deeply inverted T waves throughout leads V_1 to V_4 in this patient who was found to have profoundly elevated pulmonary artery pressures.

Similarly, the right ventricular dilatation and the resulting rotation pushes the terminal portion of the QRS vector toward the right and away from lead I, producing an S wave. Others propose the $S_1Q_3T_3$ pattern results from acute left posterior hemiblock.[6] T wave inversion may be caused by subendocardial ischemia in the right ventricle and inferior septal wall in the presence of high right-sided pressures.[7]

Axis Deviation. As noted previously, the $S_1Q_3T_3$ pattern may be in part due to a change to the QRS axis. Although right axis deviation is described as the classic axis change associated with PE, left axis deviation as well as indeterminate QRS axis changes have been reported with variable frequency.[2] Part of this variability may be related to the specific definitions of right, left, and indeterminate axis deviations. Preexisting cardiopulmonary disease may affect axis changes as well.[8]

Anterior T Wave Inversions. Inversion of the T waves in leads V_1 to V_4 has been reported to be closely related to the severity of PE (Figs. 59-3 through 59-5). Ferrari and colleagues demonstrate a relationship between T wave inversion

in the anterior leads and both the Miller index (a measure of vascular blockage derived from the ventilation–perfusion scan) and the degree of pulmonary hypertension.[9] Thus, it may be useful in risk-stratifying patients with PE (see later). The morphology of the inverted T waves is typically symmetric, and may be found in a wider anatomic range and with deeper inversion, depending on the severity of PE. An isolated inverted T wave in lead V_1 can be normal.

Several mechanisms have been proposed to explain this phenomenon, including ischemia in the setting of preexisting right coronary artery stenosis, neurohumorally mediated changes in myocardial repolarization, and myocardial shear injury from increased intramural tension and microvascular compression. Regardless of mechanism, the finding of symmetrically inverted T waves in the precordial leads often signifies profound right ventricular strain and the potential for clinical deterioration in a patient with respiratory distress and hypoxia.

Global T Wave Inversion. Global T wave inversion (Fig. 59-4) in acute PE has been reported in a case report from the literature. Although the differential diagnosis for global

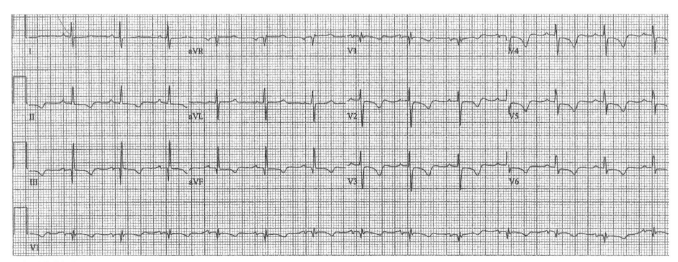

FIGURE 59-4 · Global T wave inversion. This patient was thought to have had a non–Q wave myocardial infarction because of the presence of this pattern along with elevated troponin levels. Pulmonary embolism turned out to be the lone culprit.

T wave inversion is quite broad, it is a rare finding in pulmonary embolism.

ST Segment and T Wave Changes.   In addition to the abnormalities noted previously, other nonspecific ST segment and T wave changes are frequent in PE. For example, nonspecific ST depression or elevation has been reported in up to half of all patients with PE.[2]

P Pulmonale.   P pulmonale, defined as a P wave in lead II greater than 2.5 mm in height, does occur with PE, but is also observed frequently in patients with other, more chronic

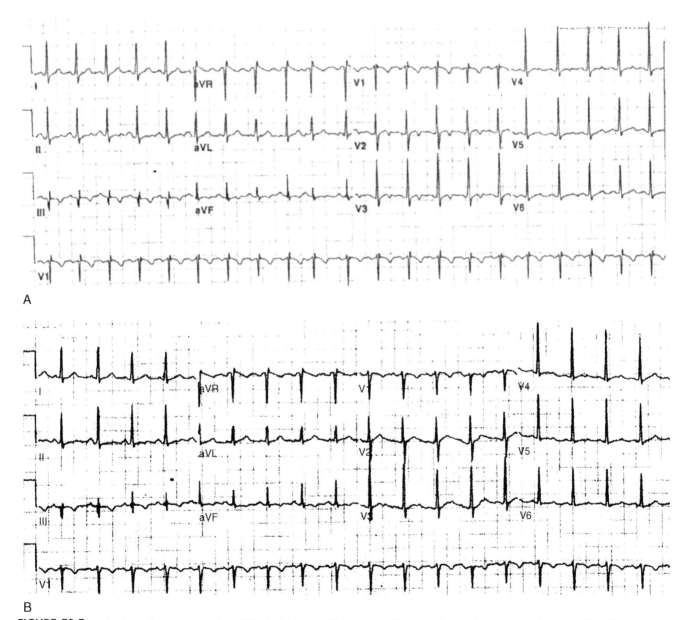

FIGURE 59-5 · Massive pulmonary embolism (PE). *A,* This patient had overt circulatory shock secondary to proximal, bilateral PEs. Note the $S_1Q_3T_3$ pattern, anterior precordial T wave, and the incomplete right bundle branch block pattern. *B,* After the infusion of tissue plasminogen activator (5 hours later), the patient reported feeling much better, his blood pressure stabilized, and his hypoxia improved. Note the resolution of the RSR′ pattern in lead V₁ and anterior T wave inversions.

59-2 • THE DANIEL ELECTROCARDIOGRAM SCORING SYSTEM TO GRADE SEVERITY OF PULMONARY EMBOLISM*

Characteristic		Present	Absent	Score
Tachycardia?		☐	☐	2
Incomplete right bundle branch block?		☐	☐	2
Complete right bundle branch block?		☐	☐	3
T wave inversion in all leads V_1 through V_4?		☐	☐	4
T wave inversion in lead V_1?				
If absent, leave blank.	<1 mm	☐	☐	0
	1–2 mm	☐	☐	1
	>2 mm	☐	☐	2
T wave inversion in lead V_2?				
If absent, leave blank.	<1 mm	☐	☐	1
	1–2 mm	☐	☐	2
	>2 mm	☐	☐	3
T wave inversion in lead V_3?				
If absent, leave blank.	<1 mm	☐	☐	1
	1–2 mm	☐	☐	2
	>2 mm	☐	☐	3
S wave in lead I?		☐	☐	0
Q wave in lead III?		☐	☐	1
Inverted T wave in lead III?		☐	☐	1
If all of $S_1Q_3T_3$ is present, add a score of 2				2
				Max = 21

*A score greater than 10 is 23.5% sensitive and 97.7% specific for a pulmonary embolism causing severe pulmonary hypertension.[3]

pulmonary diseases that increase right heart pressures. Because this finding is thought to be related to right atrial abnormality, rather than acute stretching, P pulmonale may not occur even with massive acute PE.

QRS Complex Abnormalities. Low voltage in the QRS complex in limb leads has been reported in up to 29% of patients with PE.[9] Other changes reported include a late R wave in lead aVR and slurred S wave in lead V_1 or V_2.[18]

Clinical relevance of electrocardiographic findings

Several studies have suggested a role for the ECG as a prognostic indicator in PE. Daniel et al. compiled these findings into a scoring system[10] (Table 59-2). The Daniel score was found to relate closely to the degree of pulmonary hypertension (a commonly used measure of severity) in patients with PE. In particular, a score of 10 or greater was shown to be 97.7% specific for severe pulmonary hypertension (systolic pulmonary artery pressure >50 mm Hg).

As the PE resolves after clot lysis, the ECG findings of right ventricular strain (Fig. 59-5) also resolve. Ferrari et al. reported that resolution of the anterior T wave inversion after thrombolysis is associated with an improved Miller index and lower pulmonary artery pressure at 6 days after the PE. Therefore, resolution of T wave inversion may be useful as a measure of reperfusion after thrombolysis of PE.

References

1. Courtney DM, Sasser HC, Pincus CL, Kline JA: Pulseless electrical activity with witnessed arrest as a predictor of sudden death from massive pulmonary embolism in outpatients. Resuscitation 2001;49:265.

ELECTROCARDIOGRAPHIC PEARLS

- A completely normal ECG is common in acute pulmonary embolism (PE).
- The ECG can neither diagnose nor exclude the diagnosis of PE.
- The ECG is essential in the work-up of the patient in whom PE is being considered in the differential diagnosis, primarily to exclude other causes (such as acute coronary syndrome) for the clinical presentation.

2. Chan TC, Vilke GM, Pollack M, Brady WJ: Electrocardiographic manifestations: Pulmonary embolism. J Emerg Med 2001;21:263.
3. Cutforth R, Oram S: The electrocardiogram in pulmonary embolism. Br Heart J 1958;20:41.
4. McGinn S, White PD: Acute cor pulmonale resulting from pulmonary embolism: Its clinical recognition. JAMA 1935;104:1473.
5. Panos RJ, Barish RA, Depriest WW, Groleau G: The electrocardiographic manifestations of pulmonary embolism. J Emerg Med 1988;6:301.
6. Scott RC: The s1q3 (McGinn-White) pattern in acute cor pulmonale: A form of transient left posterior hemiblock? Am Heart J 1971;82:135.
7. Gold FL, Bache RJ: Transmural right ventricular blood flow during acute pulmonary artery hypertension in the sedated dog. Circ Res 1982; 51:196.
8. Petruzzelli S, Palla A, Pieraccini F, et al: Routine electrocardiography in screening for pulmonary embolism. Respiration 1986;50:233.
9. Ferrari E, Imbert A, Chevalier T, et al: The ECG in pulmonary embolism: Predictive value of negative T waves in precordial leads—80 case reports. Chest 1997;111:537.
10. Daniel KR, Courtney DM, Kline JA: Assessment of cardiac stress from massive pulmonary embolism with 12-lead ECG. Chest 2001; 120:474.

11. Weber DM, Phillips JH Jr: A re-evaluation of electrocardiographic changes accompanying acute pulmonary embolism. Am J Med Sci 1966;251:381.

12. Smith M, Ray CT: Electrocardiographic signs of early right ventricular enlargement in acute pulmonary embolism. Chest 1970;58:205.

13. Szucs MM Jr, Brooks HL, Grossman W, et al: Diagnostic sensitivity of laboratory findings in acute pulmonary embolism. Ann Intern Med 1971;74:161.

14. Sasahara AA, Hyers TM, Cole CM, et al: The Urokinase-Pulmonary Embolism Trial (UPET): A national cooperative study. Circulation 1973;47/48(Suppl 2):II60.

15. Stein PD, Dalen JE, McIntyre KM, et al: The electrocardiogram in acute pulmonary embolism. Prog Cardiovasc Dis 1975;17:247.

16. Stein PD, Terrin ML, Hales CA, et al: Clinical, laboratory, roentgenographic, and electrocardiographic findings in patients with acute pulmonary embolism and no pre-existing cardiac or pulmonary disease. Chest 1991;100:598.

17. Sreeram N, Cheriex EC, Smeets JL, et al: Value of the 12-lead electrocardiogram at hospital admission in the diagnosis of pulmonary embolism. Am J Cardiol 1994;73:298.

18. Rodger M, Makropoulos D, Turek M, et al: Diagnostic value of the electrocardiogram in suspected pulmonary embolism. Am J Cardiol 2000;86:807.

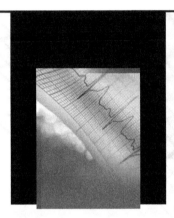

Chapter 60

Chronic Obstructive Pulmonary Disease

Chris A. Ghaemmaghami

Clinical Features

The term *chronic obstructive pulmonary disease* (COPD) is used to describe the spectrum of pulmonary diseases that are characterized by chronic airway obstruction caused primarily by emphysema, chronic bronchitis, or, most commonly, components of both. COPD affects over 52 million individuals worldwide and is the fourth leading cause of mortality in the United States. Emphysematous changes are the result of chronic inflammatory processes in the lung leading to irreversible destruction of the normal architecture of the terminal bronchi. As the disease process progresses, an overall decrease in lung compliance, prolonged expiratory flow times, and chronic lung hyperinflation are observed. Coalescence of damaged areas can lead to bullae formation and increased anatomic dead space in the lung.

Hyperinflation of the lungs results in an increased anterior–posterior diameter of the thorax and flattening and downward displacement of the diaphragm. These changes allow the anatomic position of the heart to become more vertical. In addition, because of its attachments with the great vessels, the heart makes a clockwise rotation, resulting in posterior rotation of the left ventricle and anterior rotation of the right ventricle. The pulmonary vascular bed is affected both directly and indirectly by COPD. The active destruction of lung tissue directly damages pulmonary capillaries. Chronic vasoconstriction of pulmonary arterioles and arteries occurs in response to the low alveolar oxygen tensions present throughout alveoli in the injured tissue. Over time, muscular hyperplasia in these vessels results in a further decrease in the total pulmonary vascular cross-section. The combination of the loss of capillaries and increased resistance through the medium and large pulmonary arteries results in chronic pulmonary hypertension and a pressure-overloaded state for the right atrium and ventricle. These changes can lead to right heart failure and cor pulmonale. Most of the electrocardiographic (ECG) findings related to COPD can be attributed to the chamber-altering effects of this pulmonary hypertension.

Electrocardiographic Manifestations

The greater the extent of secondary cardiac disease from COPD and cor pulmonale, the more pronounced the ECG findings. In fact, although COPD has several associated ECG abnormalities, once right ventricular hypertrophy (RVH) is demonstrated electrocardiographically, the diagnosis of chronic cor pulmonale can be made.

Right Atrial Abnormality. Pressure overload of the right atrium leads to the development of wall thickening and subsequent morphologic changes in the P waves. Termed *P pulmonale*, these changes are typically seen in the anterior precordial leads V_1 and V_2. Tall, peaked P waves are seen in the inferior limb leads, lead V_1, and occasionally lead V_2. The P waves are usually upright but may appear biphasic in lead V_1. These tall P waves measure greater than 1.5 mm in height in lead V_1 and over 2.5 mm in leads II, III, and aVF. In addition to changes in magnitude, a P wave axis change in the limb

leads can be observed, with measurements greater than 70 degrees in the frontal plane (Fig. 60-1).[1]

It is important to distinguish between right atrial abnormality (RAA) and left atrial abnormality (LAA) on the ECG because the clinical significance of each is distinct. Analysis of the P wave contour can aid in the distinction. P waves in RAA frequently have a sharp upstroke and peaked first portion. In contrast, the P wave in LAA is usually flat or notched on top, the classically described biphasic P wave in lead V_1. The P wave of RAA has a normal duration, whereas those in LAA frequently are prolonged. In addition, increased P wave height in the inferior limb leads should not be observed in isolated LAA.[1]

Right Ventricular Hypertrophy. Chronic pressure overload of the right ventricle due to increased pulmonary artery pressures tends to cause right ventricular enlargement through mechanisms of both hypertrophy and dilatation. Because the specific pathophysiologic mechanisms causing these alterations cannot reliably be determined by surface ECG, the term *RVH* is used here to denote both alterations in right ventricular structure (Fig. 60-2; see Chapter 35, Ventricular Hypertrophy).

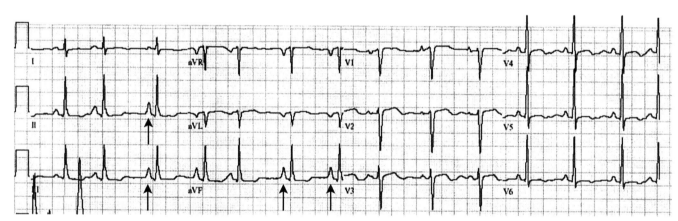

FIGURE 60-1 · **Chronic obstructive pulmonary disease (COPD) with P pulmonale.** Right atrial abnormality with peaked enlarged P waves (*arrows*), best seen in leads II, III, and aVF. Note the sharp initial deflection.

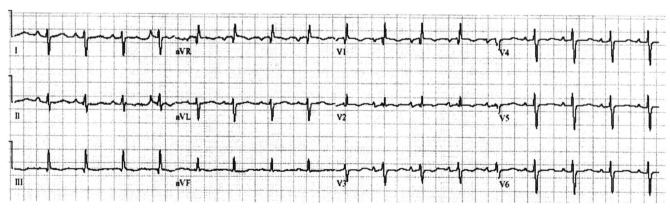

FIGURE 60-2 · **Right ventricular hypertrophy.** Note the right axis deviation, qR pattern in lead V_1, and prominent S waves in the left precordial leads.

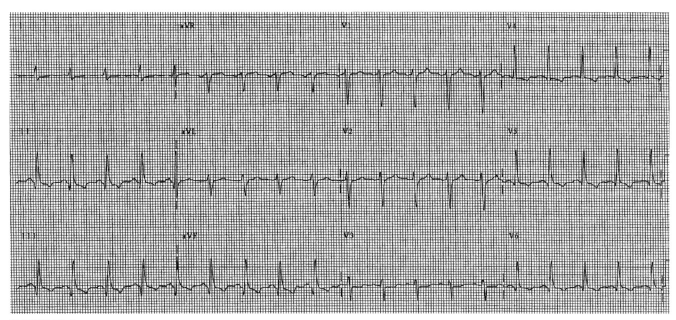

FIGURE 60-3 • **Vertical axis in a patient with chronic obstructive pulmonary disease (COPD).** Vertical axis in ECG of a 54-year-old woman with severe COPD revealing an $SV_1SV_2SV_3$ pattern.

Vertical Heart Position. In advanced COPD, the heart assumes a lowered position in the mediastinum because of depression of the diaphragm. With this depression comes a clockwise rotation of the heart leading to an anteriorly oriented right ventricle and a posteriorly oriented left ventricle.[2] Electrocardiographically, this phenomenon may cause all six precordial leads to have low-amplitude R waves and more prominent S waves (Fig. 60-3). This is known as the $SV_1SV_2SV_3$ pattern and usually is associated with a severely deviated leftward QRS axis. This morphology could be misinterpreted as an anterior wall myocardial infarction (MI).

Low-Voltage QRS Complexes. Low-voltage QRS complexes are frequently seen in the ECGs of patients with COPD. When no lead has a maximum QRS complex deflection greater than 5 mm in the limb leads and greater than 10 mm in the precordial leads, the conditions defining low voltage are present. Three primary mechanisms may account for these low-voltage QRS complexes. First, the decreased conductivity of electrical signals through emphysematous lungs decreases the magnitude of the measurable electrical potentials reaching the skin's surface. Second, the increase in thoracic anterior–posterior diameter may further reduce the measured voltage. Finally, and perhaps most important, posterior rotation of the left ventricle places the bulk of the myocardium farther away from the anterior chest wall and orients most of the electrical vector forces away from the precordial leads. This positional relationship then gives the false picture of a relatively massive right heart compared with a smaller left ventricle.

Right Axis Deviation of the QRS Complex. A frequent finding in patients with COPD is frontal plane QRS right axis deviation (RAD). QRS axes between +90 degrees and +110 degrees in the limb leads may be pathologic, but often also represent a common normal variant. RAD greater than +110 degrees is always abnormal (Fig. 60-3). The differential diagnosis for this finding includes RVH (the most frequent cause of RAD), anterior MI, acute cor pulmonale (usually secondary to pulmonary embolism), left posterior fascicular block, dextrocardia, right bundle branch block (RBBB), or reversal of the limb electrodes.

Also suggestive of COPD is the $S_1S_2S_3$ pattern when the R:S ratio is less than 1 in leads I, II, and III. This may well result in RAD.

Right Bundle Branch Block. RVH may produce RBBB and is therefore pertinent to the discussion of patients with COPD (Fig. 60-4). Unfortunately, the presence of a RBBB can mimic or mask many of the other, more subtle ECG findings associated with COPD and cor pulmonale discussed previously (see Chapter 21, Intraventricular Conduction Abnormalities).[3]

Multifocal Atrial Tachycardia. Multifocal atrial tachycardia is a tachydysrhythmia frequently associated with decompensated

---

> ### *ELECTROCARDIOGRAPHIC PEARLS*
>
> - The combination of ECG findings consistent with chronic obstructive pulmonary disease (COPD) and right ventricular hypertrophy are predictive of the presence of chronic cor pulmonale.
> - Complete right bundle branch block may mask many of the other diagnostic features seen in COPD and cor pulmonale.
> - Right axis deviation is common in COPD but may also occur in an acute anterior wall myocardial infarction and pulmonary embolism.
> - Low voltage is a finding nonspecific for COPD.

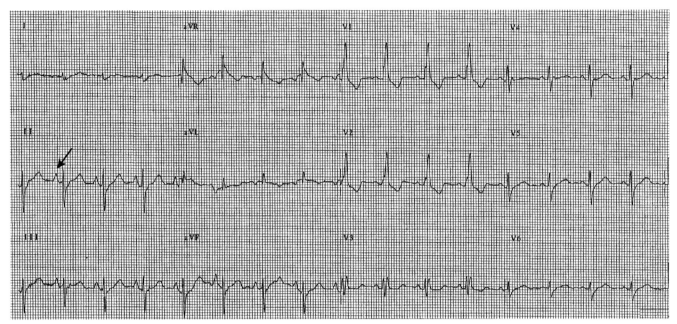

FIGURE 60-4 · **Right bundle branch block (RBBB) in a patient with chronic obstructive pulmonary disease.** Complete RBBB pattern showing rSR' pattern in leads V_1 and V_2 with QRS duration of 0.125 sec. S wave in leads I and V_6 is prolonged. Also note peaked P waves in inferior leads (*arrow*).

pulmonary disease.[4] This dysrhythmia is easily confused with atrial fibrillation because of its irregularity, and with atrial flutter or other supraventricular tachycardias.

References

1. Friedman HH: Diagnostic Electrocardiography and Vectorcardiography. New York, McGraw-Hill, 1985.

2. Scott RC: The electrocardiogram in pulmonary emphysema and cor pulmonale. Am Heart J 1961;61:843.

3. Wasserburger RH: The electrocardiographic pentalogy of pulmonary emphysema: A correlation of roentgenographic findings and pulmonary function studies. Circulation 1959;20:831.

4. McCord J: Multifocal tachycardia. Chest 1998;113:203.

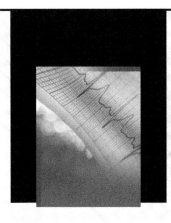

Chapter 61

Pulmonary Hypertension

Brian Korotzer

Clinical Features

Pulmonary hypertension, an abnormal blood pressure elevation in the pulmonary vascular bed, can occur acutely or chronically. Acute pulmonary hypertension is most commonly caused by pulmonary embolism. Chronic pulmonary hypertension can be caused by chronic lung diseases (chronic obstructive pulmonary disease, interstitial lung disease, pulmonary fibrosis, collagen vascular disease, and obstructive sleep apnea), chronic thromboembolic disease, left heart dysfunction (left ventricular dysfunction, mitral or aortic valve disease), hypoxia, cirrhosis, acquired immunodeficiency syndrome–related illnesses, and sickle cell anemia. Unexplained pulmonary hypertension is classified as primary pulmonary hypertension, a distinct clinical syndrome typically occurring in women of childbearing age and sometimes associated with use of anorectic drugs.[1]

Patients with pulmonary hypertension often complain of shortness of breath and dyspnea on exertion. Most of the clinical findings associated with pulmonary hypertension are due to its effect on the right ventricle and right atrium, which typically enlarge and hypertrophy in response to the increased pulmonary vascular pressure. When right ventricular hypertrophy (RVH) develops owing to chronic lung disease, the term *cor pulmonale* is applied.[2,3] Although the clinical examination is often insensitive in the detection of pulmonary hypertension, findings encountered include accentuated pulmonic component of the second heart sound, the murmur of tricuspid regurgitation, elevated jugular venous pressure, hepatojugular reflux, and lower extremity edema.[2,3]

ELECTROCARDIOGRAPHIC HIGHLIGHTS

- Right atrial abnormality/P pulmonale
- Right ventricular hypertrophy
- Right axis deviation
- Right bundle branch block (complete or incomplete)
- Right ventricular strain pattern: ST segment depression with inverted T waves in right precordial leads

---

Electrocardiographic Manifestations

There are no electrocardiographic (ECG) findings specific to pulmonary hypertension. Rather, the ECG reflects the dilation and hypertrophy of the right-sided heart chambers, including right atrial abnormality (RAA), RVH, and right ventricular strain. Because the right ventricle in normal adults is only one fourth to one third of the mass of the left ventricle, the ECG is insensitive to mild right ventricular changes because there must be at least a doubling in right ventricular mass before RVH can be detected.[3] In general, the ECG findings correlate poorly with severity of underlying pulmonary hypertension or lung disease.[2,4]

Right Atrial Abnormality. In pulmonary hypertension, RAA results in increased P wave size, with tall (>2.5 mm) P waves in leads II, III, and aVF[2–6] (Fig. 61-1). These findings are referred to as *P pulmonale*. The P wave axis may also be shifted rightward (>70 degrees).[2,3,5,6] Left atrial abnormality (LAA) can cause similar ECG changes, and it can be very difficult to distinguish RAA and LAA in some circumstances[4,6] (see Fig. 61-1).

Right Ventricular Hypertrophy. Most of the ECG changes seen in pulmonary hypertension are due to RVH. Overall, the ECG has poor sensitivity for detecting RVH, but when RVH is found on the ECG, it is highly specific. The electrical forces of the larger left ventricle dominate the normal ECG. When RVH develops from pulmonary hypertension, right-sided electrical forces can equal or even surpass those of the left ventricle, resulting in characteristic RVH ECG patterns as well as, in some cases, right axis deviation (RAD) and right bundle branch block (RBBB).

There are numerous ECG criteria for determining the presence of RVH. Typically, abnormal findings are seen in lead V_1, with prominent R, qR, or Rs waves in that lead[5] (see Figs. 61-1 and 61-2). An abnormal R wave in lead V_1 is defined as an R:S ratio greater than 1.[4] In severe RVH, the normal precordial lead patterns can be totally reversed, with tall R waves in the right precordial leads and deep S waves in the left precordial leads.[5] Secondary repolarization abnormalities, with ST segment depression and T wave inversion, may be seen in the right precordial leads as well.[4,6] RAD is supportive evidence of RVH. Often the rightward axis

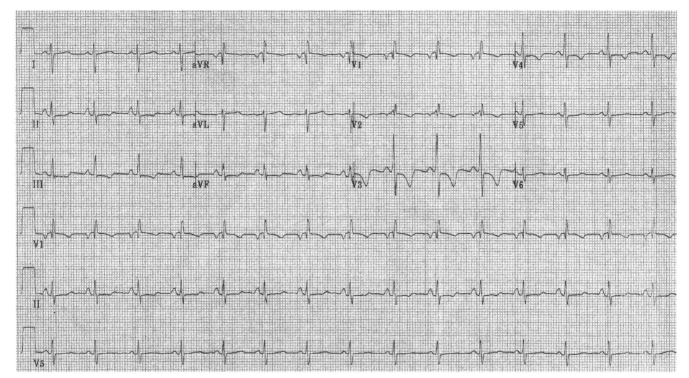

FIGURE 61-1 • **Pulmonary hypertension secondary to lupus.** There is evidence of P pulmonale with inverted P wave in lead V_1 and P wave axis of 70 degrees, and right axis deviation with QRS axis of 125 degrees. Right ventricular hypertrophy is evident by the qR pattern in leads V_1 and V_2. There is a right ventricular strain pattern with ST segment depression and T wave inversion in the right precordial leads.

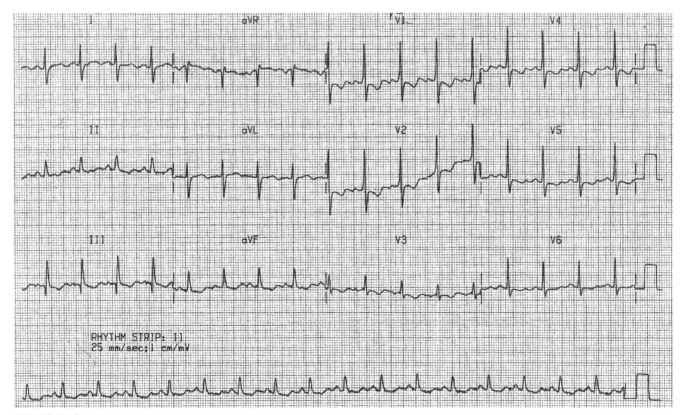

FIGURE 61-2 • **Primary pulmonary hypertension.** ECG from a 65-year-old woman with long-standing primary pulmonary hypertension demonstrating right ventricular hypertrophy with very prominent R waves in leads V_1 and V_2, and right ventricular strain pattern.

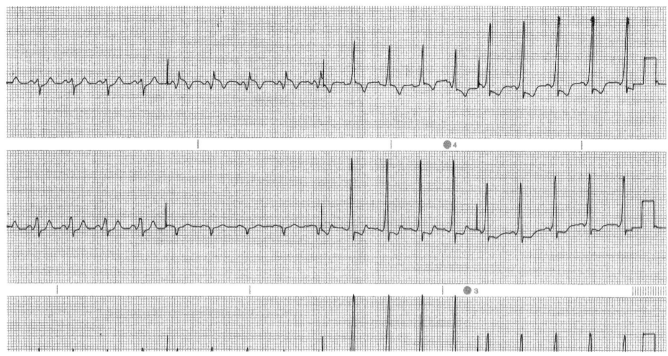

FIGURE 61-3 · **Pulmonary embolism.** ECG from a 27-year-old patient with acute pulmonary embolism showing sinus tachycardia and right ventricular hypertrophy with strain.

produces a tall R wave in lead aVR, although this by itself is not diagnostic of RVH.[4]

Right Bundle Branch Block. RBBB, either incomplete or complete, is frequently seen in RVH. Although not due to a true interruption of the right bundle branch fibers, the QRS widening occurs because of the additional time it takes the pathologically enlarged right ventricle to depolarize.[5]

Right Ventricular Strain. In cases of severe right ventricular pressure overload as seen in massive acute pulmonary embolism, there is abnormal repolarization of the right ventricular myocardium. This abnormal repolarization is manifested by ST segment depression and T wave inversion in right precordial leads[4-6] (Figs. 61-1 through 61-3). The pattern is the same as that seen in the lateral leads in left ventricular hypertrophy with strain.

References

1. Rich S: Pulmonary hypertension. In Braunwald E, Zipes DP, Libby P (eds): Heart Disease: A Textbook of Cardiovascular Medicine, 6th ed. Philadelphia, WB Saunders, 2001, p 1908.
2. McLaughlin V, Rich S: Cor pulmonale. In Braunwald E, Zipes DP, Libby P (eds): Heart Disease: A Textbook of Cardiovascular Medicine, 6th ed. Philadelphia, WB Saunders, 2001, p 1936.
3. Butler J, Agostoni PG: Cor pulmonale. In Murray JF, Nadel JA (eds): Textbook of Respiratory Medicine, 2nd ed. Philadelphia, WB Saunders, 1994.
4. Goldman MJ: Principles of Clinical Electrocardiography, 12th ed. Los Altos, Calif, Lange Medical Publishers, 1986.
5. Wagner GS: Marriott's Practical Electrocardiography, 10th ed. Philadelphia, Lippincott Williams & Wilkins, 2001.
6. O'Keefe JH, Hammill SC, Freed M: The Complete Guide to ECGs. Birmingham, Ala, Physicians' Press, 1997.

ELECTROCARDIOGRAPHIC PEARLS

- ECG findings in pulmonary hypertension reflect underlying right ventricular dilation, hypertrophy, and strain, but do not correlate with the severity of underlying lung disease or pulmonary hypertension.
- The ECG has low sensitivity in detecting right ventricular hypertrophy (RVH). However, when RVH is found on ECG, the findings are highly specific.
- The ECG criteria used to diagnose RVH are less useful in chronic obstructive pulmonary disease than in other forms of pulmonary hypertension because of the changes induced by hyperinflation.

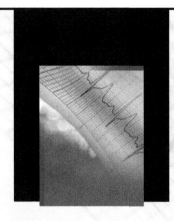

Chapter 62

Pneumothorax

Richard A. Harrigan and Bryon K. McNeil

Clinical Features

The clinical characteristics of a pneumothorax are usually the basis for suspecting and making the diagnosis. These signs and symptoms can be related to the size or type of pneumothorax present. Symptoms may include pleuritic chest pain, dyspnea, or palpitations. Objective findings can be mild or dramatic and may include hypoxia, tachypnea, tachycardia, hyperresonance and decreased breath sounds on the affected side, jugular venous distention, tracheal deviation away from the affected side, and hemodynamic compromise. The latter three findings are suggestive of tension pneumothorax. Of course, the patient should be treated immediately without obtaining proof from a chest radiograph and electrocardiograph (ECG).

Electrocardiographic Manifestations

The electrocardiographic changes associated with pneumothorax are myriad and nonspecific. Essentially, changes in voltage, QRS frontal plane axis, and ST segment morphology can be seen with a pneumothorax, but there is no change that is classically suggestive and there are no changes that are pathognomonic.

The literature on this topic is principally restricted to case reports or small case series of abnormal findings.[1–19] Because unusual cases tend to be reported, there exists a propensity for bias when reviewing the reported changes and drawing conclusions about what is typical and atypical. A case series reported in 1929 on ECG changes in 110 patients with artificial pneumothorax induced for the treatment of pulmonary tuberculosis is illustrative.[20] The report lacks detail with regard to a number of relevant changes, focusing instead on right versus left "ventricular preponderance" as an index of ventricular hypertrophy. In only 45 of these cases was a prepneumothorax ECG available for comparison; thus, reliable attribution of the findings to the pneumothorax rather than the underlying pulmonary disease is not possible. Furthermore, the reversibility of these findings after resolution of the pneumothorax is not demonstrable because these therapeutic pneumothoraces were permanent.

Left-sided pneumothorax is the best described, with rightward shift in the frontal plane QRS axis, voltage reduction, poor R wave progression, and ST segment/T wave changes[2–11,13] (Fig. 62-1). Less commonly, phasic voltage changes (variations of electrical alternans) have been described in left pneumothorax[3,8,15] (Fig. 62-2). More recently, abnormalities suggestive of atrial ischemia (PR segment elevation inferiorly) have been reported, accompanied by the aforementioned changes of axis and voltage.[16]

Right-sided pneumothorax also features findings of rightward axis deviation and decreased voltage.[6,17] Other findings with right-sided pneumothorax include tall, peaked P waves inferiorly, incomplete right bundle branch block, prominent R wave with smaller-than-expected S wave in lead V_2 mimicking posterior myocardial infarction, and the $S_1Q_3T_3$ pattern classically linked to pulmonary embolism.[6,17,19]

Bilateral pneumothoraces are infrequently reported and are limited in terms of generalization owing to the inequality of pneumothorax volume on the two sides (i.e., one side invariably has a larger defect than the other, thus favoring changes for the left or right).[1,14]

ELECTROCARDIOGRAPHIC HIGHLIGHTS

- Reduced QRS complex voltage and amplitude
- Relative change in QRS axis
- New left or right QRS frontal plane axis deviation
- Prominent R wave voltage with loss of S wave
- Phasic voltage alteration
- Changes in precordial R waves
- ST segment elevation or depression

ELECTROCARDIOGRAPHIC PEARLS

- ECG changes with pneumothorax can be subtle, even in the face of clinically significant pneumothoraces.
- ECG changes in pneumothorax are extremely nonspecific.

FIGURE 62-1 · ECG in a patient with chronic obstructive pulmonary disease and pneumothorax. In the first tracing (*A*), the patient had severe dyspnea; the second tracing (*B*) was obtained several minutes after the onset of left chest pain due to pneumothorax. Note the loss of R wave in lead I, leading to a new right axis deviation; the loss of R waves across the precordium; and emergence of new deep S waves in leads V_5 and V_6. (From Habibzadeh MA: ECG changes associated with spontaneous left-sided pneumothorax. Postgrad Med 1980;68:221–223, 226, with permission.)

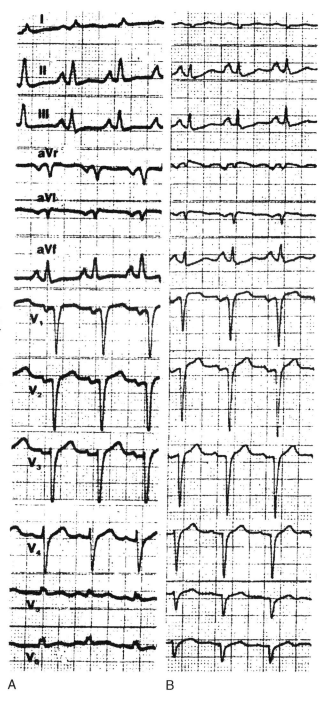

A   B

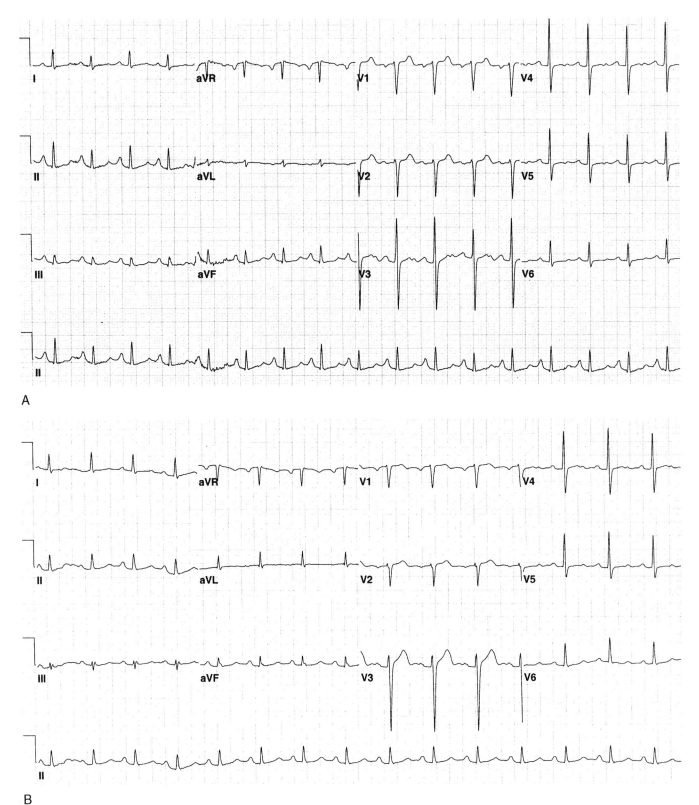

FIGURE 62-2 • ECG in a patient with left-sided pneumothorax with radiographic evidence of tension. These ECGs are from an elderly man with left-sided chest pain, who was hemodynamically stable yet manifested chest radiographic evidence of early tension, with some shift of the mediastinal structures before (*A*) and after (*B*) successful tube thoracostomy. The first tracing (*A*) demonstrates minimal evidence of right atrial strain in the inferior leads; this disappears after resolution of the pneumothorax. There is a slight rightward shift in QRS axis on the initial ECG compared with the post-thoracostomy tracing (note that the most isoelectric lead in *A* is aVL, whereas in *B* it is lead III). R wave transition zones in the precordium have also changed (although this may be due to lead placement). Finally, scrutiny of the amplitude of the QRS complexes in the first tracing (*A*) reveals phasic alteration in QRS height—clearly seen in the rhythm strip in beats 2, 9, and 12 (note also morphology of QRS in lead I [beat 2] and in lead V$_3$ [beat 12])—which disappears in the subsequent tracing.

References

1. Smith CE, Otworth JR, Kaluszyk P: Bilateral tension pneumothorax due to defective anesthesia breathing circuit filter. J Clin Anesth 1991;3:229.
2. Werne CS, Sands MJ: Left tension pneumothorax masquerading as anterior myocardial infarction. Ann Emerg Med 1985;14:164.
3. Kuritzky P, Goldfarb AL: Unusual electrocardiographic changes in spontaneous pneumothorax. Chest 1976;70:535.
4. Walston A, Brewer DL, Kitchens CS, Krook JE: The electrocardiographic manifestations of spontaneous left pneumothorax. Ann Intern Med 1974; 80:375.
5. Feldman T, January CT: ECG changes in pneumothorax. Chest 1984; 86:143.
6. Summers RS: The electrocardiogram as a diagnostic aid in pneumothorax [letter]. Chest 1973;63:127.
7. Ruo W, Rupani G: Left tension pneumothorax mimicking myocardial ischemia after percutaneous central venous cannulation. Anesthesiology 1992;76:306.
8. Kounis NG, Zavras GM, Kitrou MP, et al: Unusual electrocardiographic manifestations in conditions with increased intrathoracic pressure. Acta Cardiol 1988;43:653.
9. Habibzadeh MA: ECG changes associated with spontaneous left-sided pneumothorax. Postgrad Med 1980;68:221.
10. Diamond JR, Estes NM: ECG changes associated with iatrogenic left pneumothorax simulating anterior myocardial infarction. Am Heart J 1982;103:303.
11. Botz G, Brock-Utne JG: Are electrocardiographic changes the first sign of impending perioperative pneumothorax? Anaesthesia 1992; 47:1057.
12. Athanasopoulos C, Childers R: Q-T prolongation in acute pneumothorax. Acta Cardiol 1979;34:85.
13. Gould L, Gopalaswamy C, Chandy F, Kim BS: ECG changes after left pneumonectomy [letter]. N Engl J Med 1983;308:1481.
14. Ti LK, Lee TL: The electrocardiogram complements a chest radiograph for the early detection of pneumothorax in post-coronary artery bypass grafting patients. J Cardiothorac Vasc Anesth 1998;12:679.
15. Kozelj M, Rakovec P, Sok M: Unusual ECG variations in left-sided pneumothorax. J Electrocardiol 1997;30:109.
16. Strizik B, Forman R: New ECG changes associated with tension pneumothorax. Chest 1999;115:1742.
17. Alikhan M, Biddison JH: Electrocardiographic changes with right-sided pneumothorax. South Med J 1998;91:677.
18. Raev D: A case of spontaneous left-sided pneumothorax with ECG changes resembling acute myocardial infarction. Int J Cardiol 1996;56:197.
19. Goddard R, Scofield RH: Right pneumothorax with the $S_1Q_3T_3$ electrocardiogram pattern usually associated with pulmonary embolus. Am J Emerg Med 1997;15:310.
20. Bronfin ID, Simon S, Black LT: Electrocardiographic studies in artificial pneumothorax: A report on 110 cases. Tubercle 1929;11:114.

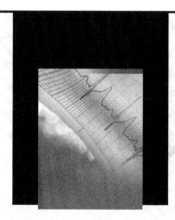

Chapter 63

Endocrine and Metabolic Disorders

David A. Wald

Numerous endocrinopathies can lead to cardiovascular dysfunction. Interactions with the cardiovascular system are often complex and usually occur as a result of direct hormone effects or indirectly as a manifestation of electrolyte abnormalities. Thyroid disease, parathyroid disorders, adrenal disease, hypothermia, and other metabolic and nutritional disorders have been associated with a number of electrocardiographic (ECG) abnormalities.

THYROID DISEASE

Clinical Features

Excess thyroid hormone, or deficiency, may have a profound effect on the cardiovascular system, and has been associated with a varying number of ECG abnormalities. Patients with

ELECTROCARDIOGRAPHIC HIGHLIGHTS

Hyperthyroidism

- Sinus tachycardia
- Atrial fibrillation

Hypothyroidism

- Bradycardia
- Low voltage
- Flattened or inverted T waves

Hyperparathyroidism

- Shortened QT interval

Hypoparathyroidism

- Prolonged QT interval

Hyperaldosteronism

- U waves
- T wave abnormalities

Primary adrenal insufficiency

- T wave abnormalities, including peaked waves if hyperkalemia is present

Pheochromocytoma

- Nonspecific ST segment/T wave abnormalities
- Sinus tachycardia

Acromegaly

- T wave abnormalities

Hypothermia

- Sinus bradycardia
- Atrial fibrillation
- Osborne waves (J waves)
- Ventricular fibrillation

Beriberi disease

- T wave abnormalities
- QT prolongation

Keshan disease

- Nonspecific ST segment/T wave abnormalities

Kwashiorkor syndrome

- Atrioventricular conduction disturbances

Carnitine deficiency

- T wave abnormalities

hyperthyroidism (i.e., thyrotoxicosis or thyroid storm) may present with varying degrees of cardiovascular, gastrointestinal, or neurologic dysfunction. The cardiovascular manifestations of a hyperthyroid state are common, and older patients are more likely to present with cardiovascular dysfunction.[1] Excess thyroid hormone has been shown to alter cardiovascular physiology by a variety of direct and indirect mechanisms.[2–5] The clinical manifestations of hyperthyroidism resemble other hyperdynamic states of sympathoadrenal stimulation. The cardiovascular manifestations of excess thyroid hormone include an enhanced cardiac output and left ventricular contractility, increased myocardial oxygen consumption

and increased coronary blood flow, a decrease in the systemic vascular resistance, and an expanded blood volume.[6,7] In patients with thyroid storm, the cardiovascular manifestations may be profound.

The cardiovascular manifestations of hypothyroidism are essentially the opposite of what is seen in hyperthyroidism. These manifestations commonly include a decrease in cardiac output resulting from a decrease in stroke volume and heart rate. The myocardial oxygen consumption is decreased, the systemic vascular resistance is increased, and there is a decrease in the circulating blood volume.[6,7] Hypothyroid patients may also complain of dyspnea on exertion and have poor exercise tolerance.

Electrocardiographic Manifestations

ECG manifestations of hyperthyroidism are common, yet no change is pathognomonic. Sinus tachycardia is the most common cardiac dysrhythmia in hyperthyroidism and occurs in 40% of patients[7,8] (Fig. 63-1). Nonspecific ST segment/T wave abnormalities are noted in 25% of patients.[9] Atrial fibrillation occurs in 10% to 22% of hyperthyroid patients[7] (Fig. 63-2). Atrial fibrillation appears to be more likely to occur in thyrotoxic patients who are men, older than 60 years of age, and have a history of hypertension or rheumatic heart disease.[7] With hyperthyroidism, there may be PR segment interval shortening. Intraventricular conduction disturbances, most commonly left anterior fascicular block or right bundle branch block (RBBB), occur in approximately 15% of patients without underlying heart disease.[9]

The ECG manifestations of hypothyroidism include sinus bradycardia, low-voltage complexes, prolonged PR intervals and QT intervals, and flattened or inverted T waves[6–8,10] (Fig. 63-3). Pericardial effusions occur in up to 30% of hypothyroid patients, and may be responsible for some of the ECG manifestations.[6,10] Atrial, intraventricular, or ventricular conduction disturbances are three times more likely to occur in patients with myxedema than in the general population.[6,9,10]

PARATHYROID DISEASE

Clinical Features

By itself, parathyroid hormone has few direct cardiovascular effects.[6] Indirectly, an excess or deficiency of parathyroid hormone affects the heart through its regulation of calcium. Primary hyperparathyroidism is often caused by a solitary adenoma (85%).[11] Hypercalcemia is the hallmark laboratory abnormality of this disorder. Although hypertension has been closely associated with hyperparathyroidism, many patients are either asymptomatic, or have vague, nonspecific complaints when diagnosed.[11] There are no specific examination findings that are pathognomonic for hyperparathyroidism.

Hypoparathyroidism is a rare condition that is usually associated with deficient parathyroid hormone secretion. In this disease, the hallmark laboratory finding is hypocalcemia. Typical findings of hypocalcemia may be present, including paresthesias of the fingers, toes, and circumoral area. In more severe cases, carpopedal spasm, laryngeal stridor, or convulsions have been noted.[11]

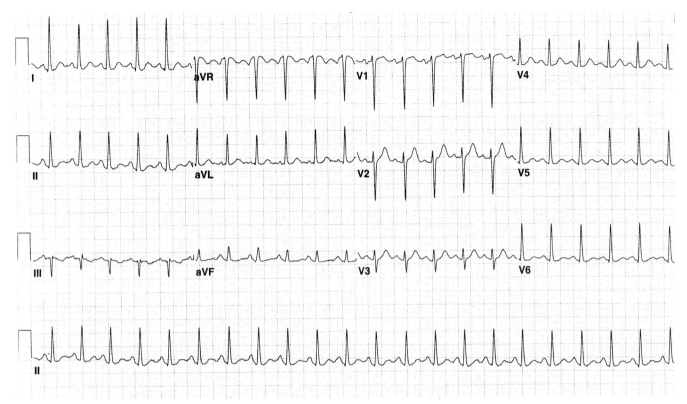

FIGURE 63-1 · **Hyperthyroidism.** This 12-lead ECG shows sinus tachycardia with nonspecific inferior T wave abnormalities in a patient with hyperthyroidism.

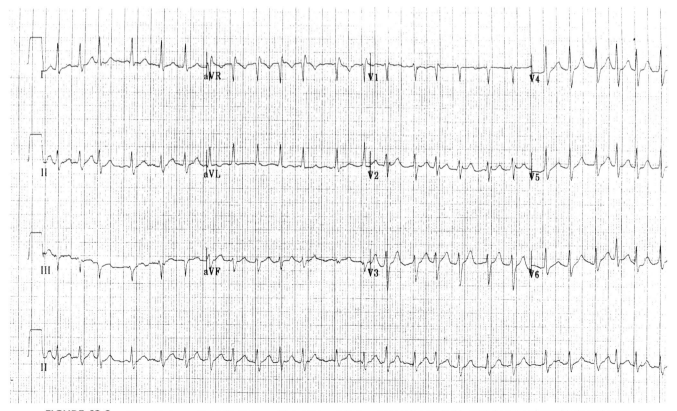

FIGURE 63-2 · **Thyroid storm.** Atrial fibrillation with a rapid ventricular response is seen in this ECG from a patient with thyroid storm.

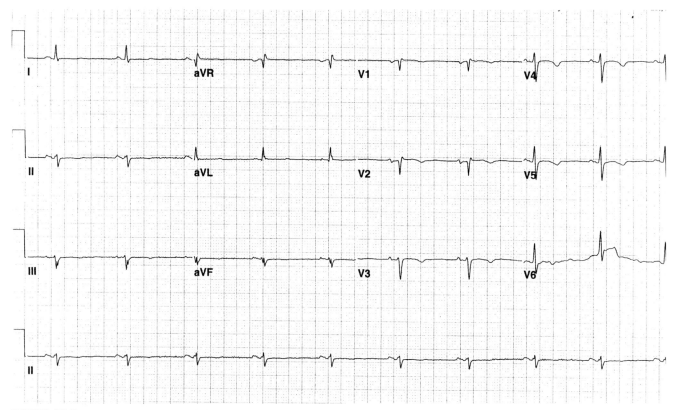

FIGURE 63-3 • **Myxedema.** This ECG is from a 57-year-old woman with myxedema, a temperature of 34.4°C (94°F), and a serum thyroid-stimulating hormone level of 19.88 mIU/mL. ECG reveals sinus bradycardia with low voltage and diffuse T wave abnormalities.

Electrocardiographic Manifestations

The ECG manifestations of patients with hyperparathyroidism occur secondary to the resultant hypercalcemia. Hypercalcemia shortens the plateau phase of the cardiac action potential and decreases the effective refractory period.[8,9] On the ECG, this is identified by a shortened QT interval (Fig. 63-4). In cases of severe hypercalcemia (calcium >16 mg/dL), the T wave can widen, which tends to increase the QT interval.[6,10]

Because of the resultant hypocalcemia associated with hypoparathyroidism, ECG manifestations include a prolongation of the QT interval (Fig. 63-5). QT interval prolongation occurs because hypocalcemia prolongs the plateau phase of the cardiac action potential[8] (see Chapter 58, Electrolyte Abnormalities).

ADRENAL DISEASE

Clinical Features

Although rare, hyperaldosteronism is considered the most common endocrine cause of hypertension, accounting for 0.5% to 2% of all patients with hypertension.[6,8,10] Excess aldosterone production by the adrenal cortex leads to enhanced sodium retention with plasma volume expansion, hypokalemia, metabolic alkalosis, and suppression of renin and angiotensin. Patients often present with moderate to severe hypertension without edema. Symptoms of hypokalemia may include muscle cramps, weakness, headaches, palpitations, or polyuria.

Adrenal insufficiency occurs as a result of decreased glucocorticoid and mineralocorticoid production. Primary adrenal insufficiency (Addison's disease) occurs when a significant portion (90%) of the adrenal gland has been destroyed.[10] The most common cause of Addison's disease is autoimmune destruction of the adrenal cortex, although many other etiologies, including adrenal hemorrhage, tuberculosis, acquired immunodeficiency syndrome, fungal infection, and metastasis, have been noted to cause this disorder.[10,11] Laboratory abnormalities commonly associated with primary adrenal insufficiency include hyponatremia, hyperkalemia, hypercalcemia, hypoglycemia, and metabolic acidosis. Isolated mineralocorticoid (aldosterone) deficiency may also be associated with hyperkalemia, but this disorder is much less commonly encountered.

Electrocardiographic Manifestations

ECG abnormalities in patients with hyperaldosteronism or primary adrenal insufficiency usually occur secondary to altered serum potassium levels. ECG manifestations of hypokalemia may be seen in patients with hyperaldosteronism. These changes often include T wave abnormalities, development of U waves (Fig. 63-6), increased P wave amplitude and duration, and ST segment depression. In addition, conduction abnormalities and various dysrhythmias may

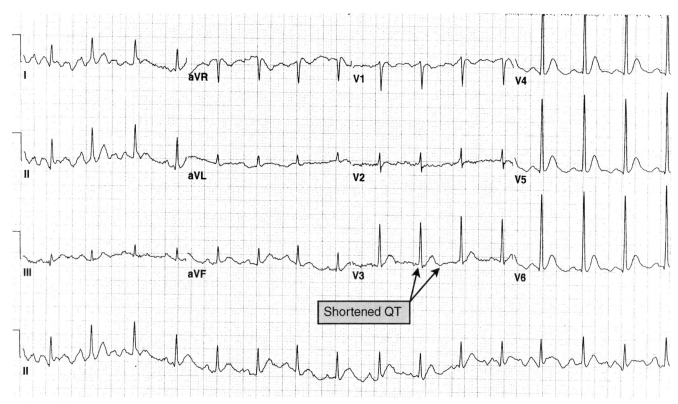

FIGURE 63-4 • **Hyperparathyroidism.** This ECG is from an 84-year-old woman with a history of primary hyperparathyroidism presenting with weakness, fatigue, and anorexia, and calcium level of 17.2 mg/dL. ECG reveals a sinus rhythm with voltage criteria for left ventricular hypertrophy, and a shortened QT interval.

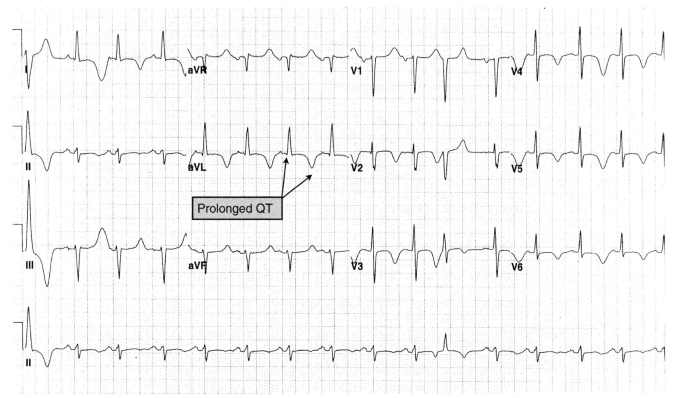

FIGURE 63-5 • **Hypoparathyroidism.** This ECG from a patient with hypoparathyroidism and a calcium level of 4.9 mg/dL reveals a sinus rhythm with occasional premature ectopic complexes, diffuse ST segment and T wave abnormalities, and a prolonged QT interval.

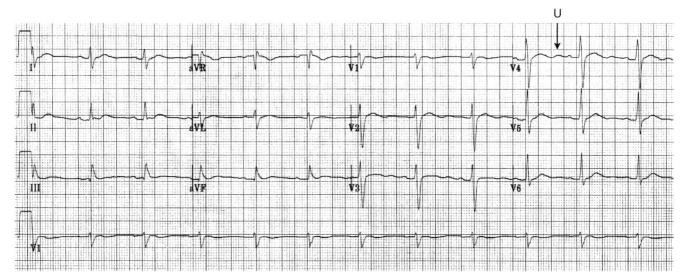

FIGURE 63-6 • **Hyperaldosteronism.** This ECG from a 22-year-old woman with hyperaldosteronism and a potassium level of 1.9 mg/dL reveals a sinus rhythm, nonspecific T wave findings, and U waves (u) seen most prominently in leads V_3 to V_5.

be seen in patients with severe hypokalemia (see Chapter 58, Electrolyte Abnormalities).

ECG abnormalities can also occur in patients with primary adrenal insufficiency. Findings may include sinus tachycardia or sinus bradycardia, and nonspecific T wave abnormalities. Conduction disturbances, most often first degree atrioventricular block, can occur in up to 20% of patients with adrenal insufficiency.[10] When hyperkalemia is prominent, a number of characteristic ECG changes may occur, including peaked T waves, flattening of the P wave, and prolongation of the PR interval and QRS complexes (see Chapter 58, Electrolyte Abnormalities).

PHEOCHROMOCYTOMA AND OTHER ENDOCRINOPATHIES

Clinical Features

Pheochromocytomas are rare, catecholamine-producing tumors that are most often located in the adrenal medulla (90%).[8,11] As a cause of hypertension, pheochromocytomas account for 0.1% to 0.2% all cases.[11] The classic triad of symptoms includes paroxysms of headache, palpitations, and diaphoresis. Hypertension is a common manifestation of this disorder; it is often labile and refractory to standard antihypertensive therapy.

The cardiovascular system is also vulnerable to excess growth hormone production associated with acromegaly. Acromegaly usually occurs as the result of a growth hormone–producing pituitary adenoma.[8] Hypertension, although not a prominent feature, is seen in 25% to 35% of patients with this disorder.[10]

Electrocardiographic Manifestations

ECG abnormalities in patients with pheochromocytoma are common. Nonspecific ECG changes include ST

segment/T wave abnormalities. Numerous dysrhythmias have been noted in these patients, including sinus tachycardia, ventricular tachycardia, torsades de pointes, or ventricular fibrillation.[8] Conduction disturbances have been reported, including both right and left bundle branch block and prolonged QT intervals.[6,8,10] Prominent U waves, peaked P waves, and ventricular strain patterns may also be seen.

ECG abnormalities may be seen in patients with excessive growth hormone production and acromegaly. These ECG findings include ST segment depression, nonspecific T wave changes, left ventricular hypertrophy, and intraventricular conduction disturbances.[6] Ventricular ectopy and atrial fibrillation or flutter can also be seen.

HYPOTHERMIA

Clinical Features

Hypothermia is defined as a core body temperature less than 35°C (95°F). The signs and symptoms are myriad. In mild cases, patients may exhibit fatigue, incoordination, shivering, and slurred speech. In moderate to severe cases, patients exhibit progressive disorientation, stupor, lethargy, and cardiac dysrhythmias leading to hypotension, progressive coma, and eventually death.

Electrocardiographic Manifestations

When patients become moderate to severely hypothermic, various ECG changes can be seen. Typical findings include slowing of the sinus rate, prolongation of the PR and QT intervals, and the appearance of the classic Osborne or J wave.[9,12] The J wave, also known as the *camel-hump sign*, is an extra deflection noted on the ECG at the junction of the QRS complex and the beginning of the ST segment take-off[12,13] (Figs. 63-7 and 63-8). Osborne waves are consistently present when the body temperature falls below 25°C.[12]

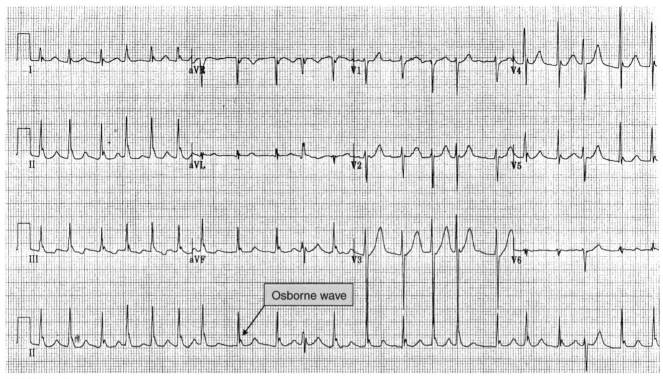

FIGURE 63-7 · Hypothermia. In a patient with hypothermia and a core body temperature of 32.2°C (90° F), the ECG demonstrates atrial fibrillation with a rapid ventricular response. Osborne waves are noted, and are most prominent in the limb leads (*arrow*).

Atrial fibrillation is also common in hypothermia, occurring in 50% to 60% of patients, appearing at a mean body temperature of 29°C; the ventricular response rate may be normal or bradycardic.[12] In severe hypothermia, marked bradycardia, asystole, and ventricular fibrillation may be seen. The myocardium may be more irritable and at greater risk for ventricular dysrhythmias and fibrillation with stimulation. In general, with core body temperature rewarming, the ECG abnormalities associated with hypothermia are transient and should resolve.

METABOLIC/NUTRITIONAL DISORDERS

Clinical Features

Nutritional deficiencies such as beriberi, Keshan disease, kwashiorkor syndrome, and carnitine deficiency can lead to a variety of cardiovascular abnormalities. Beriberi disease occurs as a result of vitamin B_1 (thiamine) deficiency and is seen in populations whose dietary staple consists of polished

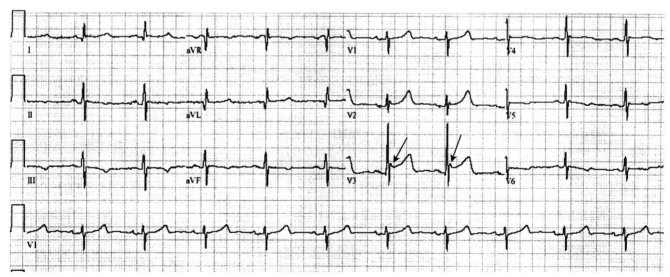

FIGURE 63-8 · Hypothermia with Osborn waves. This ECG, in a patient with a core temperature of 31.1°C (88°F), features a bradycardic rate and Osborn (or J) waves, best seen in the precordial leads (*arrows*).

ELECTROCARDIOGRAPHIC PEARLS

- ECG changes associated with various endocrine and metabolic disorders are not diagnostic of the underlying disease.
- Some ECG abnormalities associated with endocrinopathies may represent altered serum electrolyte levels.
- Various tachydysrhythmias may occur as a result of hyperthyroidism or pheochromocytoma.
- Most ECG abnormalities associated with nutritional disorders are nonspecific.

---

rice, as well as in alcoholics and individuals following fad diets.[14] Beriberi heart disease is characterized by high-output heart failure as demonstrated by an increase in cardiac index, an increase in the circulating blood volume, and a decrease in the peripheral vascular resistance. Keshan disease, which is found mainly in China, is caused by selenium deficiency. In the United States, a Keshan-like disease state may occur in patients on long-term home parenteral nutrition.[14] Findings of heart failure including cardiomegaly and pulmonary edema may be seen. Kwashiorkor syndrome, which is found mostly in Africa, results from a diet that is deficient in protein calories. In the United States, this syndrome may be seen on occasion in patients with anorexia nervosa.[14] Abnormalities in cardiac function and the conduction system of the heart can be seen in this syndrome. Various cardiac manifestations of carnitine deficiency have been reported, including a hypertrophic cardiomyopathy type with a decreased ejection fraction, a type that resembles a dilated cardiomyopathy, and an endocardial fibroelastosis type.[14]

Electrocardiographic Manifestations

The ECG manifestations of beriberi heart disease are often nonspecific and may at times be recognized retrospectively after treatment. Abnormalities include tachycardia, prolongation of the QT interval, and various T wave changes (inverted, diphasic, or depressed).[14] The T wave abnormalities occur mainly in the right-sided precordial leads.[14] Various ECG abnormalities can also be seen in patients with Keshan disease, including nonspecific ST segment/T wave changes, RBBB, and premature ventricular contractions.[14] In patients

with kwashiorkor syndrome, various atrioventricular conduction disturbances may be seen. ECG manifestations also occur as a result of carnitine deficiency. Some cases have been associated with T wave enlargement similar to that seen in hyperkalemia; other cases have been associated with T wave inversions in the anterolateral precordial leads (V_4 to V_6), or diffuse low voltage.[14] However, the most frequently identified ECG abnormality is tachycardia.

References

1. Braverman LE, Utiger RD: Introduction to thyrotoxicosis. In Braverman LE, Utiger RD (eds): Werner and Ingbar's The Thyroid: A Fundamental and Clinical Text, 6th ed. Philadelphia, JB Lippincott, 1991, pp 645–647.
2. Klein I: Thyroid hormone and the cardiovascular system. Am J Med 1990;88:631.
3. Klein I, Levey GS: The cardiovascular system in thyrotoxicosis. In Braverman LE, Utiger RD (eds): Werner and Ingbar's The Thyroid: A Fundamental and Clinical Text, 7th ed. Philadelphia, JB Lippincott, 1996, pp 607–615.
4. Magner JA, Clark W, Allenby P: Congestive heart failure and sudden death in a young woman with thyrotoxicosis. West J Med 1988; 149:86.
5. Skelton CL: The heart and hyperthyroidism. N Engl J Med 1982;307:1206.
6. Vela BS, Crawford MH: Endocrinology and the heart. In Crawford MH (ed): Current Diagnosis and Treatment in Cardiology. Norfolk, CT, Lange Medical Books, 1995, pp 411–427.
7. Chipkin SR: Lipoprotein Metabolism and Coronary Artery Disease. In Hurst JW, Alpert JS (eds): Diagnostic Atlas of the Heart. New York, Raven Press, 1994, pp 503–516.
8. Barsness GW, Feinglos MN: Endocrine systems and the heart. In Topol EJ, Califf RM, Isner JM, et al (eds): Comprehensive Cardiovascular Medicine. Philadelphia, Lippincott-Raven, 1998, pp 952–969.
9. Harumi K, Chen CY: Miscellaneous electrocardiographic topics. In Macfarlane PW, Veitch Lawrie TD (eds): Comprehensive Electrocardiography. Oxford, Pergamon Press, 1989, pp 671–728.
10. Vela BS: Endocrinology and the heart. In Crawford MH, DiMarco JP, Paulus WJ, et al (eds): Cardiology. St. Louis, Mosby, 2001, pp 4.1–4.13.
11. Spiegel AM: The parathyroid glands, hypercalcemia, and hypocalcemia. In Goldman L, Bennet JC (eds): Cecil Textbook of Medicine, 21st ed. Philadelphia, WB Saunders, 2000, pp 1398–1409.
12. Chou TC: Electrocardiography in Clinical Practice: Adult and Pediatric, 3rd ed. Philadelphia, WB Saunders, 1991, pp 503–508.
13. Cheng D: The ECG of hypothermia. J Emerg Med 2002;22:87.
14. Kawai C, Nakamura Y: The heart in nutritional disorders. In Braunwald E (ed): Atlas of Heart Disease, Vol II: Cardiomyopathies, Myocarditis, and Pericardial Disease. New York, McGraw-Hill, 1995, pp 7.1–7.18.

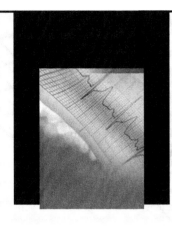

Chapter 64

Neurologic and Neuromuscular Conditions

Teresa L. Smith, Steven L. Bernstein, and Thomas P. Bleck

Suspected since antiquity, Byer and colleagues first proved a relationship between the brain and heart in 1947, demonstrating that intracranial disease processes were associated with specific electrocardiographic (ECG) abnormalities.[1] Among the most common neurologic disorders that can result in ECG changes are central nervous system (CNS) processes, such as subarachnoid hemorrhage (SAH), other forms of stroke, acute spinal cord injury, and epilepsy; as well as numerous neuromuscular diseases[2,3] (Table 64-1).

CENTRAL NERVOUS SYSTEM DISEASES

Clinical Features

The exact pathophysiologic mechanism by which certain CNS diseases produce ECG changes is not known. Animal studies have demonstrated an influence of multiple brain regions, including the brainstem, hypothalamus, amygdala, and insular cortex, on ECG findings. As an example, repetitive stimulation of the posterior hypothalamus can lead to prolongation of the QT interval, increase in T wave size, decrease

in PR interval, and ventricular tachycardia. These effects are believed mediated by the sympathetic nervous system and can be blocked by propranolol.[4]

Pathologic examinations of hearts in stroke deaths have demonstrated a particular diffuse damage to ventricular myocytes. Commonly found are hemorrhages near the conduction system, scattered areas of edematous myocytes with infiltrating inflammatory cells, interstitial hemorrhage, and myofibrillary degeneration. These pathologic changes also can be seen after intense catecholamine surges.[4]

Several theories have been postulated as to the mechanism of ECG abnormalities associated with acute cerebrovascular disease and stroke. Elevated sympathoadrenal tone causes direct excitation of sodium channels on myocytes, which may itself be dysrhythmogenic. Alternatively, the resultant calcium influx may lead to an increase in dysrhythmias. Another theory is that stroke affects the heart by altering the intrinsic cardiac sympathetic nerves, thus increasing sympathetic outflow to the myocardium. Increased central sympathetic outflow may cause coronary vasoconstriction, resulting in dysrhythmias on the basis of coronary ischemia.[4] Whatever the mechanism, acute cerebrovascular disease–associated dysrhythmias can be problematic. Their occurrence

64-1 • ELECTROCARDIOGRAPHIC CHANGES ASSOCIATED WITH SEVERAL CENTRAL NERVOUS SYSTEM PROCESSES				
ECG Change	SAH	Ischemic Stroke with CAD	Ischemic Stroke without CAD	ICH
Prolonged QT interval	71%	37%	28%	50%
T wave	25%	2%	34%	38%
ST segment abnormality	11%	25%	25%	25%
U waves	32%	25%	9%	44%
Q waves	21%	22%	9%	19%
Tachycardia	36%	22%	15%	44%
Bradycardia	12%	9%	11%	19%
Atrial fibrillation	11%	13%	0%	6%

CAD, coronary artery disease; ICH, intracerebral hemorrhage; SAH, subarachnoid hemorrhage.

ELECTROCARDIOGRAPHIC HIGHLIGHTS

The principal abnormalities in subarachnoid hemorrhage, intracerebral hemorrhage, and ischemic stroke include:
- Diffuse ST segment elevation or depression
- T waves with large positive or negative deflections
- The presence of U waves
- Prolonged QT interval segments

Dysrhythmias are also common and include:
- Bradydysrhythmias and tachydysrhythmias
- Sinus arrhythmia
- Atrial fibrillation
- Ventricular premature beats
- Ventricular tachycardia

---

is correlated with increased mortality rates in patients with ischemic stroke.

A sympathomimetic mechanism has also been postulated for the myocardial and ECG effects of SAH because these changes can be blocked by phentolamine and propranolol.[5] Similar to stroke, the presence of repolarization abnormalities corresponds to a worsened prognosis after SAH.[4,6]

Seizures and epilepsy can also result in ECG abnormalities. In focal seizures that secondarily generalize, such as a temporal lobe aura followed by a generalized tonic-clonic seizure, tachycardia coincides with or even precedes the aura.[4] This finding suggests that the rhythm abnormality is related to the epileptic discharge rather than motor activity. Studies in animals suggest that epileptic neuronal firing can cause an imbalance of sympathetic and parasympathetic discharges in the heart, which can lead to disintegration of repolarization and depolarization, making way for ectopic activity. The entity of sudden unexpected death in epileptic patients (SUDEP) tends to occur in young, healthy patients, often with

low anticonvulsant levels. Studies suggest ventricular fibrillation as the chief cardiac event in SUDEP, although autopsy is often unrevealing.[7,8]

Electrocardiographic Manifestations

Certain CNS disorders produce ECG changes, including prolongation of QT intervals, flattening, peaking, or inversion of the T wave, ST segment elevation or depression, and the development of U and Q waves. In addition, CNS disease can precipitate various dysrhythmias such as sinus bradycardia (Figs. 64-1) and tachycardia, sinus dysrhythmia, atrial fibrillation (Fig. 64-2), paroxysmal atrial tachycardia, premature ventricular contractions, atrioventricular (AV) block, and ventricular tachycardia.

The most common condition that results in ECG changes is SAH, with reported rates ranging from 60% to 70% and 90% to 100% in various studies, with life-threatening abnormalities estimated at 20%. In acute ischemic stroke, ECG abnormalities are reported in 5% to 17%.[4] Almost all patients with cervical spinal cord lesions have a bradydysrhythmia as a result of interruption of sympathetic outflow through the cord.

T Wave Abnormalities.   Common ECG abnormalities in CNS dysfunction include conspicuously increased T wave amplitudes. The T waves may be bifid and can be confused with a U wave.[9] Various neurogenic etiologies of T wave changes exist with characteristic features. Coined the "cerebrovascular accident T wave pattern," descriptions of the T wave morphology include a distinctly deep, widely splayed appearance with an outward bulge of the ascending limb, resulting in a striking asymmetry. Although most commonly observed with SAH, this pattern occurs in a variety of neural insults, including arterial occlusion, intracerebral hemorrhage, radical neck dissection, truncal vagotomy, bilateral carotid surgery, and Stokes-Adams syndrome. Explanations

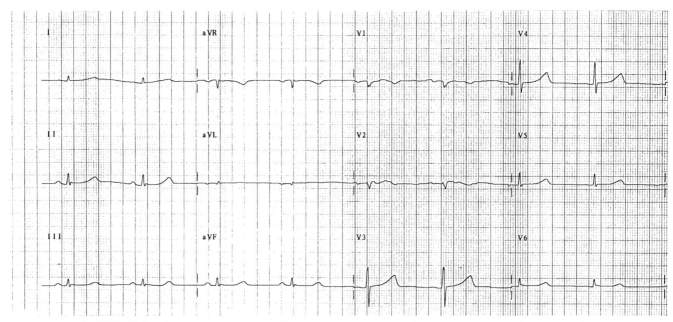

FIGURE 64-1 • **Sinus bradycardia.** This ECG from a patient with a cervical spinal cord transection shows bradycardia.

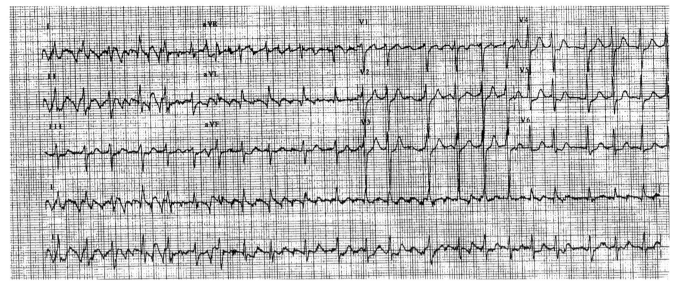

FIGURE 64-2 • Atrial fibrillation. This ECG is from a patient with Parkinson's disease and a new ischemic stroke. On day 1 post-stroke, this paroxysmal atrial fibrillation developed. Given the underlying tremor, the baseline is difficult to interpret.

for this ECG finding include increased sympathetic and vagal tone leading to aberrant repolarization, perhaps secondary to myocyte injury and contraction band necrosis.

Hypothalamic dysfunction has been implicated in the pathophysiologic process of these changes as supported by the association between T wave changes and central diabetes insipidus. In addition, T wave changes are observed in 20% to 50% of cases of SAH from rupture of posterior or anterior communicating artery aneurysms and subsequent damage to the hypothalamus[10] (Fig. 64-3).

U Waves.   Best observed in the chest leads and usually highest in lead V_3 just to the right of the QRS complex transition zone, the U wave is thought to be due to the late repolarization forces occurring during the myocyte after potential recovery period.[9] When the QT interval is prolonged, the U wave may fuse with the T wave. Positive inotropic phenomena such as catecholamine surges tend to increase the U wave amplitude[10] (Fig. 64-4).

ST Segment Changes.   In CNS processes, the ECG can show ST segment elevation or depression. These changes are also consistent with myocardial infarction and thus should be managed as such until proven otherwise (Fig. 64-5). Diffuse elevations of the ST segment can appear similar to acute pericarditis.

QT Interval Prolongation.   Prolongation of the corrected QT interval can be seen with a number of CNS diseases, particularly in patients with stroke (see Fig. 64-1).

NEUROMUSCULAR DISEASES

Clinical Features

The neuromuscular diseases are rare inherited disorders. The heart is frequently involved in these disorders, affected either by abnormalities of the myocardium or of the conduction system.

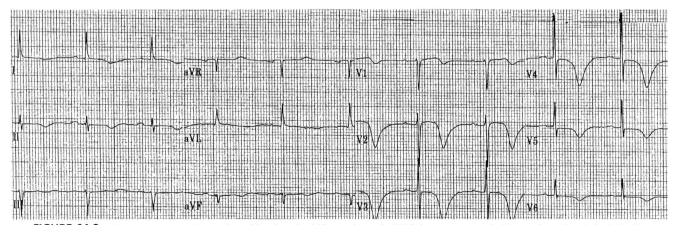

FIGURE 64-3 • T wave inversion. In a patient with subarachnoid hemorrhage, the ECG demonstrates marked T wave inversions in leads V_2-V_6.

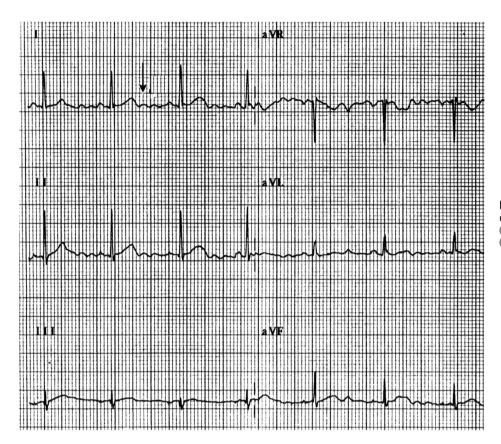

FIGURE 64-4 · **U waves in subarachnoid hemorrhage (SAH).** Small U waves (*arrow*) are present in a patient post-SAH (limb leads only).

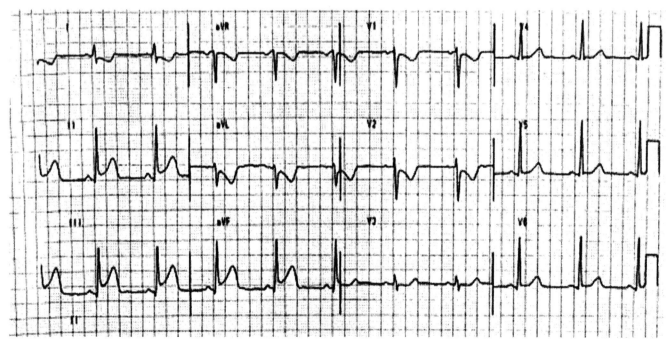

FIGURE 64-5 · **ST segment changes in brainstem hemorrhage.** This ECG shows ST segment elevation in the inferior leads with ST segment depression in the lateral and right precordial leads.

Although the clinical spectrum of a given disease between individuals may vary based on phenotypic expression, ECG findings are often remarkably consistent. We discuss the ECG abnormalities associated with Friedreich's ataxia, Duchenne muscular dystrophy (DMD), Emery-Dreifuss syndrome, Kearns-Sayre syndrome, and myotonic dystrophy.

Electrocardiographic Manifestations

Friedreich's ataxia is an autosomally inherited recessive disorder presenting in late childhood and resulting in degeneration of the spinocerebellar tracts, dorsal columns, and corticospinal tract. In patients with Friedreich's ataxia, either a hypertrophic or dilated cardiomyopathy and congestive heart failure may develop.[11] ECG findings associated with Friedreich's ataxia include PR interval shortening, right axis deviation, left ventricular hypertrophy, and inferolateral Q waves that are broad and shallow.[11]

Duchenne muscular dystrophy is an X-linked recessive disorder that manifests during childhood as weakness of gait, toe walking, and "pseudohypertrophy" of the calves due to fatty infiltration of muscle. The ECG abnormalities occur with increasing frequency in DMD as patients age and ultimately occur in almost all patients.[12] Common ECG abnormalities include sinus tachycardia and right axis deviation. The most striking abnormalities are of the QRS complex morphology and frequently include tall R waves in lead V_1 and Q waves in the lateral precordial leads.[13]

Emery-Dreifuss syndrome is an X-linked recessive muscular dystrophy characterized by contractures of the elbows, Achilles tendons, and posterior cervical musculature, and muscle wasting of the upper arms and lower leg muscles.[14] Cardiomyopathy is invariably present. ECG abnormalities in Emery-Dreifuss syndrome include sinus bradycardia with PR interval prolongation. Heart block may progress, and is a cause of sudden death in these patients.

Kearns-Sayre syndrome is a mitochondrial myopathy consisting of the triad of retinitis pigmentosa, external ophthalmoplegia, and cardiac conduction disturbances. Symptoms commonly appear in late childhood or early adolescence. Conduction abnormalities, such as RBBB, appear to be caused by fibrosis of the His bundle[15] (Fig. 64-6). In Kearns-Sayre syndrome, the ECG may show any degree of heart block, and progression to complete heart block is common.

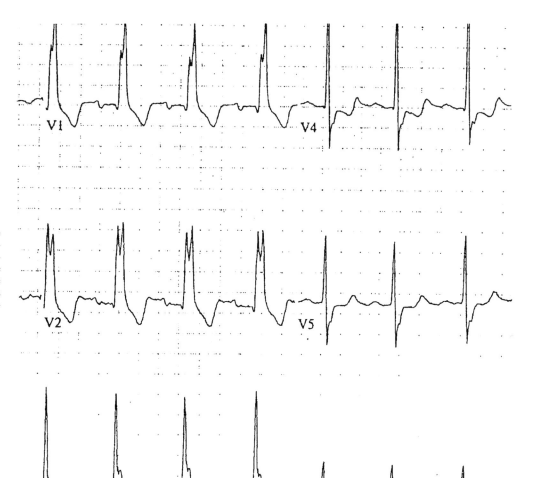

FIGURE 64-6 · Kearns-Sayre syndrome. A 12-lead ECG (precordial leads only) from a 10-year-old boy with Kearns-Sayre syndrome shows right bundle branch block. The PR interval is 0.2 sec, consistent with a borderline first-degree AVB.

ELECTROCARDIOGRAPHIC PEARLS

- ECG abnormalities in patients with acute stroke may represent true cardiac ischemia and infarction.
- The occurrence of ECG abnormalities in patients with stroke or subarachnoid hemorrhage portends a worse prognosis.
- Patients with spinal cord lesions often present with brady-dysrhythmias as a result of decreased sympathetic outflow.

Myotonic dystrophy (Steinert's disease) is an autosomal dominant disorder and is the most commonly occurring muscular dystrophy. Clinical symptoms include myotonia and progressive muscle atrophy. Cardiac involvement in this disease appears to be related to damage of the cardiac conduction system, although myocardial degeneration also occurs. ECG abnormalities commonly seen in myotonic dystrophy include first degree AV block and left anterior fascicular block. Atrial dysrhythmias and pathologic Q waves may be seen in patients with progressive disease.[16]

References

1. Byer E, Ashman R, Toth LA: Electrocardiograms with large, upright T waves and long QT intervals. Am Heart J 1947;33:796.
2. Goldstein DS: The electrocardiogram in stroke: Relationship to pathophysiologic type and comparison with prior tracings. Stroke 1979; 10:253.
3. Ramani A, Shetty U, Kundaje GN: Electrocardiographic abnormalities in cerebrovascular accidents. Angiology 1990;41:681.
4. Oppenheimer S, Norris JW: Cardiac manifestations of acute neurological lesions. In Aminoff MJ (ed): Neurology and General Medicine, 3rd ed. Philadelphia, Churchill Livingstone, 2001, pp. 196–211.
5. Neil-Dwyer G, Walter P, Cruickshank JM, et al: Effect of propranolol and phentolamine on myocardial necrosis after subarachnoid haemorrhage. BMJ 1978;2:990.
6. Svigelij V, Grad A, Kiauta T: Heart rate variability, norepinephrine and ECG changes in subarachnoid hemorrhage patients. Acta Neurol Scand 1996;94:120.
7. Leestma JE, Kalelkar MB, Teas SS: Sudden unexpected death associated with seizures: Analysis of 66 cases. Epilepsia 1984;25:84.
8. Silver FL, Norris JW, Lewis AJ, et al: Early mortality following stroke: A prospective review. Stroke 1984;15:492.
9. Lipman B, Dunn M, Massie E: Clinical Electrocardiography, 7th ed. Chicago, Year Book, 1984.
10. Surawicz B, Knilans TK: Chou's Electrocardiography in Clinical Practice: Adult and Pediatric, 5th ed. Philadelphia, WB Saunders, 2001.
11. Child JS, Perloff JK, Bach PM, et al: Cardiac involvement in Friedreich's ataxia: A clinical study of 75 patients. J Am Coll Cardiol 1986; 7:1370.
12. Nigro G, Comi LI, Politano L, Bain RJI: The incidence and evolution of cardiomyopathy in Duchenne muscular dystrophy. Int J Cardiol 1990;26:271.
13. Slucka C: The electrocardiogram in Duchenne progressive muscular dystrophy. Circulation 1968;38:933.
14. Emery AEH: Emery-Dreifuss syndrome. J Med Genet 1989;26:637.
15. Clark DS, Myerburg RJ, Morales AR, et al: Heart block in Kearns-Sayre syndrome: Electrophysiologic-pathologic correlation. Chest 1975; 68:727.
16. Olofsson B-O, Forsberg H, Andersson S, et al: Electrocardiographic findings in myotonic dystrophy. Br Heart J 1988;59:47.

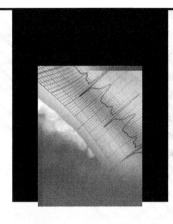

Chapter 65

Rheumatologic/Immunologic Disorders

Steven L. Bernstein and John Matjucha

Rheumatologic and immunologic disorders can present with a number of electrocardiographic (ECG) abnormalities as a direct result of the disease process or as a result of complications, such as pericarditis and pericardial effusions. This chapter reviews the ECG findings associated with sarcoidosis, rheumatoid arthritis, systemic lupus erythematosus, progressive systemic sclerosis, polymyositis/dermatomyositis, and primary vasculitides.

SARCOIDOSIS

Clinical Manifestations

Sarcoidosis is a multisystemic disease of unknown etiology. It occurs most commonly in younger patients, and more commonly in women. The most commonly affected organs are the lungs, lymphatics, and skin. Cardiac involvement has been noted in 20% to 30% of patients with sarcoidosis, but is usually clinically silent. Cardiac symptoms occur in approximately 5% of all cases.[1] The pathologic process of sarcoidosis is that of a noncaseating granuloma with a predominance of macrophages and lymphocytes. Myocardial disease is caused by formation of granulomata and subsequent scarring of cardiac tissue. Granulomata may affect any region of the myocardium or valves, but occur most commonly in the interventricular septum and left ventricular free wall.

Electrocardiographic Manifestations

The ECG abnormalities associated with sarcoidosis are varied.

T Wave Abnormalities.   Initially, T wave abnormalities may be seen, resulting from repolarization abnormalities due to local myocardial destruction and scarring. Pathologic Q waves also occur and are thought to represent more extensive cardiac involvement (Fig. 65-1).

Conduction Abnormalities.   Intraventricular and varying degrees of atrioventricular (AV) block are common. Complete heart block is the most common conduction abnormality in

patients with sarcoidosis, occurring in up to 30% of patients with cardiac involvement.[2] Bundle branch blocks may be seen, with right bundle branch block occurring more frequently. Septal involvement is associated with ventricular conduction abnormalities.

Ventricular Dysrhythmias.   Ventricular tachydysrhythmias are the second most common dysrhythmia in sarcoidosis, occurring in up to 20% of patients.[2] Ventricular tachycardia appears to become more common with more extensive ventricular involvement.[3] Cases of ventricular fibrillation have also been reported.[4]

Complete heart block and ventricular fibrillation are the most likely etiologies of sudden cardiac death.[2,5,6]

Less frequent than ventricular dysrhythmias are atrial dysrhythmias, occurring in approximately 15% of patients. Because atrial involvement by sarcoidosis is rare, the occurrence of atrial dysrhythmia is thought to be secondary to worsening left ventricular function and elevated atrial pressure and size.

RHEUMATOID ARTHRITIS

Clinical Features

Rheumatoid arthritis (RA) is a chronic inflammatory disease of unknown etiology. It most commonly presents as a polysynovitis, typically of smaller joints. Cardiac involvement occurs overall in up to 30% of patients and may involve pericardium, myocardium, and the heart valves. Pericardial effusions are found in up to 30% of patients. Most of these effusions are clinically and electrocardiographically silent. Symptoms of pericarditis occur in only 2% to 4% of patients with RA.[7,8] Vasculitis may rarely affect the coronary arteries and cause acute coronary syndromes, including acute myocardial infarction (MI). In patients who have infarction, the RA may be considered etiologic if there is other evidence of an acute or generalized vasculitis. The myocardium may be destroyed by rheumatoid granulomas.[9] Valvular involvement with rheumatoid nodules may occur.[9,10]

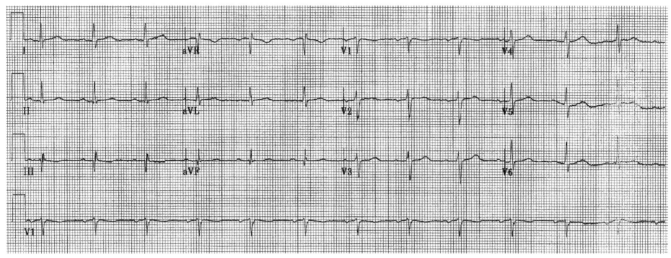

FIGURE 65-1 • **Sarcoidosis.** This ECG is from a 37-year-old man with sarcoidosis. Although there is no history of cardiac disease, inferior Q waves suggest clinically silent cardiac involvement.

Electrocardiographic Manifestations

Numerous ECG abnormalities may be seen with RA, commonly associated with complications from the disease. Manifestations include ECG findings consistent with a pericardial effusion or pericarditis, including ST segment elevation, T wave inversion, and PR segment changes. In the setting of vasculitis, ischemic ST segment and T wave abnormalities can occur in patients with involvement of the coronary vessels. In addition, AV block and other dysrhythmias may occur.

SYSTEMIC LUPUS ERYTHEMATOSUS

Clinical Features

Systemic lupus erythematosus (SLE) is an autoimmune disorder that can cause lesions in any organ. SLE may occur at any age and affects both men and women, but occurs most commonly in women of childbearing age. Cardiac manifestations of SLE include pericarditis, myocarditis, and MI. Cardiac complications are thought to arise from immune complex deposition in cardiac structures.[11,12]

In addition, patients with SLE are at increased risk for coronary artery disease.[12] Acute MI and sudden cardiac death have been described as the result of coronary arterial vasculitis.[11] The frequency of MI in patients with SLE increases with the duration of illness, suggesting that coronary atherosclerosis results from the complications of SLE.

Pericarditis is the most common cardiac complication in SLE, occurring in up to 50% of patients. It is the presenting symptom in 1% to 2% of patients.[13] Progressive myocardial involvement occurs in approximately 10% of patients.[14,15]

Electrocardiographic Manifestations

ECG findings in SLE are variable and relate to the cardiac involvement and complications of the disease. Findings of

---

ELECTROCARDIOGRAPHIC HIGHLIGHTS

Sarcoidosis
- T wave abnormalities initially
- Complete heart block in up to 30% of patients
- Ventricular dysrhythmias in up to 20% of patients

Rheumatoid arthritis
- Abnormalities, when present, most typically show myopericarditis

Systemic lupus erythematosus
- Myopericarditis
- Sinus tachycardia, atrial dysrhythmia, atrioventricular block, bundle branch block
- Neonates: complete heart block

Vasculitides
- Myopericarditis
- ST segment/T wave abnormalities

---

myocarditis include sinus tachycardia and ST segment/T wave changes. Pericardium is an electrically silent tissue, and the ECG abnormalities resulting from pericarditis are caused by superficial myocardial inflammation. Atrial dysrhythmias may occur and diffuse ST segment elevations with PR segment depression may be seen (Fig. 65-2).

Sinus tachycardia, atrial dysrhythmias, AV block, and bundle branch block have all been described in patients with SLE. However, it is yet to be shown that they result directly from SLE, rather than coexistent heart disease.[14] One exception is the neonatal lupus syndrome (NLS). This is a congenital complete heart block that occurs in a small minority of patients whose mothers have SLE and produce anti SS-A antibodies. The heart block is caused by immune complex deposition in the AV conduction system, and results in permanent fibrosis of the conducting fibers. The onset of NLS is usually from 18 to 30 weeks of gestation.[16]

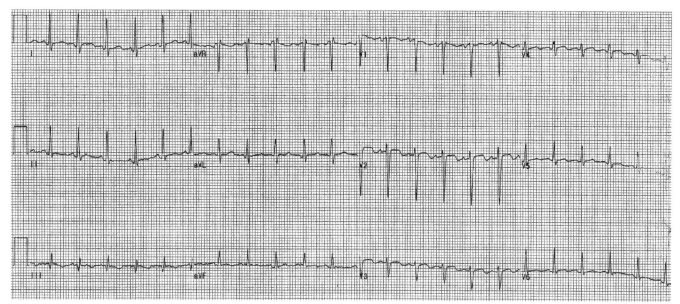

FIGURE 65-2 • Systemic lupus erythematosus (SLE). This ECG is from a 27-year-old woman who presented with fever and pleuritic chest pain and had a creatine phosphokinase level of 8000 mg/dL. A malar rash developed shortly after admission. Serologic studies confirmed the diagnosis of SLE. ECG demonstrates sinus tachycardia with nonspecific ST segment/T wave abnormalities.

PROGRESSIVE SYSTEMIC SCLEROSIS

Clinical Features

Scleroderma, or progressive systemic sclerosis (PSS), is an idiopathic multisystemic disease characterized by vascular abnormalities and fibrosis of the affected tissue. The organs affected most commonly are the skin, distal extremities, lung, heart, gastrointestinal tract, and kidney. Primary cardiac involvement results from the formation of focal areas of fibrosis in the myocardium. The pathophysiologic process of these lesions has not been definitely determined. Contraction band necrosis, a histopathologic finding suggestive of reperfusion injury, was found at autopsy in patients with PSS who died of apparent MI and who had normal coronary arteries.[17] But obliterative vasculitis or tissue necrosis due to local inflammatory response may also be causes of myocardial fibrosis.

Electrocardiographic Manifestations

The ECG demonstrates evidence of ventricular dysfunction and conduction system abnormalities that result most commonly from myocardial fibrosis. Although over 50% of patients with PSS have normal ECGs, most of these patients have fixed perfusion deficits at perfusion scanning, indicative of myocardial fibrosis. The most common ECG abnormality in PSS was evidence of AV and intraventricular conduction dysfunction (Fig. 65-3), seen in approximately 20% of affected patients.[18] Pulmonary or systemic hypertension from pulmonary or renal involvement may also cause ventricular hypertrophy. A rather broad range of other abnormalities has also been reported, including atrial and ventricular dysrhythmias as well as ST segment and T wave changes. Pericardial disease has been reported in PSS with a frequency of 7%.[19]

ECGs in patients with pericardial disease most commonly show left axis deviation and T wave abnormalities. Chronic pericardial effusions are twice as common as cases of acute pericarditis.

POLYMYOSITIS/DERMATOMYOSITIS

Clinical Manifestations

Polymyositis is characterized by muscle inflammation and resultant weakness. The proximal muscles of the shoulder and pelvic girdle are most commonly affected. Visceral organ involvement is generally thought to be uncommon. However, 30% of patients with polymyositis were found to have myocarditis at autopsy.[20]

Electrocardiographic Manifestations

ECG abnormalities occur in up to 33% of patients with polymyositis.[21] Most of these abnormalities are conduction abnormalities. The presence of ECG abnormalities does not appear to reflect the severity of polymyositis.

PRIMARY VASCULITIDES

The primary vasculitides are a heterogeneous group of disorders that cause a necrotizing vasculitis. They are distinct from the vasculitides of the connective tissue disorders.

Polyarteritis nodosa (PAN) is a necrotizing vasculitis that involves medium-sized arteries. PAN occurs more commonly in men. It typically presents with myalgias and arthralgias, hypertension, and renal insufficiency. It may present with acute MI or pericarditis.[22] ECG abnormalities may be present

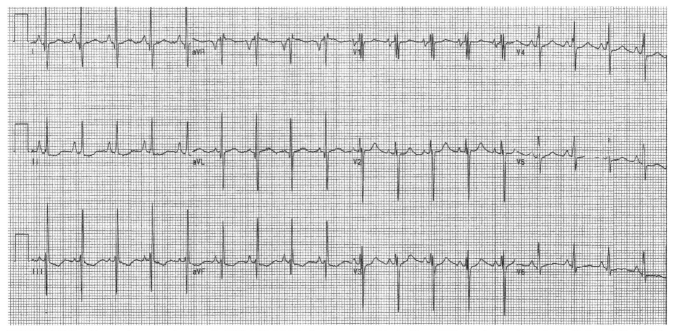

FIGURE 65-3 · **Progressive systemic sclerosis (PSS).** This ECG is from a patient with significant PSS; note incomplete right bundle branch block, right atrial abnormality, and left ventricular hypertrophy.

ELECTROCARDIOGRAPHIC PEARLS

- Ventricular dysrhythmia in a patient with sarcoidosis signifies extensive cardiac involvement.
- Myopericarditis occurs in up to half of all patients with systemic lupus erythematosus.
- Infants with neonatal lupus syndrome may present with complete heart block and require permanent pacemaker placement.
- The ECG may not distinguish acute from chronic pericardial involvement in scleroderma.
- A number of immunologic diseases can result in vasculitides of the coronary arteries, resulting in ischemia and infarct patterns on the ECG.

---

in 85% of patients with PAN. Nonspecific T wave changes occur most commonly. ECG changes consistent with pericarditis, MI, left axis deviation, and left ventricular hypertrophy have also been reported.

Takayasu's arteritis (TA) is a disease of unknown cause that affects the aortic arch and its proximal branches, causing a granulomatous panarteritis. The most common cardiac manifestation in TA is poorly controlled hypertension leading to congestive heart failure. Takayasu's arteritis usually does not involve the coronary arteries, but the coronary ostia may be affected if the aortic root is involved. Cardiac angiography reveals most of the significant lesions (71%) to be in the ostia.[23] The ECG abnormalities in these patients commonly include ST segment depression and T wave inversion. However, nearly one fourth of these patients had normal ECGs.

Behçet's disease is characterized by recurrent oral and genital ulceration with uveitis. Behçet's disease occurs more commonly in men and occurs more commonly in patients of Japanese or Mediterranean descent. Behçet's disease is associated with both retinal and systemic vasculitis. The vasculitis results in aneurysm formation and vascular occlusion.[24] The coronary arteries do not appear to become involved. Pericarditis and myocarditis may occur during exacerbations of orogenital ulcers and arthritis, and ECG findings suggestive of pericarditis have been noted.[24,25]

References

1. Wynne JBE: The cardiomyopathies and myocarditides. In Braunwald E (ed): Heart Disease: A Textbook of Cardiovascular Medicine, vol 2, 6th ed. Philadelphia, WB Saunders, 2001, p 1779.
2. Roberts WC, McAllister HA, Ferrans VJ: Sarcoidosis of the heart: A clinicopathologic study of 35 necropsy patients (group I) and review of 78 previously described necropsy patients (group II). Am J Med 1977;63:86.
3. Silverman KJ, Hutchins GM, Bulkley BH: Cardiac sarcoid: A clinicopathologic study of 84 unselected patients with systemic sarcoidosis. Circulation 1978;58:1204.
4. Winters SL, Cohen M, Greenberg S, et al: Sustained ventricular tachycardia associated with sarcoidosis: Assessment of the underlying cardiac anatomy and the prospective utility of programmed ventricular stimulation, drug therapy and an implantable antitachycardia device. J Am Coll Cardiol 1991;18:937.
5. Mitchell DN, duBois RM, Oldershaw PJ: Cardiac sarcoidosis: A potentially fatal condition that needs expert assessment [editorial]. BMJ 1997;314:320.
6. Sharma OD: Myocardial sarcoidosis: A wolf in sheep's clothing. Chest 1994;106:988.
7. Hara KS, Ballard DJ, Ilstrup DM, et al: Rheumatoid pericarditis: Clinical features and survival. Medicine (Baltimore) 1990;69:81.

8. Nomeir AM, Turner RA, Watts LE: Cardiac involvement in rheumatoid arthritis: Followup study. Arthritis Rheum 1979;22:561.

9. Pizzarello RA, Goldberg J: The heart in rheumatoid arthritis. In Utsinger PD (ed): Rheumatoid Arthritis: Etiology, Diagnosis, and Management. Philadelphia, JB Lippincott, 1985, p 431.

10. Arnett FC, Willerson JT: Connective tissue diseases and the heart. In Willerson JT, Cohn JN (eds): Cardiovascular Medicine, 2nd ed. New York, Churchill Livingstone, 2000, p 1939.

11. Korbet SM, Schwartz MM, Lewis EJ: Immune complex deposition and coronary vasculitis in systemic lupus erythematosus. Am J Med 1984;77:141.

12. Bidani AK, Roberts JL, Schwartz MM, Lewis EJ: Immunopathology of cardiac lesions in fatal systemic lupus erythematosus. Am J Med 1980;69:849.

13. Borenstein DG, Fye WB, Arnett FC, Stevens MB: The myocarditis of systemic lupus erythematosus: Association with myositis. Ann Intern Med 1978;89:619.

14. Moder KG, Miller TD, Tazelaar HD: Cardiac involvement in systemic lupus erythematosus. Mayo Clin Proc 1999;74:275.

15. Stevens MB: Systemic lupus erythematosus and the cardiovascular system: The heart. In Lahita RG (ed): Systemic Lupus Erythematosus. New York, John Wiley & Sons, 1987, p 707.

16. Buyon JP, Hiebert R, Copel J, et al: Autoimmune-associated congenital heart block: Demographics, mortality, morbidity and recurrence rates obtained from a national neonatal lupus registry. J Am Coll Cardiol 1998;31:1658.

17. Bulkley BH, Klacsmann PG, Hutchins GM: Angina pectoris, myocardial infarction and sudden cardiac death with normal coronary arteries: A clinicopathologic study of 9 patients with progressive systemic sclerosis. Am Heart J 1978;95:563.

18. Follansbee WP, Curtiss EI, Rahko PS, et al: The electrocardiogram in systemic sclerosis (scleroderma). Am J Med 1985;79:183.

19. McWhorter JE, LeRoy EC: Pericardial disease in scleroderma (systemic sclerosis). Am J Med 1974;57:566.

20. Denbow CE, Lie JT, Tancredi RG, Bunch TW: Cardiac involvement in polymyositis: A clinicopathologic study of 20 autopsied patients. Arthritis Rheum 1979;22:1088.

21. Stern L, Godbold JH, Chess Q, Kagen LJ: ECG abnormalities in polymyositis. Arch Intern Med 1984;144:2185.

22. Holsinger DR, Osmundson PJ, Edwards JE: The heart in periarteritis nodosa. Circulation 1962;25:610.

23. Amano J, Suzuki A: Coronary artery involvement in Takayasu's arteritis: Collective review and guideline for surgical treatment. J Thorac Cardiovasc Surg 1991;102:554.

24. James DG: Medical eponyms updated: 1. Behçet's disease. Br J Clin Pract 1990;44:364.

25. Lewis PD: Behçet's disease and carditis. BMJ 1964;1:1026.

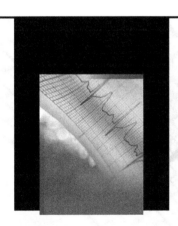

Chapter 66

Acute Rheumatic Fever

Todd J. Berger and Katherine L. Heilpern

Clinical Features

Acute rheumatic fever (ARF) is a nonsuppurative inflammatory complication of a streptococcal upper respiratory infection occurring most commonly in children 5 to 10 years of age. Streptococcal pharyngitis must precede this illness, although one third of patients do not recall having a symptomatic sore throat (but have elevated serologic markers). Although improved standards of living and availability of antibiotics have substantially decreased the prevalence of this disease in industrialized nations, it remains a common problem in developing countries, where 10% to 35% of cardiac-related hospital admissions are due to complications of rheumatic fever. In industrialized nations, ARF occurs primarily in lower socioeconomic populations where overcrowding remains a persistent problem.[1] More recently, there have been several epidemics of ARF in this country in suburban areas.[2]

ARF is diagnosed clinically because there is no test specific to this disease. Several clinical manifestations may occur, leading to the creation of the "Jones criteria" for diagnosis (see Table 66-1). There are five "major manifestations" that are pathognomonic but not entirely specific for the disease.

Of the "major manifestations," carditis is the only potentially fatal complication, although it is usually mild or even asymptomatic. It usually manifests 1 to 3 weeks after the onset of symptoms. Valvulitis, most commonly of the mitral valve, can produce regurgitation, prolapse, or stenosis with accompanying new murmurs and decreased cardiac output. Congestive heart failure, cardiomegaly, pericarditis or pericardial effusion, and myocarditis can also occur.

66-1 • JONES CRITERIA FOR DIAGNOSIS OF ACUTE RHEUMATIC FEVER

Major Manifestations
- Carditis
- Polyarthritis
- Chorea
- Erythema marginatum
- Subcutaneous nodules

Minor Manifestations
- Fever
- Arthralgias
- Elevated markers of inflammation
- Prolonged PR interval

Diagnosis requires two major or one major and two minor manifestations along with documented streptococcal infection by culture or antibody titer. Exceptions can be made when there are delayed manifestations (such as chorea or carditis) months after the initial attack, when serum markers have already gone back to baseline. Also, patients with recurrence of previously diagnosed acute rheumatic fever do not need strictly to meet the Jones criteria for diagnosis.

Electrocardiographic Manifestations

There are many electrocardiographic (ECG) abnormalities that have been associated with ARF. Most of them do not seem to correlate with the presence of carditis or the prognosis of the disease. The vast majority of ECG abnormalities resolve with resolution of the illness.[3]

Sinus Tachycardia. The most common finding is sinus tachycardia, which can be present in 90% of patients, although it is sometimes difficult to distinguish whether this is a primary abnormality or a result of fever. However, the tachycardia is often out of proportion to the fever and persists during sleep. Occasionally, sinus bradycardia and sinus dysrhythmias can also occur, especially during resolution of the attack. This finding is probably due to increased vagal tone because it resolves with atropine. Sinus node suppression with atrioventricular (AV) junctional escape rhythms has also been seen and responds to atropine as well.[4]

PR Interval Prolongation. The characteristic ECG finding for ARF is first degree AV block (Fig. 66-1). Incidence varies tremendously between studies, from 10% to 95%.

The etiology is unclear. Theories include inflammation of the AV conduction system and vasculitis of the AV nodal artery, which can cause transient ischemia or even infarction. PR interval prolongation usually responds to atropine, so increased vagal tone is likely to be involved. Although no consensus has been reached, it is thought that the presence of a first degree AV block is not specifically associated with the presence of carditis or valvulitis. It remains a "minor manifestation" for the Jones diagnostic criteria.[4]

Atrioventricular Block. Higher degree AV conduction delays are less common and usually transient. Second degree AV blocks are seen infrequently. Third degree AV block has also been noted. During the course of this disease, AV conduction delays can progress to higher degrees as the illness progresses, and similarly resolve as symptoms dissipate. AV nodal blocks do not appear to have prognostic value and rarely persist beyond the acute illness.[4]

Atrial Tachydysrhythmias. Atrial tachydysrhythmias such as atrial flutter, atrial fibrillation, and multifocal atrial tachycardia can occur. Dysrhythmias result from inflammation of the myocardium, mitral regurgitation, congestive heart failure, cardiomegaly, or pericarditis.[4]

Bundle Branch Blocks. Bundle branch blocks are very rare. The prognostic impact of the presence of bundle branch blocks in patients with ARF is unknown.[4]

QT Interval Prolongation. It is unclear if there is a significant QT interval prolongation due to ARF itself or whether it is associated with the presence of carditis. There is some evidence to support that the length of the QT interval varies with the severity of the symptoms during the course of the illness. This finding may contribute to rare cases of ventricular dysrhythmias, including torsades de pointes.

Myopericarditis. Myopericarditis can occur with ARF. Pericarditis is almost always associated with myocarditis, so its presence is associated with a poorer prognosis[4] (see Chapter 37, Myopericarditis).

Frequency of Electrocardiographic Abnormalities. The frequency of ECG abnormalities in ARF has been explored by many authorities. One study looked at the ECGs of 508 patients with ARF and reported PR interval prolongation above baseline in 364 (71.7%), second degree type I AV block in 12 (2.4%), third degree AV block in 3 (0.6%), and a junctional rhythm in 13 (2.6%).[4] Another study reviewed 232 ECGs from patients with ARF, of which 74 (31.9%) showed AV conduction abnormalities, 66 (28.4%) had PR interval

ELECTROCARDIOGRAPHIC HIGHLIGHTS

- Sinus tachycardia
- Junctional escape rhythm
- First degree atrioventricular (AV) block
- Higher degrees of AV block
- Atrial fibrillation/flutter
- Multifocal atrial tachycardia
- Myopericarditis
- Prolonged QT interval
- Bundle branch blocks
- Ventricular tachydysrhythmias

ELECTROCARDIOGRAPHIC PEARLS

- ECG findings do not correlate with the presence of carditis and are not prognostic. They usually resolve with the resolution of the disease.
- Sinus tachycardia is the most common finding. It can occur out of proportion to the fever and usually persists during sleep.
- First degree atrioventricular block is the most characteristic finding.

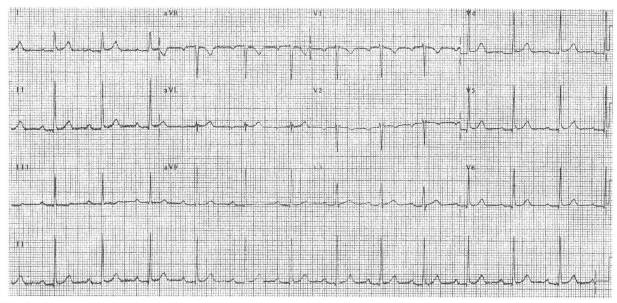

FIGURE 66-1 · **First degree atrioventricular block.** This ECG from a patient with acute rheumatic fever shows PR interval prolongation (0.24 sec) consistent with first degree heart block.

prolongation, 4 (1.7%) had second degree type I AV blocks, and 4 (1.7%) had third degree AV blocks.[2]

References

1. Chako S, Bisno AL: Acute rheumatic fever. In Furster V, Alexander RW (eds): Hurst's The Heart, 10th ed. New York, McGraw-Hill, 2001, pp 1657–1665.

2. Veasy LG, Tani LY, Hill HR: Persistence of acute rheumatic fever in the intermountain area of the United States. J Pediatr 1994;124:9.

3. Clarke M, Keith JD: Atrioventricular conduction in acute rheumatic fever. Br Heart J 1972;34:472.

4. Krishnan SC, Kushwaha SS, Josephson ME: Electrocardiographic abnormalities and arrhythmias in patients with acute rheumatic fever. In Narula J, Virmani R, Reddy KS, Tandon R (eds): Rheumatic Fever. Washington, DC, Armed Forces Institute of Pathology, 1999, pp 287–298.

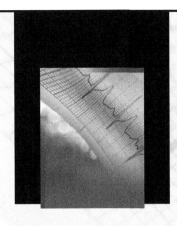

Chapter 67

Miscellaneous Infectious Syndromes: Lyme Carditis, Human Immunodeficiency Virus– Associated, and Chagas Disease

David J. Karras

LYME CARDITIS

Clinical Features

Lyme disease is caused by the spirochete *Borrelia burgdorferi* and transmitted to humans by bites from ticks of the *Ixodes* genus. The disease is prevalent in temperate regions of North America, Europe, and Asia and is endemic in large areas of the United States, particularly in the New England and mid-Atlantic states and the west coast, and most common during summer months.[1]

The clinical characteristics of Lyme disease occur in three stages, although presentation is highly variable.[2,3] Stage 1 consists of erythema migrans, a characteristic annular rash arising from the site of the tick bite, which may be accompanied by influenza-like symptoms. Stage 2, occurring days to weeks after the bite, is characterized by disseminated disease primarily involving the heart, nervous system, and joints. Months to years later, patients may progress to stage 3, with persistent arthritis, neuropathy, or dermatitis.

Electrocardiographic Manifestations

Cardiac involvement is noted in 5% to 10% of untreated patients within weeks after onset of Lyme disease.[4] Conduction disturbances are by far the most common finding.

Atrioventricular Block. Approximately 90% of patients with Lyme myocarditis manifest atrioventricular block (Fig. 67-1). The degree of block may fluctuate rapidly, sometimes within a period of minutes. Only approximately half of patients with first degree blocks progress to second or third degree blocks.[4] Based on electrophysiologic testing, these blocks occur proximal to the bundle of His. However, there have been reports of widened escape QRS complexes in

patients with third degree block, suggesting an escape focus below the atrioventricular junction.[4]

Virtually all patients with Lyme disease–related conduction abnormalities manifest first degree block at some time during their illness.[5] Although PR intervals as long as 0.42 sec have been reported, most patients have intervals in the range of 0.2 to 0.3 sec.[4] Progression to higher degree blocks is not noted in patients whose PR intervals remain under 0.3 sec. Wenckebach episodes are noted in 40% of patients with Lyme carditis. Between 40% and 50% of patients with conduction abnormalities experience periods of complete heart block associated with ventricular escape rates between 30 and 60 bpm. All patients in whom complete heart block developed had PR intervals greater than 0.3 sec. Bundle branch blocks have not been reported in association with Lyme carditis.[4]

ELECTROCARDIOGRAPHIC HIGHLIGHTS

Lyme carditis

- Rapid fluctuation between degrees of atrioventricular (AV) block
- Nonspecific ST segment abnormalities

Chagas disease

- Right bundle branch block, left anterior fascicular block, left posterior fascicular block
- Left bundle branch block
- AV block
- Atrial fibrillation
- Multifocal ventricular premature depolarizations
- Sustained ventricular tachycardia, ventricular fibrillation
- Nonspecific ST segment/T wave abnormalities
- Pathologic Q waves

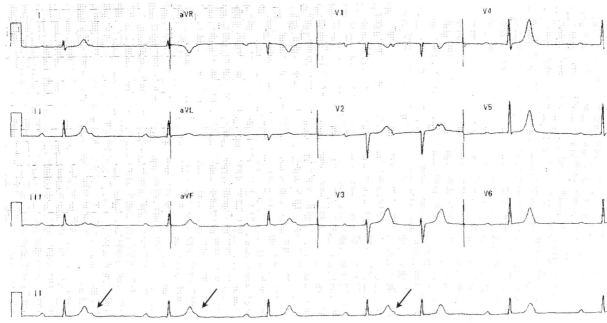

FIGURE 67-1 · **ECG of a 62-year-old man with Lyme carditis demonstrating second degree atrioventricular block.** Note the nonconducted P waves (*arrows*).

ST Segment and T Wave Abnormalities.   More than half of patients with Lyme myocarditis manifest electrocardiographic evidence of diffuse cardiac involvement.[4] Nonspecific ST segment abnormalities and T wave flattening or inversions may be noted, more commonly in the inferior and lateral leads. These abnormalities are consistent with and may be associated with other evidence of myopericarditis. These abnormalities resolve with remission of disease.

Uncommon Dysrhythmias.   There have been reports of ventricular tachycardia in association with Lyme carditis, although this appears to be uncommon.[6] There has been a single report of atrial fibrillation with rapid ventricular response in a patient whose electrocardiogram was normal during disease remission.[4]

HUMAN IMMUNODEFICIENCY VIRUS–ASSOCIATED DISEASE

Clinical Features

Cardiac dysfunction is a frequent late-stage complication of human immunodeficiency virus (HIV) infection. HIV is now recognized as a common cause of symptomatic congestive heart failure.[7] Autopsy studies have demonstrated a cardiac cause of death in approximately 10% of patients with acquired immunodeficiency syndrome (AIDS) and have noted HIV-related cardiac involvement in approximately 20% of all deaths attributed to AIDS.[8,9] The incidence of heart disease is strongly associated with the patient's CD4 lymphocyte count, with dilated cardiomyopathy particularly common among individuals with CD4 counts less than 100 cells/mL.[10]

HIV and its associated complications can lead to pericarditis, myocarditis, and endocarditis as well.

Cardiac abnormalities in patients with HIV infection may be related to direct cardiotoxic effects of the virus itself, opportunistic infections, nutritional deficiencies, and cardiotoxic medications used to treat the disease and its sequelae. HIV cardiomyopathy with left ventricular systolic dysfunction is a common finding in both symptomatic and asymptomatic patients and becomes more frequent as the disease progresses.

Toxoplasmosis is the most common opportunistic infection causing dilated cardiomyopathy in patients with AIDS. Infections with *Pneumocystis*, *Histoplasma*, *Cryptococcus*, *Mycobacterium*, cytomegalovirus, herpes simplex virus, coxsackievirus, and Epstein-Barr virus are other notable causes of myocarditis and subsequent heart failure in this population. Asymptomatic pericardial effusions are common. Finally, numerous antiretroviral, anti-infective, and chemotherapeutic agents used in the treatment of HIV infection and AIDS may cause dilated cardiomyopathy, accelerated atherogenesis, or dysrhythmias.[11]

Electrocardiographic Manifestations

It has been documented that the majority of HIV-infected individuals, including asymptomatic patients, have baseline electrocardiographic abnormalities.[11] The most common findings include nonspecific conduction defects, nonspecific repolarization changes, and supraventricular and ventricular ectopic beats.[12] However, there are no reports of specific electrocardiographic abnormalities that predominate in individuals with HIV infection or that are suggestive of AIDS-related cardiac disease.

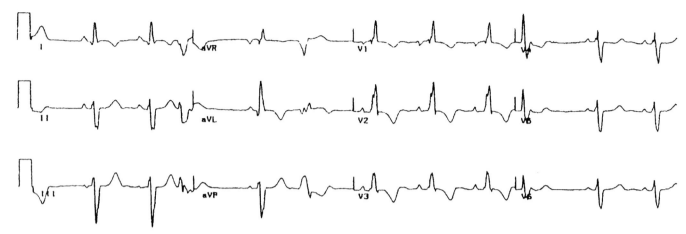

FIGURE 67-2 · **Chagas disease.** This ECG is from a patient with Chagas disease presenting with acute congestive heart failure. Note the right bundle branch block, left anterior fascicular block, and first degree atrioventricular block. (From Hagar JM, Rahimtoola SH: Chagas' heart disease. Curr Probl Cardiol 1995;20:873, with permission.)

CHAGAS DISEASE

Clinical Features

Chagas disease, or American trypanosomiasis, is a major health problem throughout most of Central and South America. The disease may appear in nonendemic areas because of emigration from endemic regions or, more rarely, by infected blood transfusion. It is estimated that approximately 18 million people in Latin America are infected with *Trypanosoma cruzi,* resulting in 45,000 deaths annually.[1] No more than one third of infected individuals, however, manifest symptoms of Chagas disease.

The causative organism is *T. cruzi,* a protozoan transmitted by blood-sucking insects known as reduviid (kissing) bugs, which bite humans, typically about the eyes, causing a local inflammatory lesion known as a *chagoma.* The parasite migrates widely throughout the body, most commonly to the heart. Acute Chagas disease is seen in fewer than 10% of infected individuals and more frequently occurs in younger patients. Acute disease may present with fever, myalgias, congestive heart failure, and hepatosplenomegaly. The heart shows marked biventricular enlargement with thinning of the myocardium and apical aneurysms. Epicardial involvement may be manifested as pericardial effusions. Although acute Chagas disease is fatal in 10% of cases, most patients recover over several months.[2] Latent Chagas disease develops after infection with *T. cruzi* regardless of whether acute disease developed.

Chronic Chagas disease becomes evident in approximately 10% of infected individuals after a latency averaging 20 years.[6] The heart is again the most common site of involvement and patients may present with right-sided heart failure, thromboembolic disease, or symptomatic dysrhythmias with dizziness, syncope, seizures, or sudden death.[13,14]

Electrocardiographic Manifestations

Conduction Abnormalities.   At least 80% of patients with Chagas heart disease have evidence of intraventricular conduction defects[4,5] (Fig. 67-2). Right bundle branch block

(RBBB) is the most common abnormality, seen in approximately half of all patients. Left anterior fascicular block and, less often, left posterior fascicular block are also seen in approximately half of patients and are frequently associated with RBBB. Left bundle branch block is seen in 5% to 10% of patients. Second degree atrioventricular block and complete heart block are also seen in under 10% of patients.[7]

Dysrhythmias.   Sinus bradycardia is noted in approximately 20% of individuals with chronic Chagas heart disease, particularly those with more advanced disease. Atrial fibrillation, usually with a slow ventricular response, is seen in approximately 10% of individuals.[3] Bradycardia–tachycardia syndromes have been described in both symptomatic and asymptomatic individuals.[8]

Multifocal ventricular premature depolarizations and self-limited episodes of ventricular tachycardia are very commonly seen. Although sustained ventricular tachycardia is most common among patients with severe ventricular dysfunction, sudden cardiac death due to ventricular fibrillation may occur in the absence of any overt evidence of congestive heart failure.[9]

Pseudoinfarct Patterns.   Nonspecific ST segment and T wave abnormalities are common in patients with chronic Chagas disease, particularly those with advanced disease. These changes appear to be closely associated with the presence of ventricular aneurysms and severe myocardial hypokinesis; they do not generally reflect acute ischemic injury.[10] ST segment elevation (or, less commonly, depression) and T wave inversions may mimic anterolateral or inferolateral myocardial infarction. Pathologic Q waves, corresponding to areas of wall motion abnormalities, are seen in up to half of patients and are most common in severe disease.

References

1. Centers for Disease Control and Prevention: Lyme disease: United States, 2000. Mor Mortal Wkly Rep CDC Surveill Summ 2002;51:29.
2. Steere AC: *Borrelia burgdorferi.* In: Mandell GL, Bennett JE, Dolin R (eds): Principals and Practice of Infectious Disease, 5th ed. Philadelphia, Churchill Livingstone, 2000, p 2504.
3. Steere AC: Lyme disease. N Engl J Med 2001;345:115.

4. Steere AC, Batsford WP, Weinberg M, et al: Lyme carditis: Cardiac abnormalities of Lyme disease. Ann Intern Med 1980;93:8.

5. van der Linde MR, Crijns HJ, de Koning J, et al: Range of atrioventricular conduction disturbances in Lyme borreliosis. Br Heart J 1990;63:162.

6. Wynne J, Braunwald E: The Cardiomyopathies and Myocarditides. In Braunwald E, Zipes DP, Libby P (eds): Heart Disease: A Textbook of Cardiovascular Medicine, 6th ed. Philadelphia, WB Saunders, 2001, p 1788.

7. Fisher SD, Lipshultz SE: Cardiovascular abnormalities in HIV-infected individuals. In Braunwald E, Zipes DP, Libby P (eds): Heart Disease: A Textbook of Cardiovascular Medicine, 6th ed Philadelphia, WB Saunders, 2001, p 2211.

8. Patel RC, Frishman WH: Cardiac involvement in HIV infection. Med Clin North Am 1996;80:1493.

9. Barbaro G, Barbarini G, DiLorenzo G: Cardiac involvement in the acquired immunodeficiency syndrome: A multicenter clinical-pathological study. AIDS Res Hum Retroviruses 1998;14:1071.

10. Currie PF, Jacob AJ, Foreman AR, et al: Heart muscle disease related to HIV infection: Prognostic implications. BMJ 1994;309:1605.

11. Barbaro G, Barbarini G, DiLorenzo G: Early impairment of systolic and diastolic function in asymptomatic HIV-positive patients: A multicenter echocardiographic and echo-Doppler study. AIDS Res Hum Retroviruses 1996;12:1559.

12. Chaisson RE, Sterling TR, Gallant JE: General clinical manifestations of human immunodeficiency virus infection. In Mandell GL, Bennett JE, Dolin R (eds): Principals and Practice of Infectious Disease, 5th ed. Philadelphia, Churchill Livingstone, 2000, p 1398.

13. McAlister HF, Klementowicz PT, Andrews C, et al: Lyme carditis: An important cause of reversible heart block. Ann Intern Med 1989;110:339.

14. Rees DJ, Keeling PJ, McKenna WJ, et al: No evidence to implicate *B. burgdorferi* in the pathogenesis of dilated cardiomyopathy in the United Kingdom. Br Heart J 1994;71:1994.

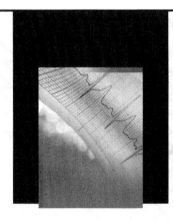

Chapter 68

Electrocardiographic Manifestations of Gastrointestinal Disease

Edward Ullman and Sonal Patel

Clinical Features

An electrocardiogram (ECG) is often obtained during the initial evaluation of patients presenting with abdominal pain or other manifestations of gastrointestinal (GI) disease. Disease states, including pancreatitis, cholecystitis, peptic ulcer disease, appendicitis, inflammatory bowel disease, and cirrhosis, have been associated with ECG abnormalities. These ECG findings can both mimic a number of primary cardiac disease states and provide clues to underlying gastrointestinal pathologic processes. Alternatively, certain GI diseases may be associated with increased risk for concurrent cardiac ischemia or infarction. In addition, malnutrition as a result of GI disease can result in electrolyte imbalances that produce a number of the abnormal ECG changes.

Electrocardiographic Manifestations

ST Segment Elevation. Although ST segment elevation (STE) in the face of abdominal pain raises concern of possible acute coronary syndrome (ACS), certain GI diseases may present with an ECG consistent with pseudoinfarction. On the other hand, certain GI diseases can increase the propensity for coronary thrombosis and true ACS as well.

Several case reports have shown STE secondary to pancreatitis with no evidence of coronary disease on cardiac catheterization or autopsy.[1,2] Possible theories behind these ECG changes include the action of proteolytic enzymes causing damage to myocytes, as well as the potential for enzymatic changes to alter platelet adhesion and lead to coronary artery thrombosis[2] (Fig. 68-1).

ELECTROCARDIOGRAPHIC HIGHLIGHTS

Pancreatitis

- Nonspecific ST segment/T wave changes
- ST segment elevation (STE)
- T wave inversions

Acute cholecystitis

- Nonspecific ST segment/T wave changes
- STE
- T wave inversion
- Bradycardia

Inflammatory bowel disease

- STE
- ECG changes associated with acute myopericarditis
- Wenckebach second degree atrioventricular block
- Complete heart block

Duodenal perforation

- T wave inversion

Cirrhosis

- QT interval prolongation

Celiac sprue

- QT interval prolongation

Patients with cholecystic disease may present with anterior ischemic patterns on their ECGs that often resolve after gallbladder removal.[3] The "biliary-cardiac reflex" is commonly cited as the cause for STE.[3,4] Gallbladder distention may lead to a vagal response, producing intermittent spasm of the coronary arteries and reducing flow through these vessels. Other case reports indicate that acute cholecystitis may manifest ECG findings of noninfarction ACS[4] (Fig. 68-2).

Other intra-abdominal conditions, such as splenic rupture, have been cited as a cause for STE and pseudoinfarct pattern on ECG.[5,6] The lack of ECG normalization despite ACS medical management can indicate the presence of a noncardiac pathologic process.[7]

Alternatively, GI disease can increase the risk for cardiac disease resulting in ST segment changes. A known complication of inflammatory bowel disease (IBD) is acute vascular thrombosis, and patients with Crohn's disease and ulcerative colitis are at an increased risk for thrombotic complications.[8] In addition, myopericarditis is a rare but reported complication of IBD.[9] Myopericarditis has been associated with mesalamine, a medication used to treat IBD.

T Wave Inversion. Various GI disorders can cause T wave inversion, resulting in a pseudoischemic ECG pattern. Several cases in the literature show T wave inversion secondary to duodenal perforation.[10] Transient deep T wave inversions during an attack of acute pancreatitis or cholecystitis have also been reported, often resolving with definitive therapy.[1,3]

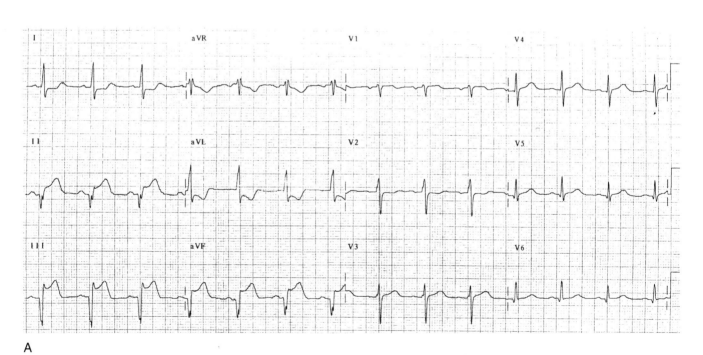

A

FIGURE 68-1 · **Patient presenting with acute pancreatitis.** *A,* Initial ECG reveals marked inferior ST segment elevation in leads II, III, and aVF, and depressions in leads I and aVL. There are also nonspecific ST segment changes in lead V_2.

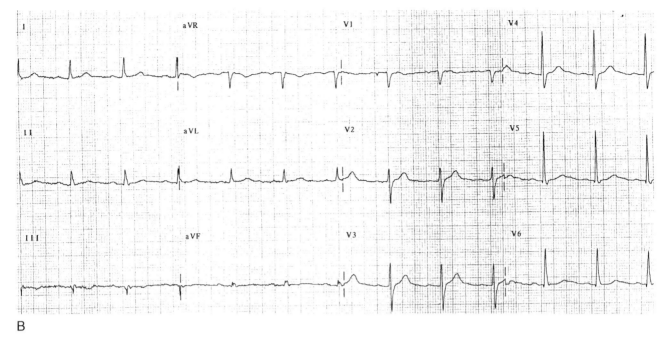

B

FIGURE 68-1 · **Patient presenting with acute pancreatitis.** *B,* ECG after resolution of acute pancreatitis reveals normalization of the pseudoinfarction pattern seen in *A.*

Bradycardia. Sinus bradycardia may occur as a vagal response to a patient's primary GI disorder or severe abdominal pain (Fig. 68-3). In addition, specific GI disorders may result in more specific causes of bradycardia. Several cases of second degree atrioventricular (AV) block as well as complete AV block have been reported with ulcerative colitis.[11] Although bile acids have been implicated in the jaundiced patient as a cause of bradycardia, recent evidence does not support this idea.[12]

QT Interval Prolongation. Initially thought to occur only in patients with severe alcoholic liver disease, QT interval prolongation may occur in any cirrhotic patient regardless of the etiology (Fig. 68-4). Although there is no consensus regarding severity of hepatic function and QT interval prolongation, there is a growing body of evidence that a correlation exists and that this finding is associated with a poorer clinical outcome. A case series has shown a statistically significant reduction of the corrected QT interval upon liver transplantation.[13]

QT interval prolongation can also be seen in states of malnutrition (such as anorexia or ileojejunal bypass), celiac sprue, and other disease states that cause hypokalemia and

hypocalcemia.[14] In one study, one third of all adults with celiac disease had QT interval prolongation.[14] Such findings may indicate a potential increased risk for ventricular dysrhythmias and sudden death.

ELECTROCARDIOGRAPHIC PEARLS

- ST segment/T wave changes associated with gastrointestinal (GI) disease may represent a true acute coronary syndrome event or a pseudoischemic pattern related to the GI disease.
- Patients with inflammatory bowel syndrome are at increased risk for thrombotic events, including acute myocardial infarction.
- The biliary-cardiac reflex is a known phenomenon that can help explain ECG changes during acute cholecystitis.
- QT interval prolongation can occur in patients presenting with cirrhosis, celiac sprue, anorexia nervosa, and other states of malnutrition that can result in electrolyte abnormalities.

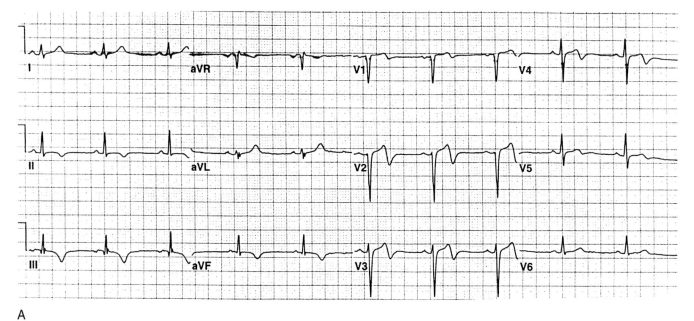

A

B

FIGURE 68-2 · **Patient presenting with cholecystitis.** *A,* Initial ECG reveals ST segment elevation in leads V$_2$, V$_3$, and V$_4$. In addition, T wave inversions are seen inferiorly in leads II, III, and aVF. *B,* ECG after cholecystectomy shows resolution of these ST segment and T wave changes.

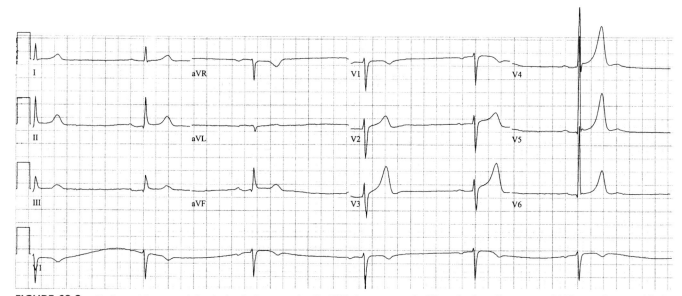

FIGURE 68-3 · **Patient with severe abdominal pain from renal colic.** ECG demonstrates significant bradycardia at a rate of 35 bpm and nonspecific ST segment findings.

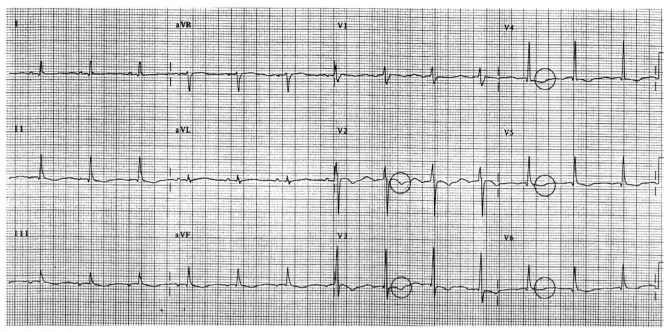

FIGURE 68-4 · ECG of patient with end-stage liver disease awaiting transplantation. Note the QT interval prolongation and diffuse ST segment depression (*circles*).

References

1. Maunter RK, Siegel LA, Giles TD, Kayser J: Electrocardiographic changes in acute pancreatitis. South Med J 1982;75:317.

2. Cafri C, Basok A, Katz A, et al: Thrombotic therapy in acute pancreatitis presenting as acute myocardial infarction. Int J Cardiol 1995;49:279.

3. Ryan ET, Pak PP, DeSanctis RW: Myocardial infarction mimicked by acute cholecystitis. Ann Intern Med 1992;116:218.

4. Krasna MJ, Flancbaum L: Electrocardiographic changes in cardiac patients with acute gallbladder disease. Am Surg 1986;52:541.

5. Reymond JM, Sztajzel J: Severe chest pain, diagnostic electrocardiogram, and ileus. Lancet 1996;348:1560.

6. Thomas I, Mathew J, Kumar VP, et al: Electrocardiographic changes in catastrophic abdominal illness mimicking acute myocardial infarction. Am J Cardiol 1987;59:1224.

7. Antonelli D, Rosenfeld T: Variant angina induced by biliary colic. Br Heart J 1987;58:417.

8. Efremidis M, Prappa E, Kardaras F: Acute myocardial infarction in a young patient during an exacerbation of ulcerative colitis. Int J Cardiol 1999;70:211.

9. Abid MA, Gitlin N: Pericarditis: An extraintestinal complication of inflammatory bowel disease. West J Med 1990;153:314.

10. Sole DP, McCabe JL, Wolfson AB: ECG changes with perforated duodenal ulcer mimicking acute cardiac ischemia. Am J Emerg Med 1996;14:410.

11. Ballinger A, Farthing MJG: Ulcerative colitis complicated by Wenckebach atrioventricular block. Gut 1992;33:1427.

12. Song E, Segal I, Hodkinson J, Kew MC: Sinus bradycardia in obstructive jaundice: Correlation with total serum bile acid concentrations. S Afr Med J 1983;64:548.

13. Mohamed R, Forsey PR, Davies MK, Neuberger JM: Effect of liver transplantation on QT interval prolongation and autonomic dysfunction in end-stage liver disease. Hepatology 1996;23:1128.

14. Corazza GR, Frisoni M, Filipponi C, et al: Investigation of QT interval in adult coeliac disease. BMJ 1992;304:1285.

Section IV

Advanced Techniques and Technologies

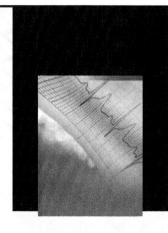

Chapter 69

Additional Lead Electrocardiograms

Robert P. Wahl, Sridevi R. Pitta, and Robert J. Zalenski

Traditionally, the electrocardiogram (ECG) contains six limb leads and six anterior chest leads. This arrangement has been the standard approach for almost half a century. However, there are anatomic locations of the heart that are not well represented by the standard 12-lead ECG, of which the posterior wall of the left ventricle and the entire right ventricle are the most clinically significant.

Sensitivity of the 12-lead ECG may be improved if additional leads are used in selected individuals. The most frequently used additional leads use posterior (V_7 to V_9) electrodes and right-sided precordial electrodes (V_{1R} to V_{6R}).[1] Posterior electrodes are placed at same horizontal level as lead V_4 at the fifth intercostal space. Lead V_7 is located at the posterior axillary line, lead V_8 at the inferior angle of scapula, and lead V_9 at the paraspinal line; lead V_7 is omitted in many cases. Right-sided lateral precordial leads are placed as the mirror image of left-sided leads (i.e., mid-clavicular line for V_{4R}, anterior axillary line for V_{5R}, and midaxillary line for V_{6R}; Fig. 69-1).

There are three clinical situations where information from additional leads can prompt changes in the management of the patient with acute myocardial infarction (AMI). First, a change in the diagnosis from an AMI with ST segment depression to an AMI with ST segment elevation (STE) may qualify a patient to receive reperfusion therapy (Fig. 69-2). Second, the recognition of patients with larger infarct size who are at higher risk of complications of AMI can lead to

more aggressive treatment strategies to optimize patient outcome. Last, the identification of patients who may have an AMI that is subtle on the standard 12-lead ECG but more evident with extra leads may reduce missed diagnoses, and allow these patients to receive revascularization therapy.

Posterior Wall Acute Myocardial Infarction

Posterior wall myocardial infarction (MI), usually involving occlusion of either the left circumflex or the right coronary artery with its posterior descending branches, is one of the most commonly missed AMI ECG patterns.[2] Posterior wall MI has been reported to represent 15% to 20% of AMIs, most associated with acute infarction of the inferior or lateral wall of the left ventricle. The diagnosis of isolated posterior wall MI, once thought to be a rare event, has now been recognized in 3% to 11% of all patients with AMI.[2]

Standard 12-lead ECG posterior wall AMI findings include the following: "horizontal" ST segment depression in leads V_1 to V_3; a tall, wide R wave in leads V_1 or V_2; an identifiable R/S ratio greater than 1 in lead V_1 or V_2; and an upright T wave in lead V_1 or V_2 (see Fig. 69-2). In the setting of horizontal ST segment depression in the right precordial leads, the presence of either a prominent R wave or upright T wave in some leads provides further ECG evidence for posterior wall AMI. In addition, the presence of STE in

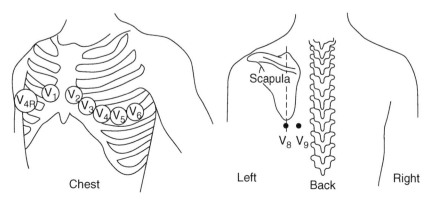

FIGURE 69-1 · Additional lead electrode placement. Electrode placement is shown for leads V_{4R} (right ventricular), V_8, and V_9 (posterior wall).

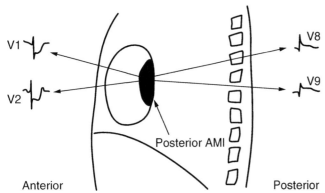

FIGURE 69-2 · Anatomic basis for ECG changes in posterior wall acute myocardial infarction (AMI). According to the standard 12-lead ECG, ST segment depression, prominent R waves, and upright T waves in leads V_1 to V_3 are indicative of posterior wall AMI and represent reciprocal changes because the endocardial surface of the posterior wall faces the anterior pre-cordial leads. From the posterior perspective view of the thorax (through posterior chest leads), ST segment elevation, Q waves, and T wave inversion represent posterior wall AMI. (Adapted from Brady WJ, Erling B, Pollack M, Chan TC. Electrocardiographic manifestations: acute posterior wall myocardial infarction. J Emerg Med 2001 May;20(4):391-401.)

the inferior or lateral leads further suggests the diagnosis (Figs. 69-3 and 69-4).

Utility of Posterior Leads. The presence of STE on additional posterior leads, particularly leads V_8 and V_9, can help identify patients with a clinical presentation suggestive of an AMI, but with only ST segment depression noted in the precordial leads of the standard 12-lead ECG (see Fig. 69-3). Zalenski et al. showed that in a patient population with high clinical suspicion for AMI, the sensitivity of STE for AMI on 12- versus 15-lead ECGs increased from 47.1% to 58.8%, respectively, with no decrease in specificity.[3] In addition, they showed a sixfold increase in the odds for meeting ECG thrombolytic therapy criteria. However, the use of additional leads did not improve the ability to diagnose AMI in emergency department (ED) patients with a normal ECG. Brady et al. found that use of 15-lead ECGs in patients presenting to the ED with chest pain did not alter the patient's ED diagnosis, ED-based therapy, or hospital disposition.[4] However, it was noted that a more complete description of myocardial injury was obtainable. Boden et al. observed that 5% of 544 patients initially presumed to have non–Q wave AMI actually had transmural infarction of the posterior wall.[5] Melendez et al. found that 3 of 46 (7%) patients with AMI had isolated changes seen in the posterior leads.[6] In a large cohort study Zalenski et al. reported 9 patients (1.7%) of 533 who had isolated STE noted in the posterior leads.[7]

Aside from data in the setting of AMI, there is also evidence to support the use of posterior ECG leads to diagnose AMI from the cardiac catheterization laboratory. Wung and Drew used a percutaneous transluminal coronary angioplasty model of posterior wall AMI to show improved sensitivity of detecting STE in the posterior leads when the left circumflex coronary artery is occluded.[8] However, they recommended adjusting the ischemic criterion from the standard 1 mm to 0.5 mm of elevation in leads V_7 to V_9 to achieve a sensitivity of 94% for detecting STE associated with occlusion of the left

circumflex artery. This finding compares with a sensitivity of 49% when 1-mm elevation is used in leads V_7 to V_9 as the threshold criterion. They noted that most patients with STE greater than 1 mm in the posterior leads also had STE identified on the standard 12-lead ECG, whereas in subjects who had STE between 0.5 and 1 mm, only a small proportion had STE identified on the standard 12-lead ECG. Of note, the maximal normal variation of the baseline did not exceed 0.2 mm in the leads. In patients with inferior AMI, those with STE in leads V_7 to V_9 represented a subgroup with larger infarct size due to posterolateral wall involvement, and a higher occurrence rate of adverse clinical events, including reinfarction, heart failure, or death.[9] The evidence is conflicting, however, because Zalenski et al. did not find patients with inferior and posterior STE to be at a higher risk of hospital complications than those with inferior STE alone.[10]

The explanation for the low voltages seen in posterior wall AMI is found by looking at the anatomy of the thorax (Fig. 69-5). The chest with fully aerated lungs is not an ideal conductor, and the heart is not in the exact middle of chest. The degree of STE in posterior leads is significantly less pronounced in patients with posterior wall AMI mainly because of the long distance between the posterior surface electrode and the posterior wall of the left ventricle (see Fig. 69-2); this greater distance, with much interposed tissue, results in resistance to current flow and produces a smaller injury current, ultimately causing STE of a lesser magnitude in many instances.

Right Ventricular Infarction

Right ventricular (RV) infarction is predominantly a complication of inferior wall AMI. Approximately one third of patients with inferior wall AMI have RV involvement, and in approximately one half of these patients, it is of hemodynamic significance.[11] In contrast, RV infarction is rarely associated with anterior wall MI. An isolated RV infarction is a rare event.

The presence of RV infarction can be difficult to recognize based on the interpretation of the standard 12-lead ECG because the RV is relatively small compared with the left ventricle, and STE in leads V_1 and V_2 due to RV infarction is suppressed by concurrent inferior wall MI. Findings suggestive of RV infarction on 12-lead ECG include STE in lead V_1, inferior STE, and maximal inferior STE in lead III.

Utility of Right Chest Leads. The most reliable ECG evidence of RV infarction is the presence of STE greater than 1 mm (0.1 mV) in the right chest leads, especially V_{4R}, when associated with STE in standard leads II, III, and aVF[12] (Figs. 69-6 and 69-7). Lead V_{4R} can distinguish patients with proximal occlusion of the right coronary artery from those with an occlusion of the distal right coronary artery or the left circumflex artery.[13] STE of 1 mm or more has a 93% sensitivity and 88% specificity for a proximal right coronary artery lesion. Morphology of the ST segment in lead V_{4R} is also helpful in identifying the occluded vessel. Distal occluded segments of the right coronary artery present with no STE in lead V_{4R}, but have an upsloping ST segment/T wave, and circumflex occlusion has a downsloping ST segment/T wave without STE in lead V_{4R}.[13]

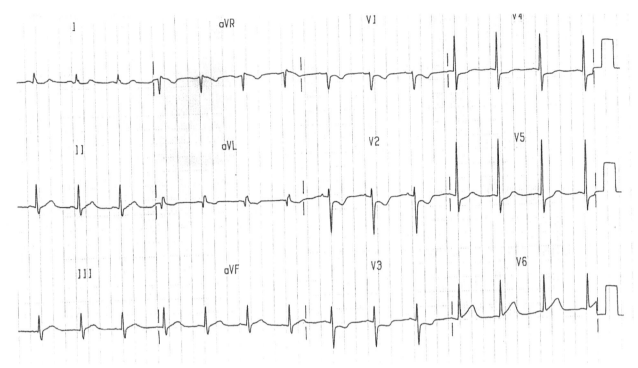

A

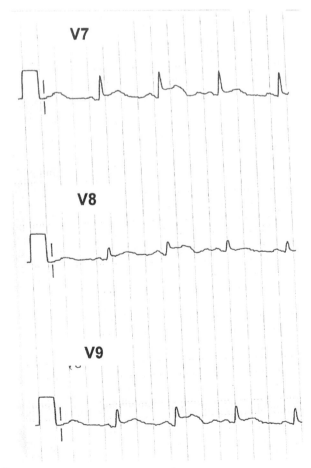

B

FIGURE 69-3 · Posterior wall acute myocardial infarction (AMI). *A,* Standard 12-lead ECG shows the reciprocal changes of ST segment depression in leads V₁ to V₃. *B,* Posterior chest leads show ST segment elevation representing posterior wall AMI.

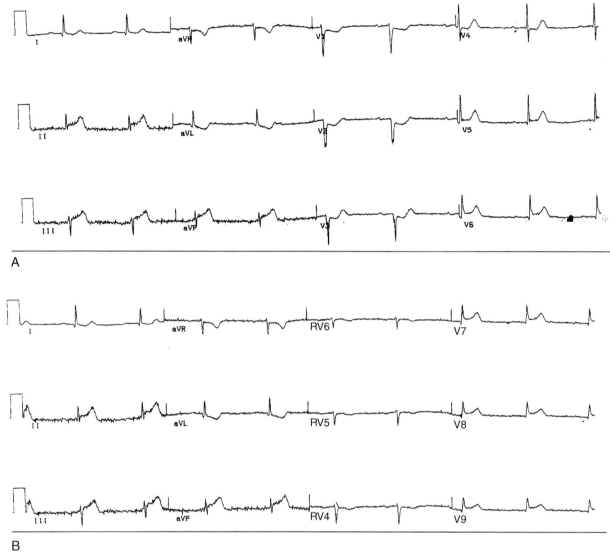

A

B

FIGURE 69-4 · **Inferolateral posterior wall acute myocardial infarction (AMI).** *A,* Twelve-lead ECG and *B,* additional-lead ECGs reveal ST segment elevation in leads II, III, aVF, and V_6 through V_9, consistent with an AMI of the inferior, lateral, and posterior walls of the left ventricle—representing a larger infarct size and associated increased complications.

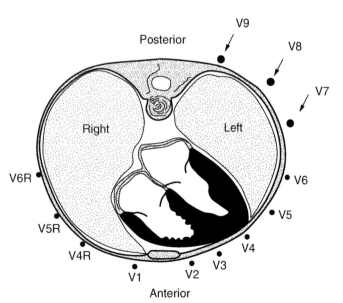

FIGURE 69-5 · **Cross-sectional view of thorax showing relation of ECG leads to heart.** (Adapted from Melendez LJ, Jones DT, and Salcedo JR. Usefulness of three additional electrocardiographic chest leads (V_7, V_8, and V_9) in the diagnosis of acute myocardial infarction. CMAJ 1978, 119:745-748.)

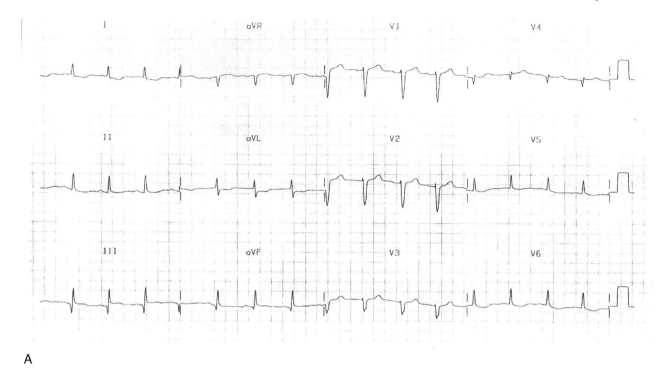

A

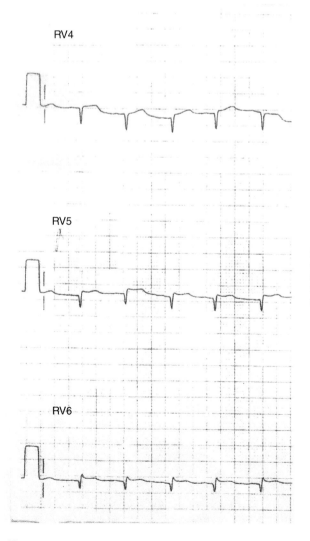

B

FIGURE 69-6 · **Inferior wall acute myocardial infarction (AMI) with right ventricular infarction.** *A,* Standard ECG reveals subtle ST segment elevation in leads III and aVF, consistent with inferior wall AMI. *B,* Right-sided ECG shows ST segment elevation in leads V_{4R} to V_{6R}, consistent with acute infarction of the right ventricle.

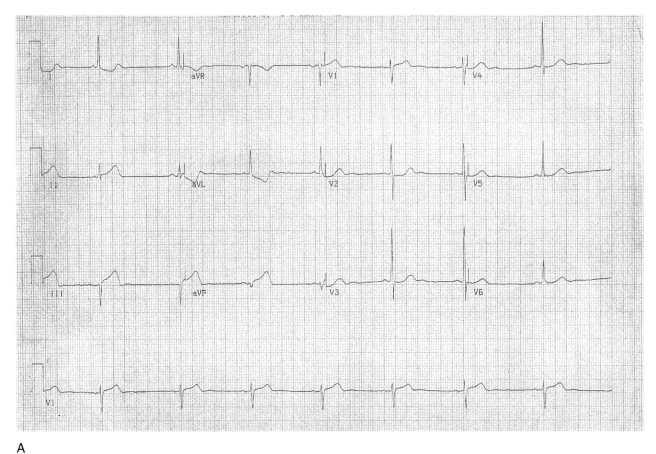

A

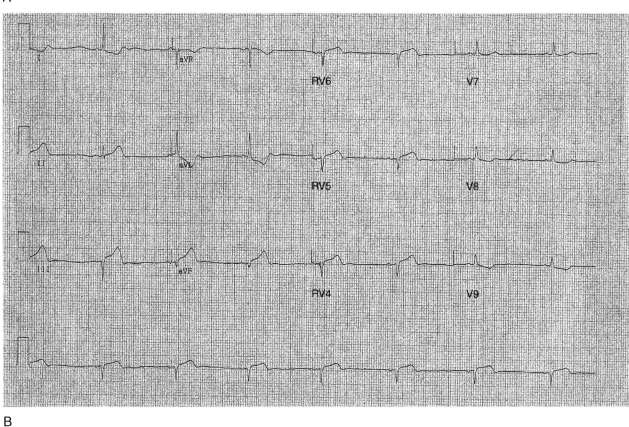

B

FIGURE 69-7 · Inferior wall acute myocardial infarction (AMI) with right ventricular infarction. *A,* ECG reveals ST segment elevation in leads II, III, and aVF, consistent with inferior wall AMI. *B,* Right-sided ECG shows ST segment elevation in leads V_{4R} to V_{6R}, demonstrating that inferior AMI is associated with right ventricular infarction, which was documented by angiography to be due to proximal right coronary artery occlusion.

Anderson and colleagues observed that the STE seen in right precordial leads in patients with extensive RV involvement decreases within 18 to 24 hours.[14]

The finding of ST segment depression in the right-sided leads may also be helpful because it too can be associated with acute RV infarction. Rechavia and colleagues reported that four of nine patients with ST segment depression in leads V_{3R} and V_{4R} had clinical findings compatible with RV infarction.[15]

Patients with RV infarction can exhibit variable clinical sequelae, ranging from no hemodynamic compromise to severe hypotension and cardiogenic shock. Significant RV ischemia can lead to acute RV failure. As a consequence, filling of the left ventricle is decreased, lowering cardiac output and resulting in hypotension. The administration of venodilating agents such as nitrates must be avoided to prevent a decrease in RV filling and worsening systemic hypotension. Volume resuscitation is the mainstay of therapy, with vasopressors initiated in those patients who fail to respond to volume loading.

Patients with STE in lead V_{4R} had a higher in-hospital mortality rate (31% versus 6%) and a higher incidence of major in-hospital complications (64% versus 28%) than patients without STE in lead V_{4R}. STE in lead V_{4R} was found to be a strong, independent predictor of major complications and in-hospital mortality in patients with inferior wall AMI.[16]

References

1. Wung SF, Drew B: Comparison of 18-lead ECG and selected body surface potential mapping leads in determining maximally deviated ST lead and efficacy in detecting acute myocardial ischemia during coronary occlusion. J Electrocardiol 1999;32(Suppl):30.
2. Brady WJ, Erling B, Pollack M, Chan TC: Electrocardiographic manifestations: Acute posterior wall myocardial infarction. J Emerg Med 2001;20:391.
3. Zalenski RJ, Cooke DC, Rydman R, et al: Assessing the diagnostic value of an ECG containing leads V_{4R}, V_8, and V_9: The 15-lead ECG. Ann Emerg Med 1993;22:786.
4. Brady WJ, Hwang V, Sullivan R, et al: A comparison of 12- and 15-lead ECGs in ED chest pain patients: Impact on diagnosis, therapy, and disposition. Am J Emerg Med 2000;18:239.
5. Boden WE, Kleiger RE, Gibson RS, et al: Electrocardiographic evolution of posterior acute myocardial infarction: Importance of early precordial ST-segment depression. Am J Cardiol 1987;59:782.
6. Melendez LJ, Jones DT, Salcedo JR: Usefulness of three additional electrocardiographic chest leads (V7, V8, and V9) in the diagnosis of acute myocardial infarction. CMAJ 1978;119:745.
7. Zalenski RJ, Rydman RJ, Sloan EP, et al: Value of posterior and right ventricular leads in comparison to the standard 12-lead electrocardiogram in evaluation of ST-segment elevation in suspected acute myocardial infarction. Am J Cardiol 1997;79:1579.
8. Wung SF, Drew BJ: New electrocardiographic criteria for posterior wall acute myocardial ischemia validated by a percutaneous transluminal coronary angioplasty model of acute myocardial infarction. Am J Cardiol 2001;87:970.
9. Matetzky S, Freimark D, Chouraqui P, et al: Significance of ST-segment elevations in posterior chest leads (V_7 to V_9) in patients with acute inferior myocardial infarction: Application for thrombolytic therapy. J Am Coll Cardiol 1998;31:506.
10. Zalenski RJ, Rydman RJ, Sloan EP, et al: ST segment elevation and the prediction of hospital life-threatening complications: The role of right ventricular and posterior leads. J Electrocardiol 1998;31(Suppl):164.
11. Fijewski TR, Pollack ML, Chan TC, Brady WJ: Electrocardiographic manifestations: Right ventricular infarction. J Emerg Med 2002; 22:189.
12. Berger PB, Ryan TJ: Inferior myocardial infarction: High-risk subgroups. Circulation 1990;81:401.
13. Braat SH, Gorgels AP, Bar FW, Wellens HJ: Value of the ST-T segment in lead V4R in inferior wall acute myocardial infarction to predict the site of coronary arterial occlusion. Am J Cardiol 1988;62:140.
14. Andersen HR, Falk E, Nielsen D: Right ventricular infarction: The evolution of ST-segment elevation and Q wave in right chest leads. J Electrocardiol 1989;22:181.
15. Rechavia E, Strasberg B, Zafrir N, et al: S-T segment depression in right-sided precordial leads during acute inferior wall infarction. Cardiology 1992;80:42.
16. Zehender M, Kasper W, Kauder E, et al: Right ventricular infarction as an independent predictor of prognosis after acute inferior myocardial infarction. N Engl J Med 1993;328:981.

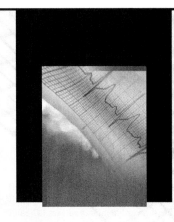

Chapter 70

Serial Electrocardiography and ST Segment Trend Monitoring

J. Lee Garvey

A single, static electrocardiogram (ECG) contains information demonstrating cardiac electrical activity during approximately 10 seconds of cardiac function. Contrast that to the course of coronary artery disease (months to years) and acute coronary syndrome (ACS; minutes to hours). Optimally, the timing of ECG sampling performed when patients present with symptoms should match the time domain of the underlying pathologic process. Repeated sampling of the 10-second standard ECG during the time period of ACS of minutes to hours supplies additional diagnostic and prognostic information. This can be accomplished manually or automatically by using hardware and software devices.

ACS results in derangement of the electrical function of the heart, most often reflected by an alteration of the ST segment. Dynamic changes in ST segment elevation or depression have been documented in the course of ischemia and acute myocardial infarction (AMI).[1-5] The typical course probably reflects varying degrees of elevation or depression, spontaneously occurring and resolving because of the underlying pathophysiologic process.[6] Because each of these processes changes over time, and also with therapeutic interventions, the resulting ST segment amplitude will show corresponding changes over a similar time frame—minute to minute, for a period of hours to days.

ST segment trend monitoring systems usually display information using typical ECG presentations. A set of up to 10 electrode wires is attached to the patient in the usual manner. Signal processing techniques are used to reduce artifactual signal and atypical beats (e.g., premature ventricular contractions). Most systems require an electrode set to be physically connected to the monitoring equipment, but telemetric systems impose fewer physical limitations on patients. Radiolucent electrode systems do not interfere with cardiac catheterization imaging.

The ST segment monitor samples typical (static) 12-lead ECGs repeatedly at a frequency of one per minute. At this rate, 1440 ECGs may be collected in a 24-hour period. Obviously, real-time human review of this number of ECGs is prohibitive. Automated analysis of ST segment amplitude of each lead for such a number of samples is a trivial task for

today's microprocessors. This rate is sufficient to capture changes in the underlying pathophysiologic processes of ischemia, and may be visually shown as a trend of ST segment change over time. ST segment trend data may be displayed for each of the 12 leads (Fig. 70-1), or as the absolute value of a summation of ST changes (Fig. 70-2).

Automated visual and auditory alarm systems call attention to situations in which ST segment changes have exceeded preset limits. Typical limits for ST segment trend analysis alarms are a change (increase or decrease) of 200 μV in a single lead, or 100 μV of change in two or more electrically contiguous leads occurring for two or three consecutive samples. This implies that the baseline ECG is compared with subsequent ECGs. Systems that use a Frank lead set (x, y, z) of orthogonal electrodes calculate and display ST segment changes as the ST vector magnitude $(ST-VM) = (STx^2 + STy^2 + STz^2)^{1/2}$ over time (Fig. 70-2). A reversible increase in $ST-VM$ of greater than 50 μV from baseline is considered abnormal.[7]

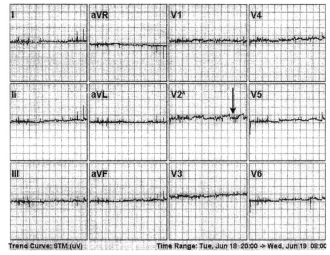

FIGURE 70-1 · **Normal trend of ST segment amplitude in each of 12 standard ECG leads over 12 hours.** *Arrow* denotes minor changes in ST segment amplitude (<100 mV) resulting from change in body position.

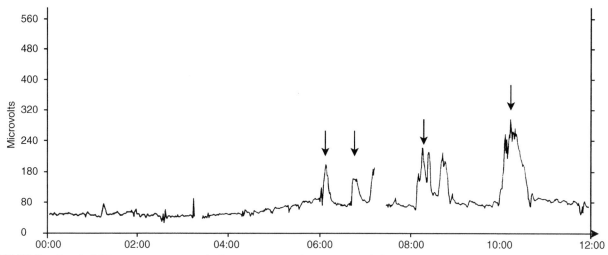

FIGURE 70-2 • **Trend of ST segment vector magnitude recorded over 12 hours.** *Arrows* indicate periods of cardiac ischemia. (Adapted from Dellborg M, Andersen K: Key factors in the identification of the high-risk patient with unstable coronary artery disease: Clinical findings, resting 12-lead electrocardiogram, and continuous electrocardiographic monitoring. Am J Cardiol 1997;80:35E, with permission.)

Clinicians must remember that ST segment amplitude is rarely isoelectric in all leads at baseline. Subsequent further changes of less than 100 μV may occur and render an ECG "diagnostic" for ACS before being detected by a system that is set to detect changes of voltage. Similarly, subtle changes in ST segment amplitude of less than 100 μV may truly reflect active ischemia. This degree of change is very difficult to detect visually, and is usually excluded from automated systems' alarm settings to increase specificity.

Changes in body position may be reflected as a change in the ST segment amplitude, particularly in the precordial leads.[8] The underlying 12-lead ECGs generally continue to show a consistent overall pattern, but QRS voltage and subsequent repolarization voltage (ST segment/T wave) may be changed. This is usually of small magnitude, but may be noticed during continuous ST segment trend monitoring (Fig. 70-1).

Alarm violations may occur when electrical noise contaminates the signal. Meticulous attention to skin preparation and lead positioning minimizes this risk. When alarms occur, trained staff should examine the ST segment trend and specific underlying 12-lead ECGs to determine the pathophysiologic or artifactual cause.

ST Segment Monitoring in the Emergency Department

It is intuitive that application of a tool (ischemia monitoring) that captures transient diagnostic changes (ST elevation or depression) that otherwise could be missed should improve the time to definitive treatment, and thus improve outcomes in ACS. The ST segment trend for a patient with "atypical symptoms" who demonstrated acute ischemia is presented in Figure 70-3. The dynamic nature of the underlying coronary artery disease is reflected in the time course of ECG changes for this patient.

In a series of 1000 patients, Fesmire et al.[9] showed that ST segment trend monitoring is useful for patients with chest pain in the emergency department (ED). In their series, ST segment magnitudes were measured every 20 seconds for at least 1 hour, and automated serial ECGs were obtained at least every 20 minutes. This cohort included the entire spectrum of patients with chest pain in the ED—from ST segment elevation AMI through those at low likelihood for ACS. This monitoring technique improved sensitivity in identifying AMI and ACS compared with the initial presentation ECG (68% versus 55% for AMI; 34% versus 27% for ACS). ACS diagnostic sensitivity improved (99.4% versus 97.1%). This monitoring technique was also used to identify patients requiring intensive anti-ischemic therapy, intensive care unit admission, and emergent cardiac catheterization; as well as to assess reperfusion therapy.

ST segment monitoring is also used as a means of surveillance for ischemia in patients in the ED considered to be at low risk for ACS.[10–12] A consensus panel[8] suggests that a total of 8 to 12 hours of continuous ST segment monitoring, in conjunction with serial sampling of blood for markers of myocardial necrosis and provocative testing for ischemia, may be an effective way to evaluate patients with chest pain in the ED.

However, although protocols for the rapid evaluation have been published,[13,14] no specific study evaluating the cost effectiveness of ST segment monitoring of patients at low risk for ACS has been reported. Moreover, because a normal or nondiagnostic ECG obtained on presentation does not exclude AMI or the presence of coronary artery disease, serial ECGs and ST segment monitoring likewise cannot be the sole means to exclude potential ACS.

Use in Assessing Coronary Artery Patency

During elective coronary angioplasty procedures, Krucoff et al.[15] studied the relation between balloon inflation and dynamic ST segment movement. ST segment changes were typically detectable in an anterior lead set with inflation in the left anterior descending artery, or in an inferior lead set with

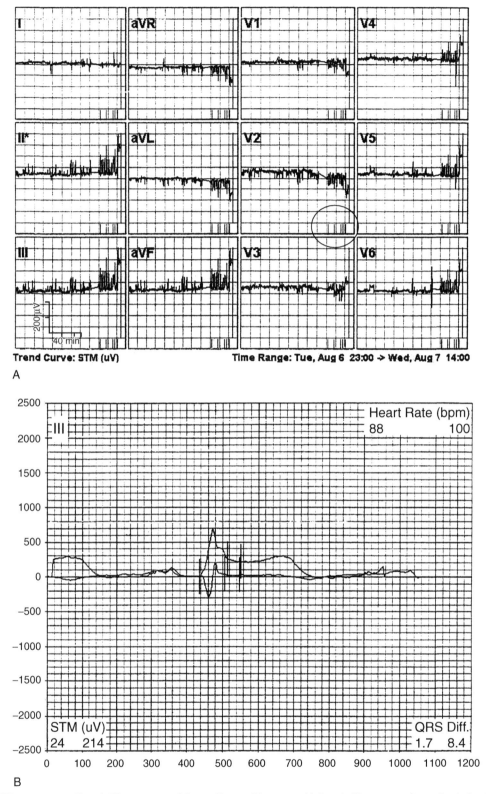

FIGURE 70-3 • **ST segment trending.** *A,* ST segment trend from a 62-year-old woman with "atypical" symptoms for cardiac ischemia. A cluster of spikes at the base of each panel notes recurrent, brief episodes of abnormal, dynamic ST segment changes documenting ischemia. *B,* Individual composite beats from lead III showing baseline ECG, and ECG at time of maximal ST segment elevation.

(Continued)

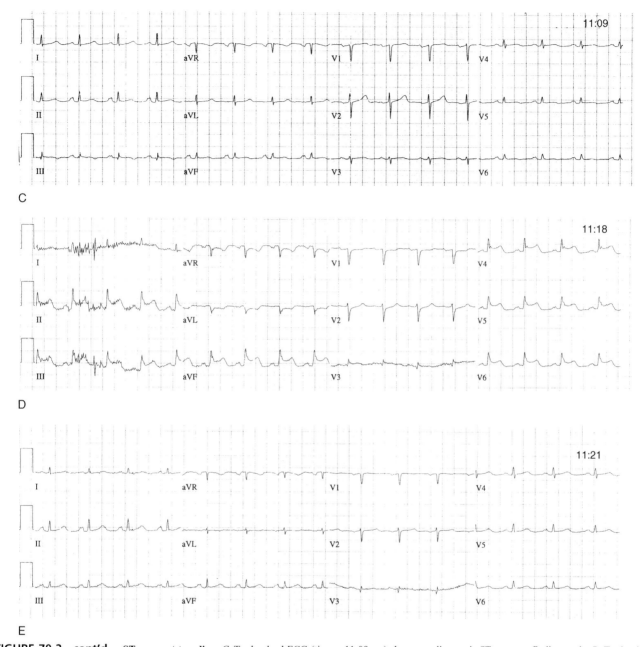

FIGURE 70-3—cont'd · **ST segment trending.** *C,* Twelve-lead ECG (time = 11:09 AM) shows nondiagnostic ST segment findings only. *D,* Twelve-lead ECG (time = 11:18 AM) is now diagnostic for ST segment elevation in inferior and lateral leads. *E,* Twelve-lead ECG (time = 11:21 AM) shows resolution of ST segment abnormalities within 3 minutes.

inflation in the right coronary artery or circumflex. Similarly, ST segment monitoring has also been used to predict infarct artery patency after pharmacologic reperfusion therapy.[16–18]

To investigate the association between early recovery from ST segment elevation and long-term mortality in patients with AMI, French et al.[17] followed 766 patients treated with fibrinolytic therapy. They found that ST segment recovery in the lead with initial maximum ST segment elevation was a predictor of long-term survival (2.5 to 10 years, $P = 0.03$ to 0.0005), but ST segment recovery, measured as the sum of all leads with ST segment changes (or elevation), was not.

Use in Perioperative and Intraoperative Settings

Cardiovascular monitoring is a cornerstone of management in the perioperative setting. Application of ST segment monitoring in an attempt to identify episodes of ischemia has been used in this setting as well.[19–21] This area is not without its own controversy and discussion.[22–24] Discordance may exist between ST segment changes (electrical) and transesophageal echocardiography (mechanical) as detectors of perioperative ischemia. In a comparison with post hoc analysis of intraoperative Holter recordings, various real-time ST segment monitors were found to be of moderate sensitivity (60% to 78%) and specificity (69% to 89%) in detecting ischemia in patients undergoing coronary artery bypass surgery.[25]

References

1. Velez J, Brady WJ, Perron AD, Garvey L: Serial electrocardiography. Am J Emerg Med 2002;20:43.
2. Fesmire FM, Smith EE: Continuous 12-lead electrocardiograph monitoring in the emergency department. Am J Emerg Med 1993;11:54.
3. Krucoff MW, Croll MA, Pope JE, et al: Continuously updated 12-lead ST-segment recovery analysis for myocardial infarct artery patency assessment and its correlation with multiple simultaneous early angiographic observations. Am J Cardiol 1993;71:145.
4. Cohn PF, Sodums MT, Lawson WE, et al: Frequent episodes of silent myocardial ischemia after apparently uncomplicated myocardial infarction. J Am Coll Cardiol 1986;8:982.
5. Klootwijk P, Cobbaert C, Fioretti P, et al: Noninvasive assessment of reperfusion and reocclusion after thrombolysis in acute myocardial infarction. Am J Cardiol 1993;72:75G.
6. Patel DJ, Knight CJ, Holdright DR, et al: Pathophysiology of transient myocardial ischemia in acute coronary syndromes: Characterization by continuous ST-segment monitoring. Circulation 1997;95:1185.
7. Dellborg M, Andersen K: Key factors in the identification of the high-risk patient with unstable coronary artery disease: Clinical findings, resting 12-lead electrocardiogram, and continuous electrocardiographic monitoring. Am J Cardiol 1997;80:35E.
8. Drew BJ, Krucoff MW: Multilead ST-segment monitoring in patients with acute coronary syndromes: A consensus statement for healthcare professionals: ST-Segment Monitoring Practice Guideline International Working Group. Am J Crit Care 1999;8:372.
9. Fesmire FM, Percy RF, Bardoner JB, et al: Usefulness of automated serial 12-lead ECG monitoring during the initial emergency department evaluation of patients with chest pain. Ann Emerg Med 1998;31:3.
10. Gibler WB, Sayre MR, Levy RC, et al: Serial 12-lead electrocardiographic monitoring in patients presenting to the emergency department with chest pain. J Electrocardiol 1993;26(Suppl):238.
11. Garvey JL: Can ST segment monitoring beat static twelve-lead ECG? In Gibler WB (ed): Pushing the Therapeutic Envelope for Emergency Cardiac Medicine: Acute Coronary Syndromes and Beyond. New York, Health Science Communications, 2001, p. 2.
12. Sarko J, Pollack CV Jr: Beyond the twelve-lead electrocardiogram: Diagnostic tests in the evaluation for suspected acute myocardial infarction in the emergency department, part I. J Emerg Med 1997;15:839.
13. Graff L, Joseph T, Andelman R, et al: American College of Emergency Physicians Information Paper: Chest pain units in emergency departments—a report from the Short-Term Observation Services Section. Am J Cardiol 1995;76:1036.
14. Gomez MA, Anderson JL, Karagounis LA, et al: An emergency department-based protocol for rapidly ruling out myocardial ischemia reduces hospital time and expense: Results of a randomized study (ROMIO). J Am Coll Cardiol 1996;28:25.
15. Krucoff MW, Loeffler KA, Haisty WKJ, et al: Simultaneous ST-segment measurements using standard and monitoring-compatible torso limb lead placements at rest and during coronary occlusion. Am J Cardiol 1994;74:997.
16. Pasceri V, Andreotti F, Maseri A: Clinical markers of thrombolytic success. Eur Heart J 1996;17(Suppl E):35.
17. French JK, Andrews J, Manda SOM, et al: Early ST-segment recovery, infarct artery blood flow, and long-term outcome after acute myocardial infarction. Am Heart J 2002;143:265.
18. Krucoff MW, Green CE, Satler LF, et al: Noninvasive detection of coronary artery patency using continuous ST-segment monitoring. Am J Cardiol 1986;57:916.
19. Slogoff S, Keats AS, David Y, Igo SR: Incidence of perioperative myocardial ischemia detected by different electrocardiographic systems. Anesthesiology 1990;73:1074.
20. McDermott MM, Lefevre F, Arron M, et al: ST segment depression detected by continuous electrocardiography in patients with acute ischemic stroke or transient ischemic attack. Stroke 1994;25:1820.
21. Kotrly KJ, Kotter GS, Mortara D, Kampine JP: Intraoperative detection of myocardial ischemia with an ST segment trend monitoring system. Anesth Analg 1984;63:343.
22. Jopling MW: Pro: Automated electrocardiogram ST-segment monitoring should be used in the monitoring of cardiac surgical patients. J Cardiothorac Vasc Anesth 1996;10:678.
23. Proctor LT, Kingsley CP: Con: ST-segment analysis—who needs it? J Cardiothorac Vasc Anesth 1996;10:681.
24. Selbst J, Comunale ME: Myocardial ischemia monitoring. Int Anesthesiol Clin 2002;40:133.
25. Leung JM, Voskanian A, Bellows WH, Pastor D: Automated electrocardiograph ST segment trending monitors: Accuracy in detecting myocardial ischemia. Anesth Analg 1998;87:4.

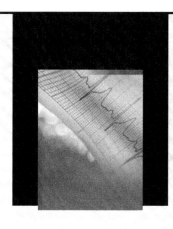

Chapter 71

The Prehospital 12-Lead Electrocardiogram

Michael J. Urban, Jeffrey D. Ferguson, M. Todd Clever,
William J. Brady, and Tom P. Aufderheide

The National Heart Attack Alert Program (National Heart Lung and Blood Institute) has set an ambitious goal of treating all patients with acute myocardial infarction (AMI) within 30 minutes of arriving at the hospital.[1] Prehospital 12-lead electrocardiograms (ECGs) allow the identification of AMI before the patient's arrival at the hospital and potentially reduce the time to definitive treatment in the largest number of patients possible.[2–7] Prehospital ECGs have demonstrated reasonable diagnostic accuracy for identification of patients with ST segment elevation (STE) AMI[8]; the rate of correct diagnosis of patients with non–acute coronary syndrome (ACS) chest pain in the out-of-hospital setting is less impressive, although still of benefit to clinicians.[8] Prehospital 12-lead ECGs provide additional potential benefits, including improved prehospital diagnostic accuracy in patients with chest pain,[8] detection of ischemia that resolves before hospital arrival,[9] assistance in identifying the cause of wide-complex tachycardias,[10–12] incorporation of diagnostic aids such as predictive instruments for acute cardiac ischemia and fibrinolytic therapy,[13–15] and triage of high-risk patients to tertiary cardiac centers[16]; prehospital therapy and transport means may also be affected by information obtained from the ECG. Both the American College of Cardiology and the American Heart Association recommend that prehospital 12-lead ECG programs should be established in urban and suburban emergency medical services (EMS) systems as a class I recommendation.[16,17]

History and Technology

In 1969, advanced prehospital cardiac care was initiated in Belfast, Northern Ireland, with use of Pantridge's mobile coronary care units.[18] In 1970, Nagel and colleagues reported the successful use and benefits of prehospital telemetry in the EMS system in Florida.[19] Single-lead telemetry with online medical control provided the technologic basis for prehospital emergency cardiac care and advanced cardiac life support in patients experiencing dysrhythmia. Unfortunately, single-lead

electrocardiography provides no diagnostic information on the other two major clinical syndromes of coronary artery disease—angina pectoris and myocardial infarction. In the mid-1980s, the introduction of portable 12-lead ECGs made the prehospital diagnosis of acute coronary syndromes a possibility. In Western Europe, physician-staffed mobile intensive care units were the first to apply this technology.[20] Similar practices in the United States have also demonstrated that carefully trained prehospital personnel can accurately and successfully interpret prehospital 12-lead ECGs under remote supervision of an on-line medical control physician in the emergency department (ED).[4,21]

Numerous systems have demonstrated that the prehospital ECG is easily and safely performed.[2,5,7,8] For example, Grim et al. verified that prehospital ECGs have identical intervals and morphologic characteristics compared with ECGs acquired in the ED.[22] Many studies have looked at the feasibility of implementing prehospital 12-lead ECG programs.[2,5,7,8] Although transmission failures occur, as an EMS system becomes more familiar with the prehospital ECG technology, the transmission failure rate decreases.[8] One study showed the transmission failure rate dropped from 33% during the first month after program implementation to only an 11% failure rate by the sixth month.[8] Several reasons can account for unsuccessful transmission, including poor transmission pathways (especially during times of peak usage), lack of proximity of EMS personnel to a cellular telephone cell, concrete and steel structures such as high-rise buildings, and operator error.

Most established urban paramedic systems can easily implement field 12-lead ECG technology. One urban system achieved a 98.7% success rate in obtaining diagnostic-quality ECGs in 94.6% of eligible prehospital patients after one 4-hour training session.[9] Because paramedics use this technology while simultaneously performing other duties, time delays are minimal. In Salt Lake City, a study of the EMS system finds no significant difference in time spent at the scene for patients randomized to field ECG versus no ECG groups.[5]

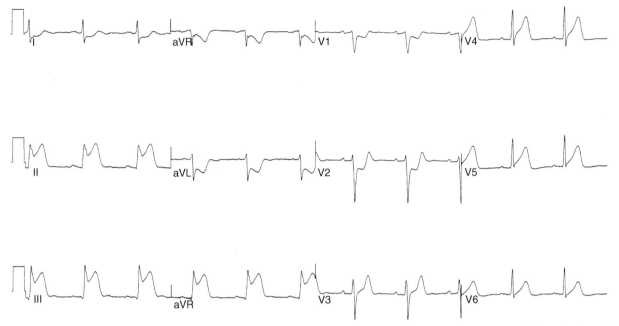

FIGURE 71-1 • **Prehospital ECG.** This is a representative example of a successfully transmitted prehospital 12-lead ECG diagnostic for an inferior posterolateral acute myocardial infarction.

Prehospital identification of fibrinolytic candidates increased scene time by an average of only 4 minutes in an urban EMS system.[2] This added time allowed for the prehospital ECG to be acquired and transmitted to a base station for physician interpretation and physician review of a 20-item paramedic fibrinolytic eligibility checklist (Figs. 71-1 and 71-2).

Impact of the Prehospital Electrocardiogram

The main role of the prehospital ECG is in the reduction of time to definitive treatment for the patient with STE AMI. Published studies have shown that by identifying the patient with AMI before his or her arrival at the hospital, prehospital 12-lead ECGs can reduce the time to reperfusion therapy by 20 to 60 minutes.[2–7] For instance, the FAST-MI Trial (Field Ambulance Study of Thrombolysis in Myocardial Infarction)[5] revealed that prehospital patients with AMI undergoing an ECG before ED arrival had significantly shorter times to hospital-based delivery of reperfusion treatments. In this trial, patients were evaluated in the field and randomized to receive either prehospital or hospital-based 12-lead ECGs. The time from hospital arrival to fibrinolytic administration in patients with AMI without prehospital ECG was 68 minutes, whereas the time from ED arrival to initiation of fibrinolysis for patients with AMI with prehospital ECGs was 48 minutes. In both treatment groups, the delays to hospital-based therapy were significantly shorter than the delay of approximately 100 minutes previously reported in a control group of patients with AMI over a 3-year period before the onset of the FAST-MI Trial.[5]

Multiple additional investigations have demonstrated similar benefit. The Myocardial Infarction Triage and Intervention—Phase I trial (the Seattle study) and the Cincinnati Heart Project used prehospital ECGs in patients with chest pain before ED arrival[6,7,23] (Table 71-1). In these studies, the administration of hospital-based thrombolysis occurred much earlier than in patients who did undergo

prehospital ECGs. For instance, the hospital-based delay to treatment with fibrinolytic therapy in the Seattle trial was reduced from 102 minutes to 46 minutes after introducing the prehospital 12-lead ECG.[7] The Cincinnati Heart Project noted a reduction in hospital time to fibrinolytic therapy from approximately 89 minutes to approximately 63 minutes over 1 year. The greatest reduction in time to treatment at the hospital was noted in patients who had undergone prehospital ECGs.[6,23] Kereiakes et al.[6] specifically compared time to hospital-based reperfusion therapy between groups based on prehospital mode of transportation. The study reported an average door-to-therapy time of 64 minutes in patients who arrived at the ED by private vehicle, 55 minutes by private (non-EMS) ambulance, 50 minutes by EMS, and 30 minutes by EMS with ECG capability. These studies demonstrate that routine transmission of the ECG from the field to the receiving hospital results in the greatest reduction of hospital-based time delays.[6,7,23]

An additional benefit of prehospital electrocardiography may be in detecting prehospital ACS that resolves before ED arrival. Paramedics often evaluate patients who are actively experiencing ACS-related symptoms that may resolve before the arrival at the hospital. Demonstrating electrocardiographic abnormality in the out-of-hospital setting may improve hospital-based evaluation in specific cases—particularly if the chest pain and related electrocardiographic changes have resolved. Alternatively, showing dynamic alteration in the ST segment/T wave also assists in establishing the diagnosis of an ACS (Fig. 71-2).

Many health care providers are concerned about the potential for scene and prehospital time delays resulting from performance of the prehospital ECG. Multiple authorities,[4,5,24,25] however, have reported minimal time delay, universally less than 4 minutes. In fact, one large, retrospective review demonstrated acceptable scene times with minimal out-of-hospital prolongation coupled with a marked reduction in mortality rate with the use of prehospital 12-lead ECGs.[3]

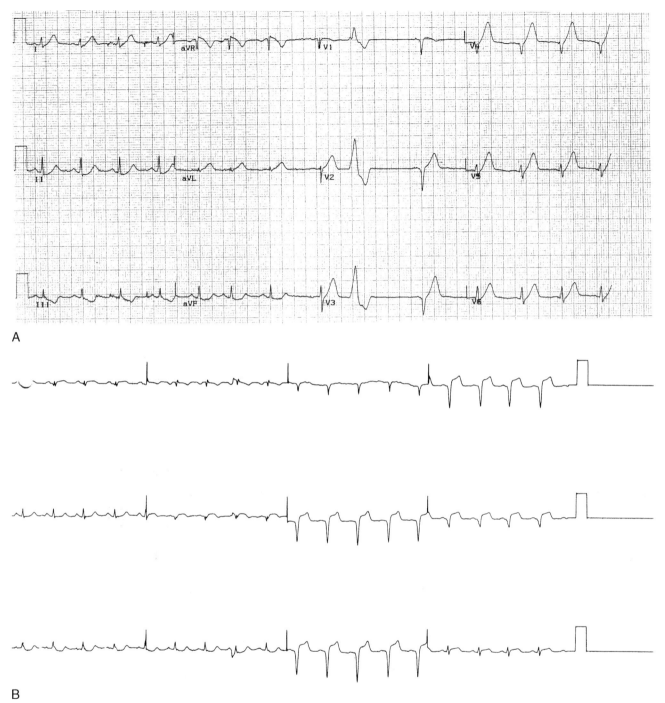

FIGURE 71-2 • **Dynamic changes seen with prehospital ECG.** *A,* This prehospital 12-lead ECG shows hyperacute T wave changes (without ST segment elevation) in leads V_2 to V_6. *B,* An initial hospital ECG shows ST elevation and Q waves in the same leads.

Prehospital patients with STE AMI are potential candidates for fibrinolysis administered by paramedics.[6-8,23,26-28] Fibrinolytic administration in this setting has been shown to be possible; in fact, a mortality benefit has been demonstrated if the time reduction is greater than 1 hour.[26-28] Obviously, the prehospital ECG not only drives this out-of-hospital medical decision making but represents the key diagnostic indication for fibrinolysis by EMS. Although unproven, it is highly likely that the patient with ACS with electrocardiographic abnormality would receive a more aggressive therapeutic approach by EMS personnel.

Although this has not been investigated, the prehospital ECG may affect patient management in terms of the destination hospital. In a patient with a diagnosis of STE AMI, an institution with rapidly available percutaneous coronary intervention may be a more medically appropriate destination; essentially, such a practice would represent a diversion to the regional "heart" hospital, analogous to the regional trauma systems established in most areas of the United States, the United Kingdom, and Western Europe. Of course, such a strategy would require preplanning among the community's hospitals, including representatives of the involved EDs, cardiologists,

71-1 • SUMMARY OF PREHOSPITAL ELECTROCARDIOGRAM AND IMPACT ON HOSPITAL-BASED REPERFUSION MANAGEMENT

Investigation (Lead Author)	ECG Interpretation	Time to Hospital Reperfusion,* Study Patients (min)	Time to Hospital Reperfusion,* Control Patients (min)	Time Difference (min)
Kereiakes[6]	Transmitted to hospital	30	50	20
Foster[4]	Interpreted by EMS	22	51	29
Karagounis[5]	Transmitted to hospital	48	68	20
Kereiakes[23]	Transmitted to hospital	36	63	27
Millar-Craig[24]	Interpreted by EMS	37	97	60
Canto[3]	Transmitted to hospital	30	40	10
Aufderheide[29]	Transmitted to hospital	46	65	19

*Defined as the time from EMS arrival at patient to receipt of hospital-based reperfusion therapy.
EMS, emergency medical services.

and EMS agencies. In another area of prehospital transport, a patient with known STE AMI geographically distant from the ED may benefit from a more rapid means of transport to the hospital, such as aeromedical evacuation. The prehospital ECG is the primary data point for such changes in management.

References

1. National Heart Attack Alert Program Coordinating Committee, 60 Minutes to Treatment Working Group: Emergency department: Rapid identification and treatment of patients with acute myocardial infarction. Ann Emerg Med 1994;23:311.

2. Aufderheide TP, Hendley GE, Thakur RK, et al: Milwaukee Prehospital Chest Pain Project—Phase I: Feasibility and accuracy of prehospital thrombolytic candidate selection. Am J Cardiol 1992;69:991.

3. Canto JG, Rogers WJ, Bowlby LJ, et al: National Registry of Myocardial Infarction 2 Investigators. The prehospital electrocardiogram in acute myocardial infarction: Is its full potential being realized? J Am Coll Cardiol 1997:29;498.

4. Foster DB, Dufendach JH, Barkdoll CM, et al: Prehospital recognition of AMI using independent nurse/paramedic 12-lead ECG evaluation: Impact on in-hospital times to thrombolysis in a rural community hospital. Am J Emerg Med 1994:12:25.

5. Karagounis L, Ipsen SK, Jessop MR, et al: Impact of field-transmitted electrocardiography on time to in-hospital thrombolytic therapy in acute myocardial infarction. Am J Cardiol 1990:66:786.

6. Kereiakes DJ, Gibler WB, Martin LH, et al: Relative importance of emergency medical system transport and the prehospital electrocardiogram on reducing hospital time delay to therapy for acute myocardial infarction: A preliminary report form the Cincinnati Heart Project. Am Heart J 1992;123:835.

7. Weaver WD, Eisenberg MS, Martin JS, et al: Myocardial Infarction Triage and Intervention Project—Phase I: Patient characteristics and feasibility of prehospital initiation of thrombolytic therapy. J Am Coll Cardiol 1990;15:925.

8. Aufderheide TP, Hendley GE, Woo J, et al: A prospective evaluation of prehospital 12-lead ECG application in chest pain patients. J Electrocardiol 1991;24S:8.

9. Aufderheide TP, Hendley GE, Thakur RK, et al: The diagnostic impact of prehospital 12-lead electrocardiography. Ann Emerg Med 1990;19:1280.

10. De Lorenzo RA: Prehospital misidentification of tachydysrhythmias: A report of five cases. J Emerg Med 1993;11:431.

11. White RD: Prehospital recognition of multifocal atrial tachycardia: Association with acute myocardial infarction. Ann Emerg Med 1992;21:753.

12. White RD: Prehospital 12-lead ECG [letter]. Ann Emerg Med 1992;21:586.

13. Aufderheide TP, Rowlandson I, Lawrence SW, et al: Test of the acute cardiac ischemia time-insensitive predictive instrument (ACI-TIPI) for prehospital use. Ann Emerg Med 1996;27:193.

14. Selker HP, Beshansky JR, Griffith JL, et al: Use of the acute cardiac ischemia time-insensitive predictive instrument (ACI-TIPI) to assist with triage of patients with chest pain or other symptoms suggestive of acute cardiac ischemia: A multicenter, controlled clinical trial. Ann Intern Med 1998;129:845.

15. Selker HP, Griffith, JL, Beshansky JR, et al: Patient-specific predictions of outcomes in myocardial infarction for real-time emergency use: A thrombolytic predictive instrument. Ann Intern Med 1997;127:538.

16. Ewy GA, Ornato JP: 31st Bethesda Conference: Emergency Cardiac Care. Task Force 1: Cardiac arrest. J Am Coll Cardiol 2000;35:832.

17. Anonymous: The Era of Reperfusion: Section 1: Acute Coronary Syndromes (Acute Myocardial Infarction). Circulation 2000; 102(Suppl I):I-172.

18. Pantridge JF, Geddes JS: A mobile intensive-care unit in the management of myocardial infarction. Lancet 1969;2:271.

19. Nagel EL, Hirshman JC, Nussenfeld SR, et al: Telemetry: Medical command in coronary and other mobile emergency care systems. JAMA 1970;214:332.

20. Aufderheide TP: Prehospital 12-lead electrocardiography and evaluation of the patient with chest pain. In Gibler WB, Aufderheide TP (eds): Emergency Cardiac Care. St. Louis, Mosby, 1994, p 38.

21. Brinsfield K, Feldman J, Bernard S, et al: Identification of ST elevation AMI on prehospital 12 lead ECG: Accuracy of unaided paramedic interpretation [abstract]. J Emerg Med 1998;16:22S.

22. Grim P, Feldman T, Martin M, et al: Cellular telephone transmission of 12-lead electrocardiograms from ambulance to hospital. Am J Cardiol 1987;60:715.

23. Kereiakes DJ, Weaver WD, Anderson JL, et al: Time delays in the diagnosis and treatment of acute myocardial infarction: A tale of eight cities. Report from the Prehospital Study Group and the Cincinnati Heart Project. Am Heart J 1990;120:773.

24. Millar-Craig MW, Joy AV, Adamowicz M, et al: Reduction in treatment delay by paramedic ECG diagnosis of myocardial infarction with direct CCU admission. Heart 1997;78:456.

25. Brown SGA, Galloway DM: Effect of ambulance 12-lead ECG recording on times to hospital reperfusion in acute myocardial infarction. Med J Aust 2000;172:81.

26. Weaver WD, Cerqueira M, Hallstrom AP, et al: Prehospital-initiated vs hospital-initiated thrombolytic therapy. The Myocardial Infarction Triage and Intervention Trial. JAMA 1993;270:1211.

27. European Myocardial Infarction Project Group (EMIP): Prehospital thrombolytic therapy in patients with suspected acute myocardial infarction. N Engl J Med 1993;329:383.

28. GREAT Group: Feasibility, safety, and efficacy of domiciliary thrombolysis by general practitioners: Grampion Region Early Anistreplase Trial. BMJ 1992;305:548.

29. Aufderheide TP, Lawrence SW, Hall KN, et al: Prehospital 12-lead electrocardiograms reduce hospital-based time to treatment in thrombolytic candidates. Acad Emerg Med 1994;1:A13.

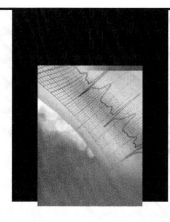

Chapter 72

The Electrocardiogram and Stress Testing

Michael C. Kontos

Patients presenting to the emergency department (ED) with chest pain or other symptoms consistent with myocardial ischemia are a common problem. Because of the limitations of the initial evaluation, most low-risk patients undergo further evaluation, either in the ED or chest pain observation unit (CPU) or as an inpatient. Because myocardial serum markers are unable to exclude ischemia or to detect early infarction, provocative testing is usually required.

The preferred method of stress testing is exercise. Besides the electrocardiographic response to stress, the additional information obtained has important diagnostic and prognostic significance. Its costs are low, the presence of a cardiologist is not routinely necessary, and it can be conveniently performed without requiring much additional space. Although imaging adds incremental diagnostic information to the exercise treadmill testing (ETT), it is unclear if this is true for low-risk patients with chest pain.[1]

Training Requirements, Personnel, Protocols, and Safety

Specific guidelines for training,[2] for clinical exercise testing laboratories,[3] and for performing and interpreting ETTs[4] have been published (Tables 72-1 and 72-2).

Although a number of protocols exist, the Bruce protocol is most commonly used.[5] In this protocol, the initial stage starts at 1.7 mph with a 5% grade. Speed and grade increase every 3 minutes up to stage 7 (5.5 mph, 20% grade). For patients in whom exercise tolerance is low, the protocol can be modified by adding two early stages (which do not include an incline).

Because the patient is exercising, the traditional electrocardiogram (ECG) lead placement must be altered. This change results in a right axis deviation, possible loss of inferior Q waves, masking of any previous inferior myocardial infarction (MI), and development of a Q wave in lead aVL. Therefore, the stress ECG should not be used in place of or for comparison with the standard 12-lead ECG.

Indications for ETT termination recommended by the American College of Cardiology include attainment of peak maximal heart rate (not universally accepted), physical exhaustion, and the development of diagnostic abnormality[4] (see Table 72-2). Some institutions terminate testing at 85% of the predicted maximal heart rate (as calculated by 220 − age). However, predicted heart rate is only an estimate, and may vary by 10 to 20 beats for an individual patient. A recent study that analyzed results from more than 18,000 patients found that (208 − [0.7 × age]) better predicted maximal heart rate, particularly for older patients.[6] Therefore, continuing the test until exhaustion or another end point is reached is recommended.

Data that should be routinely obtained during the ETT include heart rate, blood pressure, and the ECG. These should be recorded at the end of each stage of exercise, as well as

---

72-1 • CONTRAINDICATIONS TO EXERCISE TESTING

Absolute
- Acute myocardial infarction occurring within 2 days
- Unstable angina not previously stabilized by medical therapy
- Uncontrolled cardiac dysrhythmias causing symptoms or hemodynamic compromise
- Symptomatic severe aortic stenosis
- Uncontrolled symptomatic heart failure
- Acute pulmonary heart failure, pulmonary embolus, or pulmonary infarction
- Acute myocarditis or pericarditis
- Acute aortic dissection

Relative
- Left main coronary stenosis
- Moderate stenotic valvular heart disease
- Electrolyte abnormalities
- Severe arterial hypertension
- Tachydysrhythmias or bradydysrhythmias
- Hypertrophic cardiomyopathy and other forms of outflow tract obstruction
- Mental or physical impairment leading to inability to exercise adequately
- High-degree atrioventricular block

72-2 • ABSOLUTE INDICATIONS FOR TERMINATING EXERCISE TESTING

- Drop in systolic blood pressure of >10 mm Hg from baseline blood pressure despite an increase in workload, when accompanied by other evidence of ischemia
- Moderate to severe angina
- Increasing nervous system symptoms (e.g., ataxia, dizziness, or near-syncope)
- Signs of poor perfusion (cyanosis or pallor)
- Technical difficulties in monitoring ECG or systolic blood pressure
- Subject's desire to stop
- Sustained ventricular tachycardia
- ST segment elevation (>1.0 mm) in leads without diagnostic Q waves

72-3 • NORMAL AND ABNORMAL ELECTROCARDIOGRAPHIC FINDINGS IN THE EXERCISE STRESS TEST

Normal
- Shortening of PR interval
- Narrowing of QRS complex
- Shortening of QT interval
- Increase in P wave amplitude
- Development of ST segment depression (at J point with prompt return to baseline)

Abnormal

ST Segment Alterations
- Accentuated horizontal position
- Majority of significant changes occur in leads I and V_3 to V_5 (lead V_5 with greatest diagnostic sensitivity)

ST Segment Depression (STD)
- Downsloping STD with no return to baseline before T wave
- Increasing downsloping STD morphology
- Upsloping STD only in *high-risk* populations—increased sensitivity
- Upsloping STD in *lower-risk* populations—reduced specificity (not routinely used)
- Criterion—1 mm horizontal or downsloping STD
- STD in exercise and recovery phases—same diagnostic accuracy
  Note: STD confined to inferior leads usually does not represent ischemia
- STD not associated with particular coronary territory/does not localize coronary artery

ST Segment Elevation (STE)
- STE 0.08 sec after QRS complex present in three consecutive beats
- STE in leads without Q waves (highly specific)
- STE with Q waves (not specific)
- STE associated with particular coronary territory/does localize coronary artery

T and R Wave Changes
- Not diagnostic for coronary artery disease (CAD)

U Wave Inversion
- Diagnostic for CAD
- Supraventricular dysrhythmias
- Not diagnostic for CAD

Ventricular Dysrhythmias
- Diagnostic for CAD

Left Bundle Branch Block
- Worrisome for CAD
- Associated with increased mortality
- Testing should be terminated (identification of changes is no longer possible)

during recovery. The patient should be asked frequently about chest pain and other symptoms. Chest pain is usually considered an indication for stopping. However, in patients with atypical chest pain undergoing a CPU evaluation who have symptoms that have not resolved before testing, exercise can be carefully continued as long as the symptoms are mild, the ECG does not demonstrate ischemia, and no other termination end points are reached.[7]

With appropriate patient selection, exercise stress testing is safe. Overall risk is approximately 1 death per 20,000 to 50,00 tests, with nonfatal MI occurring in approximately 1 per 2500 patients tested.[8] Appropriate patient selection and supervision are crucial in reducing the risk of complications (see Table 72-1).

There are special considerations involving patients who have internal cardiac defibrillators (ICDs). Most ICDs are activated based on an upper rate cut-off; therefore, if the patient is stressed to the point that this heart rate is reached, the ICD will fire. To prevent accidental firing, testing should be terminated at a heart rate sufficiently below the rate cut-off, or the device should be temporarily deactivated.

Stress Test Interpretation

The normal ECG response to exercise includes shortening of the PR intervals, QRS complexes, and QT intervals; increase in the P wave amplitude; and ST segment depression at the J point, which usually returns to baseline. With ischemia, the ST segment becomes more horizontal or downsloping with no return to baseline before the T wave. With increasing exercise, the amount of ST segment depression downsloping may increase (Table 72-3).

The most commonly used criterion for a positive ETT is 1 mm horizontal or downsloping ST segment depression or elevation 0.08 seconds after the QRS complex present in three consecutive beats[5] (Fig. 72-1). However, the ECG response represents a continuum of abnormality, and, as with any diagnostic test, there is a large overlap of test results in patients with and without coronary disease. Changing the diagnostic criteria alters sensitivity and specificity. For example, if an abnormal ETT response is changed to 2 mm, specificity improves (i.e., fewer false-positive results), but sensitivity is reduced (i.e., increased false-negative results). This alteration may prove desirable in certain situations, such as asymptomatic patients in whom the pretest probability is low.

ST segment depression on the stress ECG is not associated with a particular coronary territory and does not localize the coronary artery. Most of the significant ECG changes occur in leads I and V_3 to V_5, with lead V_5 having the highest diagnostic sensitivity.[4,9] ST segment depression confined to the inferior leads usually does not represent ischemia.[10] Use of upsloping ST segment depression is associated with increased sensitivity in high-risk populations, but in lower-risk populations significantly reduces specificity, and therefore should not be used routinely.[4] ST segment depression occurring in recovery has the same diagnostic accuracy as ST segment depression that initially occurs in exercise.

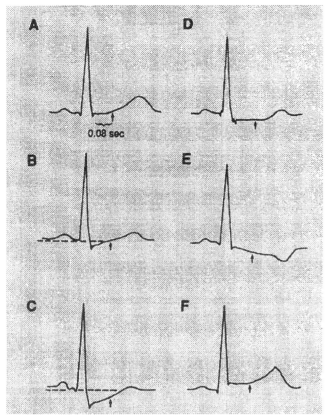

FIGURE 72-1 • **ST segment responses to exercise.** *A,* Normal. *B,* Junctional depression that returns to baseline within 80 msec. *C,* Junctional depression that remains below baseline at 80 msec. *D,* Horizontal ST segment depression. *E,* Downsloping ST segment depression. *F,* ST segment elevation. *B* and *C* are considered nondiagnostic responses. *D, E,* and *F* are ischemic responses to exercise. (Adapted from Tavel ME: Stress testing in cardiac evaluation: Current concepts with emphasis on the ECG review. Chest 2001;119;907, with permission.)

In a meta-analysis of stress ECG studies (147 studies, 24,074 patients),[11,12] the overall sensitivity was 68% and specificity was 77% for significant coronary artery disease. These studies may be limited by selection bias because the ETT studies were performed only in patients who underwent coronary angiography. Inclusion of studies in which all patients agreed to have both coronary angiography and stress testing resulted in a lower sensitivity of 50% but a higher specificity of 90%. This observation is consistent with the results of most ED CPU evaluation studies, in which most patients had negative studies.

Other ECG stress-induced abnormalities include ST segment elevation, T wave changes, and U wave inversion. Stress-induced ST segment elevation in leads without Q waves is highly specific for ischemia and is associated with high-grade proximal coronary stenosis (Fig. 72-2). In contrast to depression, ST segment elevation often localizes ischemia to a specific coronary territory. It is uncommon, occurring in less than 5% of patients undergoing stress testing. The etiology of ST segment elevation in leads with Q waves is controversial, but is thought to be due to wall motion abnormalities and dyskinesis of the underlying left ventricle.[13,14] It is more common in patients with previous anterior, rather than

inferior infarctions,[15] and is usually associated with significant left ventricular dysfunction.[16,17]

T and R wave changes are relatively nonspecific for coronary disease. U wave inversion has been reported to be a specific, but insensitive sign of ischemia, and may occur in the absence of other ischemic changes.[5] The development of supraventricular dysrhythmias during stress testing is relatively uncommon, and is not diagnostic for ischemic heart disease.[18] Exercise-induced left bundle branch block (LBBB) is also rare, occurring in less than 0.5% of tests.[19] It is associated with a twofold increase in mortality rate.[19] Testing should be terminated because identification of ischemic changes is no longer possible.

Electrocardiographic Confounders

The presence of significant baseline ST segment changes (such as with left ventricular hypertrophy [LVH], LBBB, ventricular paced rhythms, and Wolff-Parkinson-White syndrome) may make the stress ECG uninterpretable, necessitating the addition of imaging for detecting myocardial ischemia. The stress ECG remains interpretable in patients with right bundle branch block, except for leads V_1 to V_3. ST segment depression occurring in other leads has the same significance as when the resting ECG is normal. The presence of LVH, both with and without baseline ST segment changes, is associated with increased incidence of false-positive results. Other causes of false-positive results include hypokalemia[20] and digoxin.[21]

The degree, duration, and timing of ST segment depression are important. A positive ETT (i.e., ST segment depression) is more likely to be a true positive if it is associated with exercise-induced chest pain, occurs at a low exercise level (stage 2 or 6 minutes on the Bruce protocol), is greater than 2 mm in depth, or persists for more than 8 minutes into recovery (Table 72-3 and Fig. 72-3). These variables have been associated with an increased incidence of multivessel or left main coronary artery disease.[22,23] In contrast, false-positive ETTs are usually associated with ST segment depression only at peak exercise, with quick resolution in recovery[24] (Fig. 72-4). Patients who are able to exercise to stage 4 of the Bruce protocol have an excellent prognosis, regardless of whether the stress ECG result is positive.[23]

Patient-Related Variables

A number of patient-related variables can affect diagnostic accuracy. These include medications, the pretest probability of disease, sex, and exercise capacity. ETT sensitivity is reduced in patients who do not obtain a high enough heart rate, which is frequent in those taking beta-adrenergic blocking agents. Sensitivity is also reduced in patients with single-vessel and left circumflex coronary artery disease.

Both sensitivity and specificity of ETT are lower in women. Sensitivity is reduced because there is a lower prevalence of severe coronary disease, and the ability to exercise to maximum aerobic capacity may be lower.[25] There are several different hypotheses for the lower specificity, such as hormonal effects,[26] but the most likely explanation is the lower pretest probability of coronary artery disease in women.[27] However, in the large Coronary Artery Surgery study, there

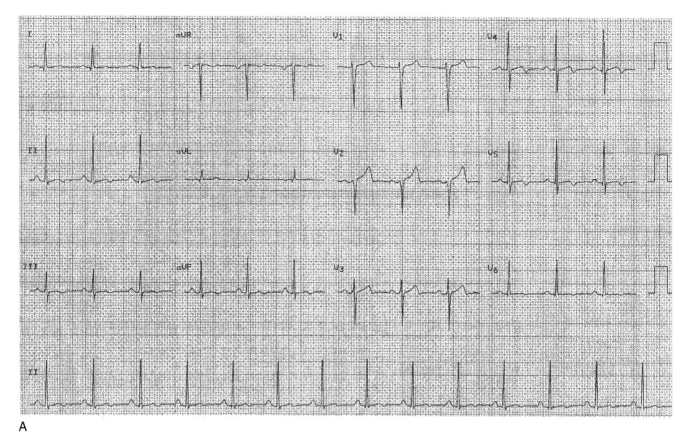

A

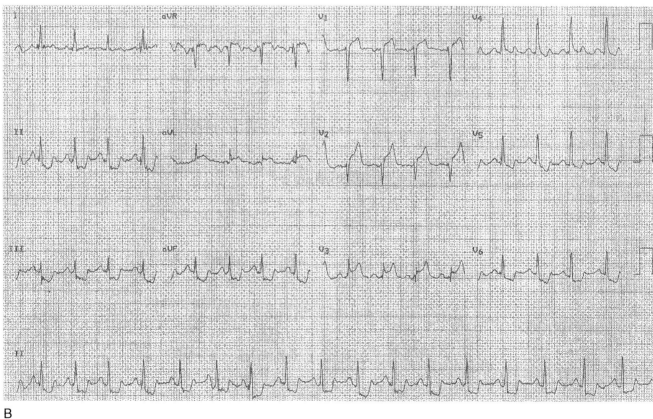

B

FIGURE 72-2 • **ST segment changes with exercise.** *A,* Initial ECG showed nonspecific T wave changes in leads V_4 and V_5. *B,* After 4 minutes of exercise, anterior ST segment elevation developed in leads V_1 to V_3; also note the ST segment depression in leads II, III, aVF, V_5, and V_6. Subsequent coronary angiography demonstrated a 95% proximal right coronary artery stenosis.

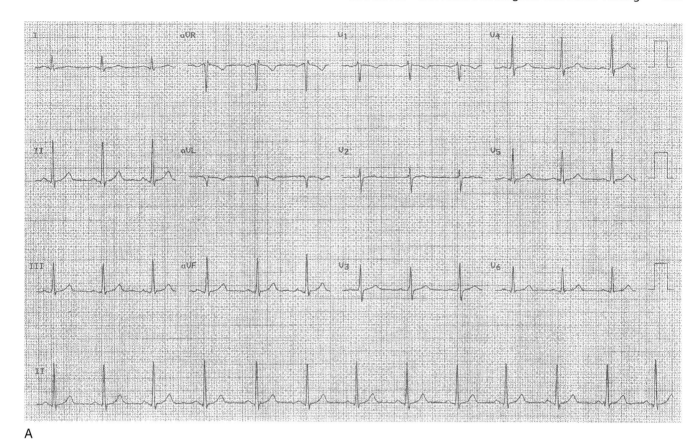

A

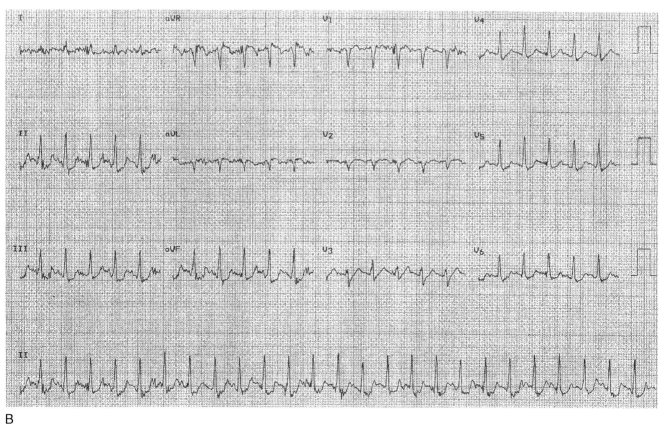

B

FIGURE 72-3 • **True-positive ST segment depression with exercise.** Baseline ECG was normal *(A)*. After exercise for 5 minutes, the exercise stress test was stopped because of chest pain and shortness of breath. Peak exercise ECG demonstrated mild ST segment depression in leads II, III, aVF, V₅, and V₆ *(B)*.

(Continued)

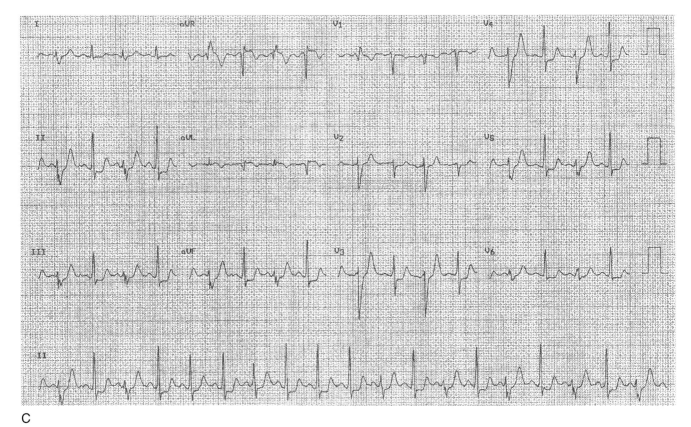

C

FIGURE 72-3—cont'd · **True-positive ST segment depression with exercise recovery phase ECG demonstrates more prominent ST segment depressions.** *(C)*, Subsequent coronary angiography demonstrated significant coronary artery disease.

was no difference in ETT specificity or sensitivity after men and women were matched for age and extent of coronary artery disease.[27] Therefore, ETT still has an important role in evaluating women with chest pain, and should still be considered in those with a normal or near-normal baseline ECG.[4]

Prognostic variables other than the ECG include blood pressure response to exercise, poor exercise capacity, and failure to increase heart rate.

Stress Testing in the Emergency Department–Based Chest Pain Unit

Specific recommendations on performing ETT after a CPU evaluation have been published by the American Heart Association.[1] Patients should be low risk, with less than a 7% risk of having MI, and have undergone an assessment with serial ECGs and myocardial markers over an 8- to 12-hour period. Patients with ischemic chest pain should not be stressed. Testing should be performed using symptom-limited, maximal testing, rather than a predetermined heart rate end point. Patients requiring stress imaging because they cannot exercise or have an uninterpretable baseline ECG, or those who fail to reach the target heart rate, should ideally remain hospitalized until the evaluation is completed.

The first large reported study of early ETT performed as part of a CPU evaluation was reported by Gibler and colleagues.[28] A total of 1010 patients underwent a 9-hour rule-out protocol in their heart ED. At the end of the evaluation,

791 patients (78%) underwent symptom-limited ETT, of whom 782 had either negative or nondiagnostic tests, resulting in a specificity of 99.4%. False-positive results were present in five of the nine positive tests. There were no complications related to ETT, and only two patients who had a negative evaluation had cardiac events in the subsequent 30 days.

Other studies have confirmed the safety of using early symptom-limited ETT in low-risk patients with chest pain.[7,29,30] Because of differences in selection criteria, the proportion of patients who have positive tests has varied from 1%[28] to approximately 15% to 20%.[7,30] A consistent finding among these studies is that approximately half of all positive ETTs turn out to be true-positive results.

Alternatives that shorten the observation period further have been reported. Investigators have used immediate ETT in low-risk patients presenting to the ED.[7,30,31] In this protocol, patients considered at low risk for chest pain based on the absence of ischemic ECG changes underwent ETT using a modified Bruce protocol. No significant complications were reported in a total of 1000 patients who underwent immediate ETT. Overall, tests were negative in two thirds of patients, positive in 13%, and nondiagnostic in 23%. Patients with negative and nondiagnostic ETTs were discharged directly from the ED. Only one patient with a negative ETT had an MI within the following 30 days. Expanding immediate ETT to patients with known coronary disease, using identical selection criteria, resulted in similar results, with very low incidence of adverse events.[31]

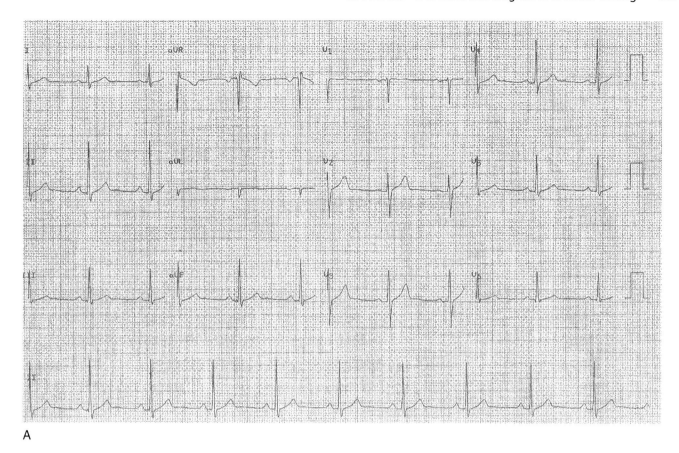

A

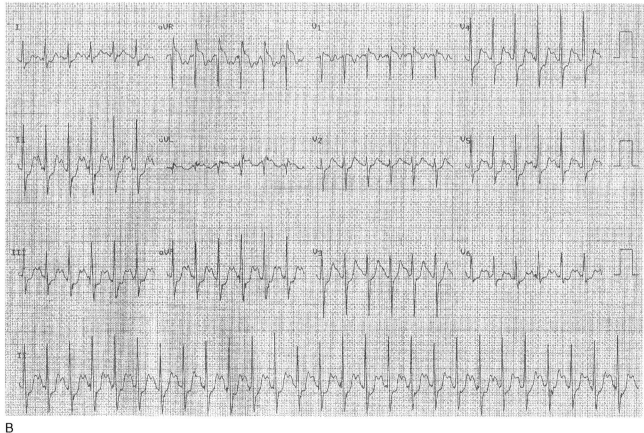

B

FIGURE 72-4 • **False-positive ST segment depression at peak exercise.** Baseline ECG was normal *(A)*. The patient exercised for over 10 minutes, stopping for fatigue. Upsloping ST segment depression was present at peak exercise in leads III, V₄, and V₅, with horizontal ST segment depression in lead V₆ *(B)*.

(Continued)

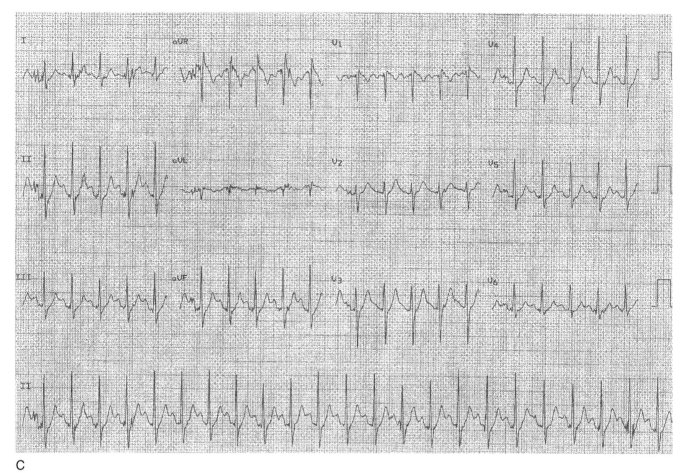

C

FIGURE 72-4—cont'd • **False-positive ST segment depression at peak exercise.** These changes almost resolved within 30 seconds in recovery *(C)*. Repeat testing using myocardial perfusion imaging demonstrated normal perfusion at peak exercise.

Immediate ETT is subject to a number of limitations. It should be applied only to carefully selected patients, who are low risk by all criteria. Close supervision is required, given the potential risk of stressing patients with ongoing MI. The test should be terminated once significant ST segment changes occur. Although no significant complications were reported in these studies, the safety of performing ETT in patients with unrecognized ischemia has not been clearly demonstrated.

For the significant minority of patients who have nondiagnostic tests, what further evaluation needs to be performed is unclear. Recommendations are that these patients should be hospitalized until the evaluation has been completed.[1] However, Amsterdam and colleagues found that routine discharge from the ED was associated with a low rate of MI or death.[7] This was confirmed by Diercks and colleagues.[32] Although the event rate was higher than in those with negative tests, most of the events were revascularization procedures.[7,32]

References

1. Stein RA, Chaitman BR, Balady GJ, et al: Safety and utility of exercise testing in emergency room chest pain centers. Circulation 2000;102:1463.
2. Rodgers GP, Ayanian JZ, Balady G, et al: American College of Cardiology/American Heart Association Clinical Competence Statement on Stress Testing: A report of the American College of Cardiology/American Heart Association/American College of Physicians–American Society of Internal Medicine Task Force on Clinical Competence. J Am Coll Cardiol 2000;36:1441.
3. Pina IL, Balady GJ, Hanson P, et al: Guidelines for clinical exercise testing laboratories: A statement for healthcare professionals from the Committee on Exercise and Cardiac Rehabilitation, American Heart Association. Circulation 1995;91:912.
4. Gibbons RJ, Balady GJ, Beasley JW, et al: ACC/AHA guidelines for exercise testing: A report of the American College of Cardiology/American Heart Association Task Force on Practice Guidelines (Committee on Exercise Testing). J Am Coll Cardiol 1997;30:260.
5. Chaitman BR: Exercise stress testing. In Braunwald E, Zipes DP, Libby P (eds): Heart Disease: A Textbook of Cardiovascular Medicine, 6th ed. Philadelphia, WB Saunders, 2001, p 129.
6. Tanaka H, Monahan KD, Seals DR: Age-predicted maximal heart rate revisited. J Am Coll Cardiol 2001;37:153.
7. Amsterdam EA, Kirk JD, Diercks DB, et al: Immediate exercise testing to evaluate low-risk patients presenting to the emergency department with chest pain. J Am Coll Cardiol 2002;40:251.
8. Stuart RJ, Ellestad MH: National survey of exercise stress testing facilities. Chest 1980;77:94.
9. Viik J, Lehtinen R, Turjanmaa V, et al: Correct utilization of exercise electrocardiographic leads in differentiation of men with coronary artery disease from patients with a low likelihood of coronary artery disease using peak exercise ST-segment depression. Am J Cardiol 1998;81:964.
10. Miranda CP, Liu J, Kadar A, et al: Usefulness of exercise-induced ST-segment depression in the inferior leads during exercise testing as a marker for coronary artery disease. Am J Cardiol 1992;69:303.

11. Gianrossi R, Detrano R, Mulvihill D, et al: Exercise-induced ST depression in the diagnosis of coronary artery disease: A meta-analysis. Circulation 1989;80:87.

12. Detrano R, Gianrossi R, Froelicher V: The diagnostic accuracy of the exercise electrocardiogram: A meta-analysis of 22 years of research. Prog Cardiovasc Dis 1989;32:173.

13. Manvi KN, Ellestab MH: Elevated ST segments with exercise in ventricular aneurysm. J Electrocardiol 1972;5:317.

14. Haines DE, Beller GA, Watson DD, et al: Exercise-induced ST segment elevation 2 weeks after uncomplicated myocardial infarction: Contributing factors and prognostic significance. J Am Coll Cardiol 1987;9:996.

15. DeFeyter PJ, Majid PA, van Eenige MJ, et al: Clinical significance of exercise-induced ST segment elevation. Br Heart J 1981;46:84.

16. Paine RD, Dye LE, Roitman DI, et al: Relation of graded exercise test findings after myocardial infarction to extent of coronary artery disease and left ventricular dysfunction. Am J Cardiol 1978;42:716.

17. Ho JL, Lin LC, Yen RF, et al: Significant of dobutamine-induced ST-segment elevation and T-wave pseudonormalization in patients with Q-wave myocardial infarction: Simultaneous evaluation by dobutamine stress echocardiography and thallium-201 SPECT. Am J Cardiol 1999;84:125.

18. Maurer MS, Shefrin EA, Fleg JL: Prevalence and prognostic significance of exercise-induced supraventricular tachycardia in apparently healthy volunteers. Am J Cardiol 1995;75:788.

19. Grady TA, Chiu AC, Snader CE, et al: Prognostic significant of exercise-induced left bundle-branch block. JAMA 1998;279:153.

20. Georgopoulos AJ, Proudfit WL, Page IH: Effect of exercise on electrocardiograms of patients with low serum potassium. Circulation 1961;23:567.

21. Sketch MH, Mooss AN, Butler ML, et al: Digoxin-induced positive exercise tests: Their clinical prognostic significance. Am J Cardiol 1981;48:655.

22. Colby J, Hakki AH, Iskandrian AS, et al: Hemodynamic, angiographic and scintigraphic correlations of positive exercise electrocardiograms: Emphasis on strongly positive exercise electrocardiograms. J Am Coll Cardiol 1983;2:21.

23. McNeer JF, Margolis JR, Lee KL, et al: The role of the exercise test in the evaluation of patients for ischemic heart disease. Circulation 1978;57:64.

24. Tavel ME: Stress testing in cardiac evaluation: Current concepts with emphasis on the ECG review. Chest 2001;119:907.

25. Pryor DB, Shaw L, Harrell FE, et al: Estimating the likelihood of severe coronary artery disease. Am J Med 1991;90:553.

26. Morise AP, Dalai JN, Duval RD: Frequency of oral estrogen replacement therapy in women with normal and abnormal exercise electrocardiograms and normal coronary arteries by angiogram. Am J Cardiol 1993;72:1197.

27. Weiner DA, Ryan TJ, McCabe CH, et al: Exercise stress testing: Correlations among history of angina, ST-segment response and prevalence of coronary-artery disease in the Coronary Artery Surgery Study (CASS). N Engl J Med 1979;301:230.

28. Gibler WB, Runyon JP, Levy RC, et al: A rapid diagnostic and treatment center for patients with chest pain in the emergency department. Ann Emerg Med 1995;25:1.

29. Mikhail MG, Smith FA, Gray M, et al: Cost-effectiveness of mandatory stress testing in chest pain center patients. Ann Emerg Med 1997;29:88.

30. Kirk JD, Turnipseed S, Lewis WR, Armsterdam EA: Evaluation of chest pain in low-risk patients presenting to the emergency department: The role of immediate exercise testing. Ann Emerg Med 1998;32:1.

31. Lewis WR, Amsterdam EA, Turnipseed S, Kirk JD: Immediate exercise testing of low risk patients with known coronary artery disease presenting to the emergency department with chest pain. J Am Coll Cardiol 1999;33:1843.

32. Diercks DB, Gibler WB, Liu T, et al: Identification of patients at risk by graded exercise testing in an emergency department chest pain center. Am J Cardiol 2000;86:289.

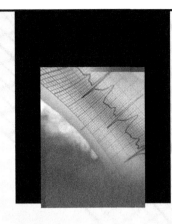

Chapter 73

QT Dispersion

Tom P. Aufderheide and Melody C. Graves

QT dispersion is defined as the difference between the longest QT interval and the shortest QT interval, as calculated in each lead of a 12-lead electrocardiogram (ECG). QT dispersion values when measured in each lead of a standard 12-lead ECG have been used for identifying ischemic patients, helping to confirm the absence of ischemia, predicting the likelihood of sudden death, and determining the efficacy of therapeutic interventions.

The QT interval is a measure of ventricular repolarization; prolonged QT intervals occur in ischemic tissue, whereas shorter QT intervals occur in healthy tissue.[1-6] For example, in the setting of acute myocardial infarction (AMI), a lateral infarction would produce normal QT intervals in leads V_1 to V_4 and prolonged QT intervals in leads V_5, V_6, I, and aVL. By contrast, the absence of ischemia throughout the ventricular myocardium would produce normal repolarization in all leads with little difference between the longest and shortest QT intervals. Furthermore, because injured myocardium repolarizes more slowly than normal cells, some areas of myocardium have shortened refractory periods relative to adjacent areas. This imbalance causes reentry points for ventricular dysrhythmias such as ventricular tachycardia or ventricular fibrillation.[7]

QT Dispersion Determination

Manual derivation of QT dispersion requires determination of the difference between the maximum and minimum QT interval lengths on a 12-lead ECG, and involves using either calipers or a ruler to determine the longest and shortest QT interval. Manual calculation has a number of disadvantages. Time is required to complete all measurements and to derive the QT dispersion value, limiting its clinical utility.[8] Additional disadvantages include intraobserver and interobserver variabilities[8-10] as well as difficulties in identifying the beginning and end points for the QT interval.

To determine QT dispersion, exact determination of Q wave onset (onset of QRS complex) and T wave end (return of T wave to isoelectric point) is critical to obtain precise measurements. Variable T wave morphology (flattened, biphasic, or fused), the presence of U waves, lack of an appropriate

number of measurable leads, and dysrhythmias may preclude QT interval measurement.[11]

An alternative to calculating T wave end is determining T wave peak. As the highest point on the arc of the T wave, it can be used instead of T wave end in calculating QT dispersion in each ECG lead. This can be helpful because the T wave peak may be more accurately measured, depending on the T wave morphology. Disadvantages of T wave peak calculations include flat and biphasic waves that may make measurements difficult or impossible. Either QT end or QT peak measurements must be used for measurements in all ECG leads to derive an accurate QT dispersion value. Although determination of the QT interval may not be possible in all leads, a minimum of eight leads is necessary for calculation of QT dispersion[12] (Fig. 73-1).

Automated or computer-generated programs have been devised to overcome the disadvantages of manual measurement, prevent interobserver and intraobserver variability, and provide the clinician with an immediately available automated calculation to maximize clinical utility[5,13,14] (Fig. 73-2). These programs hold great potential for use in the clinical setting.[8-10,14] Like manual measurement, automated measurement can still be limited by variable T wave morphology, the presence of U waves, lack of an appropriate number of measurable leads, ECG interference, and dysrhythmias.

QT dispersion values vary depending on manual versus automated calculation, and the patient population studied. In general, normal QT dispersion values are considered to no greater than 35 msec, with significantly higher measurements occurring in patients with cardiac disease (AMI, acute coronary syndrome [ACS], congestive heart failure).[7,14] Although normal and abnormal values can be defined for specific patient populations, QT dispersion values for individual patients may overlap the normal and abnormal ranges (Table 73-1).[7]

Clinical Application

QT dispersion holds the potential to assist the emergency physician in triage and risk stratification of patients with chest pain.[5,14,15] One retrospective database analysis using a computerized QT end and QT peak dispersion software

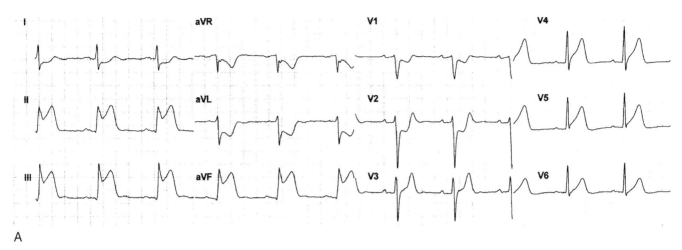

A

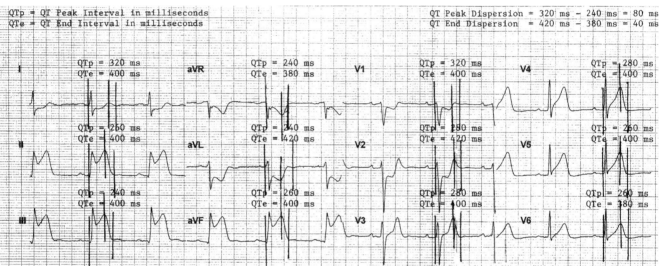

B

FIGURE 73-1 • **Manual QT dispersion calculation.** QT dispersion has been calculated here both by T wave end and T wave peak methods. *Hash marks* represent the onset of the QT interval and either T wave peak or T wave end. *A,* ECG without calculation. *B,* ECG with calculation.

73-1 • QT DISPERSION

- Manual or automated QT interval is measured in each lead of the 12-lead ECG
- There are two types of QT intervals (the same QT interval must be measured in each lead of the 12-lead ECG for a valid measurement):
  - QT end: onset of the QRS complex to end of the T wave, or
  - QT peak: onset of the QRS interval to the peak of the T wave
- QT dispersion is determined by subtracting the shortest from the longest QT interval
- The QT interval may be impossible to measure because of:
  - T wave morphology
  - ECG artifact
  - Dysrhythmias (atrial fibrillation, atrial flutter, tachycardias, paced rhythms, and second or third degree heart block)
- A minimum of eight leads is necessary for calculation of QT dispersion
- Automated QT dispersion programs obviate intraobserver and interobserver variability found with manual calculations
- Significantly increased QT dispersion has been demonstrated in patients with acute coronary syndrome, chronic ischemic heart disease, and heart failure
- Clinical use of QT dispersion is limited by the lack of a standardized method of measurement, limitations in measurement due to T wave morphology, ECG interference and dysrhythmias, and lack of prospective validation of clinical benefit

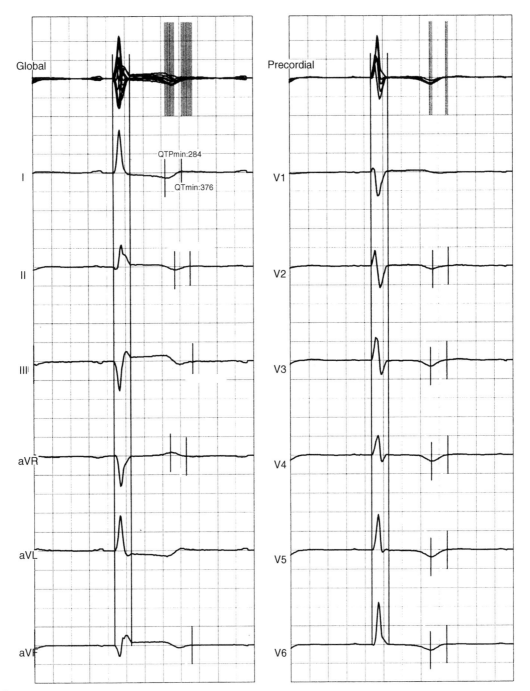

FIGURE 73-2 · Automated QT dispersion calculation. QT dispersion has been automatically calculated by a computerized QT dispersion analysis program. *Hash marks* represent the onset of the QT interval and either T wave end or T wave peak. (Courtesy of Joel Xue, PhD, General Electric Medical Information Technology, Milwaukee, Wisconsin.)

demonstrated significant differences in QT dispersion values between patients with ACS and nonischemic chest pain.[14] By combining automated QT dispersion measurements, automated detection of ST segment deviations, and physician ECG interpretation, this retrospective study demonstrated a 35% increase in sensitivity for detection of AMI and a 55% increase for detection of acute cardiac ischemia. In a retrospective study, 586 patients without ischemic ECG changes and normal initial cardiac enzymes were entered into a chest pain observation unit. Patients who ultimately proved to have AMI had mean QT dispersion values of 44.6 ± 18.5 msec

compared with 10.5 ± 13.8 msec for patients without AMI ($P < 0.05$).[15] These studies supported a potential clinical role for QT dispersion in detecting patients with ACS in the emergency department setting.

QT dispersion holds the potential to determine noninvasively the effectiveness of acute interventions in patients with AMI. Patients successfully reperfused after fibrinolytic therapy, angioplasty, or coronary artery bypass grafting have significantly lower QT dispersion values after the intervention.[11] QT dispersion may also help identify patients at high risk for sudden death. Patients with stable and unstable angina, AMI, or heart failure who have significantly increased QT dispersion are at greater risk for sudden cardiac death from ventricular dysrhythmias.[7,14,16] The effects of antidysrhythmic medication on QT dispersion have also been evaluated and hold promise for optimizing medical therapy for patients with cardiovascular heart disease. Patients taking beta-adrenergic blocking agents, angiotensin-converting enzyme inhibitors, angiotensin II receptor blocking agents, and calcium channel antagonists have been shown to have lowered QT dispersion values, which may explain the pharmacologic action and benefit of these agents for patients with AMI, angina, hypertension, and congestive heart failure.[11]

References

1. Mirvis DM: Spatial variation of QT interval in normal persons and patients with acute myocardial infarction. J Am Coll Cardiol 1985; 5:625.

2. Van de Loo A, Arendts W, Hohnloser SH: Variability of QT dispersion measurements in the surface electrocardiogram in patients with acute myocardial infarction and in normal subjects. Am J Cardiol 1994; 74:1113.

3. Higham PD, Furniss SS, Campbell RW: QT dispersion and components of the QT interval in ischemia and infarction. Br Heart J 1995;73:32.

4. Moreno FL, Villanueva T, Karagounis LA, et al: Reduction in QT interval dispersion by successful thrombolytic therapy in acute myocardial infarction. Circulation 1994;71:508.

5. Endoh Y, Kasanuki H, Ohnishi S, et al: Influence of early coronary reperfusion on QT interval dispersion after acute myocardial infarction. Pacing Clin Electrophysiol 1997;20:1646.

6. Yunus A, Gillis AM, Traboulsi M, et al: Effect of coronary angioplasty on precordial QT dispersion. Am J Cardiol 1997;79:1339.

7. Davey P: QT interval and mortality from coronary artery disease. Prog Cardiovasc Dis 2000;42:359.

8. Savelieva I, Yi G, Guiu X, et al: Agreement and reproducibility of automatic versus manual measurement of QT interval and QT dispersion. Am J Cardiol 1998;81:471.

9. Ahnve S: Errors in the visual determination of corrected QT (QTc) interval during myocardial infarction. J Am Coll Cardiol 1985;5:699.

10. Murray A, McLaughlin NB, Bourke JP, et al: Error in manual measurement of QT intervals. Br Heart J 1994;71:386.

11. Malik M, Batchvarov VN: Measurement, interpretation and clinical potential of QT dispersion. J Am Coll Cardiol 2000;36:1749.

12. Sahu P, Lim PO, Struthers AD: QT dispersion in medicine: Electrophysiological holy grail or fool's gold. QJM 2000;93:425.

13. Aufderheide TP, Rowlandson I, Lawrence SW, et al: Test of the acute cardiac ischemia time-insensitive predictive instrument (ACI-TIPI) for prehospital use. Ann Emerg Med 1996;27:193.

14. Aufderheide TP, Xue, Q, Dhala AA, et al: The added diagnostic value of automated QT-dispersion measurements and automated ST-segment deviations in the electrocardiographic diagnosis of acute cardiac ischemia. J Electrocardiol 2000;42:329.

15. Shah CP, Thakur RK, Reisdorff EJ, et al: QT dispersion may be a useful adjunct for detection of myocardial infarction in the chest pain center. Am Heart J 1998;136:496.

16. Hohnloser SH: Effect of coronary ischemia on QT dispersion. Prog Cardiovasc Dis 2000;42:351.

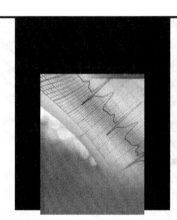

Chapter 74

Electrocardiographic Predictive Instruments

Tom P. Aufderheide and Christopher R. George

Many predictive instruments and clinical decision aids have been developed to help clinicians accurately recognize acute cardiac ischemia (ACI) and to risk stratify these patients. Predictive instruments are based on logistic regression predictive models that use electrocardiographic and clinical characteristics at presentation to identify patients at risk for ACI; in addition, they may compute the probability of a patient having ACI or a specific outcome. They have the potential to increase the accuracy and speed of patient triage and reduce health care costs for patients presenting with chest pain or similar symptoms.[1] Their use can help in correctly identifying high-risk patients for early and aggressive treatment, as well as reliably identifying low-risk patients who can be appropriately discharged for follow-up in an outpatient setting.

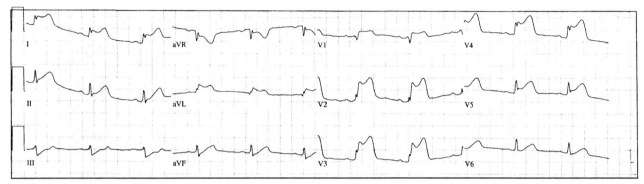

Vent. rate	65	BPM	Normal sinus rhythm
PR interval	152	ms	Low voltage QRS, consider pulmonary disease, pericardial effusion, or normal variant
QRS duration	92	ms	ST elevation consider anterolateral injury or acute infarct
QT/QTc	408/424	ms	** ** ** ** * ACUTE MI * ** ** ** **
P–R–T axes	24 28	34	Abnormal ECG
			No previous ECGs available

FIGURE 74-1 • **Standard ECG.** This is an example of a computer interpretation of ***ACUTE MI*** with ST segment elevation and reciprocal changes.

Predictive instruments and clinical decision aids can help physicians with decision making but are designed only to supplement, not replace, clinical judgment.

Initial Electrocardiogram

The initial electrocardiogram (ECG) can be used as a predictive instrument. A 1999 study of the Global Utilization of Streptokinase and Tissue Plasminogen Activator for Occluded Coronary Arteries (GUSTO)-IIb trial data stratified patients into groups based on the presenting ECG characteristics. Categories included ST segment elevation (STE) of 0.05 mV or greater in two contiguous leads (28% of patients), ST segment depression greater than 0.05 mV (35%), a combination of elevation and depression (15%), or isolated T wave inversion greater than 0.1 mV (22%). The patient groups of STE or both elevation and depression had confirmed acute myocardial infarction (AMI) 81% and 89% of the time, respectively, and the 30-day incidence of death was 9.4% and 12.4%, respectively. In comparison, only 32% of patients with T wave inversion had enzymatic evidence of AMI, with a 30-day mortality rate of only 5.5%.[2] In 1996, Goldman et al. reported a strategy for predicting the need for intensive care for patients presenting to the emergency department (ED) with chest pain. Using retrospective data analysis, clinical and ECG criteria were identified as predictors of major complications such as cardiac arrest, emergency cardioversion, cardiogenic shock, intubation, or recurrent ischemic chest pain requiring mechanical revascularization within 72 hours. The study showed that ECG abnormalities are the most important predictors of major complications within 24 hours of presentation. Patients with STE or Q waves not known to be old had a relative risk of 13 to 17 of having a major complication within 72 hours, whereas those with ST segment depression or T wave inversion not known to be old had a relative risk of 5.1 to 6.8.[3] This predictor was applied to a separate data set with similar findings, but has not yet been used in a prospective trial.

Algorithms and Computer Interpretation

There are many computerized algorithms to help with the interpretation of ECGs. The GE Marquette Medical Information Technology (12-SL) computerized ECG interpretation is a representative example (Fig. 74-1). It includes an assessment of rhythm, rate, axis, and an interpretation of S-T and T wave abnormalities. When specified ECG criteria are met, the computer displays an interpretation, such as "***Acute MI ***." A 1991 study found the positive predictive value for determining AMI to be 94% for computer ECG interpretation, and 86% for physician interpretation. Conversely, the negative predictive values were 81% and 85%, respectively.[4] A 1998 study by Goldman et al. demonstrated the effectiveness of a computer protocol to predict MI in patients with chest pain in the ED. After deriving the protocol from a set of clinical data, the protocol was then prospectively tested in 4770 patients at both university and community hospitals. The specificity of the protocol for detecting the presence of MI is similar to that of physicians (88% and 87.8%, respectively), although the sensitivity is slightly better (74% versus 71%).[5]

There is a continuous effort to improve computerized algorithms for the detection of AMI. In fact, there may be significant differences in ECG manifestations between men and women experiencing AMI. For example, a study showed that when a computerized algorithm using neural networking to incorporate sex and age data was used, the sensitivity of detection of inferior AMI in women improved from 49% to 54%, while maintaining 98% specificity for patients with noncardiac chest pain.[6]

ACI-TIPI

The Acute Cardiac Ischemia Time-Insensitive Predictive Instrument (ACI-TIPI) displays a percentage prediction on the ECG representing the probability for acute coronary syndrome. When obtaining the ECG, the user adds certain specific clinical data such as the patient's age and sex and the

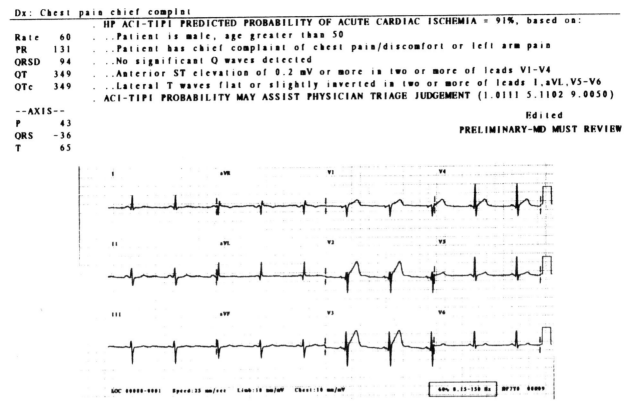

FIGURE 74-2 · Acute Cardiac Ischemia Time-Insensitive Predictive Instrument (ACI-TIPI) example. In the ACI-TIPI, the probability of ischemia and the primary reasons for this prediction are printed above the ECG. This takes into consideration age, sex, and if chest or left arm pain is the chief complaint, as well as the computer interpretation of various ECG characteristics.

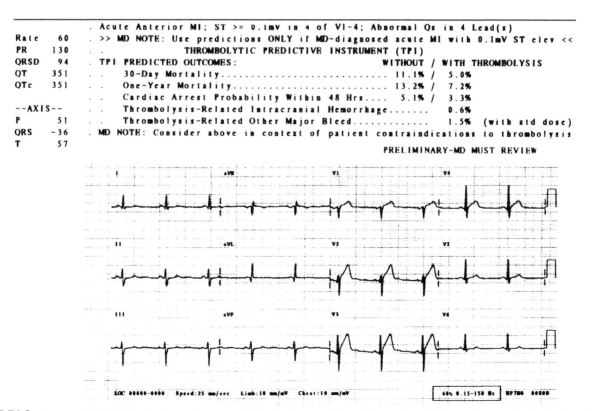

FIGURE 74-3 · Fibrinolytic Predictive Instrument example. The Fibrinolytic Predictive Instrument is applied to patients meeting ECG criteria for acute myocardial infarction and takes into consideration a number of clinical and ECG factors to compute probabilities of five adverse outcomes with and without administration of fibrinolytic therapy.

presence or absence of chest or left arm pain as the chief complaint on presentation. These data are combined with ECG characteristics such as the presence of Q waves and ST segment or T wave abnormalities.[7] The ACI-TIPI score is the probability of acute ischemia and is displayed as a percentage at the top of the ECG (Fig. 74-2).

A 1998 multicenter, controlled clinical trial verified the effectiveness of the ACI-TIPI.[7] This study showed that the ACI-TIPI is associated with reduced hospitalization for patients without cardiac ischemia and for those with stable angina, thereby decreasing the false-positive diagnoses and avoiding unnecessary admissions. These findings are most significant for less experienced physicians.[7] Admission rates for patients with AMI or unstable angina did not change with use of the ACI-TIPI, regardless of the level of physician training. The authors estimate that the results of the trial would correspond nationally to 204,000 fewer hospitalizations, 112,000 fewer cardiac care unit admissions, and a savings of $278 million annually.[7] Further studies involving the ACI-TIPI have shown that it can increase the speed of ED triage.[8] The ACI-TIPI has also been retrospectively validated for prehospital use.[9]

Fibrinolytic Predictive Instrument

The Fibrinolytic Predictive Instrument provides predictions of outcomes for patients with AMI with and without the use of fibrinolytic therapy. This is based on computer-interpreted ECG characteristics and a number of clinical factors (Fig. 74-3). It was designed to help clinicians weigh the likely risks of the use of fibrinolytics in specific patients. It gives predictions on five adverse outcomes with and without the use of fibrinolytics: 30-day and 1-year mortality, and risk of cardiac arrest, stroke, and major bleeding. As with the ACI-TIPI, these predictions are displayed as a percentage and listed at the top of the ECG. The Fibrinolytic Predictive Instrument was developed as a logistic regression–based predictive instrument, and then validated on a separate retrospective data set.[10] A prospective study evaluating the benefits of its use is in progress.

References

1. Aufderheide TP, Brady WI: Electrocardiography in the patient with myocardial ischemia or infarction. In Gibler WB, Aufderheide TP (eds): Emergency Cardiac Care, vol 1. St. Louis, Mosby–Year Book, 1994, p 171.
2. Estes NA 3rd, Salem DN: predictive value of the electrocardiogram in acute coronary syndromes. JAMA 1999;281:753.
3. Goldman L, Cook EF, Johnson PA, et al: Prediction of the need for intensive care in patients who come to the EDs with acute chest pain. N Engl J Med 1996;34:1498.
4. Kudenchuk PJ, Ho MT, Weaver WD, et al: Accuracy of computer-interpreted electrocardiography in selecting patients for thrombolytic therapy. MITI Project Investigators. J Am Coll Cardiol 1991;17:1486.
5. Goldman L, Cook EF, Brand DA, et al: A computer protocol to predict MI in ED patients with chest pain. N Engl J Med 1998;318:797.
6. Xue J, Taha B, Reddy S, et al: A new method to incorporate age and gender into the criteria for the detection of acute inferior MI. J Electrocardiol 2001;34(Suppl 2001):229.
7. Selker HP, Beshansky JR, Griffith JL, et al: Use of the Acute Cardiac Ischemia Time-Insensitive Predictive Instrument (ACI-TIPI) to assist with triage of patients with chest pain or other symptoms suggestive of acute cardiac ischemia. Ann Intern Med 1998;129:845.
8. Sarasin FP, Reymond JM, Griffith JL, et al: Impact of the Acute Cardiac Ischemia Time-Insensitive Predictive Instrument (ACI-TIPI) on the speed of triage decision making for ED patients presenting with chest pain: A controlled clinical trial. J Gen Intern Med 1994;9:187.
9. Aufderheide TP, Rowlandson I, Lawrence SW, et al: Test of the Acute Cardiac Ischemia Time-Insensitive Predictive Instrument (ACI-TIPI) for prehospital use. Ann Emerg Med 1996;27:193.
10. Selker HP, Griffith JL, Beshansky JR, et al: Patient-specific predictions of outcomes in MI for real-time emergency use: A thrombolytic predictive instrument. Ann Intern Med 1997;127:538.

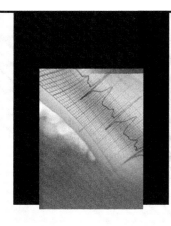

Chapter 75

Electrocardiographic Body Surface Mapping

Joseph P. Ornato

The standard 12-lead electrocardiogram (ECG) has been the principal tool used to diagnose ST segment elevation myocardial infarction (STEMI) in real time at the bedside since the 1940s, yet has significant limitations in the evaluation of patients suspected of having an acute coronary syndrome (ACS). The sensitivity of a single 12-lead ECG for diagnosing acute MI (AMI) or unstable angina is relatively poor.[1] This is, in part, because leads do not cover the lateral, true posterior, and right ventricular locations comprehensively. Body surface mapping, a computer-assisted, multiple-lead ECG tool, is emerging as a supplement to conventional electrocardiography.

Early Body Surface Mapping Technology

In 1920, Pardee described ST segment elevation as an important element of the early ECG pattern in patients with AMI.[2] Body surface mapping uses multiple leads, ranging from 40 to as many as 120 leads, to sample the ECG activity over a much larger portion of the torso than the traditional 12-lead ECG. The earliest body surface mapping systems plotted the degree of ST segment elevation or depression on a two-dimensional (i.e., "flat") representation of the torso. Using such primitive maps, early investigators were able to diagnose the location and extent of AMI in animal models.[3]

In the 1970s, precordial ECG mapping was found to be useful in predicting the amount of myocardial damage (as determined by histologic appearance and the creatine phosphokinase activity of myocardial biopsy specimens obtained 24 hours after coronary artery occlusion) that would result after experimental induction of MI in an animal model.[4] Soon thereafter, investigators began to speculate that the sum of the ST segments recorded from multiple precordial leads could be used to assess changes in myocardial injury in man.[5] In 1975, Muller et al. confirmed that there was a close correlation between direct measures of myocardial cell damage and the sum of the precordial ST segment elevations in dogs instrumented for simultaneous recording of epicardial and 30-lead precordial ECGs.[6]

Soon thereafter, investigators began to show that this technique could also be used to diagnose the location and extent of AMI in humans.[7-13] Toyama et al. showed that the area of myocardial damage identified with a body surface map correlated well with results of thallium-201 scintigraphic imaging in patients with AMI.[12] Ikeda et al. showed that a body surface mapping was superior to both the ECG and the vectorcardiogram for detecting true posterior MI.[10] This technique was also found to be of value in diagnosing AMI in the presence of left bundle branch block.[14]

Until recently, body surface mapping was limited by the inability of computer technology to process multiple leads simultaneously and display the results in a simple-to-interpret, intuitive format. Computer processing limitations necessitated the use of two-dimensional, static, black-and-white displays (Fig. 75-1). Interpretation of the resultant maps was difficult and required a great deal of knowledge and training. As a result, this technology found its principal use in the hands of researchers and never became a practical, bedside, clinical device.

The 80-Lead Body Surface Mapping Electrocardiographic System

Modern body surface mapping can be used in patients with ACS to (1) determine the location and size of the MI, (2) select a reperfusion therapy, and (3) monitor the efficacy of treatment. At present, the most mature diagnostic platform available for clinical use in the United States is the PRIME ECG 80-lead body surface mapping system (Meridian Medical Technologies, Baltimore, MD).

The 80-lead body surface mapping ECG system uses 80 leads (64 on the chest and 16 on the back) to collect data (Fig. 75-2). The 80-lead body surface mapping ECG system leads are screen-printed in conductive silver ink onto a disposable vest made up of clear plastic strips that combine at the base to form a single connection. The vest is applied by removing a paper backing to reveal self-adhesive hydrogel pads at each electrode site. The strips can be positioned and

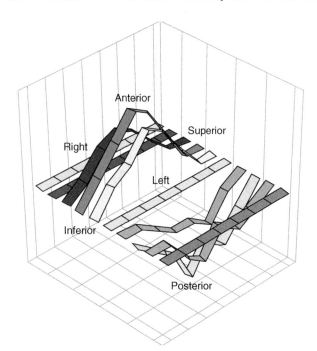

FIGURE 75-1 · **An example of early body surface mapping display format.**

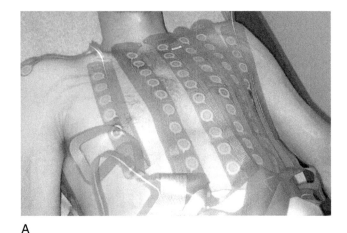

FIGURE 75-2 · **Application of the 80-lead body surface mapping ECG electrodes.** *A,* Front; *B,* back.

secured in 5 to 7 minutes, just a few minutes longer than the time needed to acquire a standard 12-lead ECG.

After the strips are in place, the vest is connected to the 80-lead body surface mapping ECG's computer diagnostic unit, and data collection begins. All 80 leads are recorded simultaneously. The device measures the degree of ST segment elevation or depression in each of the leads and uses algorithms to develop a three-dimensional representation of the human torso on a computer screen. The torso remains green in color if there is no significant ST segment elevation or depression (as would be the case in a normal, healthy individual; Fig. 75-3, see color insert). Deviations from the 95% confidence interval for normal values at each point on the human chest and abdomen are represented on the screen in red (ST segment elevation) or blue (ST segment depression). The degree of ST segment elevation or depression is represented by the color intensity.

Examples of 80-lead body surface mapping ECG recordings from various AMI locations are shown in Figure 75-4 (see color insert). Anterior wall infarction (Fig. 75-4A) is noted as a patch of red color on the anterior chest, typically with reciprocal, blue ST segment depression over the back. Inferior wall infarction (Fig. 75-4B) is noted as a patch of red across the inferior abdomen, often with reciprocal ST segment depression (blue) anteriorly or laterally. Posterior involvement (Fig. 75-4C) is noted as a patch of red over the back, and right ventricular involvement (Fig. 75-4D) is noted as a red area over the right chest and in the right axilla.

Clinical Comparison of the Body Map with Conventional Electrocardiography

Menown et al. compared the ability of an early version of the 80-lead body surface mapping ECG system with a standard 12-lead ECG to classify correctly 314 patients with chest pain.[15] This early version of the 80-lead body surface mapping ECG system correctly classified 123/160 patients with

MI (sensitivity 77%) as having an infarction and 131/154 patients without MI (specificity 85%) as not having an MI.

Since then, much progress has been made in refining the diagnostic criteria for differentiating a normal tracing from normal variants, cardiac ischemia, MI, and a host of other ECG abnormalities. As a result of this progress, major software enhancements have been made in the system diagnostic computer algorithm. Using the latest version of the 80-lead body surface mapping ECG system, Ornato et al. conducted a prospective, multicenter, international evaluation of whether the 80-lead body surface mapping ECG system could detect more acute STEMI cases than standard 12-lead ECGs in patients with chest pain presenting to hospital emergency departments.[16] The 80-lead body surface mapping ECG demonstrated superior diagnostic capability in posterior, right ventricular, septal, and inferior MI.[16] In another study, Menown et al. performed an 80-lead body surface mapping ECG and a standard 12-lead ECG on 62 patients with inferior wall MI.[17] Body surface mapping better classified patients

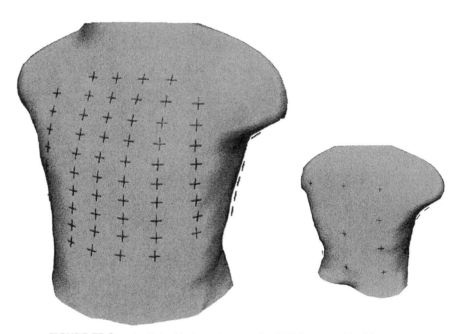

FIGURE 75-3 • An 80-lead body surface mapping ECG in a normal healthy person.

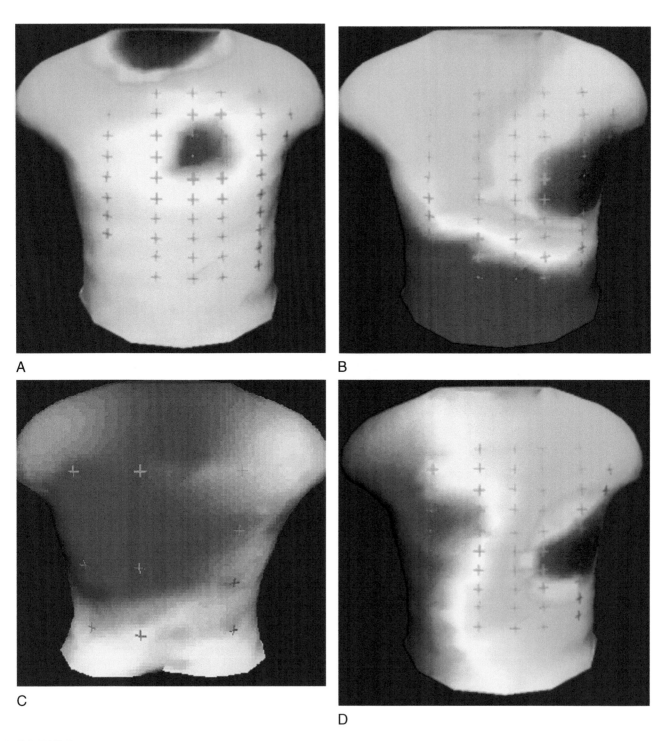

FIGURE 75-4 • **An 80-lead body surface mapping ECG in various acute myocardial infarction locations.** *A,* Anterior AMI. *B,* Inferior AMI. *C,* Posterior AMI. *D,* RV AMI.

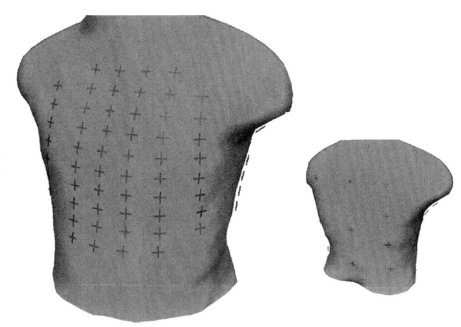

FIGURE 75-3 • An 80-lead body surface mapping ECG in a normal healthy person. (See color insert.)

with inferior wall MI accompanied by right ventricular or posterior wall involvement compared with right ventricular or posterior chest leads.

A number of other potential uses for the 80-lead body surface mapping ECG system are emerging. The device can detect reperfusion after treatment with fibrinolytic drugs, and subsequent potential reocclusion. In a study comparing the ability of the 80-lead body surface mapping ECG system and the standard 12-lead ECG to detect reperfusion after fibrinolytic therapy in patients with AMI, the 80-lead body surface mapping ECG system identified 97% of patients who

achieved reperfusion and 100% of those who did not based on coronary angiographic results as the gold standard.[18] The 12-lead ECG identified only 59% of patients who achieved reperfusion and only 50% of those who did not.

The 80-lead body surface mapping ECG system can also detect AMI accurately despite the presence of left bundle branch block.[19] Studies are under way to define better its use in diagnosing patients with an ACS and during stress testing.

Relatively preliminary studies suggest that modern body surface mapping technology has the potential to be a more sensitive test than the standard 12-lead ECG for detecting STEMI.

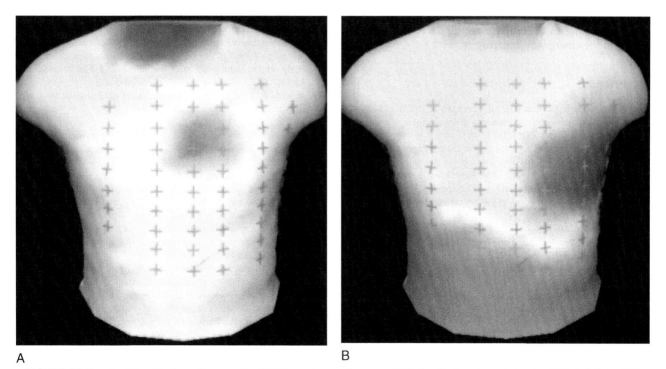

A   B

FIGURE 75-4 • **An 80-lead body surface mapping ECG in various acute myocardial infarction locations.** *A,* Anterior AMI. *B,* Inferior AMI.

(Continued)

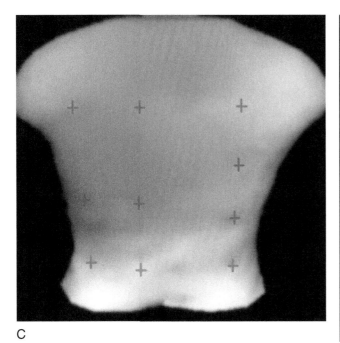

C

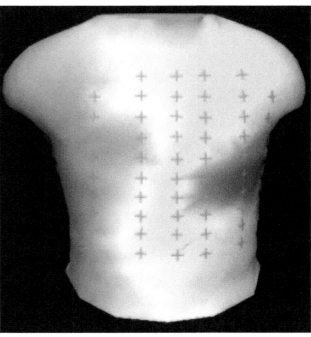

D

FIGURE 75-4—cont'd · **An 80-lead body surface mapping ECG in various acute myocardial infarction locations.** *C*, Posterior AMI. *D*, RV AMI. (See color insert.)

The two technologies appear to have similar specificity. Body maps make it relatively easy to diagnose STEMI, even when it occurs in locations that are difficult to detect on the standard 12-lead ECG (posterior, lateral, and right ventricular walls). Thus far, the greatest value of body surface mapping is that it is easy to learn to use. The modern systems generate high-quality, color computer images that are as easy to interpret as watching color Doppler radar on television. Although this technology appears to offer great promise, it is still relatively early in its development and refinement. Further study is under way to define the ultimate usefulness of body surface mapping in the emergency department.

References

1. Brady WJ, Hwang V, Sullivan R, et al: A comparison of 12- and 15-lead ECGs in ED chest pain patients: Impact on diagnosis, therapy, and disposition. Am J Emerg Med 2000;18:239.
2. Pardee HEB: An electrocardiographic sign of coronary artery obstruction. Arch Intern Med 1920;26:244.
3. Sugiyama S, Wada M, Sugenoya J, et al: Experimental study of myocardial infarction through the use of body surface isopotential maps: Ligation of the anterior descending branch of the left coronary artery. Am Heart J 1977;93:51.
4. Maroko PR, Kjekshus JK, Sobel BE, et al: Factors influencing infarct size following experimental coronary artery occlusions. Circulation 1971;43:67.
5. Maroko PR, Libby P, Covell JW, et al: Precordial S-T segment elevation mapping: An atraumatic method for assessing alterations in the extent of myocardial ischemic injury. The effects of pharmacologic and hemodynamic interventions. Am J Cardiol 1972;29:223.
6. Muller JE, Maroko PR, Braunwald E: Evaluation of precordial electrocardiographic mapping as a means of assessing changes in myocardial ischemic injury. Circulation 1975;52:16.
7. Braunwald E, Maroko PR: ST-segment mapping: Realistic and unrealistic expectations. Circulation 1976;54:529.
8. Askenazi J, Maroko PR, Lesch M, Braunwald E: Usefulness of ST segment elevations as predictors of electrocardiographic signs of necrosis in patients with acute myocardial infarction. Br Heart J 1977;39:764.
9. Toyama S, Suzuki K, Takahashi T, Yamashita Y: Epicardial isopotential mapping from body surface isopotential mapping in myocardial infarction. J Electrocardiol 1985;18:277.
10. Ikeda K, Kubota I, Tonooka I, et al: Detection of posterior myocardial infarction by body surface mapping: A comparative study with 12 lead ECG and VCG. J Electrocardiol 1985;18:361.
11. Tonooka I, Kubota I, Watanabe Y, et al: Isointegral analysis of body surface maps for the assessment of location and size of myocardial infarction. Am J Cardiol 1983;52:1174.
12. Toyama S, Suzuki K, Koyama M, et al: The body surface isopotential mapping of the QRS wave in myocardial infarction: A comparative study of the scintigram with thallium-201. J Electrocardiol 1982; 15:241.
13. Yamada K: Experimental basis and clinical application of body surface isopotential map. Jpn J Med 1985;24:283.
14. Musso E, Stilli D, Macchi E, et al: Body surface maps in left bundle branch block uncomplicated or complicated by myocardial infarction, left ventricular hypertrophy or myocardial ischemia. J Electrocardiol 1987;20:1.
15. Menown IB, Patterson RS, MacKenzie G, Adgey AA: Body-surface map models for early diagnosis of acute myocardial infarction. J Electrocardiol 1998;31(Suppl):180.
16. Ornato JP, Menown IB, Riddell JW, et al, for the PRIME Investigators: 80-Lead body map detects acute ST-elevation myocardial infarction missed by standard 12-lead electrocardiography. J Am Coll Cardiol 2002;39:332A.
17. Menown IB, Allen J, Anderson JM, Adgey AA: Early diagnosis of right ventricular or posterior infarction associated with inferior wall left ventricular acute myocardial infarction. Am J Cardiol 2000;85:934.
18. Menown IB, Allen J, Anderson JM, Adgey AA: Noninvasive assessment of reperfusion after fibrinolytic therapy for acute myocardial infarction. Am J Cardiol 2000;86:736.
19. Menown IB, Mackenzie G, Adgey AA: Optimizing the initial 12-lead electrocardiographic diagnosis of acute myocardial infarction. Eur Heart J 2000;21:275.

Index

Note: Page numbers followed by the letter f refer to figures and those followed by t refer to tables.

Printed and bound by CPI Group (UK) Ltd, Croydon, CR0 4YY

03/10/2024

01040311-0015